NURSE PRACTITIONER

Certification Examination
And Practice Preparation

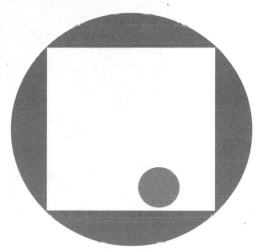

THIRD EDITION

NURSE PRACTITIONER
Certification Examination And Practice Preparation

Margaret A. Fitzgerald, DNP, FNP-BC, NP-C, FAANP, CSP
President, Fitzgerald Health Education Associates, Inc.
North Andover, Massachusetts
Family Nurse Practitioner
Greater Lawrence Family Health Center
Lawrence, MA

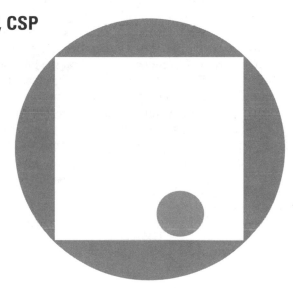

F.A. Davis Company • Philadelphia

F. A. Davis Company
1915 Arch Street
Philadelphia, PA 19103
www.fadavis.com

Printed in the United States of America

Last digit indicates print number: 10 9 8 7 6 5

Publisher, Nursing: Joanne Patzek DaCunha, RN, MSN
Director of Content Development: Darlene D. Pedersen, MSN, APRN, BC
Project Editor: Kim Mackey, Tyler R. Baber
Design & Illustration Manager: Carolyn O'Brien

As new scientific information becomes available through basic and clinical research, recommended treatments and drug therapies undergo changes. The author(s) and publisher have done everything possible to make this book accurate, up to date, and in accord with accepted standards at the time of publication. The author(s), editors, and publisher are not responsible for errors or omissions or for consequences from application of the book, and make no warranty, expressed or implied, in regard to the contents of the book. Any practice described in this book should be applied by the reader in accordance with professional standards of care used in regard to the unique circumstances that may apply in each situation. The reader is advised always to check product information (package inserts) for changes and new information regarding dose and contraindications before administering any drug. Caution is especially urged when using new or infrequently ordered drugs.

To my aunt, Helen M. Laffey, RN (1913–1996)
A Boston public health nurse who delivered some of the first
polio vaccines given in the city of Boston, cared for the victims of
the great Cocoasnut Grove Fire, and took me along on rounds
when I was a young child.
To my grandchildren, Mouhammed, Maggie, Aissatou,
Sebastian, Tidiane, Iris, and Isabel, with lots of love from Nana

Acknowledgments

This book represents a sum of the efforts of many people.

I thank my family, especially my husband and business partner Marc Comstock, for their support as they lived through this experience.

I thank the staff of Fitzgerald Health Education Associates, Inc. for sharing me with this project for many months.

I thank the patients and staff of the Greater Lawrence (MA) Family Health Center as they continue to serve as a source of inspiration as I developed this book.

I thank Joanne DaCunha, and the F.A. Davis staff for their ongoing encouragement.

Last but not least, I thank the thousands of nurse practitioners who, over the years, have attended the Fitzgerald Health Education Associates, Inc. Nurse Practitioner Certification and Practice Preparation courses. Your eagerness to learn, thirst for knowledge, and dedication to success continue to inspire me. It is indeed a privilege to be part of your professional development.

Introduction

This book represents a perspective on learning and practice developed during my years of practice at the Greater Lawrence (MA) Family Health Center as well as a nurse practitioner (NP) and family practice residency faculty member and professional speaker. In addition, my experience in the years of helping thousands of NPs achieve professional success through conducting NP Certification and Practice Preparation Courses influenced the development and presentation of the information held within.

The scope of practice of the nurse practitioner is wide, encompassing the care of the young, the old, the sick, and the well. This book has been developed to help the nurse practitioner develop the knowledge and skills to successfully enter NP practice as well as achieve certification, an important landmark in professional achievement.

This book is not intended to be a comprehensive primary care text, but rather a source to reinforce learning and a guide for the development of the information base needed for NP practice. The reader is encouraged to answer the questions given in each section and then check on the accuracy of response. The discussion section is intended to enhance learning through highlighting the essentials of primary care NP practice. The numerous tables can serve as a quick-look resource not only as the NP prepares for entry to practice and certification but also in the delivery of ongoing care.

MARGARET A. FITZGERALD,
DNP, FNP-BC, NP-C, FAANP, CSP
PRESIDENT
FITZGERALD HEALTH EDUCATION ASSOCIATES, INC.
NORTH ANDOVER, MA
FAMILY NURSE PRACTITIONER, ADJUNCT FACULTY,
FAMILY PRACTICE RESIDENCY
GREATER LAWRENCE (MA) FAMILY HEALTH CENTER

Table of Contents

1

Health Promotion and Disease Prevention

1. An example of a primary prevention measure for a 78-year-old man with chronic obstructive pulmonary disease is:

    A. reviewing the use of prescribed medications.
    B. ensuring adequate illumination in the home.
    C. checking pulmonary function.
    D. performing a digital rectal examination and fecal occult blood test (FOBT).

2. Which of the following is an example of a primary prevention activity in a 76-year-old woman with osteoporosis?

    A. bisphosphonate therapy
    B. calcium supplementation
    C. home survey to identify fall hazards
    D. use of a back brace

3. Secondary prevention measures for a 78-year-old man with chronic obstructive pulmonary disease include:

    A. checking stool for occult blood.
    B. administering influenza vaccine.
    C. obtaining a serum theophylline level.
    D. advising about appropriate use of car passenger restraints.

4. Tertiary prevention measures for a 69-year-old woman with heart failure include:

    A. administering antipneumococcal vaccine.
    B. adjusting therapy to minimize dyspnea.
    C. surveying skin for precancerous lesions.
    D. reviewing safe handling of food.

5. Which of the following provides passive immunity?

    A. hepatitis B immune globulin (HBIG)
    B. measles, mumps, and rubella (MMR) vaccine
    C. pneumococcal conjugate vaccine
    D. influenza vaccine

6. Active immunity is defined as:

    A. resistance developed in response to an antigen.
    B. immunity conferred by an antibody produced in another host.
    C. the resistance of a group to an infectious agent.
    D. defense against disease acquired naturally by the infant from the mother.

ANSWERS

1.	B	2.	C	3.	A
4.	B	5.	A	6.	A

DISCUSSION

Primary prevention measures include activities provided to individuals to prevent the onset or acquisition of a given disease. The goal of primary prevention measures is to spare individuals the suffering, burden, and cost associated with the clinical condition. Examples include health-protecting education and counseling, such as encouraging the use of car restraints and bicycle helmets and providing information on accident and fall prevention.

Immunizations and chemoprophylaxis are also examples of primary prevention measures. Active immunization through the use of vaccines provides long-term protection from disease. The use of vaccines is preferred to passive immunization through the use of immune globulin (IG) because IG use provides only temporary protection. In herd or community immunity, a significant portion of a given population has immunity against an infectious agent; the likelihood that the susceptible portion of the group would become infected is minimized (Figure 1–1).

Secondary prevention measures include activities provided to identify and treat asymptomatic persons who have risk factors for a given disease or in preclinical

See full color images of this topic on DavisPlus at http://davisplus.fadavis.com | Keyword: Fitzgerald

Preventive Services Recommended by the USPSTF

The U.S. Preventive Services Task Force (USPSTF) recommends that clinicians discuss these preventive services with eligible patients and offer them as a priority. All these services have received an "A" (strongly recommended) or a "B" (recommended) grade from the Task Force.

For definitions of all grades used by the USPSTF, see Appendix A (beginning on P. 206). The full listings of all USPSTF recommendations for adults and children are in Section 2 (beginning on P. 9) and Section 3 (beginning on P. 179).

Recommendation	Adults		Special Populations	
	Men	Women	Pregnant Women	Children
Abdominal Aortic Aneurysm, Screening[1]	✓			
Alcohol Misuse Screening and Behavioral Counseling Interventions	✓	✓	✓	
Aspirin for the Primary Prevention of Cardiovascular Events[2]	✓	✓		
Bacteriuria, Screening for Asymptomatic			✓	
Breast Cancer, Chemoprevention[3]		✓		
Breast Cancer, Screening[4]		✓		
Breast and Ovarian Cancer Susceptibility, Genetic Risk Assessment and BRCA Mutation Testing[5]		✓		
Breastfeeding, Behavioral Interventions to Promote[6]		✓	✓	
Cervical Cancer, Screening[7]		✓		
Chlamydial Infection, Screening[8]		✓	✓	
Colorectal Cancer, Screening[9]	✓	✓		
Dental Caries in Preschool Children, Prevention[10]				✓
Depression, Screening[11]	✓	✓		
Diabetes Mellitus in Adults, Screening for Type 2[12]	✓	✓		
Diet, Behavioral Counseling in Primary Care to Promote a Healthy[13]	✓	✓		
Gonorrhea, Screening[14]		✓	✓	
Gonorrhea, Prophylactic Medication[15]				✓
Hepatitis B Virus Infection, Screening[16]			✓	
High Blood Pressure, Screening	✓	✓		
HIV, Screening[17]	✓	✓	✓	✓
Iron Deficiency Anemia, Prevention[18]				✓
Iron Deficiency Anemia, Screening[19]			✓	
Lipid Disorders, Screening[20]	✓	✓		
Obesity in Adults, Screening[21]	✓	✓		
Osteoporosis in Postmenopausal Women, Screening[22]		✓		
Rh (D) Incompatibility, Screening[23]			✓	
Sickle Cell Disease, Screening[24]				✓
Syphilis Infection, Screening[25]	✓	✓	✓	
Tobacco Use and Tobacco-Caused Disease, Counseling[26]	✓	✓	✓	
Visual Impairment in Children Younger than Age 5 Years, Screening[27]				✓

Figure 1–1 Preventive services recommended by the U.S. Preventive Services Task Force (USPSTF).

[1]One-time screening by ultrasonography in men aged 65 to 75 who have ever smoked.

[2]Adults at increased risk for coronary heart disease.

[3]Discuss with women at high risk for breast cancer and at low risk for adverse effects of chemoprevention.

[4]Mammography every 1-2 years for women 40 and older.

[5]Refer women whose family history is associated with an increased risk for deleterious mutations in *BRCA1* or *BRCA2* genes for genetic counseling and evaluation for *BRCA* testing.

[6]Structured education and behavioral counseling programs.

[7]Women aged 21-65 who have been sexually active and have a cervix.

[8]Sexually active women 24 and younger and other asymptomatic women at increased risk for infection. Asymptomatic pregnant women 24 and younger and others at increased risk.

[9]Men and women 50 and older.

[10]Prescribe oral fluoride supplementation at currently recommended doses to preschool children older than 6 months whose primary water source is deficient in fluoride.

[11]In clinical practices with systems to assure accurate diagnoses, effective treatment, and follow-up.

[12]Adults with hypertension or hyperlipidemia.

[13]Adults with hyperlipidemia and other known risk factors for cardiovascular and diet-related chronic disease.

[14]Sexually active women, including pregnant women 25 and younger, or at increased risk for infection.

[15]Prophylactic ocular topical medication for all newborns against gonococcal ophthalmia neonatorum.

[16]Pregnant women at first prenatal visit.

[17]All adolescents and adults at increased risk for HIV infection and all pregnant women.

[18]Routine iron supplementation for asymptomatic children aged 6 to 12 months who are at increased risk for iron deficiency anemia.

[19]Routine screening in asymptomatic pregnant women.

[20]Men 35 and older and women 45 and older. Younger adults with other risk factors for coronary disease. Screening for lipid disorders to include measurement of total cholesterol and high-density lipoprotein cholesterol.

[21]Intensive counseling and behavioral interventions to promote sustained weight loss for obese adults.

[22]Women 65 and older and women 60 and older at increased risk for osteoporotic fractures.

[23]Blood typing and antibody testing at first pregnancy-related visit. Repeated antibody testing for unsensitized Rh (D)-negative women at 24-28 weeks gestation unless biological father is known to be Rh (D) negative.

[24]Newborns.

[25]Persons at increased risk and all pregnant women.

[26]Tobacco cessation interventions for those who use tobacco. Augmented pregnancy-tailored counseling to pregnant women who smoke.

[27]To detect amblyopia, strabismus, and defects in visual acuity.

Figure 1–1 cont'd

disease. Examples include screening examinations for pre-clinical evidence of cancer, such as mammography and cervical examination with Papanicolaou test. Other examples of secondary prevention activities include screening for clinical conditions with a protracted asymptomatic period, such as blood pressure measurement to detect hypertension and lipid profile to detect hyperlipidemia (Table 1–1).

Tertiary prevention measures are part of the management of a person with an established disease. The goal is to minimize disease-associated complications and the negative health effects of the conditions. Examples include medications and lifestyle modification to normalize blood glucose levels in individuals with diabetes mellitus and in conjunction with the treatment of heart failure, aimed at improving or minimizing disease-related symptoms.

Discussion Source

http://www.ahrq.gov/clinic/uspstfix.htm, Agency for Healthcare Research and Quality: United States Preventive Services Task Force (USPSTF) Recommendations, accessed 8/21/09.

QUESTIONS

7. When advising a patient about injectable influenza immunization, the nurse practitioner (NP) considers the following about the vaccine:

   A. Its use is contraindicated during pregnancy.
   B. Its use is limited to children older than 6 years.
   C. It contains live virus.
   D. Its use is recommended for virtually all children age 6 months to 18 years.

8. A middle-aged man with chronic obstructive pulmonary disease who is about to receive injectable influenza vaccine should be advised that:

   A. it is more than 90% effective in preventing influenza.
   B. its use is contraindicated in the presence of eczema.
   C. localized reactions such as soreness and redness at the site of the immunization are fairly common.
   D. a short, intense flu-like syndrome typically occurs after immunization.

TABLE 1–1
Secondary Prevention Principles

Principle	Comment
Prevalence sufficient to justify screening	Routine mammography in women but not men
Health problem has significant effect on quality or quantity of life	Target diseases for secondary prevention include hypertension, type 2 diabetes mellitus, dyslipidemia, and certain cancers
Target disease has a long asymptomatic period. The natural history of the disease, or how the disease unfolds without intervention, is known	Treatment is available for the target disease. Providing treatment alters the disease's natural history
A population acceptable screening test is available	The test should be safe, available at a reasonable cost, and have reasonable sensitivity and specificity

Source: http://www.surgeongeneral.gov/library/mentalhealth/chapter2/sec5.html, Overview of prevention, accessed 1/21/10.

9. A 44-year-old woman with asthma presents asking for a "flu shot." She is currently taking ciprofloxacin for treatment of a urinary tract infection, does not have a fever, and is feeling better. You inform her that she:

   A. should return for the immunization after completing her antibiotic therapy.
   B. would likely develop a significant reaction if immunized today.
   C. can receive the immunization today.
   D. is not a candidate for influenza vaccine.

10. Which of the following statements best describes amantadine or rimantadine use in the care of patients with or at risk for influenza?

   A. Significant resistance to select strains of influenza limits the usefulness of these medications.
   B. The primary action of these therapies is in preventing influenza A during outbreaks.
   C. These therapies are active against influenza A and B.
   D. The use of these products is an acceptable alternative to influenza vaccine.

11. Which of the following statements best describes zanamivir (Relenza) or oseltamivir (Tamiflu) use in the care of patients with or at risk for influenza?

   A. Initiation of therapy early in acute influenza illness can help minimize the severity of disease when the disease is caused by a nonresistant viral strain.
   B. The primary indication is in preventing influenza A during outbreaks.
   C. The drugs are active only against influenza B.
   D. The use of these medications is an acceptable alternative to influenza vaccine.

12. When advising a patient about immunization with the influenza vaccine nasal spray vaccine, the NP considers the following:

   A. Its use is acceptable during pregnancy.
   B. Its use is limited to children younger than 6 years.
   C. It contains live, attenuated virus.
   D. This is the preferred method of influenza protection for individuals with severe allergic reaction to egg and egg products.

13. Approximately ____% of health-care providers receive influenza immunization annually.

   A. less than 20
   B. 40
   C. 60
   D. more than 80

14. The most common mode of influenza virus transmission is via:

   A. contact with a contaminated surface.
   B. respiratory droplet.
   C. saliva contact.
   D. skin-to-skin contact.

15. In an immunocompetent adult, the length of incubation for the influenza virus is on average:

   A. less than 24 hours.
   B. 1 to 4 days.
   C. 4 to 7 days.
   D. more than 1 week.

ANSWERS

7.	D	**8.**	C	**9.**	C
10.	A	**11.**	A	**12.**	C
13.	B	**14.**	B	**15.**	B

DISCUSSION

An individual who presents with an abrupt onset of symptoms including fever, myalgia, headache, malaise, nonproductive cough, sore throat, and rhinitis typically has uncomplicated influenza illness, more commonly known as "the flu." Children with influenza commonly have acute otitis media, nausea, and vomiting. Although the worst symptoms in most uncomplicated cases resolve in about 1 week, the cough and malaise often persist for 2 or more weeks. Individuals with ongoing health problems such as pulmonary or cardiac disease, young children, and pregnant women also have increased risk of influenza-related complications including pneumonia. Rarely, influenza virus infection also has been associated with encephalopathy, transverse myelitis, myositis, myocarditis, pericarditis, and Reye syndrome.

Influenza viruses spread from person to person largely via respiratory droplet from an infected person, primarily through cough or sneeze. In an immunocompetent adult, the influenza virus has a short incubation period, with a range of 1 to 4 days (average of 2 days). Adults pass the illness on 1 day before the onset of symptoms and continue to remain infectious for approximately 5 days after the onset of the illness. Children remain infectious for 10 or more days after the onset of symptoms and can shed the virus before the onset of symptoms. People who are immunocompromised can remain infectious for up to 3 weeks.

Historically, the risks for complications, hospitalizations, and deaths from influenza are higher among adults older than 65 years, young children, and individuals of any age with certain underlying health conditions than among healthy older children and younger adults. In children younger than 5 years, hospitalization rates for influenza-related illness have ranged from approximately 500/100,000 for children with high-risk medical conditions to 100/100,000 for children without high-risk medical conditions. Hospitalization rates for influenza-related illness among children younger than 24 months are comparable to rates reported among adults older than 65 years. Influenza strains such as novel H1N1, an influenza A virus also known as swine flu, and H5N1, an influenza A virus also known as avian flu, seem to cause a greater disease burden in younger adults.

Considering these factors, influenza, regardless of the viral strain, is not just a bad cold, but rather a potentially serious illness with significant morbidity and mortality risk across the life span. Even in the absence of complications, this viral illness typically causes many days of incapacitation and suffering and the risk of death. The influenza vaccines are about 70% to 80% effective in preventing influenza or reducing the severity of the disease. The injectable vaccine does not contain live virus and is not shed; there is no risk of transmitting an infectious agent to household contacts. Mild to moderate illness or current antimicrobial therapy is not a contraindication to any immunization, including the administration of the influenza vaccine.

Injectable trivalent influenza vaccine (TIV), more commonly called the "flu shot," can be used during pregnancy and is recommended for all pregnant women. The timing of TIV administration is based largely on the vaccine's availability because a formulation based on predicted influenza strains is produced annually. This vaccine can be given to infants 6 months old and older.

Immunization rates against influenza for individuals with chronic illness are typically the highest, although with considerable room for improvement. Certain groups have very low immunization rates and should be targeted for improvement. These include persons who live with or care for persons at high risk for influenza-related mortality and morbidity. Persons who provide essential community services should be considered for vaccination to minimize disruption of essential activities during influenza outbreaks. Students and other persons in institutional or other group-living situations should be encouraged to receive vaccine to minimize the risk of an outbreak in a relatively closed community. As supply allows, vaccination providers should administer influenza vaccine to any person who wishes to reduce the likelihood of becoming ill with influenza or transmitting influenza to others.

Currently, health-care providers have a 40% immunization rate against influenza. The Advisory Committee on Immunization Practices (ACIP), sponsored by the Centers for Disease Control and Prevention (CDC), recommends that health-care administrators consider the level of vaccination coverage among health-care personnel to be one measure of a patient safety quality program, and implement policies to encourage vaccination of health-care personnel (e.g., obtaining signed statements from health-care personnel who decline influenza vaccination). A strategy of universal influenza vaccination is a laudable public health goal, one that has been advocated by public health authorities and would likely be achievable with increased vaccine supplies and increased public awareness of the disease's possible consequences.

The nasal spray flu vaccine, also known as live attenuated influenza vaccine (LAIV) (FluMist), differs from the injectable TIV. Administered via a well-tolerated nasal mist, LAIV offers an easily administered, noninjection method of influenza immunization. LAIV contains influenza viruses that are sufficiently weakened as to be incapable of causing disease, but with enough strength to stimulate a protective immune response. The viruses in the LAIV are cold-adapted and temperature-sensitive. As a result, the viruses can grow in the nose and throat, but not in the lower respiratory tract where the temperature is higher. LAIV is approved for use in healthy people 2 to 49 years old. Individuals who should not receive LAIV include children younger than 2 years; adults older than 50 years; patients with a medical condition that places them at high risk for complications from influenza, including chronic heart disease, chronic lung disease such as asthma or reactive airways disease, diabetes or kidney failure, and immunosuppression; children or adolescents receiving long-term high-dose aspirin therapy; people with a history of Guillain-Barré syndrome; pregnant women; and people with a history of allergy to any of the components of LAIV or to eggs. Adverse effects of LAIV include nasal irritation and discharge, muscle aches, sore throat, and fever.

In the Northern Hemisphere, the optimal time to receive any influenza vaccine is usually in October or November, about 1 month before the anticipated onset of the flu season; this timing is reversed in the Southern Hemisphere. Children younger than 9 years who are receiving initial influenza immunization need two doses of vaccine separated by 4 or more weeks with TIV and 6 or more weeks with LAIV.

In the United States, four antiviral drugs are approved by the Food and Drug Administration (FDA) for use against influenza: amantadine (Symmetrel), rimantadine (Flumadine), zanamivir (Relenza), and oseltamivir (Tamiflu). The adamantane derivatives (amantadine and rimantadine) are approved only for treatment and prevention of influenza A, whereas the neuraminidase inhibitor drugs (zanamivir and oseltamivir) are approved for use in influenza A and influenza B. Ongoing CDC viral surveillance has shown high levels of resistance of influenza A viruses to amantadine and similar medications. Because of this significant level of resistance, amantadine and rimantadine have not been recommended for use in more recent U.S. flu seasons. Less resistance to the antiviral drugs oseltamivir and zanamivir has been noted in North America, but higher levels have been noted in Asia and other parts of the world. The health-care provider should keep well informed on these developments.

Zanamivir and oseltamivir are used to treat influenza A and B infections caused by susceptible viral strains; treatment with either of these drugs can shorten the time a person infected with influenza feels ill by approximately 1 day, if treatment is started during the first 2 days of illness. Zanamivir is inhaled and can cause bronchospasm, especially in patients with asthma or other chronic lung disease. The adverse effects of oseltamivir are largely gastrointestinal; the risk of nausea and vomiting is significantly reduced if the medication is taken with food.

Although many antiviral medications carry indications for the postexposure prevention of influenza, all have a less favorable adverse reaction profile than influenza vaccine; these products are also significantly more expensive. Active immunization against influenza A and B by administering the flu shot or intranasal spray is the preferred method of disease prevention.

Discussion Sources

Centers for Disease Control and Prevention. http://www.cdc.gov/flu/avian/, Avian influenza (bird flu), accessed 8/25/09.

Centers for Disease Control and Prevention. http://www.cdc.gov/flu/, Seasonal flu, accessed 8/26/09.

Centers for Disease Control and Prevention. http://www.cdc.gov/h1n1flu/general_info.htm, H1N1 flu (swine flu): General information, accessed 8/25/09.

http://www.cdc.gov/mmwr/preview/mmwrhtml/rr5606a1.htm, Prevention and control of influenza: Recommendations of the Advisory Committee on Immunization Practices (ACIP), accessed 8/26/09.

QUESTIONS

16. When considering an adult's risk for measles, mumps, and rubella (MMR), the NP considers the following:

    A. Patients born before 1957 have a high likelihood of immunity because of a history of natural infection.

    B. Considerable mortality and morbidity occur with all three diseases.

    C. Most cases in the United States occur in infants.

    D. The use of the vaccine is often associated with protracted arthralgia.

17. Which of the following is true about the MMR vaccine?

    A. It contains inactivated virus.

    B. Its use is contraindicated in patients with a history of egg allergy.

    C. Revaccination of an immune person is associated with risk of allergic reaction.

    D. Two doses at least 1 month apart are recommended for young adults who have not been previously immunized.

18. A 22-year-old man is starting a job in a college health center and needs proof of German measles, measles, and mumps immunity. He received childhood immunizations and supplies documentation of MMR vaccination at age 1.5 years. Your best response is to:

    A. obtain rubella rubeola and mumps titers.

    B. give MMR immunization now.

    C. advise him to obtain IG if he has been exposed to measles or rubella.

    D. advise him to avoid individuals with skin rashes.

19. Concerning the MMR vaccine, which of the following is true?

    A. The link between use of MMR vaccine and childhood autism has been firmly established.

    B. There is no credible scientific evidence that MMR use increases the risk of autism.

    C. The use of the combined vaccine is associated with increased autism risk, but giving the vaccine's three components as separate vaccines minimizes this risk.

    D. The vaccine contains thimerosal, a mercury derivative.

ANSWERS

16.	A	**17.**	D
18.	B	**19.**	B

DISCUSSION

The MMR vaccine contains live but weakened (attenuated) virus. Two immunizations 1 month apart are recommended for adults born after 1957 because adults born before then are considered immune as a result of having had these diseases (native or wild infection); vaccine against these three formerly common illnesses was unavailable until the 1960s. As with all vaccines, giving additional doses to patients with an unclear immunization history is safe (see Figure 1–2 for adult immunization schedules).

Rubella typically causes a relatively mild, 3- to 5-day illness with little risk of complication to the person infected. When rubella is contracted during pregnancy, however, the effects on the fetus can be devastating. Immunizing the entire population against rubella protects unborn children from the risk of contracting congenital rubella syndrome. Measles can cause severe illness with serious sequelae, including encephalitis and pneumonia; sequelae of mumps include orchitis.

In the past, a history of egg allergy was considered a contraindication to receiving MMR vaccine. The vaccine now seems to be safe in people with egg allergy. Patients with a history of life-threatening allergic reaction to neomycin or gelatin should not receive MMR. The MMR vaccine is safe to use during lactation, but its use during pregnancy is discouraged because of the theoretical but unproven risk of congenital rubella syndrome from the live virus contained in the vaccine. MMR vaccine is well tolerated; there have been rare reports of mild, transient adverse reactions such as rash and sore throat.

At the request of the CDC and the National Institutes of Health (NIH), the Institute of Medicine and National Academy of Sciences conducted a review of all the evidence related to the MMR vaccine and autism. This independent panel examined completed studies, ongoing studies, published medical and scientific articles, and expert testimony to assess whether or not there was a link between autism and the MMR vaccine. The groups concluded that the evidence reviewed did not support an association between autism and the MMR vaccine. Although the preservative thimerosal, a mercury derivative, has been mentioned as a possible autism contributor, the MMR vaccine licensed for use in the United States does not contain this preservative.

Discussion Sources

Centers for Disease Prevention and Control. http://www.cdc.gov/vaccines/vpd-vac/combo-vaccines/mmr/faqs-mmr-hcp.htm, MMR vaccine: Questions and answers, accessed 8/21/09.

Centers for Disease Prevention and Control. http://www.cdc.gov/ncbddd/autism/faq_vaccines.htm, Autism information center, accessed 8/21/09.

QUESTIONS

20. When advising a patient about antipneumococcal immunization, the NP considers the following about the vaccine:

    A. It contains inactivated bacteria.

    B. Its use is contraindicated in individuals with asthma.

    C. It protects against community-acquired pneumonia caused by atypical pathogens.

    D. Its use is seldom associated with significant adverse reactions.

21. Of the following, who is at greatest risk for invasive pneumococcal infection?

    A. a 68-year-old man with chronic obstructive pulmonary disease

    B. a 34-year-old woman who underwent splenectomy after a motor vehicle accident

    C. a 50-year-old man with a 15-year history of type 2 diabetes

    D. a 75-year-old woman with decreased mobility caused by rheumatoid arthritis

22. All of the following patients received a dose of antipneumococcal vaccine 5 years ago. Who is not a candidate for receiving a second dose of antipneumococcal immunization?

    A. a 45-year-old man with chronic bronchitis

    B. a 72-year-old woman with hypertension

    C. a 35-year-old man with a history of asthma

    D. a 58-year-old woman with immunosuppression

Recommended adult immunization schedule, by vaccine and age group — United Sates, 2010

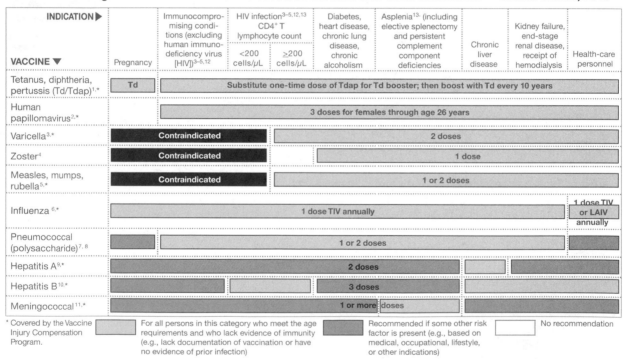

VACCINE AGE GROUP ▶	19–26 years	27–49 years	50–59 years	60–64 years	≥ 65 years
Tetanus, diphtheria, pertussis (Td/Tdap)[1,*]	Substitute one-time dose of Tdap for Td booster; then boost with Td every 10 years				Td booster every 10 years
Human papillomavirus[2,*]	3 doses (females)				
Varicella[3,*]	2 doses				
Zoster[4]					1 dose
Measles, mumps, rubella[5,*]	1 or 2 doses			1 dose	
Influenza[6,*]	1 dose annually				
Pneumococcal (polysaccharide)[7, 8]	1 or 2 doses				1 dose
Hepatitis A[9,*]	2 doses				
Hepatitis B[10,*]	3 doses				
Meningococcal[11,*]	1 or more doses				

* Covered by the Vaccine Injury Compensation Program.

[ ] For all persons in this category who meet the age requirements and who lack evidence of immunity (e.g., lack documentation of vaccination or have no evidence of prior infection)

[ ] Recommended if some other risk factor is present (e.g., based on medical, occupational, lifestyle, or other indications)

[ ] No recommendation

Vaccines that might be indicated for adults based on medical and other indications — United States, 2010

INDICATION ▶ VACCINE ▼	Pregnancy	Immunocompromising conditions (excluding human immunodeficiency virus [HIV])[3–5,12]	HIV infection[3–5,12,13] CD4+ T lymphocyte count <200 cells/μL	HIV infection CD4+ T lymphocyte count ≥200 cells/μL	Diabetes, heart disease, chronic lung disease, chronic alcoholism	Asplenia[13.] (including elective splenectomy and persistent complement component deficiencies	Chronic liver disease	Kidney failure, end-stage renal disease, receipt of hemodialysis	Health-care personnel
Tetanus, diphtheria, pertussis (Td/Tdap)[1,*]	Td	Substitute one-time dose of Tdap for Td booster; then boost with Td every 10 years							
Human papillomavirus[2,*]		3 doses for females through age 26 years							
Varicella[3,*]	Contraindicated			2 doses					
Zoster[4]	Contraindicated			1 dose					
Measles, mumps, rubella[5,*]	Contraindicated			1 or 2 doses					
Influenza[6,*]	1 dose TIV annually								1 dose TIV or LAIV annually
Pneumococcal (polysaccharide)[7, 8]		1 or 2 doses							
Hepatitis A[9,*]		2 doses							
Hepatitis B[10,*]		3 doses							
Meningococcal[11,*]		1 or more doses							

* Covered by the Vaccine Injury Compensation Program.

[ ] For all persons in this category who meet the age requirements and who lack evidence of immunity (e.g., lack documentation of vaccination or have no evidence of prior infection)

[ ] Recommended if some other risk factor is present (e.g., based on medical, occupational, lifestyle, or other indications)

[ ] No recommendation

NOTE: The above recommendations must be read along with the footnotes on pages Q3–Q4 of this schedule.

1. Tetanus, diphtheria, and acellular pertussis (Td/Tdap) vaccination

Tdap should replace a single dose of Td for adults aged 19–64 years who have not received a dose of Tdap previously.

Adults with uncertain or incomplete history of primary vaccination series with tetanus and diphtheria toxoid-containing vaccines should begin or complete a primary vaccination series. A primary series for adults is 3 doses of tetanus and diphtheria toxoid-containing vaccines; administer the first 2 doses at least 4 weeks apart and the third dose 6–12 months after the second; Tdap can substitute for any one of the doses of Td in the 3-dose primary series. The booster dose of tetanus and diphtheria toxoid-containing vaccine should be administered to adults who have completed a primary series and if the last vaccination was received ≥10 years previously. Tdap or Td vaccine may be used, as indicated.

If a woman is pregnant and received the last Td vaccination ≥10 years previously, administer Td during the second or third trimester. If the woman received the last Td vaccination <10 years previously, administer Tdap

Figure 1–2 Recommended immunization schedule by vaccine and age group—United States, 2009.

during the immediate postpartum period. A dose of Tdap is recommended for postpartum women, close contacts of infants aged <12 months, and all health-care personnel with direct patient contact if they have not previously received Tdap. An interval as short as 2 years from the last Td vaccination is suggested; shorter intervals can be used. Td may be deferred during pregnancy and Tdap substituted in the immediate postpartum period, or Tdap can be administered instead of Td to a pregnant woman.

Consult the ACIP statement for recommendations for giving Td as prophylaxis in wound management.

2. Human papillomavirus (HPV) vaccination

HPV vaccination is recommended at age 11 or 12 years with catch-up vaccination at ages 13 through 26 years.

Ideally, vaccine should be administered before potential exposure to HPV through sexual activity; however, females who are sexually active should still be vaccinated consistent with age-based recommendations. Sexually active females who have not been infected with any of the four HPV vaccine types (types 6, 11, 16, 18, all of which HPV4 prevents) or any of the two HPV vaccine types (types 16 and 18, both of which HPV2 prevents) for receive the full benefit of the vaccination. Vaccination is less beneficial for females who have already been infected with one or more of the HPV vaccine types. HPV4 or HPV2 can be administered to persons with a history of genital warts, abnormal Papanicolaou test, or positive HPV DNA test, because these conditions are not evidence of prior infection with all vaccine HPV types.

HPV4 may be administered to males aged 9 through 26 years to reduce their likelihood of acquiring genital warts. HPV4 would be most effective when administered before exposure to HPV through sexual contact.

A complete series for either HPV4 or HPV2 consists of 3 doses. The second dose should be administered 1–2 months after the first dose; the third does should be administered 6 months after the first dose.

Although HPV vaccination is not specifically recommended for persons with the medical indications described in Figure 2, "Vaccines that might be indicated for adults based on medical and other indications," it may be administered to these persons because the HPV vaccine is not a live-virus vaccine. However, the immune response and vaccine efficacy might be less for persons with the medical indications described in Figure 2 than in persons who do not have the medical indications described or who are immunocompetent. Health-care personnel are not at increased risk because of occupational exposure and should be vaccinated consistent with age-based recommendations.

3. Varicella vaccination

All adults without evidence of immunity to varicella should receive 2 doses of single-antigen varicella vaccine if not previously vaccinated or the second dose if they have received only 1 dose, unless they have a medical contraindication. Special consideration should be given to those who 1) have close contact with persons at high risk for severe disease (e.g., health-care personnel and family contacts of persons with immunocompromising conditions) or 2) are at high risk for exposure or transmission (e.g., teachers; child-care employees; residents and staff members of institutional settings, including correctional institutions; college students; military personnel; adolescents and adults living in households with children; nonpregnant women of childbearing age; and international travelers).

Evidence of immunity to varicella in adults includes any of the following: 1) documentation of 2 doses of varicella vaccine at least 4 weeks apart; 2) U.S.-born before 1980 (although for health-care personnel and pregnant women, birth before 1980 should not be considered evidence of immunity); 3) history of varicella based on a diagnosis or verification of varicella by a health-care provider (for a patient reporting a history of or having an atypical case, a mild case, or both, health-care providers should seek either an epidemiologic link with a typical varicella case or to a laboratory-confirmed case or evidence of laboratory confirmation, if it was performed at the time of acute disease); 4) history of herpes zoster based on diagnosis or verification of herpes zoster by a health-care provider; or 5) laboratory evidence of immunity or laboratory confirmation of disease.

Pregnant women should be assessed for evidence of varicella immunity. Women who do not have evidence of immunity should receive the first dose of varicella vaccine upon completion or termination of pregnancy and before discharge from the health-care facility. The second dose should be administered 4–8 weeks after the first does.

4. Herpes zoster vaccination

A single dose of zoster vaccine is recommended for adults aged ≥60 years regardless of whether they report a prior episode of herpes zoster. Persons with chronic medical conditions may be vaccinated unless their condition constitutes a contraindication.

5. Measles, mumps, rubella (MMR) vaccination

Adults born before 1957 generally are considered immune to measles and mumps.

Measles component: Adults born during or after 1957 should receive 1 or more doses of MMR vaccine unless they have 1) a medical contraindication; 2) documentation of vaccination with 1 or more doses of MMR vaccine; 3) laboratory evidence of immunity; or 4) documentation of physician-diagnosed measles.

A second dose of MMR vaccine, administered 4 weeks after the first dose, is recommended for adults who 1) have been recently exposed to measles or are in an outbreak setting; 2) have been vaccinated previously with killed measles vaccine; 3) have been vaccinated with an unknown type of measles vaccine during 1963–1967; 4) are students in postsecondary educational institutions; 5) work in a health-care facility; or 6) plan to travel internationally.

Mumps component: Adults born during or after 1957 should receive 1 dose of MMR vaccine unless they have 1) a medical contraindication; 2) documentation of vaccination with 1 or more doses of MMR vaccine; 3) laboratory evidence of immunity; or 4) documentation of physician-diagnosed mumps.

A second dose of MMR vaccine, administered 4 weeks after the first dose, is recommended for adults who 1) live in a community experiencing a mumps outbreak and are in an affected age group; 2) are students in postsecondary educational institutions; 3) work in a health-care facility; or 4) plan to travel internationally.

Rubella component: 1 dose of MMR vaccine is recommended for women who do not have documentation of rubella vaccination, or who lack laboratory evidence of immunity. For women of childbearing age, regardless of birth year, rubella immunity should be determined, and women should be counseled regarding congenital rubella syndrome. Women who do not have evidence of immunity should receive MMR vaccine upon completion or termination of pregnancy and before discharge from the health-care facility.

Health-care personnel born before 1957: For unvaccinated health-care personnel born before 1957 who lack laboratory evidence of measles, mumps, and/or rubella immunity or laboratory confirmation of disease, health-care facilities should consider vaccinating personnel with 2 doses of MMR vaccine at the appropriate interval (for measles and mumps) and 1 dose of MMR vaccine (for rubella), respectively.

During outbreaks, health-care facilities should recommend that unvaccinated health-care personnel born before 1957, who lack laboratory evidence of measles, mumps, and/or rubella immunity or laboratory confirmation of disease, receive 2 doses of MMR vaccine during an outbreak of measles or mumps, and 1 dose during an outbreak of rubella.

Complete information about evidence of immunity is available at http://www.cdc.gov/vaccines/recs/provisional/default.htm.

6. Seasonal influenza vaccination

Vaccinate all persons aged ≥50 years and any younger persons who would like to decrease their risk for influenza. Vaccinate persons aged 19 through 49 years with any of the following indications.

Medical: Chronic disorders of the cardiovascular or pulmonary systems, including asthma; chronic metabolic diseases (including diabetes mellitus); renal or hepatic dysfunction, hemoglobinopathies, or immunocompromising conditions (including immunocompromising conditions caused by medications or HIV); cognitive, neurologic, or neuromuscular disorders; and pregnancy during the influenza season. No data exist on the risk for severe or complicated influenza disease among person with asplenia; however, influenza is a risk factor for secondary bacterial infections that can cause severe disease among persons with asplenia.

Occupational: All health-care personnel, including those employed by long-term care and assisted-living facilities, and caregivers of children aged <5 years.

Other: Residents of nursing homes and other long-term care and assisted-living facilities; persons likely to transmit influenza to persons at high risk (e.g.; in-home household contacts and caregivers of children aged <5 years, persons aged ≥50 years, and persons of all ages with high-risk conditions).

Healthy, nonpregnant adults aged <50 years without high-risk medical conditions who are not contacts of severely immunocompromised persons in special-care units may receive either intranasally administered live, attenuated influenza vaccine (FluMist) or inactivated vaccine. Other persons should receive the inactivated vaccine.

7. Pneumococcal polysaccharide (PPSV) vaccination

Vaccinate all persons with the following indications.

Medical: Chronic lung disease (including asthma); chronic cardiovascular diseases; diabetes mellitus; chronic liver diseases, cirrhosis; chronic alcoholism; functional or anatomic asplenia (e.g., sickle cell disease or

Figure 1–2 cont'd

splenectomy [if elective spletnectomy is planned, vaccinate at least 2 weeks before surgery]); immunocompromising conditions (including chronic renal failure or nephrotic syndrome); and cochlear implants and cerebrospinal fluid leaks. Vaccinate as close to HIV diagnosis as possible.

Other: Residents of nursing homes or long-term care facilities and persons who smoke cigarettes. Routine use of PPSV is not recommended for American Indians/Alaska Natives or persons aged <65 years unless they have underlying medical conditions that are PPSV indications. However, public health authorities may consider PPSV for American Indians/Alaska Natives and persons aged 50 through 64 years who are living in areas where the risk for invasive pneumococcal disease is increased.

8. Revaccination with PPSV

One-time revaccination after 5 years is recommended for persons with chronic renal failure or anatomic asplenia; functional or anatomic asplenia (e.g., sickle cell disease or splenectomy); and for persons with immunocompromising conditions. For persons aged ≥65 years, one-time revaccination is recommended if they were vaccinated ≥5 years previously and were aged <65 years at the time of primary vaccination.

9. Hepatitis A vaccination

Vaccinate persons with any of the following indications and any person seeking protection from hepatitis A virus (HAV) infection.

Behavioral: Men who have sex with men and persons who use injection drugs.

Occupational: Persons working with HAV-infected primates or with HAV in a research laboratory setting.

Medical: Persons with chronic liver disease and persons who receive clotting factor concentrates.

Other: Persons traveling to or working in countries that have high or intermediate endemicity of hepatitis A (a list of countries is available at http://www.cdc.gov/travel/contentdiseases.aspx).

Unvaccinated persons who anticipate close personal contact (e.g., household contact or regular babysitting) with an international adoptee from a country of high or intermediate endemicity during the first 60 days after arrival of the adoptee in the United States should consider vaccination. The first dose of the 2-dose hepatitis A vaccine series should be administered as soon as adoption is planned, ideally >2 weeks before the arrival of the adoptee.

Single-antigen vaccine formulations should be administered in a 2-dose schedule at either 0 and 6–12 months (Havrix), or 0 and 6–18 months (Vaqta). If the combined hepatitis A and hepatitis B vaccine (Twinrix) is used, administer 3 doses at 0, 1, and 6 months; alternatively, a 4-dose schedule, administered on days 0, 7, and 21–30 followed by a booster dose at month 12 may be used.

10. Hepatitis B vaccination

Vaccinate persons with any of the following indications and any person seeking protection from hepatitis B virus (HBV) infection.

Behavioral: Sexually active persons who are not in a long-term, mutually monogamous relationship (e.g., persons with more than one sex partner during the previous 6 months); persons seeking evaluation or treatment for a sexually transmitted disease (STD); current or recent injection-drug users; and men who have sex with men.

Occupational: Health-care personnel and public-safety workers who are exposed to blood or other potentially infectious body fluids.

Medical: Persons with end-stage renal disease, including patients receiving hemodialysis; persons with HIV infection; and persons with chronic liver disease.

Other: Household contacts and sex partners of persons with chronic HBV infection; clients and staff members of institutions for persons with developmental disabilities; and international travelers to countries with high or intermediate prevalence of chronic HBV infection (a list of countries is available at http://www.cdc.gov/travel/contentdiseases.aspx).

Hepatitis B vaccination is recommended for all adults in the following settings: STD treatment facilities; HIV testing and treatment facilities; facilities providing drug-abuse treatment and prevention services; health-care settings targeting services to injection-drug users or men who have sex with men; correctional facilities; end-stage renal disease programs and facilities for chronic hemodialysis patients; and institutions and nonresidential day-care facilities for persons with developmental disabilities.

Administer or complete a 3-dose series of hepatitis B vaccine to those persons not previously vaccinated. The second dose should be administered 1 month after the first dose;, the third dose should be administered at least 2 months after the second dose (and at least 4 months after the first dose). If the combined hepatitis A and hepatitis B vaccines (Twinrix) is used, administer 3 doses at 0, 1, and 6 months; alternatively, a 4-dose schedule, administered on days 0, 7, and 21–30 followed by a booster dose at month 12 may be used.

Adult patients receiving hemodialysis or with other immunocompromising conditions should receive 1 dose of 40μg/mL (Recombivax HB) administered on a 3-dose schedule or 2 doses of 20μg/mL (Engerix-B) administered simultaneously on a 4-dose schedule at 0, 1, 2, and 6 months.

11. Meningococcal vaccination

Meningococcal vaccine should be administered to persons with the following indications.

Medical: Adults with anatomic or functional asplenia, or persistent following indications.

Other: First-year college students living in dormitories; microbiologists routinely exposed to isolates of *Neisseria meningitidis*; military recruits; and persons who travel to or live in countries in which meningococcal disease is hyperendemic or epidemic (e.g., the "meningitis belt" of sub-Saharan Africa during the dry season [December through June]), particularly if their contact with local populations will be prolonged. Vaccination is required by the government of Saudi Arabia for all travelers to Mecca during the annual Hajj.

Meningococcal conjugate vaccine (MCV4) is preferred for adults with any of the preceding indications who are aged ≤55 years; meningococcal polysaccharide vaccine (MPSV4) is preferred for adults aged ≥56 years. Revaccination with MCV4 after 5 years is recommended for adults previously vaccinated with MCV4 or MPSV4 who remain at increased risk for infection (e.g., adults with anatomic or functional asplenia. Persons whose only risk factor is living in on-campus housing are not recommended to receive an additional dose.

12. Immunocompromising conditions

Inactivated vaccines generally are acceptable (e.g., pneumococcal, meinigococcal, influenza [inactivated influenza vaccine]) and live vaccines generally are avoided in persons with immune deficiencies or immunocompromising conditions. Information on specific conditions is available at http://www.cdc.gov/vaccines/pubs/acip-list.htm.

13. Selected conditions for which *Haemophilus influenzae* type b (Hib) vaccine may be used

Hib vaccine generally is not recommended for persons aged ≥5 years. No efficacy data are available on which to base a recommendation concerning use of Hib vaccine for older children and adults. However, studies suggest good immunogenicity in patients who have sickle cell disease, leukemia, or HIV infection or who have had a splenectomy. Administering 1 dose of Hib vaccine to these high-risk persons who have not previously received Hib vaccine is not contraindicated.

These schedules indicate the recommended age groups and medical indications for which administration of currently licensed vaccines is commonly indicated for adults aged ≥19 years, as of January 1, 2009. Licensed combination vaccines may be used whenever any components of the combination are indicated and when the vaccine's other components are not contraindicated. For detailed recommendations on all vaccines, including those that are used primarily for travelers or are issued during the year, consult the manufacturers' package inserts and the complete statements from the Advisory Committee on Immunization Practices (ACIP) (**http://www.cdc.gov/vaccines/ pubs/acip-list.htm**).

Report all clinically significant post vaccination reactions to the Vaccine Adverse Event Reporting System (VAERS)> Reporting forms and instructions on filing a VAERS report are available at **http://www.vaers.hhs.gov** or by telephone, 800-822-7967.

Information on how to file a Vaccine Injury Compensation Program claim is available at http://www.hrsa.gov/vaccinecompensation or by telephone, 800-338-2382. To file a claim for vaccine injury, contact the U.S. Court of Federal Claims, 717 Madison Place, N.W., Washington, D.C. 20005; telephone, 202-357-6400.

Additional information about the vaccines in this schedule, extent of available data, and contraindications for vaccination is available at **http://www.cdc.gov/vaccines** or from the CDC-INFO Contact Center at 800-CDC-INFO (800-232-4636) in English and Spanish, 24 hours a day, 7 days a week.

Use of trade names and commercial sources for identification only and does not imply endorsement by the U.S. Department of Health and Human Services.

The recommendations in this schedule were approved by ACIP, the American Academy of Family Physicians, the American College of Obstetricians and Gynecologists, and the American College of Physicians.

Department of Health and Human Services • Centers for Disease Control and Prevention

---

Figure 1–2 cont'd

Recommended immunization schedule for persons aged 0 through 6 years — United States, 2010
(for those who fall behind or start late, see the catch-up schedule)

Vaccine ▼ Age ▶	Birth	1 month	2 months	4 months	6 months	12 months	15 months	18 months	19–23 months	2–3 years	4–6 years
Hepatitis B[1]	HepB	HepB			HepB						
Rotavirus[2]			RV	RV	RV[2]						
Diphtheria, Tetanus, Pertussis[3]			DTaP	DTaP	DTaP	see footnote 3	DTaP				DTaP
Haemophilus influenzae type b[4]			Hib	Hib	Hib[4]	Hib					
Pneumococcal[5]			PCV	PCV	PCV	PCV				PPSV	
Inactivated Poliovirus			IPV	IPV	IPV						IPV
Influenza[6]					Influenza (Yearly)						
Measles, Mumps, Rubella[7]						MMR		see footnote 8			MMR
Varicella[8]						Varicella		see footnote 9			Varicella
Hepatitis A[9]						HepA (2 doses)				HepA Series	
Meningococcal[10]										MCV	

Range of recommended ages for all children except certain high-risk groups

Range of recommended ages for certain high-risk groups

This schedule includes recommendations in effect as of December 15, 2009. Any dose not administered at the recommended age should be administered at a subsequent visit, when indicated and feasible. The use of a combination vaccine generally is preferred over separate injections of its equivalent component vaccines. Considerations should include provider assessment, patient preference, and the potential for adverse events. Providers should consult the relevant Advisory Committee on Immunization Practices statement for detailed recommendations: **http://www.cdc.gov/vaccines/pubs/acip-list.htm**. Clinically significant adverse events that follow immunization should be reported to the Vaccine Adverse Event Reporting System (VAERS) at **http://www.vaers.hhs.gov** or by telephone, 800-822-7967.

1. **Hepatitis B vaccine (HepB).** (Minimum age: birth)
   At birth:
   - Administer monovalent HepB to all newborns before hospital discharge.
   - If mother is hepatitis B surface antigen (HBsAg)-positive, administer HepB and 0.5 mL of hepatitis B immune globulin (HBIG) within 12 hours of birth.
   - If mother's HBsAg status is unknown, administer HepB within 12 hours of birth. Determine mother's HBsAg status as soon as possible and, if HBsAg-positive, administer HBIG (no later than age 1 week).
   After the birth dose:
   - The HepB series should be completed with either monovalent HepB or a combination vaccine containing HepB. The second dose should be administered at age 1 or 2 months. Monovalent HepB vaccine should be used for doses administered before age 6 weeks. The final dose should be administered no earlier than age 24 weeks.
   - Infants born to HBsAg-positive mothers should be tested for HBsAg and antibody to HBsAg 1 to 2 months after completion of at least 3 doses of the HepB series, at age 9 through 18 months (generally at the next well-child visit).
   - Administration of 4 doses of HepB to infants is permissible when a combination vaccine containing HepB is administered after the birth dose. The fourth dose should be administered no earlier than age 24 weeks.
2. **Rotavirus vaccine (RV).** (Minimum age: 6 weeks)
   - Administer the first dose at age 6 through 14 weeks (maximum age: 14 weeks 6 days). Vaccination should not be initiated for infants aged 15 weeks 0 days or older.
   - The maximum age for the final dose in the series is 8 months 0 days.
   - If Rotarix is administered at ages 2 and 4 months, a dose at 6 months is not indicated.
3. **Diphtheria and tetanus toxoids and acellular pertussis vaccine (DTaP).** (Minimum age: 6 weeks)
   - The fourth dose may be administered as early as age 12 months, provided at least 6 months have elapsed since the third dose.
   - Administer the final dose in the series at age 4 through 6 years.
4. **Haemophilus influenzae type b conjugate vaccine (Hib).** (Minimum age: 6 weeks)
   - If PRP-OMP (PedvaxHIB or Comvax [HepB-Hib]) is administered at ages 2 and 4 months, a dose at age 6 months is not indicated.
   - TriHiBit (DTaP/Hib) and Hiberix (PRP-T) should not be used for doses at ages 2, 4, or 6 months for the primary series but can be used as the final dose in children aged 12 months through 4 years.
5. **Pneumococcal vaccine.** (Minimum age: 6 weeks for pneumococcal conjugate vaccine [PCV]; 2 years for pneumococcal polysaccharide vaccine [PPSV])
   - PCV is recommended for all children aged younger than 5 years. Administer 1 dose of PCV to all healthy children aged 24 through 59 months who are not completely vaccinated for their age.
   - Administer PPSV 2 or more months after last dose of PCV to children aged 2 years or older with certain underlying medical conditions, including a cochlear implant. See *MMWR* 1997;46(No. RR-8).

6. **Inactivated poliovirus vaccine (IPV)** (Minimum age: 6 weeks)
   - The final dose in the series should be administered on or after the fourth birthday and at least 6 months following the previous dose.
   - If 4 doses are administered prior to age 4 years a fifth dose should be administered at age 4 through 6 years. See *MMWR* 2009;58(30):829–30.
7. **Influenza vaccine (seasonal).** (Minimum age: 6 months for trivalent inactivated influenza vaccine [TIV]; 2 years for live, attenuated influenza vaccine [LAIV])
   - Administer annually to children aged 6 months through 18 years.
   - For healthy children aged 2 through 6 years (i.e., those who do not have underlying medical conditions that predispose them to influenza complications), either LAIV or TIV may be used, except LAIV should not be given to children aged 2 through 4 years who have had wheezing in the past 12 months.
   - Children receiving TIV should receive 0.25 mL if aged 6 through 35 months or 0.5 mL if aged 3 years or older.
   - Administer 2 doses (separated by at least 4 weeks) to children aged younger than 9 years who are receiving influenza vaccine for the first time or who were vaccinated for the first time during the previous influenza season but only received 1 dose.
   - For recommendations for use of influenza A (H1N1) 2009 monovalent vaccine see *MMWR* 2009;58(No. RR-10).
8. **Measles, mumps, and rubella vaccine (MMR).** (Minimum age: 12 months)
   - Administer the second dose routinely at age 4 through 6 years. However, the second dose may be administered before age 4, provided at least 28 days have elapsed since the first dose.
9. **Varicella vaccine.** (Minimum age: 12 months)
   - Administer the second dose routinely at age 4 through 6 years. However, the second dose may be administered before age 4, provided at least 3 months have elapsed since the first dose.
   - For children aged 12 months through 12 years the minimum interval between doses is 3 months. However, if the second dose was administered at least 28 days after the first dose, it can be accepted as valid.
10. **Hepatitis A vaccine (HepA).** (Minimum age: 12 months)
    - Administer to all children aged 1 year (i.e., aged 12 through 23 months). Administer 2 doses at least 6 months apart.
    - Children not fully vaccinated by age 2 years can be vaccinated at subsequent visits.
    - HepA also is recommended for older children who live in areas where vaccination programs target older children, who are at increased risk for infection, or for whom immunity against hepatitis A is desired.
11. **Meningococcal vaccine.** (Minimum age: 2 years for meningococcal conjugate vaccine [MCV4] and for meningococcal polysaccharide vaccine [MPSV4])
    - Administer MCV4 to children aged 2 through 10 years with persistent complement component deficiency, anatomic or functional asplenia, and certain other conditions placing them at high risk.
    - Administer MCV4 to children previously vaccinated with MCV4 or MPSV4 after 3 years if first dose administered at age 2 through 6 years. See *MMWR* 2009; 58:1042–3.

The Recommended Immunization Schedules for Persons Aged 0 through 18 Years are approved by the **Advisory Committee on Immunization Practices** (http://www.cdc.gov/vaccines/recs/acip), the **American Academy of Pediatrics** (http://www.aap.org), and the **American Academy of Family Physicians** (http://www.aafp.org).
Department of Health and Human Services • Centers for Disease Control and Prevention

Figure 1–2 cont'd

Recommended immunization schedule for persons aged 7 through 18 years — United States, 2010
(for those who fall behind or start late, see the catch-up schedule)

Vaccine ▼ Age ▶	7–10 years	11–12 years	13–18 years	
Tetanus, Diphtheria, Pertussis[1]		Tdap	Tdap	Range of recommended ages for all children except certain high-risk groups
Human Papillomavirus[2]	see footnote 2	HPV (3 doses)	HPV Series	
Meningococcal[3]	MCV	MCV	MCV	
Influenza[4]	Influenza (Yearly)			Range of recommended ages for catch-up immunization
Pneumococcal[5]	PPSV			
Hepatitis A[6]	HepA Series			
Hepatitis B[7]	HepB Series			Range of recommended ages for certain high-risk groups
Inactivated Poliovirus[8]	IPV Series			
Measles, Mumps, Rubella[9]	MMR Series			
Varicella[10]	Varicella Series			

This schedule includes recommendations in effect as of December 15, 2009. Any dose not administered at the recommended age should be administered at a subsequent visit, when indicated and feasible. The use of a combination vaccine generally is preferred over separate injections of its equivalent component vaccines. Considerations should include provider assessment, patient preference, and the potential for adverse events. Providers should consult the relevant Advisory Committee on Immunization Practices statement for detailed recommendations: **http://www.cdc.gov/vaccines/pubs/acip-list.htm**. Clinically significant adverse events that follow immunization should be reported to the Vaccine Adverse Event Reporting System (VAERS) at **http://www.vaers.hhs.gov** or by telephone, 800-822-7967.

1. **Tetanus and diphtheria toxoids and acellular pertussis vaccine (Tdap).** (Minimum age: 10 years for Boostrix and 11 years for Adacel).
   - Administer at age 11 or 12 years for those who have completed the recommended childhood DTP/DTaP vaccination series and have not received a tetanus and diphtheria toxoid (Td) booster dose.
   - Persons aged 13 through 18 years who have not received Tdap should receive a dose.
   - A 5-year interval from the last Td dose is encouraged when Tdap is used as a booster dose; however, a shorter interval may be used if pertussis immunity is needed.
2. **Human papillomavirus vaccine (HPV).** (Minimum age: 9 years)
   - Two HPV vaccines are licensed: a quadrivalent vaccine (HPV4) for the prevention of cervical, vaginal and vulvar cancers (in females) and genital warts (in females and males), and a bivalent vaccine (HPV2) for the prevention of cervical cancers in females.
   - HPV vaccines are most effective for both males and females when given before exposure to HPV through sexual contact.
   - HPV4 or HPV2 is recommended for the prevention of cervical precancers and cancers in females.
   - HPV4 is recommended for the prevention of cervical, vaginal and vulvar precancers and cancers and genital warts in females.
   - Administer the first dose to females at age 11 or 12 years.
   - Administer the second dose 1 to 2 months after the first dose and the third dose 6 months after the first dose (at least 24 weeks after the first dose).
   - Administer the series to females at age 13 through 18 years if not previously vaccinated.
   - HPV4 may be administered in a 3-dose series to males aged 9 through 18 years to reduce their likelihood of acquiring genital warts.
3. **Meningococcal conjugate vaccine (MCV4).**
   - Administer at age 11 or 12 years, or at age 13 through 18 years if not previously vaccinated.
   - Administer to previously unvaccinated college freshmen living in a dormitory.
   - Administer MCV4 to children aged 2 through 10 years with persistent complement component deficiency, anatomic or functional asplenia, or certain other conditions placing them at high risk.
   - Administer to children previously vaccinated with MCV4 or MPSV4 who remain at increased risk after 3 years (if first dose administered at age 2 through 6 years) or after 5 years (if first dose administered at age 7 years or older). Persons whose only risk factor is living in on-campus housing are not recommended to receive an additional dose. See *MMWR* 2009;58:1042–3.
4. **Influenza vaccine (seasonal).**
   - Administer annually to children aged 6 months through 18 years.
   - For healthy nonpregnant persons aged 7 through 18 years (i.e., those who do not have underlying medical conditions that predispose them to influenza complications), either LAIV or TIV may be used.
   - Administer 2 doses (separated by at least 4 weeks) to children aged younger than 9 years who are receiving influenza vaccine for the first time or who were vaccinated for the first time during the previous influenza season but only received 1 dose.
   - For recommendations for use of influenza A (H1N1) 2009 monovalent vaccine. See *MMWR* 2009;58(No. RR-10)
5. **Pneumococcal polysaccharide vaccine (PPSV).**
   - Administer to children with certain underlying medical conditions, including a cochlear implant. A single revaccination should be administered after 5 years to children with functional or anatomic asplenia or an immunocompromising condition. See *MMWR* 1997;46(No. RR-8).
6. **Hepatitis A vaccine (HepA).**
   - Administer 2 doses at least 6 months apart.
   - HepA is recommended for children aged older than 23 months who live in areas where vaccination programs target older children, who are at increased risk for infection, or for whom immunity against hepatitis A is desired.
7. **Hepatitis B vaccine (HepB).**
   - Administer the 3-dose series to those not previously vaccinated.
   - A 2-dose series (separated by at least 4 months) of adult formulation Recombivax HB is licensed for children aged 11 through 15 years.
8. **Inactivated poliovirus vaccine (IPV).**
   - The final dose in the series should be administered on or after the fourth birthday and at least 6 months following the previous dose.
   - If both OPV and IPV were administered as part of a series, a total of 4 doses should be administered, regardless of the child's current age.
9. **Measles, mumps, and rubella vaccine (MMR).**
   - If not previously vaccinated, administer 2 doses or the second dose for those who have received only 1 dose, with at least 28 days between doses.
10. **Varicella vaccine.**
   - For persons aged 7 through 18 years without evidence of immunity (see *MMWR* 2007;56[No. RR-4]), administer 2 doses if not previously vaccinated or the second dose if only 1 dose has been administered.
   - For persons aged 7 through 12 years, the minimum interval between doses is 3 months. However, if the second dose was administered at least 28 days after the first dose, it can be accepted as valid.
   - For persons aged 13 years and older, the minimum interval between doses is 28 days.

The Recommended Immunization Schedules for Persons Aged 0 through 18 Years are approved by the **Advisory Committee on Immunization Practices (http://www.cdc.gov/vaccines/recs/acip), the American Academy of Pediatrics (http://www.aap.org), and the American Academy of Family Physicians (http://www.aafp.org).**
Department of Health and Human Services • Centers for Disease Control and Prevention

Figure 1–2   cont'd

Catch-up immunization schedule for persons aged 4 months through 18 years who start late or who are more than 1 month behind — United States, 2010

The table below provides catch-up schedules and minimum intervals between doses for children whose vaccinations have been delayed. A vaccine series does not need to be restarted, regardless of the time that has elapsed between doses. Use the section appropriate for the child's age.

Vaccine	Minimum Age for Dose 1	Minimum Interval Between Doses			
		Dose 1 to Dose 2		Dose 3 to Dose 4	Dose 4 to Dose 5
PERSONS AGED 4 MONTHS THROUGH 6 YEARS					
Hepatitis B [1]	Birth	4 weeks	8 weeks (and at least 16 weeks after first dose)		
Rotavirus [2]	6 wks	4 weeks	4 weeks [2]		
Diphtheria, Tetanus, Pertussis [3]	6 wks	4 weeks	4 weeks	6 months	6 months [3]
Haemophilus influenzae type b [4]	6 wks	4 weeks if first dose administered at younger than age 12 months / 8 weeks (as final dose) if first dose administered at age 12-14 months / No further doses needed if first dose administered at age 15 months or older	4 weeks [4] if current age is younger than 12 months / 8 weeks (as final dose) [4] if current age is 12 months or older and first dose administered at younger than age 12 months and second dose administered at younger than age 15 / No further doses needed if previous dose administered at age 15 months or older	8 weeks (as final dose) This dose only necessary for children aged 12 months through 59 months who received 3 doses before age 12 months	
Pneumococcal [5]	6 wks	4 weeks if first dose administered at younger than age 12 months / 8 weeks (as final dose for healthy children) if first dose administered at age 12 months or older or current age 24 through 59 months / No further doses needed for healthy children if first dose administered at age 24 months or older	4 weeks if current age is younger than 12 months / 8 weeks (as final dose for healthy children) if current age 12 months or older / No further doses needed for healthy children if previous dose administered at age 24 months or older	8 weeks (as final dose) This dose only necessary for children aged 12 months through 59 months who received 3 doses before age 12 months or for high-risk children who received 3 doses at any age	
Inactivated Poliovirus [6]	6 wks	4 weeks	4 weeks	4 weeks [6]	
Measles, Mumps, Rubella [7]	12 mos	4 weeks			
Varicella [8]	12 mos	3 months			
Hepatitis A [9]	12 mos	6 months			
PERSONS AGED 7 THROUGH 18 YEARS					
Tetanus, Diphtheria/ Tetanus, Diphtheria, Pertussis [10]	7 yrs [10]	4 weeks	4 weeks if first dose administered at younger than age 12 months / 6 months if first dose administered at age 12 months or older	6 months if first dose administered at younger than age 12 months	
Human Papillomavirus [11]	9 yrs	Routine dosing intervals are recommended [11]			
Hepatitis A [9]	12 mos	6 months			
Hepatitis B [1]	Birth	4 weeks	8 weeks (and at least 16 weeks after first dose)		
Inactivated Poliovirus [6]	6 wks	4 weeks	4 weeks	6 months	
Measles, Mumps, Rubella [7]	12 mos	4 weeks			
Varicella [8]	12 mos	3 months if the person is younger than age 13 years / 4 weeks if the person is aged 13 years or older			

1. **Hepatitis B vaccine (HepB).**
   - Administer the 3-dose series to those not previously vaccinated.
   - A 2-dose series (separated by at least 4 months) of adult formulation Recombivax HB is licensed for children aged 11 through 15 years.
2. **Rotavirus vaccine (RV).**
   - The maximum age for the first dose is 14 weeks 6 days. Vaccination should not be initiated for infants aged 15 weeks 0 days or older.
   - The maximum age for the final dose in the series is 8 months 0 days.
   - If Rotarix was administered for the first and second doses, a third dose is not indicated.
3. **Diphtheria and tetanus toxoids and acellular pertussis vaccine (DTaP).**
   - The fifth dose is not necessary if the fourth dose was administered at age 4 years or older.
4. ***Haemophilus influenzae* type b conjugate vaccine (Hib).**
   - Hib vaccine is not generally recommended for persons aged 5 years or older. No efficacy data are available on which to base a recommendation concerning use of Hib vaccine for older children and adults. However, studies suggest good immunogenicity in persons who have sickle cell disease, leukemia, or HIV infection, or who have had a splenectomy; administering 1 dose of Hib vaccine to these persons who have not previously received Hib vaccine is not contraindicated.
   - If the first 2 doses were PRP-OMP (PedvaxHIB or Comvax), and administered at age 11 months or younger, the third (and final) dose should be administered at age 12 through 15 months and at least 8 weeks after the second dose.
   - If the first dose was administered at age 7 through 11 months, administer the second dose at least 4 weeks later and a final dose at age 12 through 15 months.
5. **Pneumococcal vaccine.**
   - Administer 1 dose of pneumococcal conjugate vaccine (PCV) to all healthy children aged 24 through 59 months who have not received at least 1 dose of PCV on or after age 12 months.
   - For children aged 24 through 59 months with underlying medical conditions, administer 1 dose of PCV if 3 doses were received previously or administer 2 doses of PCV at least 8 weeks apart if fewer than 3 doses were received previously.
   - Administer pneumococcal polysaccharide vaccine (PPSV) to children aged 2 years or older with certain underlying medical conditions, including a cochlear implant, at least 8 weeks after the last dose of PCV. See *MMWR* 1997;46(No. RR-8).
6. **Inactivated poliovirus vaccine (IPV).**
   - The final dose in the series should be administered on or after the fourth birthday and at least 6 months following the previous dose.

- A fourth dose is not necessary if the third dose was administered at age 4 years or older and at least 6 months following the previous dose.
- In the first 6 months of life, minimum age and minimum intervals are only recommended if the person is at risk for imminent exposure to circulating poliovirus (i.e., travel to a polio-endemic region or during an outbreak).
7. **Measles, mumps, and rubella vaccine (MMR).**
   - Administer the second dose routinely at age 4 through 6 years. However, the second dose may be administered before age 4, provided at least 28 days have elapsed since the first dose.
   - If not previously vaccinated, administer 2 doses with at least 28 days between doses.
8. **Varicella vaccine.**
   - Administer the second dose routinely at age 4 through 6 years. However, the second dose may be administered before age 4, provided at least 3 months have elapsed since the first dose.
   - For persons aged 12 months through 12 years, the minimum interval between doses is 3 months. However, if the second dose was administered at least 28 days after the first dose, it can be accepted as valid.
   - For persons aged 13 years and older, the minimum interval between doses is 28 days.
9. **Hepatitis A vaccine (HepA).**
   - HepA is recommended for children aged older than 23 months who live in areas where vaccination programs target older children, who are at increased risk for infection, or for whom immunity against hepatitis A is desired.
10. **Tetanus and diphtheria toxoids vaccine (Td) and tetanus and diphtheria toxoids and acellular pertussis vaccine (Tdap).**
    - Doses of DTaP are counted as part of the Td/Tdap series
    - Tdap should be substituted for a single dose of Td in the catch-up series or as a booster for children aged 10 through 18 years; use Td for other doses.
11. **Human papillomavirus vaccine (HPV).**
    - Administer the series to females at age 13 through 18 years if not previously vaccinated.
    - Use recommended routine dosing intervals for series catch-up (i.e., the second and third doses should be administered at 1 to 2 and 6 months after the first dose). The minimum interval between the first and second doses is 4 weeks. The minimum interval between the second and third doses is 12 weeks, and the third dose should be administered at least 24 weeks after the first dose.

Information about reporting reactions after immunization is available online at **http://www.vaers.hhs.gov** or by telephone, **800-822-7967**. Suspected cases of vaccine-preventable diseases should be reported to the state or local health department. Additional information, including precautions and contraindications for immunization, is available from the National Center for Immunization and Respiratory Diseases at **http://www.cdc.gov/vaccines** or telephone, **800-CDC-INFO (800-232-4636)**. Department of Health and Human Services • Centers for Disease Control and Prevention

Figure 1–2 cont'd

ANSWERS

20. D   **21.** B   **22.** B

DISCUSSION

Pneumococcal disease, caused by the gram-positive diplococcus *Streptococcus pneumoniae,* results in significant mortality and morbidity. The antipneumococcal vaccine contains purified polysaccharide from 23 of the most common *S. pneumoniae* strains. These strains account for 90% of the bacteremic disease associated with the pathogen. The pneumococcal vaccine protects against invasive disease such as meningitis and septicemia associated with pneumonia and disease caused by *S. pneumoniae*; this organism is the leading cause of death from community-acquired pneumonia (CAP) in the United States.

In a retrospective study, the 23-valent pneumococcal polysaccharide vaccine was found to reduce the risk of hospitalization for pneumonia by 38% in a cohort of high-risk, elderly patients. In addition, pneumococcal vaccination was associated with reduced mortality, complications, and length of stay in hospitalized older adults (65 years or older) with CAP. Pneumococcal polysaccharide vaccine use has also been associated with a significantly reduced risk of pneumococcal bacteremia. This immunization is ineffective, however, against pneumonia and invasive disease caused by other infectious agents, including *Mycoplasma pneumoniae*; *Chlamydophila* (formerly *Chlamydia*) *pneumoniae*; *Legionella* species; and select gram-negative respiratory pathogens such as *Haemophilus influenzae, Moraxella catarrhalis,* and *Klebsiella pneumoniae.* Medical indications for this vaccine include chronic lung disease (including asthma), chronic cardiovascular diseases, diabetes mellitus, chronic liver disease including cirrhosis, chronic alcoholism, chronic renal failure or nephrotic syndrome, functional or anatomic asplenia (e.g., sickle cell disease or splenectomy [if elective splenectomy is planned, vaccinate at least 2 weeks before surgery]), immunocompromising conditions, cochlear implants, and cerebrospinal fluid leaks. A patient with HIV infection should receive antipneumococcal vaccine as soon as the diagnosis is made. Other individuals for whom vaccination is indicated include residents of nursing homes or other long-term care facilities, smokers, and all adults 65 years or older regardless of health status.

A one-time antipneumococcal revaccination after 5 years is recommended for persons with chronic renal failure or nephrotic syndrome, functional or anatomic asplenia (e.g., sickle cell disease or splenectomy), and immunocompromising conditions. For persons aged 65 years and older, one-time revaccination is recommended if the person was vaccinated 5 or more years previously and was younger than 65 years at the time of primary vaccination. This immunization, with initial and repeat vaccination, is generally well tolerated (Table 1–2).

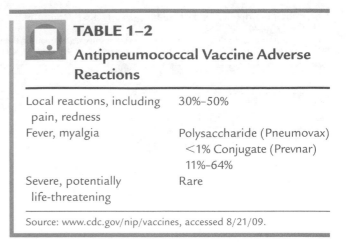

TABLE 1–2
Antipneumococcal Vaccine Adverse Reactions

Local reactions, including pain, redness	30%–50%
Fever, myalgia	Polysaccharide (Pneumovax) <1% Conjugate (Prevnar) 11%–64%
Severe, potentially life-threatening	Rare

Source: www.cdc.gov/nip/vaccines, accessed 8/21/09.

Discussion Sources

Centers for Disease Control and Prevention. http://www.cdc.gov/vaccines/vpd-vac/pneumo/default.htm, Pneumococcal vaccination, accessed 8/26/09.

Centers for Disease Control and Prevention. Recommended adult immunization schedule—United States, 2009. *MMWR Morb Mortal Wkly Rep.* 2008;57(53).

QUESTIONS

23. Concerning hepatitis B virus (HBV) vaccine, which of the following is true?

    A. The vaccine contains live, whole HBV.
    B. Adults should routinely have anti–hepatitis B surface antibody titers measured after three doses of vaccine.
    C. The vaccine should be offered during treatment for sexually transmitted diseases in unimmunized adults.
    D. Serologic testing for hepatitis B surface antigen (HBsAg) should be done before hepatitis B vaccination is initiated in adults.

24. In which of the following groups is routine HBsAg screening recommended?

    A. hospital laboratory workers
    B. recipients of hepatitis B vaccine series
    C. pregnant women
    D. college students

25. You see a woman who has been sexually involved with a man newly diagnosed with acute hepatitis B. She has not received hepatitis B vaccine in the past. You advise her that she should:

    A. start a hepatitis B immunization series.
    B. limit the number of sexual partners.
    C. be tested for hepatitis B surface antibody (HBsAb).
    D. receive hepatitis B immune globulin (HBIG) and hepatitis B immunization series.

26. Hepatitis B vaccine should not be given to a person with a history of anaphylactic reaction to:

A. egg.
B. baker's yeast.
C. neomycin.
D. streptomycin.

27. Risks associated with chronic hepatitis B include all of the following except:

A. hepatocellular carcinoma.
B. cirrhosis.
C. continued infectivity.
D. systemic hypertension.

ANSWERS

23.	C	24.	C	25.	D
26.	B	27.	D		

DISCUSSION

Hepatitis B is caused by a small double-stranded DNA virus that contains an inner core protein of hepatitis B core antigen and an outer surface of HBsAg. The virus is usually transmitted through an exchange of blood and body fluids. Acute hepatitis B is a serious illness that can lead to hepatic failure. Approximately 5% of patients with acute hepatitis B develop chronic hepatitis B; chronic hepatitis B is a potent risk factor for hematoma or primary hepatocellular carcinoma and hepatic cirrhosis. A person with chronic hepatitis B continues to be able to transmit the virus, while appearing clinically well.

Hepatitis B infection can be prevented by limiting exposure to blood and body fluids and through immunization. Recombinant hepatitis B vaccine, which does not contain live virus, is well tolerated, but is contraindicated in the persons who have a history of anaphylactic reaction to baker's yeast (Table 1–3).

Infants who become infected perinatally with HBV have an estimated 25% lifetime chance of developing hepatocellular carcinoma or cirrhosis. As a result, all pregnant women should be screened for HBsAg at the first prenatal visit, regardless of HBV vaccine history. The HBV vaccine is not 100% effective; in addition, woman may have carried HBV before becoming pregnant.

About 90% to 95% of individuals who receive the HBV vaccine develop HBsAb (anti-HBs) after three doses, implying protection from the virus. As a result, routine testing for the presence of HBsAb after immunization is not recommended. HBsAb testing should be considered, however, to confirm the development of HBV protection in individuals with high risk for infection (e.g., some health-care workers,

TABLE 1–3
Immunization Contraindications

Anaphylactic Reaction History	Immunization to Avoid
Neomycin	IPV, MMR, varicella
Streptomycin, polymyxin B, neomycin	IPV, vaccinia (smallpox)
Baker's yeast	Hepatitis B
Egg	Influenza vaccine (nasal spray, injected)
Gelatin, neomycin	Varicella zoster
Gelatin	MMR

Source: www.cdc.gov/vaccines/recs/vac-admin/contraindications. htm, accessed 8/28/09.

injection drug users, sex workers) and individuals at risk for poor immune response (e.g., dialysis patients, immunosuppressed patients).

Booster doses of HBV vaccine are recommended only in certain circumstances. For hemodialysis patients, the need for booster doses should be assessed by annual testing for antibody to HBsAg (anti-HBs or HBsAb). A booster dose should be administered when anti-HBs levels decline to less than 10 mIU/mL. For other immunocompromised persons (e.g., HIV-infected persons, hematopoietic stem-cell transplant recipients, and persons receiving chemotherapy), the need for booster doses has not been determined. When anti-HBs levels decline to less than 10 mIU/mL, annual anti-HBs testing and booster doses should be considered for individuals with an ongoing risk for exposure. Ongoing serologic surveillance in the immunocompetent population is not recommended, however.

Postexposure prophylaxis is effective in preventing HBV infection. In a person who has written documentation of a complete HBV vaccine series and who did not receive postvaccination testing, a single vaccine booster dose should be given with a nonoccupational known HBsAg-positive exposure source. A person who is in the process of being vaccinated but who has not completed the vaccine series should receive the appropriate dose of HBIG and should complete the vaccine series. Unvaccinated persons should receive HBIG and hepatitis B vaccine as soon as possible after exposure, preferably within 24 hours. Testing for HIV, hepatitis A, and hepatitis C should also be offered; where applicable, postexposure prophylaxis should be offered. Owing to the complexity of care, intervention for the person with occupational exposure should be done in consultation with experts in the area.

Discussion Sources

A comprehensive immunization strategy to eliminate transmission of hepatitis B virus infection in the United States: recommendations of the Advisory Committee on Immunization

Practices. Part I: Immunization of infants, children, and adolescents. *MMWR Morb Mortal Wkly Rep*. 2005;54(No. RR-16). Centers for Disease Control and Prevention.
http://www.cdc.gov/hepatitis/HBV/HBVfaq.htm#general, Hepatitis B FAQs for health professionals, accessed 8/21/09.

QUESTIONS

28. Which of the following best describes how smallpox is transmitted?

   A. direct deposit of infective droplets
   B. surface contact
   C. blood and body fluids
   D. vertical transmission

29. Smallpox disease includes which of the following characteristics?

   A. usually mild disease
   B. lesions that erupt over several days
   C. loss of contagiousness when vesicles form
   D. lesions all at the same stage during the eruptive phase of the illness

30. Smallpox vaccine contains:

   A. live vaccinia virus.
   B. a virus fragment.
   C. dead smallpox virus.
   D. an antigenic protein.

ANSWERS

28.   A   29.   D   30.   A

DISCUSSION

Smallpox is a serious, contagious, and sometimes fatal infectious disease caused by the variola virus. There are a variety of clinical forms, of which variola major is the most common and severe form, carrying a fatality rate of around 30%. Smallpox in its naturally occurring form was globally eradicated after a successful worldwide vaccination program; the last U.S. case of smallpox was in 1949, and the last naturally occurring case in the world was in Somalia in 1977. As a result, routine vaccination for the general public was stopped in the United States in 1972. Laboratory stockpiles of the variola virus do exist, however, and could be used as a bioterrorism agent.

Smallpox is typically spread from person to person via direct deposit of infective droplets onto the nasal, oral, or pharyngeal mucosal membrane or in the alveoli of the lungs; direct and fairly prolonged face-to-face contact is required. Smallpox is sometimes contagious during the onset of fever (prodrome phase), but it becomes most contagious with the onset of rash. At this stage, the infected person is usually very sick and not able to move around in the community. The infected person is contagious until the last smallpox scab falls off. Less commonly, smallpox can be spread through direct contact with infected bodily fluids or contaminated objects such as bedding or clothing. Rarely, smallpox has been spread by virus carried in the air in enclosed settings such as buildings, buses, and trains. Smallpox cannot be transmitted to humans by insects or animals, and animals cannot become ill with the disease.

Exposure to the virus is followed by an incubation period of about 7 to 17 days, during which the individual does not have any symptoms and the disease is not contagious. The prodromal stage lasts 2 to 4 days, during which the individual has a temperature of 101°F to 104°F (38.3°C to 40°C), malaise, headache, body aches, and sometimes vomiting. The individual is likely contagious at this time, but is typically too sick to carry on normal activities. In the next stage, the rash appears first as small red spots on the tongue and in the mouth that develop into open sores that spread large amounts of the virus into the mouth and throat. The individual becomes most contagious at this time. The rash appears on the skin, starting on the face and spreading first to the arms and legs and then to the hands and feet. Usually the rash spreads to all parts of the body within 24 hours, and the temperature typically decreases. By day 3 of the rash, the skin lesions become raised, and, by day 4, the lesions fill with a thick, opaque fluid and become umbilicated. The temperature often increases again until the lesions crust over, in about another 5 days. About 1 week later, the crusts begin to fall off, usually leaving a pitted scar. The individual remains contagious until all of the crusts have fallen off.

Although smallpox and varicella cause vesicular lesions, the clinical presentation of smallpox differs considerably from that of varicella (chickenpox). In varicella, the lesions typically erupt over days and are at various stages; some are vesicular, whereas some older lesions may be starting to crust over. In smallpox, all the skin lesions are usually at the same stage.

Smallpox treatment is largely supportive; no smallpox-specific therapy is currently available. An individual with suspected smallpox must be swiftly isolated. The NP should be aware of which local experts and governmental authorities need to be notified for a suspected case of smallpox.

In anticipation of possible exposure via bioterrorism, smallpox vaccination has been offered to or required of selected health and defense personnel, such as first responders, emergency health-care providers, and members of the military. Vaccination within 3 days of smallpox exposure prevents or significantly lessens the severity of smallpox symptoms in most people, whereas vaccination 4 to 7 days after exposure likely offers some protection from disease or may modify the severity of disease. The U.S. government has stockpiled enough vaccine to vaccinate every person in the United States in the event of a smallpox emergency.

Made from a live smallpox-related virus called vaccinia, the vaccine is given through a unique immunization method: A two-pronged needle is dipped into the vaccine solution. When removed, the needle retains a droplet of the vaccine. The needle is then used to prick the skin numerous times in a few seconds, producing a few drops of blood and some local discomfort. A red, itchy bump develops at the vaccine site in 3 to 4 days; this progresses to a large draining pustule over the next few days. During the second week, the blister begins to dry up, and a scab forms. The scab falls off in the third week, leaving a small scar. Until the scab falls off, the vaccine recipient can shed the vaccinia virus. This virus does not cause smallpox, but infection with this agent can result in serious cutaneous illnesses, such as generalized vaccinia and eczema vaccinatum. As a result, the vaccination site must be cared for to prevent the vaccinia virus from spreading. As with most vaccines, mild reactions include a few days of arm soreness and body aches. Fever is occasionally reported. The NP needs to be aware of current recommendations for smallpox vaccine candidates and vaccine contraindications.

Discussion Source

Centers for Disease Control and Prevention.
http://www.bt.cdc.gov/agent/smallpox, Smallpox, accessed 8/21/09.

QUESTIONS

31. Which of the following statements is correct about the varicella vaccine?

    A. It contains killed varicella-zoster virus.
    B. Its use is associated with an increase in reported cases of shingles.
    C. It should be offered to older adults who have a childhood history of chickenpox.
    D. Although highly protective against invasive varicella disease, mild cases of chickenpox have been reported in immunized individuals.

32. For which of the following patients should an NP order varicella antibody titers?

    A. a 14-year-old with an uncertain immunization history
    B. a health-care worker who reports having had varicella as a child
    C. a 22-year-old woman who received two varicella immunizations 6 weeks apart
    D. a 72-year-old with shingles

33. A woman who has been advised to receive varicella-zoster immune globulin (VZIG) asks about its risks. You respond that IG is a:

    A. synthetic product that is well tolerated.
    B. pooled blood product that often transmits infectious disease.
    C. blood product obtained from a single donor.
    D. pooled blood product with an excellent safety profile.

ANSWERS

31.	D	32.	B	33.	D

DISCUSSION

Varicella-zoster virus (VZV) causes the highly contagious, systemic disease commonly known as chickenpox. Naturally occurring or wild varicella infection usually confers lifetime immunity. Reinfection is rarely seen in immunocompromised patients, however. More often, reexposure causes an increase in antibody titers without causing disease. Although most cases are seen in children younger than 18 years, the greatest rate of mortality from varicella is in adults 30 to 49 years old.

The VZV can lie dormant in sensory nerve ganglia. Later reactivation causes shingles, a painful, vesicular-form rash in a dermatomal pattern. About 15% of individuals who have had chickenpox develop shingles during their lifetime. Shingles rates are markedly reduced in individuals who have received varicella vaccine compared with individuals who have had chickenpox. VZV is present in the vesicles seen in shingles. If an individual without varicella immunity comes in contact with shingles skin lesions, that individual could contract chickenpox. An individual with shingles cannot transmit shingles, however, to another person.

Evidence of immunity to varicella includes documentation of age-appropriate vaccination with varicella vaccine, laboratory evidence of immunity or laboratory confirmation of disease, birth in the United States before 1980, or the diagnosis or verification of a history of varicella disease or herpes zoster by a health-care provider. Among adults born before 1980 with an unclear or negative varicella history, most are also seropositive. Confirming varicella immunity through varicella titers, even in the presence of a history of varicella infection, should be done in health-care workers because of their risk of exposure and potential transmission of the disease.

The varicella vaccine is administered in children after the first birthday with a repeat dose usually given between ages 4 and 6 years. Older children and adults with no history of varicella infection or previous immunization should receive two immunizations 4 to 8 weeks apart. In particular, health-care workers, family contacts of immunocompromised patients, and day-care workers should be targeted for varicella vaccine, as should adults who are in environments with high risk of varicella transmission, such as college dormitories, military barracks, and long-term care facilities. Pregnant women should be assessed for evidence of varicella immunity. Women who do not have evidence of immunity should receive the first dose of varicella vaccine on completion or termination of pregnancy and before discharge from the health-care facility. The second dose should be administered 4 to 8 weeks after the first dose. The vaccine is highly protective against severe, invasive varicella. Mild cases of chickenpox may be reported after immunization, however. Because this is a live, attenuated virus vaccine, it should be used with caution in certain clinical situations (Table 1–4).

For healthy children and adults without evidence of immunity, vaccination within 3 to 5 days of exposure to varicella is beneficial in preventing or modifying the disease. Studies have shown that vaccination administered within 3 days of exposure to rash is 90% or greater effective in preventing varicella, whereas vaccination within 5 days of exposure to rash is approximately 70% effective in preventing varicella and 100% effective in modifying severe disease. For individuals without evidence of immunity who have contraindications for vaccination, but are at risk for severe disease and complications, use of VZIG is recommended for postexposure prophylaxis. VZIG, as with all forms of IG, provides temporary, passive immunity to infection. IG is a pooled blood product with an excellent safety profile. The NP should check current recommendation about postexposure prophylaxis.

Discussion Source

Centers for Disease Prevention and Control. http://www.cdc.gov/vaccines/vpd-vac/varicella/default.htm#clinical, Vaccine-preventable disease: Varicella, accessed 8/21/09.

QUESTIONS

34. An 18-year-old man has no primary tetanus immunization series documented. Which of the following represents the immunization needed?
    A. three doses of diphtheria, tetanus, and acellular pertussis (DTaP) vaccine 2 months apart
    B. tetanus IG now and two doses of tetanus-diphtheria (Td) vaccine 1 month apart
    C. Tetanus, diphtheria, acellular pertussive (Tdap) vaccine now with a dose of Td vaccine in 1 and 6 months
    D. Td vaccine as a single dose

35. Which wound presents the greatest risk for tetanus infection?
    A. a puncture wound obtained while gardening
    B. a laceration obtained while trimming beef
    C. a human bite
    D. an abrasion obtained by falling on a sidewalk

36. A 50-year-old man with hypertension and dyslipidemia presents for a primary care visit. He states, "It has been at least 10 years since my last tetanus shot." He should be immunized with:
    A. Td.
    B. Tetanus IG.
    C. Tdap.
    D. None of the above, owing to his concomitant health problems.

ANSWERS

34. C   35. A   36. C

TABLE 1–4
Live Attenuated Virus Vaccine Precautions

Live Attenuated Virus Vaccine Examples	Precautions for Use in Special Populations
MMR (measles, mumps, rubella) Varicella (chickenpox) Intranasal influenza virus vaccine (FluMist) Varicella zoster (shingles)	Pregnancy because of theoretical risk of passing virus to fetus. Immune suppression, except HIV, because of risk, likely theoretical, of becoming ill with virus. With HIV infection, live virus vaccines usually not given with CD4 T lymphocyte cell counts less than 200 cell/uL. See adult immunization guidelines for further information.

DISCUSSION

Tetanus infection is caused by *Clostridium tetani*, an anaerobic, gram-positive, spore-forming rod. This organism is found in soil, particularly if it contains manure. The organism enters the body through a contaminated wound, causing a life-threatening systemic disease characterized by painful muscle weakness and spasm (lockjaw). Diphtheria, caused by *Corynebacterium diphtheriae*, a gram-negative bacillus, is typically transmitted from person to person or through contaminated liquids such as milk. This organism causes severe respiratory tract infection, including the appearance of pseudomembranous pharyngitis.

In the developed world, tetanus and diphtheria are uncommon infections because of widespread immunization. Since protective titers wane over time, and adults are frequently lacking in up-to-date immunization, most cases of tetanus occur in adults older than 50 years.

A primary series of three tetanus vaccine injections sets the stage for long-term immunity. A booster tetanus dose every 10 years is recommended, but protection is probably present for 20 to 30 years after a primary series. Using Td vaccine rather than tetanus toxoid for primary series and booster doses in adulthood assists in keeping diphtheria immunity as well (see Figure 1–2). Early childhood tetanus and diphtheria immunizations also include acellular pertussis vaccine, providing protection for this highly contagious cough-transmitted illness. A single dose of Tdap during adulthood provides additional protection from pertussis. For adults receiving initial immunization, a series of three vaccine doses is needed. Two of the three can be Td, and one should be Tdap.

The use of tetanus and diphtheria with or without acellular pertussis immunizations is well tolerated and produces few adverse reactions. A short-term, localized area of redness and warmth is quite common and is not predictive of future problems with tetanus immunization. At the time of wound-producing injury, tetanus IG affords temporary protection for individuals who have not received tetanus immunization.

Discussion Source

Centers for Disease Control and Prevention. http://www.cdc.gov/ncidod/dbmd/diseaseinfo/diptheria_t.htm, Vaccine preventable disease: Diphtheria, accessed 8/28/09.

Centers for Disease Control and Prevention. http://www.cdc.gov/vaccines/vpd-vac/tetanus/default.htm, Vaccine preventable disease: Tetanus, accessed 8/28/09.

Centers for Disease Control and Prevention. http://www.cdc.gov/vaccines/vpd-vac/child-vpd.htm, Vaccine preventable disease: Pertussis, accessed 8/28/09.

QUESTIONS

37. The most common source of hepatitis A virus (HAV) infection is:
    A. needle sharing.
    B. raw shellfish.
    C. contaminated drinking water.
    D. intimate person-to-person contact.

38. When answering questions about HAV vaccine, the NP considers that it:
    A. contains live virus.
    B. should be offered to adults who frequently travel to developing countries.
    C. is contraindicated for use in children.
    D. confers lifelong protection after a single injection.

39. Usual treatment for an adult with acute hepatitis A includes:
    A. interferon-alfa.
    B. ribavirin.
    C. acyclovir.
    D. supportive care.

ANSWERS

37. C   38. B   39. D

DISCUSSION

Hepatitis A infection is caused by HAV, a small RNA virus. Transmitted primarily by fecal-contaminated drinking water and food supplies, hepatitis A is typically a self-limiting infection with a very low mortality rate. Although eating raw shellfish that grew in contaminated water can be problematic, fecal-contaminated water supplies are the most common source of infection. In developing countries with limited pure water, most children contract this disease by age 5 years. In North America, adults 20 to 39 years old account for nearly 50% of the reported cases. The local public health department should be consulted for advice when an outbreak of HAV infection occurs.

All children and some high-risk groups should be immunized against HAV. Candidates for immunization include individuals who reside in or travel to areas where the disease is endemic, food handlers, sewage workers, animal handlers, day-care attendees and workers, long-term care residents and workers, and military and laboratory personnel. Injection drug users may also benefit from the vaccine. HAV is rarely transmitted sexually or from needle sharing; rather, injection drug users often live in conditions that facilitate the oral-fecal transmission of HAV. In addition, coinfection with hepatitis A and C, with hepatitis A and B, or acute hepatitis A in addition to a chronic liver disease may lead to a rapid deterioration in hepatic function. Individuals with chronic hepatitis B or C or any chronic liver disease should be immunized against HAV. Individuals who have clotting-factor disorders and are receiving clotting-factor concentrates who have not had hepatitis A should also be immunized.

Two doses of vaccine are given 6 to 12 months apart to ensure an enhanced immunologic response. HAV vaccine, which does not contain live virus, is usually well tolerated without systemic reaction.

Discussion Sources

Centers for Disease Control and Prevention. http://www.cdc.gov/
NCIDOD/DISEASES/hepatitis/a, National Center for
HIV/AIDS, Viral Hepatitis, STD, and TB Prevention: Viral
hepatitis A, accessed 8/18/09.
(See also Figures 1–1 and 1–2.)

QUESTIONS

40. Which of the following statements is true about poliovirus infection?

    A. It is transmitted via the fecal-oral route.
    B. Rates of infection among household contacts are about 30%.
    C. Sporadic outbreaks continue to occur in North America.
    D. It is transmitted via aerosol and droplets.

41. A 30-year-old man with HIV lives with his two preschool-aged children. Which of the following statements best represents advice you should give him about immunizing his children?

    A. Immunizations should take place without concern for his health status.
    B. The children should not receive influenza vaccine.
    C. MMR vaccine should not be given.
    D. The children should not receive poliovirus immunization.

ANSWERS

40.   A   41.   A

DISCUSSION

Polioviruses are highly contagious and capable of causing paralytic, life-threatening infection. The infection is transmitted by the fecal-oral route. Rates of infection among

household contacts can be as high as 96%. Since 1994, North and South America have been declared free of indigenous poliomyelitis, however, largely because of the efficacy of the poliovirus immunization. The vaccine is available in two forms: a live-virus vaccine that is given orally (oral polio vaccine [OPV]) and an injectable vaccine that contains inactivated poliovirus (IPV). When OPV is used, a small amount of weakened virus is shed via the stool. This shedding presents household members with possible exposure to poliovirus, resulting in a rare risk of paralytic poliomyelitis (vaccine-associated paralytic poliomyelitis [VAPP]). Because of VAPP risk, OPV is no longer used in the United States, but it is used in other countries. IPV, containing inactivated virus, use poses no such risk.

Discussion Source

Centers for Disease Control and Prevention.
    http://www.cdc.gov/vaccines/vpd-vac/polio/default.htm#vacc,
    Vaccine preventable disease: Polio, accessed 8/18/09.

QUESTIONS

42. When working with middle-aged man with a body mass index of 33 on weight reduction, an NP considers that one of the first actions should be to:

    A. add an exercise program while minimizing the need for dietary changes.
    B. ask the patient about what he believes contributes to his weight problem.
    C. refer the patient to a nutritionist for diet counseling.
    D. ask for a commitment to lose weight.

43. A sedentary, obese 52-year-old woman is diagnosed with hypertension and states, "It is going to be too hard to diet, exercise, and take these pills." What is the least helpful response to her statement?

    A. "Try taking your medication when you brush your teeth."
    B. "You really need to try to improve your health."
    C. "Tell me what you feel will get in your way of improving your health."
    D. "Could you start with reducing the amount of salt in your diet?"

ANSWERS

42.   B   43.   B

DISCUSSION

Possessing information about methods for preventing disease and maintaining health is an important part of patient education. Knowledge alone does not ensure a change in behavior, however. NPs need to consider many factors in patient counseling and education (Box 1–1).

Discussion Source

Trinite T, Loveland-Cherry C, Marion L. The U.S. Preventive Services Task Force: an evidence-based prevention resource for nurse practitioners. *J Am Acad Nurse Pract*. 2009;21: 301–306.

BOX 1–1

Orderly Approach to Patient Education and Counseling

- Assess the patient's knowledge base about factors contributing to the problem.
- Evaluate the contribution of the patient's belief system to the problem.
- Ask the patient about perceived barriers to action and supporting factors.
- Match teaching to the patient's perception of the problem.
- Inform the patient about the purpose and benefit of an intervention.
- Give the patient an anticipated time of onset of effect of a therapy.
- Suggest small rather than large changes in behavior.
- Give accurate, specific information.
- Consider adding new positive behaviors, r than attempting to discontinue established behaviors.
- Link desired behavior with established behavior
- Give a strong, personalized message about t seriousness of health risk.
- Ask for a commitment from the patient.
- Use a combination of teaching strategies, such as visual, oral, and written methods.
- Strive for an interdisciplinary approach to patient education and counseling, with all members of the team giving the same message.
- Maintain frequent contact with the patient t monitor progress.
- Expect gains and periodic setbacks.

Source: Freda MC: http://www.medscape.com/viewarticle/ 478283_1, Issues in patient education, 2004, accessed 8/2

QUESTIONS

44. Which of the following is the most effective method of cancer screening?
    - **A.** skin examination
    - **B.** fecal occult blood test (FOBT)
    - **C.** pelvic examination
    - **D.** chest radiograph

45. Which of the following is a recommended method of annual colorectal cancer screening for a 62-year-old man?
    - **A.** digital rectal examination
    - **B.** in-office FOBT
    - **C.** at-home FOBT
    - **D.** sigmoidoscopy

46. According to the American Cancer Society recommendations, which of the following men should be considered for prostate cancer screening?
    - **A.** a 46-year-old African-American man
    - **B.** a 49-year-old man of Asian ancestry
    - **C.** an 86-year-old man with end-stage renal failure
    - **D.** a 38-year-old man with a recent history of acute prostatitis

47. Which of the following types of cancer screening is not routinely recommended in a 55-year-old woman?
    - **A.** breast
    - **B.** skin
    - **C.** endometrium
    - **D.** colorectal

ANSWERS

44.	A	**45.**	C
46.	A	**47.**	C

DISCUSSION

Cancer screening is an important part of providing comprehensive health care. Adherence to current, nationally recognized guidelines is an important part of effective clinical practice (Table 1–5).

TABLE 1–5

American Cancer Society Cancer Detection Guidelines

Cancer Site	Population	Test or Procedure	Comment
Breast	Women, age ≥20 years	Breast self-examination (BSE)	Beginning in their early 20s, women should be told about the benefits and limitations of BSE. The importance of prompt reporting of any new breast symptoms to a health professional should be emphasized. Women who choose to do BSE should receive instruction and have their technique reviewed on the occasion of a periodic health examination. It is acceptable for women to choose not to do BSE or to do BSE irregularly
		Clinical breast examination (CBE)	For women in their 20s and 30s, it is recommended that CBE be part of a periodic health examination, preferably at least every 3 years. Asymptomatic women ≥40 years should continue to receive a clinical breast examination as part of a periodic health examination, preferably annually
		Mammography	Begin annual mammography at age 40 years
		MRI	Women at high risk (>20% lifetime risk) should get an MRI and a mammogram every year. Women at moderately increased risk (15%–20% lifetime risk) should talk with their health-care providers about the benefits and limitations of adding MRI screening to their yearly mammogram. Yearly MRI screening is not recommended for women whose lifetime risk of breast cancer is <15%
Colorectal	Men and women, age ≥50 years	Fecal occult blood test (FOBT) or fecal immunochemical test (FIT), *or*	Annual, starting at age 50 years. FOBT as it is sometimes done in health-care providers' offices, with the single stool sample collected on a fingertip during a digital rectal examination, is not an adequate substitute for the recommended at-home procedure of collecting two samples from three consecutive specimens. Toilet-bowl FOBT tests also are not recommended. Compared with guaiac-based tests for the detection of occult blood, immunochemical tests are more patient-friendly, and are likely to be equal or better in sensitivity and specificity. There is no justification for repeating FOBT in response to an initial positive finding. Colonoscopy should be done if test results are positive
		Stool DNA test	Stool DNA test (sDNA), interval uncertain, starting at age 50 years. Colonoscopy should be done if results are positive
		Flexible sigmoidoscopy, *or*	Every 5 years, starting at age 50 years
		Double contrast barium enema (DCBE), *or*	DCBE every 5 years, starting at age 50 years
		Colonoscopy	Colonoscopy every 10 years, starting at age 50 years
		CT colonography	CT colonography (virtual colonoscopy) every 5 years

TABLE 1–5

American Cancer Society Cancer Detection Guidelines—cont'd

		Additional recommendations	Patients should talk to their health-care provider about earlier or more frequent screening if they have the following colorectal risk factors: a personal history of colorectal cancer or adenomatous polyps, Crohn's disease or ulcerative colitis, a strong family history (first-degree relative [parent, sibling, or child] <60 years old or in two or more first-degree relatives of any age) of colorectal cancer or polyps, or a known family history of hereditary colorectal cancer syndromes such as familial adenomatous polyposis (FAP) or hereditary nonpolyposis colon cancer (HNPCC)
Prostate	Men, age ≥50 years	Digital rectal examination (DRE) and prostate-specific antigen test (PSA)	The American Cancer Society (ACS) does not support routine testing for prostate cancer at this time. ACS does believe that health-care professionals should discuss the potential benefits and limitations of prostate cancer early detection testing with men before any testing begins. This discussion should include an *offer* for testing with the PSA test and the DRE annually, starting at age 50 years, for men who have a life expectancy of at least 10 more years. Men at high risk (African-American men and men with a strong family history of one or more first-degree relatives [father, brothers] diagnosed before age 65) should begin testing at age 45. Men at even higher risk, owing to multiple first-degree relatives affected at an early age, could begin testing at age 40. Depending on the results of this initial test, no further testing might be needed until age 45. Information should be provided to men about the benefits and limitations of testing so that an informed decision about testing can be made with the clinician's assistance
Cervical	Women	Pap test	Cervical cancer screening should begin approximately 3 years after a woman begins having vaginal intercourse, but no later than 21 years of age. Screening should be done every year with conventional Pap tests or every 2 years using liquid-based Pap tests. At or after age 30 years, women who have had three normal test results in a row may get screened every 2–3 years with cervical cytology (either conventional or liquid-based Pap test) alone, or every 3 years with a human papillomavirus DNA test plus cervical cytology. Women ≥70 years old who have had three or more normal Pap tests and no abnormal Pap tests in the last 10 years may choose to stop cervical cancer screening. Women who have had a total hysterectomy may also choose to stop cervical cancer screening, unless the surgery was done as a treatment for cervical cancer or precancer. Women who have had a hysterectomy without the removal of the cervix should continue to follow the standard guidelines.

Continued

TABLE 1–5

American Cancer Society Cancer Detection Guidelines—cont'd

		Women who have certain risk factors such as diethylstilbestrol (DES) exposure before birth, HIV infection, or a weakened immune system because of organ transplant, chemotherapy, or long-term steroid use should continue to be screened annually
Endometrial	Women, at menopause	At the time of menopause, all women should be informed about risks and symptoms of endometrial cancer and strongly encouraged to report any unexpected bleeding or spotting to their health-care provider
		For women with or at high risk for HNPCC, annual screening should be offered for endometrial cancer with endometrial biopsy beginning at age 35
Cancer-related checkup	**Men and women, age ≥20 years**	On the occasion of a periodic health examination, the cancer-related checkup should include health counseling, and depending on a person's age and gender, might include examinations for cancers of the thyroid, oral cavity, skin, lymph nodes, testes, and ovaries, and for some nonmalignant (non cancerous) diseases

Source: http://www.cancer.org/docroot/ped/content/ped_2_3x_acs_cancer_detection_guidelines_36.asp, American Cancer Society Cancer Detection Guidelines, accessed 8/30/09.

QUESTIONS

48. The components of brief intervention for treating tobacco use include:

    A. Ask, Advise, Assess, Assist, Arrange.
    B. Advise, Intervene, Counsel, Follow up, Prescribe.
    C. Document, Counsel, Caution, Describe, Demonstrate.
    D. Advise, Describe, Confer, Prescribe, Document.

49. Brief intervention that provides motivation to quit tobacco use should be:

    A. used at every clinical visit that the tobacco user has, regardless of reason for the visit.
    B. offered when the tobacco user voices concern about the health effects of smoking.
    C. applied primarily during visits for conditions that are clearly related to or exacerbated by tobacco use, such as respiratory tract disease.
    D. when the clinician is conducting a comprehensive health assessment, such as with the annual physical examination.

50. The use of FDA-approved pharmacologic intervention in tobacco use:

    A. makes little difference in smoking cessation rates.
    B. reliably increases long-term smoking abstinence rates.
    C. is helpful but generally poorly tolerated.
    D. poses a greater risk to health than continued tobacco use.

51. You see a 48-year-old patient who started taking varenicline (Chantix) 4 weeks ago to aid in smoking cessation. Which of the following is the most important question to ask during today's visit?

    A. "How many cigarettes a day are you currently smoking?"
    B. "On a scale of 0 to 10, how strong is your desire to smoke?"
    C. "Have you noticed any changes in your mood?"
    D. "Are you having any trouble sleeping?"

ANSWERS

48.   A   49.   A   50.   B
51.   C

DISCUSSION

Tobacco use poses a tremendous health hazard. Tobacco-related diseases result in a significant burden to public health and health-care costs. Tobacco dependence is a chronic disease that often requires repeated intervention and multiple attempts to quit. Effective treatments exist, however, that can significantly increase rates of long-term abstinence. Treating tobacco use and dependence guidelines from the Agency for Healthcare Research and Quality (AHRQ) offer the following recommendations for smoking cessation.

Clinicians and health-care delivery systems must consistently identify and document tobacco use status and treat every tobacco user seen in a health-care setting. Brief tobacco dependence treatment is effective. Clinicians should offer every patient who uses tobacco at least the brief treatments shown to be effective. An example of a brief intervention includes the "5 As": Ask, Advise, Assess, Assist, Arrange (Table 1–6). This strategy should be employed with all tobacco users, including individuals with no current desire to quit because this can serve as a motivating factor in future attempts to discontinue tobacco use.

Individual, group, and telephone counseling are helpful, and their effectiveness increases with treatment intensity. Two components of counseling—practical counseling (problem solving/skills training) and social support—are especially effective, and clinicians should use these when counseling patients making a quit attempt. Telephone quit line counseling has been shown to be effective with diverse populations and has broad reach. Clinicians and health-care delivery systems should ensure patient access to quit lines and promote quit line use.

Tobacco dependence treatments are effective across a broad range of populations. Clinicians should encourage every patient willing to make a quit attempt to use the counseling treatments and appropriate medications. Numerous effective medications are available for tobacco dependence, and clinicians should encourage their use by all patients attempting to quit smoking—except when medically contraindicated or with specific populations for which there is insufficient evidence of effectiveness (i.e., pregnant women, smokeless tobacco users, light smokers, and adolescents). These medications include nicotine replacement therapy (NRT) (e.g., patch, gum, inhaler, nasal spray, and lozenge) and medications to reduce the desire to smoke (bupropion [Zyban, Wellbutrin] and varenicline [Chantix]).

The use of these medications reliably increases long-term smoking abstinence rates. Generally, the risk associated with the use of these medications is less than that associated with continued tobacco use. Adverse effects occasionally attributed to the use of smoking cessation medications are sometimes actually a result of nicotine withdrawal. The FDA added a warning, however, regarding the use of varenicline. Specifically, depressed mood, agitation, changes in behavior, suicidal ideation, and suicide have been reported in patients attempting to quit smoking while using varenicline. Patients should tell their health-care provider about any history of psychiatric illness before starting this medication; clinicians should also ask about mental health history before starting this medication. Close monitoring for changes in mood and behavior should follow.

TABLE 1–6
Five As

Ask about tobacco use	Identify and document tobacco use status for every patient at every visit
Advise to quit	In a clear, strong, and personalized manner, urge every tobacco user to quit
Assess willingness to make a quit attempt	Is the tobacco user willing to make a quit attempt at this time?
Assist in quit attempt	For the patient willing to make a quit attempt, offer medication and provide or refer for counseling or additional treatment to help the patient quit
	For patients unwilling to quit at the time, provide interventions designed to increase future quit attempts
Arrange follow-up	For the patient willing to make a quit attempt, arrange for follow-up contacts, beginning within the first week after the quit date
	For patients unwilling to make a quit attempt at the time, address tobacco dependence and willingness to quit at next clinic visit

Source: http://www.ncbi.nlm.nih.gov/books/bv.fcgi?rid=hstat2.section.29645#29648, AHQR supported clinical practice guidelines: Treating tobacco use and dependence: 2008 update, accessed 1/22/09.

Counseling and medication are effective when used by clinicians as solo interventions for treating tobacco dependence. The combination of counseling and medication is more effective, however, than either alone. Clinicians should encourage all individuals making a quit attempt to use counseling and medication. For an individual who is not interested in quitting, motivational intervention is often helpful and should be provided at every clinical visit.

Treatments for tobacco dependence are clinically effective and highly cost-effective relative to interventions for other clinical disorders. Providing insurance coverage for these treatments increases quit rates. Insurers and purchasers should ensure that all insurance plans include the counseling and medication identified as effective in the AHRQ guidelines as covered benefits.

Discussion Source

http://www.ncbi.nlm.nih.gov/books/bv.fcgi?rid=hstat2.section.29645 #29648, AHQR supported clinical practice guidelines: Treating tobacco use and dependence: 2008 update, accessed 8/22/09.

2
Neurologic Disorders

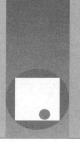

1. Assessing vision and visual fields involves testing cranial nerve (CN):
   - **A.** I.
   - **B.** II.
   - **C.** III.
   - **D.** IV.

2. You perform an extraocular movement test on a middle-aged patient. He is unable to move his eyes upward and inward. This indicates a possibility of paralysis of CN:
   - **A.** II.
   - **B.** III.
   - **C.** V.
   - **D.** VI.

3. Loss of corneal reflex is in part seen in dysfunction of CN:
   - **A.** III.
   - **B.** IV.
   - **C.** V.
   - **D.** VI.

ANSWERS

| 1. | B | 2. | B | 3. | C |

DISCUSSION

Knowledge of the CNs is critical for performing an accurate neurologic assessment. Because these are paired nerves arising largely from the brainstem, a unilateral CN dysfunction is common, often reflecting a problem in the ipsilateral cerebral hemisphere.

Cranial Nerve Mnemonic

A commonly used mnemonic for identifying and remembering the cranial nerves is: *On Old Olympus Towering Tops, A Finn And German Viewed Some Hops.* The details of the cranial nerves are as follows:

- CN I—Olfactory: You have one nose, where CN I resides. Its function contributes to the sense of smell.
- CN II—Optic: You have two eyes, where you will find CN II. Function of this CN is vital to vision and visual fields and, in conjunction with CN III, pupillary reaction.
- CN III—Oculomotor: CN III, the eye (*oculo-*) movement (*motor*) nerve, works with CNs III, IV, and VI (*abducens,* which helps the eyeball abduct or move). The actions of these CNs are largely responsible for the movement of the eyeball and eyelid.
- CN IV—Trochlear: This nerve innervates the superior oblique muscle of the eye.
- CN V—Trigeminal: Three (*tri*) types of sensation (temperature, pain, and tactile) come from this three-branched nerve that covers three territories of the face. For normal corneal reflexes to be present, the afferent limb of the first division of CN V and the effect limb of CN VII need to be intact.
- CN VI—Abducens
- CN VII—Facial: Dysfunction of this nerve gives the characteristic findings of Bell's palsy (facial asymmetry, droop of mouth, absent nasolabial fold, impaired eyelid movement).
- CN VIII—Auditory or vestibulocochlear: When this nerve does not function properly, hearing (auditory) or balance is impaired (vestibulocochlear). The Rinne test is part of the evaluation of this CN.
- CN IX—Glossopharyngeal: The name of this CN provides a clue that its function affects the tongue (*glosso*) and throat (*pharynx*). Along with CN X, the function of this nerve is critical to swallowing, palate elevation, and gustation.
- CN X—Vagus: This CN is involved in parasympathetic regulation of multiple organs, including sensing aortic pressure and regulating blood pressure, slowing heart rate, and regulating taste and digestive rate.

- CN XI—Accessory or spinal root of the accessory: Function of this CN can be tested by evaluating shoulder shrug and lateral neck rotation.
- CN XII—Hypoglossal: Function of this CN is tested by noting movement and protrusion of the tongue.

Discussion Source

http://www.med.yale.edu/caim/cnerves/, Cranial nerves, accessed 8/22/09.

QUESTIONS

4. You examine a 29-year-old woman who has a sudden onset of right-sided facial asymmetry. She is unable to close her right eyelid tightly, frown, or smile on the affected side. Her examination is otherwise unremarkable. This presentation likely represents paralysis of CN:

    A. III.
    B. IV.
    C. VII.
    D. VIII.

5. Which represents the most appropriate diagnostic test for the patient in the previous question?

    A. complete blood cell count with white blood cell (WBC) differential
    B. Lyme disease antibody titer
    C. computed tomography (CT) scan of the head with contrast medium
    D. blood urea nitrogen and creatinine levels

6. In prescribing prednisone for a patient with Bell palsy, the nurse practitioner (NP) considers that its use:

    A. has not been shown to be helpful in improving outcomes in this condition.
    B. should be initiated as soon as possible after the onset of facial paralysis.
    C. is likely to help minimize ocular symptoms.
    D. may prolong the course of the disease.

ANSWERS

4. C   5. B   6. B

DISCUSSION

Bell palsy is an acute paralysis of CN VII (in the absence of brain dysfunction) that is seen without other signs and symptoms. ♂ Because this condition can be a complication of Lyme disease, appropriate antibody testing should be obtained

in a patient presenting with CN VII palsy. Rapid plasma reagin (RPR)/Venereal Disease Research Laboratory (VDRL) test and human immunodeficiency virus (HIV) screening should also be considered. Neuroimaging is not needed, however, because a unilateral CN dysfunction is not consistent with the typical clinical presentation of an intracranial neoplasm.

Systemic corticosteroid therapy has been shown to limit the length and severity of the paralysis. This therapy is most effective when started early in the disease and is of no use if begun more than 10 days after the onset of symptoms. Acyclovir use in patients with Bell palsy is associated with some controversy and variations in clinical outcome, but is often given because herpes simplex or varicella-zoster virus is hypothesized to be a possible cause of the disease. Supportive care to help avoid ocular and oral injury and counseling about the natural history of the disease are critical. With ocular involvement, consultation with an eye care professional should be obtained.

Discussion Sources

Gilden DH, Tyler KL. Bell's palsy—is glucocorticoid treatment enough? *N Engl J Med.* 2007;357:1653–1655.
Lo B. http://emedicine.medscape.com/article/791311-print, eMedicine: Bell palsy, accessed 8/22/09.
Sullivan FM, Swan IRC, Donnan PT, et al. Early treatment with prednisolone or acyclovir in Bell's palsy. *N Engl J Med.* 2007;357:1598–1607.

QUESTIONS

7. A 40-year-old patient presents with a 5-week history of recurrent headaches that awaken him during the night. The pain is severe, lasts about 1 hour, and is located behind his left eye. Additional symptoms include lacrimation and nasal discharge. His physical examination is within normal limits. This clinical presentation is most consistent with:

    A. migraine without aura.
    B. migraine with aura.
    C. cluster headache.
    D. increased intracranial pressure (ICP).

8. A 22-year-old woman presents with a 3-year history of recurrent, unilateral, pulsating headaches with vomiting and photophobia. The headaches, which generally last 3 hours, can be aborted by resting in a dark room. She can usually tell that she is going to get a headache. She explains, "I see little 'squiggles' before my eyes for about 15 minutes." Her physical examination is unremarkable. This presentation is most consistent with:

    A. tension-type headache.
    B. migraine without aura.
    C. migraine with aura.
    D. cluster headache.

9. Prophylactic treatment for migraine headaches includes the use of:
   A. propranolol.
   B. ergot derivative.
   C. naproxen sodium.
   D. enalapril.

10. You are examining a 55-year-old woman who has a history of angina pectoris and migraine. Which of the following agents represents the best choice of acute headache (abortive) therapy for this patient?
    A. verapamil
    B. ergotamine
    C. ibuprofen
    D. sumatriptan

11. With migraine, which of the following statements is true?
    A. Migraine with aura is the most common form.
    B. Most migraineurs are in ongoing health care for the condition.
    C. The condition is equally common in men and women.
    D. The pain is typically described as pulsating.

12. In tension-type headache, which of the following is true?
    A. Photophobia is seldom reported.
    B. The pain is typically described as "pressing" in quality.
    C. The headache is usually unilateral.
    D. Physical activity usually makes the discomfort worse.

13. Treatment options in cluster headache include the use of:
    A. nonsteroidal anti-inflammatory drugs (NSAIDs).
    B. oxygen.
    C. the triptans.
    D. all of the above therapies.

14. Which of the following agents has the most rapid analgesic onset?
    A. naproxen (Naprosyn, Aleve)
    B. liquid ibuprofen (Motrin, Advil)
    C. diclofenac (Voltaren)
    D. enteric-coated naproxen (Naproxen EC)

15. Limitations of use of butalbital with acetaminophen and caffeine (Fioricet) include its:
    A. energizing effect.
    B. gastrointestinal (GI) upset profile.
    C. high rate of rebound headache if used frequently.
    D. excessive cost.

16. The use of neuroleptics such as prochlorperazine (Compazine) and promethazine (Phenergan) in migraine therapy should be limited to less than three times per week because of their:
    A. addictive potential.
    B. extrapyramidal movement risk.
    C. ability to cause rebound headache.
    D. sedative effect.

17. With appropriately prescribed headache prophylactic therapy, the patient should be informed to expect:
    A. virtual resolution of headaches.
    B. no fewer, but less severe headaches.
    C. approximately 50% reduction in the number of headaches.
    D. that lifelong therapy is advised.

18. A 48-year-old woman presents with a monthly 4-day premenstrual migraine headache, poorly responsive to triptans and analgesics, and accompanied by vasomotor symptoms (hot flashes). The clinician considers prescribing all of the following except:
    A. continuous monophasic oral contraceptive.
    B. phasic oral contraceptive with a 7-day-per-month withdrawal period.
    C. estrogen patch use during the premenstrual week.
    D. triptan prophylaxis.

19. A first-line prophylactic treatment option for the prevention of tension-type headache is:
    A. nortriptyline.
    B. lisinopril.
    C. carbamazepine.
    D. valproate.

20. A 68-year-old man presents with new onset of headaches. He describes the pain as bilateral frontal to occipital and most severe when he arises in the morning and when coughing. He feels much better by mid-afternoon. The history is most consistent with headache caused by:
    A. vascular compromise.
    B. increased ICP.
    C. brain tumor.
    D. tension-type with atypical geriatric presentation.

ANSWERS

7.	C	8.	C	9.	A
10.	C	11.	D	12.	B
13.	D	14.	B	15.	C
16.	B	17.	C	18.	B
19.	A	20.	B		

DISCUSSION

The primary headaches, including migraine, tension-type, and cluster headache, are the most common chronic pain syndromes seen in primary care practice (Table 2–1). Development of the appropriate diagnosis is critical to caring for patients with headache (Table 2–2). Despite the existence of specific criteria, clinicians frequently misdiagnose migraine. One reason for error is the nature of these diagnostic criteria. The International Headache Society (IHS) criteria do not include all symptoms frequently observed in episodes of migraine. Consequently, migraine associated with muscle or neck pain, which is not an IHS migraine diagnostic criterion, is often diagnosed as tension-type headache, and migraine associated with nasal symptoms such as rhinorrhea and nasal congestion, also not included as IHS diagnostic criteria, is diagnosed as a "sinus" headache. In both cases, these headaches are usually migraine in nature.

Headache rarely can be the presenting symptom of a serious illness. The key points to consider in assessing a patient with headache are presented in Box 2–1 and Table 2–3. The question of whether to obtain neuroimaging with head CT or magnetic resonance imaging (MRI) to evaluate for underlying disease often arises in the care of a patient with nonacute primary headache. In the absence of a normal neurologic examination, the results of neuroimaging yield little additional information, but add significantly to health-care cost (Table 2–4).

Migraine without aura affects about 80% of persons with migraine. On careful questioning, many patients report a migraine warning, however, such as agitation, jitteriness, disturbed sleep, or unusual dreams (see Table 2–2 for diagnostic criteria). Migraine with aura is found in about 20% of patients with migrainous disorders. The aura is a recurrent neurologic symptom that arises from the cerebral cortex or brainstem. Typically, the aura develops over 5 to 20 minutes, lasts less than 1 hour, and is accompanied or followed by migraine. Patients who have migraines with aura do not have more severe headaches than patients without aura, but the former patients are more likely to be offered a fuller range of therapies. Patients without aura may be misdiagnosed as having tension-type headaches and are often not offered headache therapies specifically suited for migraines, such as the triptans.

Although much of headache care is focused on the relief and prevention of migraine, tension-type headaches are a significant source of suffering and lost function (see Table 2–2 for diagnosis). Abortive treatment options include the use of acetaminophen; NSAIDs; and combination products such as butalbital with acetaminophen and acetaminophen, aspirin, and caffeine. Prophylactic therapies are highly effective at limiting the number and frequency of tension-type headache. Consideration should also be given for coexisting migraine and tension-type headache; in this situation, triptan use is often helpful.

Cluster headaches, also known as migrainous neuralgia, are most common in middle-aged men, particularly men with heavy alcohol and tobacco use. Although cluster is the only primary headache type more common in men than women, more recent study reveals that the condition is likely underdiagnosed in women. Sometimes called the "suicide headache" because of the severity of the associated pain, cluster headache occurs periodically in clusters (hence its name) of several weeks, with associated lacrimation and rhinorrhea. Treatment includes reduction of triggers, such as tobacco and alcohol use, and initiation of prophylactic therapy and appropriate abortive therapy (triptans, high-dose NSAIDs, and high-flow oxygen).

Headache treatment is aimed at identifying and reducing headache triggers. Lifestyle modification is a highly effective and often underused headache therapy (Tables 2–5 and 2–6). In addition, abortive therapy should be offered. Prophylactic therapy, aimed at limiting the number and severity of future headaches, is also often indicated. Rescue therapy is used when abortive therapy is ineffective in providing headache relief.

When a migraine abortive agent is chosen, a number of considerations should be kept in mind. These medications are available in many forms (i.e., oral, parenteral, nasal spray,

---

BOX 2–1

Helpful Observations in Patients with Acute Headache

■ History of previous identical headaches
■ Intact cognition
■ Supple neck
■ Normal neurologic examination results
■ Improvement in symptoms while under observation and treatment

---

TABLE 2–1

Headache: Primary versus Secondary

Primary Headache	Secondary Headache
Not associated with other diseases, likely complex interplay of genetic, developmental, and environmental risk factors	Associated with or caused by other conditions, generally does not resolve until specific cause is diagnosed and addressed
Migraine, tension-type, cluster	Intracranial issue such as brain tumor, bleeding, inflammation, or any condition that causes increased intracranial pressure

TABLE 2–2

Primary Headache: Clinical Presentation and Diagnosis

Headache Type	Headache Characteristics
Tension-type headache	Lasts 30 minutes to 7 days (usually 1–24 hours) with two or more of the following characteristics • Pressing, nonpulsatile pain • Mild to moderate in intensity • Usually bilateral location • Notation of 0–1 of the following (>1 suggests migraine): nausea, photophobia, or phonophobia Female:male ratio 5:4
Migraine without aura	Lasts 4–72 hours with two or more of the following characteristics • Usually unilateral location, although occasionally bilateral • Pulsating quality, moderate to severe in intensity • Aggravation by normal activity such as walking, or causes avoidance of these activities During headache, one or more of the following • Nausea/vomiting, photophobia, phonophobia Female:male ratio 3:1 Positive family history in 70%–90%
Migraine with aura	Migraine-type headache occurs with or after aura • Focal dysfunction of cerebral cortex or brainstem causes one or more aura symptoms to develop over 4 minutes, or two or more symptoms occur in succession • Symptoms include feeling of dread or anxiety, unusual fatigue, nervousness or excitement, GI upset, visual or olfactory alteration • No aura symptom should last >1 hour. If this occurs, an alternative diagnosis should be considered Positive family history in 70%–90%
Cluster headache	Tendency of headache to occur daily in groups or clusters, hence the name cluster headache Clusters usually last several weeks to months, then disappear for months to years • Usually occur at characteristic times of year, such as vernal and autumnal equinox with one to eight episodes per day, at the same time of day. Common time is ~1 hour into sleep; the pain awakens the person (hence the term "alarm clock" headache) • Headache is often located behind one eye with a steady, intense ("hot poker in the eye" sensation), severe pain in a crescendo pattern lasting 15 minutes to 3 hours, with most in the range of 30–45 minutes. Pain intensity has helped earn the condition the name "suicide headache." Most often occurs with ipsilateral autonomic sign such as lacrimation, conjunctival injection, ptosis, and nasal stuffiness Female:male ratio ~1:3 to 1:8 (depending on source) Family history of cluster headache present in ~20%

Source: Standards of Care for Headache Diagnosis and Treatment. Chicago, National Headache Foundation, 2004.

rectal suppository). Migraine is also present in many forms. A thoughtful match between the presentation of typical migraine and the form of medication is helpful. Following are some examples:

• Oral products generally take ½ to 1 hour before there is significant relief of migraine pain. These products are best suited for patients with migraine who have a slowly developing headache with minimum GI distress. As with all migraine therapies, oral medications should be used as soon as possible after the onset of symptoms. The use of oral products to manage migraine is the least expensive option and facilitates patient self-care.

• Injectable products (e.g., sumatriptan (Imitrex) and dihydroergotamine (D.H.E. 45, Migranal) have a rapid onset of action, usually within 15 to 30 minutes. These products are best suited for patients with rapidly progressing migraines accompanied by significant GI upset. Sumatriptan is available as a self-injector for patient administration. Dihydroergotamine is usually given intravenously for severe migraine along with parenteral hydration.

TABLE 2–3
Headache "Red Flags"

Consider diagnosis other than primary headache if headache "red flags" are present
- **S**ystemic symptoms
  - Fever, weight loss or secondary headache risk factors such as HIV, malignancy, pregnancy, anticoagulation
- **N**eurologic signs, symptoms
  - Any newly acquired neurologic finding including confusion, impaired alertness or consciousness, nuchal rigidity, hypertension, papilledema, CN dysfunction, abnormal motor function
- **O**nset
  - Sudden, abrupt, or split-second, the "thunderclap" headache
  - Onset of headache with exertion, sexual activity, coughing, sneezing
    - Suggests subarachnoid hemorrhage, sudden onset increased ICP
- **O**nset (age at onset of headache)
  - Older (>50 years) and younger (<5 years)
- **P**revious headache history
  - First headache in adult ≥30 years
    - Primary headache pattern usually established in youth/young adult years
  - New onset of different headache
    - Change in attack frequency, severity, or clinical features including progressive headache without headache-free period

Source: Dodick DW. Clinical clues and clinical rules: primary vs secondary headache. *Adv Stud Med.* 2003;3:S550–S555.

TABLE 2–4
Evidence-Based Guidelines in the Primary Care Setting: Neuroimaging in Patients with Nonacute Headache

Significantly increased odds of finding abnormality on neuroimaging
- Rapidly increasing headache frequency
- History
  - Dizziness or lack of coordination
  - Subjective numbness or tingling
  - Headache causing awakening from sleep
  - Headache worse with Valsalva maneuver
  - Accelerating, new-onset headache
- Abnormal neurologic examination
- Increasing age
  - More likely nonacute finding such as old infarct, atrophy

Unlikely to correlate with abnormal neuroimaging; neuroimaging unlikely to yield helpful clinical information
  - Neurologic examination normal
  - Long-standing history of similar headache
  - "Worst headache of my life"

Consensus-based principles
- Testing should be avoided if it would not lead to a change in management
- Not recommended if individual no more likely than general population to have significant abnormality
- Testing not normally recommended as population policy, although may make sense at individual level (e.g., with patient or provider fear)

Source: http://www.aan.com/professionals/practice/pdfs/gl0088.pdf, American Academy of Neurology evidence-based guidelines in the primary care setting: Neuroimaging in nonacute headache, accessed 8/22/09.

TABLE 2–5

Potential Lifestyle Triggers Influencing the Onset or Severity of Migraine Symptoms

Menses, ovulation, or pregnancy
Birth control/hormone replacement (progesterone) therapy
Illness
Intense or strenuous activity/exercise
Sleeping too much/too little/jet lag
Fasting/missing meals
Bright or flickering lights
Excessive or repetitive noises
Odors/fragrances/tobacco smoke
Weather/seasonal changes
High altitudes
Medications
Stress/stress letdown

Source: http://www.guideline.gov/summary/summary.aspx?ss=15&doc_id=6578&nbr=4138 accessed 8/22/09.

TABLE 2–6

Potential Dietary Triggers Influencing the Onset or Severity of Migraine Symptoms

Sour cream
Ripened cheeses (cheddar, Stilton, Brie, Camembert)
Sausage, bologna, salami, pepperoni, summer sausage, hot dogs
Pizza
Chicken liver, paté
Herring (pickled or dried)
Any pickled, fermented, or marinated food
Monosodium glutamate (MSG) (soy sauce, meat tenderizers, seasoned salt)
Freshly baked yeast products, sourdough bread
Chocolate
Nuts or nut butters
Broad beans, lima beans, fava beans, snow peas
Onions
Figs, raisins, papayas, avocados, red plums
Citrus foods
Bananas
Caffeinated beverages (tea, coffee, cola)
Alcoholic beverages (wine, beer, whiskey)
Aspartame/phenylalanine-containing foods or beverages

Source: http://www.guideline.gov/summary/summary.aspx?ss=15&doc_id=6578&nbr=4138, accessed 8/22/09.

Injectables are usually the most expensive treatment option, and using these products sometimes means that a patient with migraine requires a provider visit to facilitate the medication's use. Certain triptans (sumatriptan [Imitrex] and zolmitriptan [Zomig]) and dihydroergotamine (Migranal) are available as nasal sprays, have a similarly rapid onset of action, and are tolerable in the presence of GI upset. Analgesics (aspirin, acetaminophen) or antiemetics (prochlorperazine [Compazine] and promethazine [Phenergan]) have a slightly longer onset of action, but can be used for pain control or treatment of GI upset.

- Triptans act as selective serotonin receptor agonists and work at the 5-HT1D serotonin receptor site, allowing an increased uptake of serotonin. Because of potential vasoconstrictor effect, their use is contraindicated in patients with Prinzmetal angina or established or high risk for coronary artery disease, in pregnant women, and in individuals who have recently used ergots. Because of the risk of serotonin syndrome, a condition of excessive availability of this neurotransmitter, triptans should be used with caution with monoamine oxidase inhibitors (MAOIs) or high-dose selective serotonin reuptake inhibitors. Although triptans are specifically labeled for use only in migraine, some patients with severe tension-type headache benefit from their use, which lends further support to the hypothesis that there is a shared mechanism in migraine and tension-type headache. Adding an analgesic such as an NSAID to the use of a triptan yields improved pain control in many migraineurs. An example of a combined triptan/NSAID product is Treximet (sumatriptan with naproxen sodium).

- Ergotamines act as 5-HT1A and 5-HT1D receptor agonists and do not alter cerebral blood flow. Because of potential vasoconstrictor effect, their use should be avoided in the presence of coronary artery disease and pregnancy. Ergotamines are available in various forms, including oral and sublingual tablets, suppositories, injectables, and nasal sprays; examples include dihydroergotamine mesylate [Migranal, D.H.E. 45] and ergotamine tartrate with caffeine [Cafergot]). These products are helpful in the treatment of migraine, but not tension-type headache.

- NSAIDs can be highly effective in tension-type and migraine headache. These products inhibit prostaglandin and leukotriene synthesis and are most helpful when used at the first sign of headache, when GI upset is not a significant issue. The National Health Foundation Guidelines advise the use of rapid-onset NSAIDs such as ibuprofen in high doses with booster doses. Plain naproxen (Naprosyn) has a relatively slow onset of analgesic activity, whereas naproxen sodium (Aleve, Anaprox) use is associated with a significantly more rapid onset of pain relief. Acetaminophen and aspirin can also provide relief in migraine and tension-type headache, but provide less analgesic effect.

- Fioricet is a combination medication consisting of caffeine, butalbital, and acetaminophen. Caffeine enhances the analgesic properties of acetaminophen, and butalbital's barbiturate action enhances select neurotransmitter action, helping to relieve migraine and tension-type headache pain. With infrequent use, this product offers an inexpensive and generally well-tolerated headache treatment. Frequent or excessive use of Fioricet should be discouraged because of the potential for barbiturate dependency from butalbital and analgesic rebound headache from the acetaminophen component of the product.

- Midrin is a multidrug product that includes a vasoconstrictor (isometheptene mutate), analgesic (acetaminophen), and relaxant (65 mg of dichloralphenazone). This medication should be used in multiple doses at the beginning of a migraineur tension-type headache. Caution should be used when vasoconstriction is contraindicated.
- Excedrin Migraine is an over-the-counter aspirin, acetaminophen, and caffeine combination product that is approved by the U.S. Food and Drug Administration (FDA) for migraine therapy and is effective in tension-type headache. Its advantages include ease of patient access to the product, excellent side-effect profile, and low cost. Excessive acetaminophen use can lead to analgesic rebound headache.
- Neuroleptics are a class of medications historically used to treat major mental health problems; this class of drugs is also known as the first-generation antipsychotics. Examples of neuroleptics are prochlorperazine (Compazine) and promethazine (Phenergan). Because of their antiemetic effect, these products are occasionally used as adjuncts in migraine therapy. Because these drugs generally are highly sedating, using them in the clinician's office may make it difficult for patients to return home. Use should be limited to 3 days a week because of the risk of extrapyramidal movements (EPMs). Other antiemetics used in migraine include ondansetron (Zofran), a nonsedating, albeit expensive, option that is helpful if the patient needs to return quickly to work or other responsibilities. Metoclopramide (Reglan), a prokinetic agent that is generally well tolerated with infrequent use, is helpful in relieving milder GI symptoms; this drug should not be used on a daily basis because of EPM risk.
- Use of systemic corticosteroids is helpful with intractable or severe migraine and in cluster headache. Owing to the well-known adverse effects of this drug class, corticosteroid use for this purpose is not recommended more often than once a month. Examples of corticosteroid types and doses include prednisone 20 mg qid × 2 days and a Medrol Dosepak (a prepackaged 6-day methylprednisolone course with a rapid taper).
- Opioids such as hydrocodone, oxycodone, and codeine can provide analgesia and are often prescribed for migraine rescue. These products are sedating and potentially habituating, in addition to being substances of abuse.

Use of prophylactic therapy for migraine, tension-type, or cluster headache should be considered if abortive headache therapy is used frequently or if inadequate symptom relief is obtained from appropriate use of these therapies. The goal of headache prophylactic therapy is a minimum of a 50% reduction in number of headaches in about two-thirds of all patients, along with easier-to-control headaches that respond more rapidly to standard therapies

and likely require less medication. Most agents work through blockade of the 5HT2 receptor, and 1 to 2 months of use is needed before an effect is seen. Before headache prophylaxis is initiated, headache-provoking medications, such as estrogen, progesterone, and vasodilators, must be eliminated or limited. Lifestyle modification to minimize headache risk is also critical.

Secondary headaches are caused by an underlying disease process, often with increased ICP. The headache in increased ICP is usually reported as worst on awakening, which is when brain swelling is the worst. The pain is less intense as the day progresses and as the pressure lessens, in contrast to a tension-type headache, which usually worsens as the day goes on. Because intervention is guided by the underlying cause, establishing the appropriate diagnosis in all forms of secondary headache is critical.

Discussion Sources

Robbins L. http://www.headachedrugs.com/pdf/HA-2008.pdf, Headache 2008-2009, 2008, accessed 8/23/09.

Ruoff G, Urban G. Treatment of primary headache: Patient education. In: *Standards of Care for Headache Diagnosis and Treatment*. Chicago, IL: National Headache Foundation; 2004:22–26.

QUESTIONS

21. An 18-year-old college freshman is brought to the student health center with a chief complaint of a 3-day history of progressive headache and intermittent fever. On physical examination, he has positive Kernig and Brudzinski signs. The most likely diagnosis is:

    A. viral encephalitis.
    B. bacterial meningitis.
    C. acute subarachnoid hemorrhage.
    D. chronic epidural hematoma.

22. A 19-year-old college sophomore has documented meningococcal meningitis. You speak to the school health officers about the risk to the other students on campus. You inform them that:

    A. the patient does not have a contagious disease.
    B. all students are at significant risk regardless of their degree of contact with the infected person.
    C. only intimate partners are at risk.
    D. individuals with household-type or more intimate contact are considered to be at risk.

23. When evaluating the person who has bacterial meningitis, the NP expects to find cerebrospinal fluid (CSF) results of:

    A. low protein.
    B. predominance of lymphocytes.
    C. glucose at about 30% of serum levels.
    D. low opening pressure.

24. When evaluating a patient who has aseptic or viral meningitis, the NP expects to find CSF results of:
    A. low protein.
    B. predominance of lymphocytes.
    C. glucose at about 30% of serum levels.
    D. low opening pressure.

25. Which of the following describes the Kernig sign?
    A. Neck pain occurs with passive flexion of one hip and knee, which causes flexion of the contralateral leg.
    B. Passive neck flexion in a supine patient results in flexion of the knees and hips.
    C. Elicited with the patient lying supine and the hip flexed 90 degrees, it is present when extension of the knee from this position elicits resistance or pain in the lower back or posterior thigh.
    D. Headache worsens when the patient is supine.

26. Physical examination findings in papilledema include:
    A. arteriovenous nicking.
    B. macular hyperpigmentation.
    C. optic disk bulging.
    D. pupillary constriction.

27. Which of the following organisms is a gram-negative diplococcus?
    A. *Streptococcus pneumoniae*
    B. *Neisseria meningitidis*
    C. *Staphylococcus aureus*
    D. *Haemophilus influenzae*

28. During an outbreak of meningococcal meningitis, all of the following can be used as chemoprophylaxis except:
    A. a single dose of ceftriaxone.
    B. multiple doses of rifampin.
    C. multiple doses of amoxicillin.
    D. a single dose of meningococcal conjugate vaccine (MCV4 or Menactra).

ANSWERS

21.	B	22.	D	23.	C
24.	B	25.	C	26.	C
27.	B	28.	C		

DISCUSSION

Meningitis is an infection of the meninges, CSF, and ventricles. The disease is typically defined further by its cause, such as bacterial (pyogenic), viral (aseptic), fungal, or other cause.

In bacterial meningitis, the causative pathogens differ according to patient age and certain risk characteristics. Bacterial seeding usually occurs via hematogenous spread, where organisms can enter the meninges through the bloodstream from other parts of the body; the pathogen likely was asymptomatically carried in the nose and throat. Another mechanism of acquisition is local extension from another infection, such as acute otitis media or bacterial rhinosinusitis. Congenital problems and trauma can provide a pathway via facial fractures or malformation (e.g., cleft lip or palate). Common pathogens in bacterial meningitis in adults include *Streptococcus pneumoniae* (gram-positive diplococci), *Neisseria meningitidis* (gram-negative diplococci), *Staphylococcus* species (gram-positive cocci), and *Haemophilus influenzae* (gram-negative coccobacilli).

The clinical presentation of bacterial meningitis in an adult usually includes the classic triad of fever, headache, and nuchal rigidity, or stiff neck. As with most forms of infectious disease, however, atypical presentation in older adults is common. In particular, nuchal rigidity and fever are often absent. Encephalitis is more likely viral in origin and usually manifests with fewer meningeal signs.

To eliminate or support the diagnosis of meningitis, lumbar puncture with CSF evaluation should be part of the evaluation of a febrile adult or child who has altered findings on neurologic examination. Pleocytosis, defined as a WBC count of more than 5 cells/mm³ of CSF, is an expected finding in meningitis caused by bacterial, viral, tubercular, fungal, or protozoan infection; an elevated CSF opening pressure is also a nearly universal finding. The typical CSF response in bacterial meningitis includes a WBC median count of 1200 cells/mm³ of CSF with 90% to 95% neutrophils; additional findings are a reduced CSF glucose amount below the normal level of about 40% of the plasma level, and an elevated CSF protein level. In viral or aseptic meningitis, CSF results include normal glucose level, normal to slightly elevated protein levels, and lymphocytosis. Further testing to ascertain the causative organism is warranted. Head CT or MRI should be considered before lumbar puncture is performed.

Brudzinski and Kernig signs, suggestive of nuchal rigidity and meningeal irritation, are often positive in children 2 years or older and adults with meningitis. The Brudzinski sign is elicited when passive neck flexion in a supine patient results in flexion of the knees and hips. The Kernig sign is elicited with the patient lying supine and the hip flexed at 90 degrees. A positive sign is present when extension of the knee from this position elicits resistance or pain in the lower back or posterior thigh. Papilledema, or optic disk bulging, or absence of venous pulsations on funduscopic examination indicates increased ICP. Less common presenting symptoms include vomiting, seizures, and altered consciousness. In meningitis caused by *N. meningitidis,* a purpuritic or petechial rash is noted in about 50% of patients. Patients with viral meningitis usually have less severe symptoms that have a gradual onset; skin rash is uncommon.

The issue of meningitis contagion needs to be addressed. *N. meningitidis,* an organism normally carried in about 5%

to 10% of healthy adults and 60% to 80% of individuals in closed populations, such as military recruits, is transmitted through direct contact or respiratory droplets from infected people. Meningococcal disease most likely occurs within a few days of acquisition of a new strain, before the development of specific serum antibodies. Individuals acquire the infection if they are exposed to virulent bacteria and have no protective bactericidal antibodies. Smoking and concurrent upper respiratory tract viral infection diminish the integrity of the respiratory mucosa and increase the likelihood of invasive disease. The incubation period of the organism averages 3 to 4 days (range 1 to 10 days), which is the period of communicability. Bacteria can be found for 2 to 4 days in the nose and pharynx and for up to 24 hours after starting antibiotics. Public health authorities should be contacted when a person presents with suspected or documented bacterial meningitis.

Vaccination against the organism can be used for close contacts of patients with meningococcal disease resulting from A, C, Y, or W135 serogroups to prevent secondary cases. No effective vaccine exists to protect individuals from meningococcal meningitis caused by serogroup B. Widespread or universal chemoprophylaxis is not recommended during a meningococcal meningitis outbreak. Chemoprophylaxis should be considered for individuals in close contact, including household-type contact where there is a potential for sharing glassware and dishes, with patients in an endemic situation, but has limited efficacy interrupting transmission during an epidemic. Options include a single dose of oral ciprofloxacin or intramuscular ceftriaxone. An alternative is four oral doses of rifampin over 2 days.

Immunization against *N. meningitidis* can also be used in an outbreak; this option is helpful against current and future outbreaks. In the United States, two vaccines against the organism are available: meningococcal polysaccharide vaccine (MPSV4 or Menomune-A/C/Y/W-135) and meningococcal conjugate vaccine (MCV4 or Menactra). Both vaccines can prevent four types of meningococcal disease, including two of the three types most common in the United States (serogroup C, Y, and W-135) and a type that causes epidemics in Africa (serogroup A); protection from all possible meningococcal strains is not provided by the vaccines.

MCV4 is recommended for all children at their routine preadolescent visit (11 to 12 years old). For children who have never received MCV4 previously, a dose is recommended at high school entry. Other individuals at increased risk for whom routine vaccination is recommended are college freshmen living in dormitories, microbiologists who are routinely exposed to meningococcal bacteria, U.S. military recruits, individuals who are functionally or surgically asplenic, individuals with immune system disorder, people who are likely to travel to countries that have an outbreak of meningococcal disease, and people who might have been exposed to meningitis during an outbreak. MCV4 is the preferred vaccine for individuals 11 to 55 years old in these risk groups, but MPSV4 can be used if MCV4 is unavailable.

MPSV4 should be used for children 2 to 10 years old and adults older than 55 years who are at risk.

Meningitis caused by most other agents is a result of a patient rather than contagion factor; that is, the meningitis is a result of extension of an existing illness such as bacterial sinusitis and otitis media. Treatment of a patient with meningitis includes supportive care and the use of the appropriate anti-infective agents. Ceftriaxone with or without vancomycin or ampicillin or both is usually the treatment of choice in patients with suspected bacterial meningitis, pending bacterial sensitivity results. Acyclovir is an option in aseptic meningitis, pending identification of the offending virus. Prudent clinical practice requires keeping abreast of current trends in causative pathogens and microbial resistance.

Discussion Sources

Centers for Disease Control and Prevention. http://www.cdc.gov/meningitis/bacterial/faqs.htm, Meningococcal disease: Frequently asked questions, 2009, accessed 8/23/09.

Centers for Disease Control and Prevention. http://www.cdc.gov/meningitis/viral/viral-faqs.htm, Viral (aseptic) meningitis, accessed 8/23/09.

Gondim F, Singh M, Croul S. http://emedicine.medscape.com/article/1165557, eMedicine: Meningococcal meningitis, accessed 8/23/09.

QUESTIONS

29. A 34-year-old woman has recently been diagnosed with multiple sclerosis (MS). When providing primary care for this patient, you consider that MS:

 A. has a predictable course of progressive decline in intellectual and motor function.
 B. manifests with a classic pattern of myalgia, blurred vision, and ataxia.
 C. is often seen with a variable pattern of exacerbation and remissions.
 D. is accompanied by classic central nervous system lesions detectable on skull films.

30. Treatment options in MS to attenuate disease progression include:

 A. interferon beta-1b.
 B. methylprednisolone.
 C. ribavirin.
 D. phenytoin.

31. Which of the following is most consistent with findings in patients with Parkinson disease?

 A. rigid posture with poor muscle tone
 B. masklike facies and continued cognitive function
 C. tremor at rest and bradykinesia
 D. excessive arm swinging with ambulation and flexed posture

32. Treatment options in Parkinson disease include all of the following except:

   A. levodopa.
   B. chlorpromazine.
   C. ropinirole.
   D. pramipexole.

33. Surgical intervention such as deep brain stimulation can be helpful in the management of Parkinson disease–related symptoms:

   A. in early disease as a first-line therapy.
   B. when medication therapy is not tolerated or helpful.
   C. related to memory loss.
   D. only as a last resort when all other options have been exhausted.

ANSWERS

29.	C	30.	A	31.	C
32.	B	33.	B		

DISCUSSION

MS, a recurrent, chronic demyelinating disorder of the central nervous system, is a disease characterized by episodes of focal neurologic dysfunction, with symptoms occurring acutely, worsening over a few days, and lasting weeks, followed by a period of partial to full resolution. Common symptoms include weakness or numbness of a limb, monocular visual loss, diplopia, vertigo, facial weakness or numbness, sphincter disturbances, ataxia, and nystagmus. MS is usually classified into two forms: (1) relapsing, remitting MS (RRMS), in which episodes resolve with good neurologic function between exacerbations and minimal to no cumulative defects, and which accounts for approximately 85% of patients with the condition, and (2) primary progressive MS, in which episodes do not fully resolve, and there are cumulative defects. Most patients with RRMS enter a stage referred to as secondary progressive MS.

The initial diagnosis of MS is often difficult to make because the signs of recurrent fatigue, muscle weakness, and other nonspecific signs and symptoms are often attributed to other diseases or simply to stress and fatigue. MRI can reveal demyelinating plaques, a typical finding in MS. Characteristic CSF findings include pleocytosis with predominance of monocytes and abnormal protein levels, including a modest increase in total protein, a markedly increased gamma-globulin fraction, a high immunoglobulin G index, presence of oligoclonal bands, and an increase in myelin basic protein. Abnormal visual evoked potential testing can contribute to the development of the diagnosis. As with other conditions that have a complex origin and complicated course, expert consultation should be sought when diagnosing suspected MS and caring for the patient with the condition.

MS treatment generally falls into three categories: therapy for relapses, long-term disease-modifying medications, and symptomatic management. Triggers for exacerbations are varied, but often include onset of common infectious disease such as urinary tract infection; however, most exacerbations have no identifiable trigger. Treatment of exacerbations includes treatment of the underlying precipitating illness, if present, and systemic high-dose corticosteroids. Because most exacerbations improve without specific therapy, disagreement exists as to the utility of this treatment. This therapy seems to shorten the course of most exacerbations, but does not seem to have an impact on long-term disease progression. Some clinicians opt for lower dose corticosteroid therapy with variable results.

Immunomodulatory therapy with interferon beta-1b (Betaseron) or interferon beta-1a (Avonex) has been shown to reduce significantly the frequency of exacerbations and long-term disability in RRMS. Immunosuppressive therapy with mitoxantrone (Novantrone) also has some utility in reducing the rate of progression. Natalizumab (Tysabri) is a monoclonal antibody with considerable clinical efficacy in treating MS, but it carries a warning about progressive multifocal leukoencephalopathy, a rare, destructive brain infection, associated with its use. Symptom management therapies are aimed at the specific needs of the individual patient and often include nondrug interventions, such as physical and occupational therapy, and management of urologic problems such as altered bladder function. Expert consultation should be sought while providing care for the complex health-care needs of patients with MS.

Parkinson disease is a slowly progressive movement disorder that is largely caused by an alteration in dopamine-containing neurons of the pars compacta of the substantia nigra. Age at onset is usually in the sixth decade and older, but the onset can occur in much younger adults.

The diagnosis of Parkinson disease is made by clinical evaluation and consists of a combination of six cardinal features: tremor at rest, rigidity, bradykinesia (slowness in the execution of movement), flexed posture, loss of postural reflexes, and masklike facies. At least two of these, one being tremor at rest or bradykinesia, must be present. Classically, an individual with Parkinson disease holds the arms rigidly at the sides with little movement during ambulation; forward falls are common. The parkinsonian gait usually consists of a series of rapid small steps; to turn, patients must take several small steps, moving forward and backward.

Because Parkinson disease is characterized by an alteration in the dopaminergic pathway, dopamine agonists such as ropinirole (Requip) and pramipexole (Mirapex) are usually the early disease treatment of choice, in part because of a proposed neuroprotective effect and a better adverse-effect profile than levodopa. Levodopa, a metabolic precursor of dopamine, continues to be used to minimize symptoms, but tends to be less effective with more adverse effects as the disease progresses; most patients who take levodopa for more than 5 to 10 years develop dyskinesia. Levodopa is often given with carbidopa in the fixed-dose combination known as Sinemet.

Amantadine (Symmetrel) is an antiviral drug with time-limited (usually less than 1 year) antiparkinsonian benefits, but can be used in later stages of the disease to help reduce dyskinesias. Catechol O-methyltransferase (COMT) inhibitors including tolcapone (Tasmar) and entacapone (Comtan) are clinically helpful because these medications increase the half-life of levodopa by reducing its metabolism. Monoamine oxidase-B (MAO-B) inhibitors such as selegiline also help increase levodopa's half-life by reducing its metabolism. Apomorphine (Apokyn) is an injectable-only dopamine agonist that can be used in advanced Parkinson disease as a rescue therapy for the treatment of hypomobility or "off" periods. Other medications used in the treatment of Parkinson disease include anticholinergics, such as benztropine, to help with tremor; however, this class of drugs is well known to cause dry mouth, urinary retention, and altered mentation, particularly in older adults. In view of the complexity of prescribing Parkinson disease medications, the prescriber should be well versed in these products and seek expert consultation.

As Parkinson disease progresses, patients often develop variability in response to treatment, known as motor fluctuations, often referred to as "on" and "off" periods. During an "on" period, a person can move with relative ease. An "off" period describes times when a person has more difficulty with movement; this can be manifested either by significant difficulty in initiating movement or with uncontrolled body movements including dyskinesia. A common time for a person with Parkinson disease to experience an "off" period is toward the end of a levodopa dosing period, when the drug seems to be "wearing off." This problem can usually be managed with medication adjustment. If this approach is not helpful, surgical treatment offers another form of treatment for uncontrolled writhing movement (choreiform movement or dyskinesia) of the body or a limb.

For most people with Parkinson disease, "off" periods and dyskinesias can be managed with changes in medications. When medication adjustments do not improve mobility, however, or when medications cause significant side effects, surgical treatment can be considered. Pallidotomy can be helpful in tremor, rigidity, bradykinesia, and levodopa-induced dyskinesias. Deep brain stimulation surgery for Parkinson disease is helpful in making the "off" state more like movement in the "on" state, and is helpful in the reduction of levodopa-induced dyskinesias. As with other therapies, expert consultation should be sought, and all options should be thoroughly discussed with the patient before pursuing surgical intervention.

Discussion Sources

Dangond F. http://emedicine.medscape.com/article/1146199, eMedicine: Multiple sclerosis, accessed 8/23/09.

Fox R. Multiple sclerosis. In: Rakel R, Bope E, eds. *Conn's Current Therapy 2009*. Philadelphia, PA: Saunders; 2009:932–940.

National Parkinson Foundation. http://www.parkinson.org/NETCOMMUNITY/Page.aspx?pid=226&srcid=216, Parkinson primer, accessed 8/23/09.

Pahwa R, Lyons K. Parkinsonism. In: Rakel R, Bope E, eds, *Conn's Current Therapy 2009*. Philadelphia, PA: Saunders; 2009:954–958.

QUESTIONS

34. Which of the following best describes patient presentation during an absence (petit mal) seizure?
    A. blank staring lasting 3 to 50 seconds, accompanied by impaired level of consciousness
    B. awake state with abnormal motor behavior lasting seconds
    C. rigid extension of arms and legs, followed by sudden jerking movements with loss of consciousness
    D. abrupt muscle contraction with autonomic signs

35. Which of the following best describes patient presentation during a simple partial seizure?
    A. blank staring lasting 3 to 50 seconds, accompanied by impaired level of consciousness
    B. awake state with abnormal motor behavior lasting seconds
    C. rigid extension of arms and legs, followed by sudden jerking movements with loss of consciousness
    D. abrupt muscle contraction with autonomic signs

36. Which of the following best describes patient presentation during a tonic-clonic (grand mal) seizure?
    A. blank staring lasting 3 to 50 seconds, accompanied by impaired level of consciousness
    B. awake state with abnormal motor behavior lasting seconds
    C. rigid extension of arms and legs, followed by sudden jerking movements with loss of consciousness
    D. abrupt muscle contraction with autonomic signs

37. Which of the following best describes patient presentation during a myoclonic seizure?
    A. blank staring lasting 3 to 50 seconds, accompanied by impaired level of consciousness
    B. awake state with abnormal motor behavior lasting seconds
    C. rigid extension of arms and legs, followed by sudden jerking movements with loss of consciousness
    D. brief, jerking contractions of arms, legs, trunk, or all of these.

38. Treatment options for an adult with seizures include all of the following agents except:

    A. carbamazepine.
    B. phenytoin.
    C. gabapentin.
    D. trandolapril.

39. A patient taking phenytoin can exhibit a drug interaction when concurrently taking:

    A. theophylline.
    B. famotidine.
    C. acetaminophen.
    D. aspirin.

ANSWERS

34.	A	**35.**	B	**36.**	C
37.	D	**38.**	D	**39.**	A

DISCUSSION

The type of seizure directs the treatment of a seizure disorder. Knowledge of the presentation of common forms of seizures is critical (Table 2–7).

Numerous standard seizure therapies, including phenytoin, carbamazepine, clonazepam, ethosuximide, and valproic acid, and newer antiepileptic drugs (AEDs), such as gabapentin, lamotrigine, and topiramate, are now available. Expert knowledge of the indications and adverse reactions of these medications is needed before AED therapy is initiated or continued.

Certain AEDs, including phenytoin and carbamazepine, are narrow therapeutic index (NTI) drugs. A certain amount of such drugs is therapeutic, and just slightly more than this amount is potentially toxic. Conversely, a slightly lower dose might not be therapeutic. Other NTI drugs include warfarin, theophylline, and digoxin. Many of these drugs have high levels of protein binding and significant use of hepatic enzymatic pathways for drug metabolism, such as cytochrome

TABLE 2–7

Description of Common Seizure Disorders

Seizure Type	Description of Seizure	Comments
Absence (petit mal)	Blank staring lasting 3–50 seconds accompanied by impaired level of consciousness	Usual age of onset 3–15 years
Myoclonic	Awake state or momentary loss of consciousness with abnormal motor behavior lasting seconds to minutes; one or more muscle groups causing brief jerking contractions of the limbs and trunk, occasionally flinging patient	Difficult to control; at least half also have tonic-clonic seizures. Usual age of onset 2–7 years
Tonic-clonic (grand mal)	Rigid extension of arms and legs followed by sudden jerking movements with loss of consciousness; bowel and bladder incontinence common with postictal confusion	Onset at any age; in adults, new onset may be found in brain tumor, post–head injury, alcohol withdrawal
Simple partial or focal seizure (jacksonian)	Awake state with abnormal motor, sensory, autonomic, or psychic behavior; movement can affect any part of body, localized or generalized	Typical age of onset 3–15 years
Complex partial	Aura characterized by unusual sense of smell or taste, visual or auditory hallucinations, stomach upset; followed by vague stare and facial movements, muscle contraction and relaxation, and autonomic signs; can progress to loss of consciousness	Onset at any age

Source: Epilepsy Foundation: http://www.epilepsyfoundation.org/about/types/types/index.cfm, Seizures and syndromes, accessed 8/22/09.

P-450. Phenytoin is highly (greater than 90%) protein bound; when taken with other highly protein-bound drugs, it can potentially be displaced from its protein-binding site, leading to increased free phenytoin and a risk of toxicity. Carbamazepine and phenytoin can increase the metabolic capacity of hepatic enzymes, which leads to more rapid metabolism of the drug and reduced levels of this and other drugs. Phenytoin use increases theophylline clearance by increasing CYP 450 enzyme activity. Concomitant use of theophylline and phenytoin can lead to altered phenytoin pharmacokinetics. The net result is that when phenytoin and theophylline are given together, levels of both drugs can decrease by 40%. When taken with birth control pills, carbamazepine induces estrogen metabolism, potentially leading to contraceptive failure. The prescriber should be familiar with the drug interactions of all AEDs and monitor therapeutic levels and for adverse reactions.

Discussion Sources

Indiana University School of Medicine Division of Clinical Pharmacology. http://medicine.iupui.edu/clinpharm/DDIs/ClinicalTable.asp, P450 drug interaction table: Abbreviated clinically relevant table, accessed 8/23/09.

St. Louis E, Granner M. Seizure and epilepsy in adolescents and adults. In: Rakel R, Bope E, eds. *Conn's Current Therapy 2009*. Philadelphia, PA: Saunders; 2009:898–906.

Zupana M. Seizure and epilepsy in infants and children. In: Rakel R, Bope E, eds. *Conn's Current Therapy 2009*. Philadelphia, PA: Saunders; 2009:907–915.

QUESTIONS

40. Risk factors for transient ischemic attack (TIA) include all of the following except:

   A. atrial fibrillation.
   B. carotid artery disease.
   C. oral contraceptive use.
   D. pernicious anemia.

41. A TIA is characterized as an episode of reversible neurologic symptoms that can last:

   A. 1 hour.
   B. 6 hours.
   C. 12 hours.
   D. 24 hours.

42. When caring for a patient with a recent TIA, you consider that:

   A. long-term antiplatelet therapy is likely indicated.
   B. this person has a relatively low risk of future stroke.
   C. women present with this disorder more often than men.
   D. rehabilitation will be needed to minimize the effects of the resulting neurologic insult.

43. Which of the following is the most common cause of stroke?

   A. Cerebral ischemia
   B. Embolus of cardiac origin
   C. Subarachnoid hemorrhage
   D. Subdural hematoma

44. to 50. When considering the diagnosis of acute stroke, which of the following can be part of the presentation? (Answer yes or no.)

___ **44.** partial loss of visual field

___ **45.** unilateral hearing loss

___ **46.** facial muscle paralysis

___ **47.** vertigo

___ **48.** diplopia

___ **49.** headache

___ **50.** ataxia

ANSWERS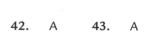

40. D	**41.** D	**42.** A	**43.** A
44. Yes	**45.** Yes	**46.** Yes	**47.** Yes
48. Yes	**49.** Yes	**50.** Yes	

DISCUSSION

A TIA is an acute neurologic event in which all signs and symptoms, including numbness, weakness, and flaccidity, and visual changes, ataxia, or dysarthria, resolve usually within minutes, but certainly by 24 hours after onset. If changes persist beyond 24 hours, the diagnosis of stroke should be considered. TIA should be considered a "stroke warning." Risk factors include carotid artery and other forms of atherosclerosis; structural cardiac problems, such as valvular problems that lead to increased risk of embolization; and hypercoagulable conditions, such as antiphospholipid antibody and oral contraceptive use. Intervention includes minimizing risk factors through lifestyle modification (e.g., smoking cessation; diet; exercise; cardiovascular and cerebrovascular disease risk reduction such as aggressive treatment of dyslipidemia, hypertension, and diabetes mellitus) and long-term antiplatelet therapy.

Acute stroke is often thought of as manifesting with sudden-onset unilateral limb weakness and motor dysfunction. Although these findings are often part of the clinical presentation, other findings, such as changes in hearing and vision, seizure, and head and neck pain, are often noted (Table 2–8).

About 80% of strokes are due to cerebral ischemia, about 15% are due to cerebral hemorrhage, and 5% are due to

TABLE 2–8
Acute Stroke Presentation

Sign/Symptom	Clinical Presentation
Alteration in consciousness	Stupor
	Confusion
	Agitation
	Memory loss
	Delirium
	Seizures
	Coma
Headache	Intense or unusually severe, often with sudden onset, usually described as having different characteristics compared with patient's typical primary headache
	Altered level of consciousness or neurologic deficit
	Unusual or severe neck or facial pain
Aphasia	Incoherent speech or difficulty understanding speech
Facial weakness or asymmetry	Paralysis of facial muscles (e.g., when patient speaks or smiles)
	May be on same side (ipsilateral) or opposite side (contralateral) to limb paralysis
Altered coordination	Incoordination, weakness, paralysis, or sensory loss of one or more limbs (usually one half of the body and in particular the hand)
	Ataxia (poor balance, clumsiness, or difficulty walking)
Visual loss	Monocular or binocular
	Report of partial loss of the field
Miscellaneous	Vertigo
	Diplopia
	Unilateral hearing loss
	Nausea, vomiting
	Photophobia
	Phonophobia

With suspected stroke, neuroimaging should be obtained. Head CT is helpful in identifying acute cerebral hemorrhage, whereas MRI is a more sensitive test in the acute phase of ischemic stroke. CT or MR angiography is helpful in showing stenosis or occlusion in the brain-supplying vessels. Carotid ultrasound, echocardiogram, and other imaging may help to identify or rule out concomitant and contributing conditions.
Source: Internet Stroke Center: http://www.strokecenter.org/education/ais_evaluation/lt_rt_hemisphere.htm, Emergency stroke evaluation and diagnosis, accessed 8/22/09.

subarachnoid hemorrhage; in younger adults, carotid artery dissection can cause stroke, accounting for about 5% of all strokes. Acute stroke should be thought of as a "brain attack," in which a portion of the brain is acutely ischemic, a potentially reversible condition if blood flow is reestablished. If blood flow is not restored, the ischemic tissue will be compromised, and the ischemia evolves into a cerebral infarction, often with devastating long-term consequences. If acute stroke is suspected, the patient must undergo emergency neuroimaging and be evaluated for thrombolytic or revascularization therapy in the appropriate health-care setting.

Because atherosclerosis is a major contributor to stroke risk, prevention of the condition should be aimed at reducing atherosclerotic risk through control of hypertension, dyslipidemia, and diabetes mellitus. Patients with a history of TIA or ischemia are also at high risk for another cerebrovascular event, myocardial infarction, and sudden cardiac death, and benefit from aggressive measures to reduce atherosclerotic risk. Secondary prevention against ischemic stroke and TIA should include antiplatelet therapy with aspirin or aspirin with extended-release dipyridamole (Aggrenox); if these options are not tolerated or in the presence of peripheral arterial or multivessel atherosclerotic disease, clopidogrel (Plavix) should be prescribed. These agents inhibit platelet activation through different mechanisms of action. When TIA or stroke originates from cardiac embolus, oral anticoagulation (warfarin) therapy, with a goal international normalized ratio of 2.0 to 3.0, should be provided.

Discussion Source

Diener H-C. Ischemic cerebrovascular disease. In: Rakel R, Bope E, eds. *Conn's Current Therapy 2009*. Philadelphia, PA: Saunders; 2009:893–895.

Internet Stroke Center. http://www.strokecenter.org/education/ais_evaluation/lt_rt_hemisphere.htm, Emergency stroke evaluation and diagnosis, accessed 8/22/09.

Saxena R, Koudstaal PJ. Anticoagulants versus antiplatelet therapy for preventing stroke in patients with nonrheumatic atrial fibrillation and a history of stroke or transient ischemic attack. *Cochrane Database Syst Rev.* 2004;(4):CD000187.

QUESTIONS

51. to 55. Identify the following as most likely associated with delirium or dementia:

____ **51.** Insidious onset over months to years

____ **52.** Acute onset of change in mental status

____ **53.** Associated with use of medications with anticholinergic effect

____ **54.** Treatment includes use of *N*-methyl-D-aspartate (NMDA) receptor antagonist

____ **55.** Mental status potentially returns to baseline with recovery.

56. The most common etiology of delirium is:
  A. cerebral ischemia.
  B. acute infection.
  C. Alzheimer disease.
  D. ingestion of a neurotoxin.

57. The most common etiology of dementia is:
  A. multi-infarct disease.
  B. Alzheimer disease.
  C. acute infection.
  D. history of head injury.

58. When discussing the use of a cholinesterase inhibitor with a 72-year-old woman with early-stage Alzheimer-type dementia and her family, you report that:
  A. This medication will help return memory to her preillness baseline.
  B. The risk associated with the use of this medication outweighs its benefits.
  C. This medication will likely afford clear, although minor and time-limited benefits.
  D. The medication should have been started earlier to help prevent the change in cognition.

ANSWERS

51.	Dementia	**52.**	Delirium	**53.**	Delirium
54.	Dementia	**55.**	Delirium	**56.**	B
57.	B	**58.**	C		

DISCUSSION

Delirium is a condition in which the patient exhibits an acute onset, over hours to a few days, of reduced ability to maintain attention to external stimuli and shift attention appropriately to new stimuli. The result is disorganized thinking. Two or more of the following are usually noted: an altered level of consciousness from baseline; memory impairment; perceptual disturbance, such as hallucinations; altered sleep; change in psychomotor activity; and disorientation to time, place, and person. Delirium is not a diagnosis, but rather a clinical state caused by an underlying health problem. Following is the *DELIRIUMS* mnemonic, which can serve as a helpful memory aid regarding the most common causes of delirium.

- *D*rugs—When any medication is added or dose is adjusted. Particularly problematic medications include anticholinergics (tricyclic antidepressants [TCAs], first-generation antihistamines), neuroleptics (haloperidol, others), opioids (in particular, meperidine), long-acting benzodiazepines (diazepam, clonazepam), and alcohol.
- *E*motional (mood disorders, loss), *E*lectrolyte disturbance.
- *L*ow PO_2 (hypoxemia from CAP, COPD, PE, MI), *L*ack of drugs (withdrawal from alcohol, other habituating substances).
- *I*nfection—Urinary tract infection and community-acquired pneumonia are the most common infectious causes of delirium.
- *R*etention of urine or feces, *R*educed sensory input (blindness, deafness, darkness, change in surroundings).
- *I*ctal or postictal state—Alcohol withdrawal is a common reason for an isolated first seizure in an older adult.
- *U*ndernutrition—Protein/calorie, vitamin B_{12} or folate deficiency, dehydration including postoperative volume disturbance.
- *M*etabolic (poorly controlled diabetes mellitus, undertreated or untreated hypothyroidism or hyperthyroidism), *M*yocardial problems (myocardial infarction, heart failure, dysrhythmia).
- *S*ubdural hematoma—Can be as a result of relatively minor head trauma to brain atrophy, fragile vessels.

The evaluation of a patient with delirium should be focused on defining its underlying cause. A thorough health history including social and home assessment and a physical examination should be conducted. A standardized evaluation of mental status must be included in the evaluation. The evaluation of the patient with mental status change starts with a comprehensive health history and physical examination. Diagnostic testing should be focused to reveal the diagnosis of the underlying etiology with potentially reversible conditions (Table 2–9).

Delirium treatment is aimed at assessing patients at greatest risk to help avoid its occurrence. When delirium occurs, treatment is focused on the condition's underlying cause. Mental status should return to baseline with recovery,

TABLE 2–9

Evaluation of the Person With Mental Status Change

The evaluation of the patient with mental status change starts with a comprehensive health history and physical examination. Diagnostic testing should be focused to reveal the underlying etiology with potentially reversible conditions

Definite	As Directed by Patient Presentation
BUN, Cr	Brain imaging (CT vs. MRI)
Glucose	PET scan
Calcium	Toxic screen
Sodium	CXR
Hepatic enzymes	ESR
Vitamin B$_{12}$/folate	HIV
TSH	Additional studies as needed
RPR	
CBC with WBC differential	
UA, U C & S	
ECG	

Source: Rolak R: Neurology Secrets, 4th ed. St. Louis, Elsevier, 2005.

TABLE 2–10

Dementia Etiology

Dementia Type	Comment
Alzheimer-type	60%–80%
Vascular (multi-infarct) dementia	10%–20%
Parkinson disease	5%
Miscellaneous causes	HIV, dialysis encephalopathy, neurosyphilis, normal pressure hydrocephalus, others

Source: Flacker J. Delirium. In: Rakel R, Bope E, eds. *Conn's Current Therapy 2009*. Philadelphia, PA: Saunders; 2009:1118–1120.

although ongoing research suggests that perhaps this recovery is incomplete in some individuals. In about two-thirds of all patients with delirium, the condition resolves within 1 week of its onset.

Dementia is defined by a chronic loss of intellectual or cognitive function of sufficient severity to interfere with social or occupational function; this condition is a symptom of an underlying diagnosis (Table 2–10). In dementia, mental status changes can evolve insidiously over months or years with a gradually worsening course. The most common causes of dementia are Alzheimer-type and multi-infarct or vascular dementia (Table 2–11). The evaluation of a person with suspected dementia is similar to assessment in delirium; the two conditions often overlap and can mimic each other. In addition to behavior and supportive therapies, patients with dementia often benefit from the use of a cholinesterase inhibitor such as donepezil (Aricept), tacrine (Cognex), rivastigmine (Exelon), or NMDA-receptor antagonist such as memantine (Namenda). These classes of medications have different mechanisms of action and can be given together and have a demonstrated, although minor and time-limited, effect in dementia care (Table 2–12); the use of these products to prevent dementia is currently not supported.

Discussion Sources

Flacker J. Delirium. In: Rakel R, Bope E, eds. *Conn's Current Therapy 2009*. Philadelphia, PA: Saunders; 2009:1118–1120.

Gordon MP, Fitten LJ. Alzheimer's disease. In: Rakel R, Bope E, eds. *Conn's Current Therapy 2009*. Philadelphia, PA: Saunders; 2009:881–887.

TABLE 2–11

Delirium versus Dementia

	Delirium	Dementia
ETIOLOGY	Precipitated by acute underlying cause such as an acute illness	Various causes
ONSET	Abrupt onset, over hours to days, usually a precise date, rapidly progressive change in mental status	Insidious onset that cannot be related to a precise date, gradual change in mental status
DURATION	Duration hours to days	Duration months to years
REVERSIBLE	Usually reversible to baseline mental status when underlying illness resolved	Chronically progressive and irreversible
SLEEP DISTURBANCE	Disturbed sleep-wake cycle with hour-to-hour variability	Disturbed sleep-wake cycle, but lacks hour-to-hour variability, often day-night reversal
PSYCHOMOTOR	Change in psychomotor activity, either hyperactive or hypoactive	No psychomotor changes until later in disease
PERCEPTUAL DISTURBANCES	Perceptual disturbances including hallucinations	No perceptual disturbances until later disease
SPEECH	Speech content incoherent, confused with a wide variety of often inappropriately used words such as misnamed persons and items	Speech content sparse, progressing to mute in later disease

Note: Delirium and dementia often coexist. The diagnosis of delirium must be considered in the presence of a sudden-onset change in mental status in the individual with dementia.

Sources: Pierson C: Older patients. In Goolsby MJ, Grubbs L (eds): Advanced Assessment: Interpreting Findings and Formulating Differential Diagnoses. Philadelphia, FA Davis, 2005, pp. 477-507; www.merck.com/mrkshared/mmg/sec5/ch39/ch39a.jsp, Merck manual: Delirium and dementia, accessed 8/30/09.

TABLE 2–12

American Academy of Neurology Standards for Care in Alzheimer-type Dementia (AD)

Strategy	Comment
To slow decline in AD	Vitamin E 1000 IU twice daily or selegiline 5 mg twice daily. No added benefit to using both products The use of NSAIDs and postmenopausal hormone therapy has not been supported for this purpose
In mild to moderate stage disease, the use of cholinesterase inhibitors is considered to be the mainstay of treatment	Cholinesterase inhibitors (donepezil [Aricept], rivastigmine [Exelon], galantamine [Razadyne]) have clear, although minor and time-limited benefits by increasing availability of cholinesterase. This small effect is clinically significant
In moderate to severe AD, further studies of multiple interventions are needed	Approved for use in moderate to severe AD, NMDA receptor antagonist memantine (Namenda), through its effect on glutamate, helps to create an environment that allows for storage and retrieval of information. Also used in earlier disease with cholinesterase inhibitor donepezil
Consider non–AD-related (noncognitive) reasons for behavioral issues such as behavioral disturbances	Evaluate for depression, pain, infection, and other clinical conditions commonly found in older adults

Source: www.aan.com/professionals/practice/pdfs/dementia_guideline.pdf, AAN guideline summary for clinicians: Detection, diagnosis and management of dementia, accessed 8/30/09.

3

Skin Disorders

1 to 12. Match the following descriptions to the correct lesion or distribution name.

_____ **1.** multiple lesions blending together
_____ **2.** flat discoloration less than 1 cm in diameter
_____ **3.** circumscribed area of skin edema
_____ **4.** narrow linear crack into epidermis, exposing dermis
_____ **5.** vesicle-like lesion with purulent content
_____ **6.** flat discoloration greater than 1 cm in diameter
_____ **7.** raised lesion, larger than 1 cm, may be same or different color from the surrounding skin
_____ **8.** netlike cluster
_____ **9.** loss of epidermis and dermis
_____ **10.** loss of skin markings and full skin thickness
_____ **11.** skin thickening usually found over pruritic or friction areas
_____ **12.** in a ring formation

A. ulcer
B. atrophy
C. fissure
D. reticular
E. wheal
F. pustule
G. patch
H. plaque
I. macule
J. confluent or coalescent
K. annular
L. lichenification

ANSWERS

1. J, confluent or coalescent
2. I. macule
3. E. wheal
4. C. fissure

5. F. pustule
6. G. patch
7. H. plaque
8. D. reticular

9. A. ulcer
10. B. atrophy
11. L. lichenification
12. K. annular

DISCUSSION

Identification of common dermatologic lesions is important to safe clinical practice (Table 3–1).

Discussion Source

Mangione S. The skin. In: Mangione S, ed. *Physical Diagnosis Secrets*. 2nd ed. Philadelphia, PA: Mosby Elsevier; 2008:63–125.

QUESTIONS

13. How many grams of a topical cream or ointment are needed for a single application to the hands?

A. 1
B. 2
C. 3
D. 4

See full color images of this topic on DavisPlus at http://davisplus.fadavis.com | Keyword: Fitzgerald

TABLE 3–1

Skin Lesions

Lesion	Description	Example
COMMON PRIMARY SKIN LESIONS		
Macule	Flat discoloration, usually <1 cm in diameter	Freckle
Patch	Flat area of skin discoloration, larger than a macule	Vitiligo
Papule	Raised lesion, <1 cm, may be same or different color from the surrounding skin	Raised nevus
Vesicle	Fluid-filled, <1 cm	Varicella
Plaque	Raised lesion, >1 cm, may be same or different color from surrounding skin	Psoriasis
Purpura	Lesions caused by red blood cells leaving circulation and becoming trapped in skin	Petechiae, ecchymosis
Pustule	Vesicle-like lesion with purulent content	Impetigo, acne
Wheal	Circumscribed area of skin edema	Hive
Nodule	Raised lesion, >1 cm, usually mobile	Epidermal cyst
Bullae	Fluid-filled, ≥1 cm	Blister with second-degree burn
COMMON SECONDARY SKIN LESIONS		
Excoriation	Marks produced by scratching	Seen in areas of pruritic skin diseases
Lichenification	Skin thickening resembling callus formation	Seen in areas of recurrent scratching
Fissure	Narrow linear crack into epidermis, exposing dermis	Split lip, athlete's foot
Erosion	Partial focal loss of epidermis; heals without scarring	Area exposed after bullous lesion opens
Ulcer	Loss of epidermis and dermis; heals with scarring	Pressure sore
Scale	Raised, flaking lesion	Dandruff, psoriasis
Atrophy	Loss of skin markings and full skin thickness	Area treated excessively with higher potency corticosteroids
TERMS DESCRIBING PATTERNS OF SKIN LESIONS		
Annular	In a ring	Erythema migrans in Lyme disease
Confluent or coalescent	Multiple lesions blending together	Multiple skin conditions
Reticular	Netlike cluster	Multiple skin conditions
Dermatomal	Along a neurocutaneous dermatome	Herpes zoster
Linear	In streaks	Poison ivy

Source: Mangione S. The skin. In: Mangione S, ed. *Physical Diagnosis Secrets*. 2nd ed. Philadelphia, PA: Mosby Elsevier; 2008:63–125.

14. How many grams of a topical cream or ointment are needed for a single application to an arm?

    A. 1
    B. 2
    C. 3
    D. 4

15. How many grams of a topical cream or ointment are needed for a single application to the entire body?

    A. 10 to 30
    B. 30 to 60
    C. 60 to 90
    D. 90 to 120

ANSWERS

13. B **14.** C **15.** B

DISCUSSION

Knowledge of the amount of a cream or ointment needed to treat a dermatologic condition is an important part of the prescriptive practice (Table 3–2). Prescribers often write prescriptions for an inadequate amount of a topical medication with insufficient numbers of refills, possibly creating a situation in which treatment fails because of an inadequate length of therapy.

Discussion Source

Arndt K, Hsu J. *Manual of Dermatologic Therapeutics.* 7th ed. Philadelphia, PA: Lippincott Williams & Wilkins; 2007.

QUESTIONS

16. You write a prescription for a topical agent and anticipate the greatest rate of absorption when it is applied to the:

- **A.** palms of the hands.
- **B.** soles of the feet.
- **C.** face.
- **D.** abdomen.

17. You prescribe a topical medication and want it to have maximum absorption, so you choose the following vehicle:

- **A.** gel
- **B.** lotion
- **C.** cream
- **D.** ointment

ANSWERS

16. C **17.** D

DISCUSSION

The safe prescription of a topical agent for patients with dermatologic disorders requires knowledge of the best vehicle for the medication. Certain parts of the body, notably the face, axillae, and genital area, are quite permeable, allowing greater absorption of medication than less permeable areas, such as the extremities and trunk. In particular, the thickness of the palms of the hands and soles of the feet creates a barrier so that relatively little topical medication is absorbed when applied to these sites. Cutaneous drug absorption is typically inversely proportional to the thickness of the stratum corneum. Hydrocortisone absorption from the forearm is less than one-third of the amount that is absorbed from the forehead.

In general, the less viscous the vehicle containing a topical medication, the less of the medication is absorbed. As a result, medication contained in a gel or lotion is absorbed in smaller amounts than medication contained in a cream or ointment. Besides enhancing absorption of the therapeutic agent, creams and ointments provide lubrication to the region, often a desirable effect in the presence of xerosis or lichenification.

Discussion Source

Robertson D. Mailbach H. Dermatologic pharmacology. In: Katzung, B, *Katsung's Basic and Clinical Pharmacology.* 10th ed. New York, NY: McGraw-Hill Medical; 2006:991–1008.

 TABLE 3–2
Topical Medication-Dispensing Formula

	Amount Needed for One Application	Amount Needed in Twice-a-Day Application for 1 Week	Amount Needed in Twice-a-Day Application for 1 Month
Hands, head, face, anogenital region	2 g	28 g	120 g (4 oz)
One arm, anterior or posterior trunk	3 g	42 g	180 g (6 oz)
One leg	6 g	84 g	320 g (12 oz)
Entire body	30–60 g	420–840 g (14–28 oz)	1.8–3.6 kg (60–120 oz or 3.75–7.5 lb)

Source: Arndt K, Hsu J. *Manual of Dermatologic Therapeutics.* 7th ed. Philadelphia, PA: Lippincott Williams & Wilkins; 2007.

QUESTIONS

18. One of the mechanisms of action of a topical cortico-steroid preparation is as:

    A. an antimitotic.
    B. an exfoliant.
    C. a vasoconstrictor.
    D. a humectant.

19. To enhance the potency of a topical corticosteroid, the prescriber recommends that the patient apply the preparation:

    A. to dry skin by gentle rubbing.
    B. and cover with an occlusive dressing.
    C. before bathing.
    D. with an emollient.

20. Which of the following is the least potent topical corti-costeroid?

    A. betamethasone dipropionate 0.1% (Diprosone)
    B. clobetasol propionate 0.05% (Cormax)
    C. hydrocortisone 2.5%
    D. fluocinonide 0.05% (Lidex)

ANSWERS

| 18. | C | 19. | B | 20. | C |

DISCUSSION

Corticosteroids are a class of drugs often used to treat inflammatory and allergic dermatologic disorders. Although corticosteroids reduce inflammatory and allergic reactions through numerous mechanisms (including immunosup-pressive and inflammatory properties), their relative poten-cy is based on vasoconstrictive activity; that is, the most potent topical steroids, such as betamethasone (class 1), have significantly greater vasoconstricting action than the least potent agents, such as hydrocortisone (class 7) (Table 3–3).

Discussion Sources

Robertson D, Mailbach H. Dermatologic pharmacology. In: Katzung B, *Katzung's Basic and Clinical Pharmacology*. 10th ed. New York, NY: McGraw-Hill Medical; 2006:991–1008.

Stringer J. Adrenocortical hormones. In: *Basic Concepts in Pharmacology*. 3rd ed. New York, NY: McGraw-Hill Medical; 2006:225–229

TABLE 3–3

Examples of Topical Corticosteroid Potency

LOW POTENCY

Hydrocortisone (0.5%, 1%, 2.5%)
Fluocinolone acetonide 0.01% (Synalar)
Triamcinolone acetonide 0.025% (Aristocort)
Fluocinolone acetonide 0.025% (Synalar)
Hydrocortisone butyrate 0.1%
Hydrocortisone valerate 0.2% (Westcort)
Triamcinolone acetonide 0.1%

MIDRANGE POTENCY

Betamethasone dipropionate, augmented, 0.05% (Diprolene AF cream)
Mometasone furoate 0.1% (Elocon ointment)

HIGH POTENCY

Fluocinolone acetonide 0.2% (Synalar-HP)
Desoximetasone 0.25% (Topicort)
Fluocinonide 0.05% (Lidex)

SUPER-HIGH POTENCY

Betamethasone dipropionate, augmented, 0.05% (Diprolene gel, ointment)
Clobetasol propionate 0.05% (Temovate)
Halobetasol propionate 0.05% (Ultravate 0.05%)

Source: Barankin B., Anatoli F. Topical Steroids, In Derm Notes: Philadelphia: F. A. Davis Company. Pp 33-35.

QUESTIONS

21. Antihistamines exhibit therapeutic effect by:

    A. inactivating circulating histamine.
    B. preventing the production of histamine.
    C. blocking activity at histamine receptor sites.
    D. acting as a procholinergic agent.

22. A possible adverse effect with the use of a first-generation antihistamine such as diphenhydramine in an 80-year-old man is:

    A. urinary retention.
    B. hypertension.
    C. tachycardia.
    D. urticaria.

23. Which of the following medications is likely to cause the most sedation?
    A. chlorpheniramine
    B. cetirizine
    C. fexofenadine
    D. loratadine

ANSWERS

21. C   22. A   23. A

DISCUSSION

Antihistamines prevent action of formed histamine, a potent inflammatory mediator, and can be used to control acute symptoms of itchiness and allergy. All antihistamines work by blocking histamine-1 (H_1) receptor sites, preventing the action of histamine.

Systemic antihistamines are usually divided into two groups: standard or first-generation products, such as diphenhydramine (Benadryl) or chlorpheniramine (Chlor-Trimeton), and newer or second-generation products, such as loratadine (Claritin), desloratadine (Clarinex), cetirizine (Zyrtec), fexofenadine (Allegra), and levocetirizine (Xyzal). The first-generation antihistamines readily cross the blood-brain barrier, causing sedation; as a result, these medications should used with appropriate caution and should not be taken during activities when risk of accident or injury is significant. Their anticholinergic activity can result in drying of secretions, visual changes, and urinary retention, the last-mentioned most often a problem for older men with benign prostatic hyperplasia. The use of first-generation antihistamines by older adults, particularly in higher doses as a sleep aid, can result in negative cognitive effects. The second-generation antihistamines do not easily cross the blood-brain barrier, which results in lower rates of sedation. With little anticholinergic effect, the use of a product such as loratadine is likely to provide less drying of nasal secretions compared with diphenhydramine use, but also less negative effect on cognition, particularly in older adults.

Discussion Source

Robertson D, Mailbach H. Dermatologic pharmacology. In: Katzung B, *Katzung's Basic and Clinical Pharmacology*. 10th ed. New York, NY: McGraw-Hill Medical; 2006:991–1008.

QUESTIONS

24. Clinical features of bullous impetigo include:
    A. intense itch.
    B. vesicular lesions.
    C. dermatomal pattern.
    D. systemic symptoms such as fever and chills.

25. The likely causative organisms of nonbullous impetigo in a 6-year-old child include:
    A. *H. influenzae* and *S. pneumoniae*.
    B. group A streptococcus and *S. aureus*.
    C. *M. catarrhalis* and select viruses.
    D. *P. aeruginosa* and select fungi.

26. The spectrum of antimicrobial activity of mupirocin (Bactroban) includes:
    A. primarily gram-negative organisms.
    B. select gram-positive organisms.
    C. *Pseudomonas* species and anaerobic organisms.
    D. only organisms that do not produce beta-lactamase.

27. An oral antimicrobial option for the treatment of methicillin-sensitive *S. aureus* includes all of the following except:
    A. amoxicillin.
    B. dicloxacillin.
    C. cephalexin.
    D. cefadroxil.

28. Which of the following is an oral antimicrobial option for the treatment of a commonly acquired methicillin-resistant *S. aureus* cutaneous infection?
    A. amoxicillin
    B. dicloxacillin
    C. cephalexin
    D. trimethoprim-sulfamethoxazole

29. You see a kindergartner with impetigo and advise that she can return ____ hours after initiating effective antimicrobial therapy.
    A. 24
    B. 48
    C. 72
    D. 96

ANSWERS

24.	B	25.	B	26.	B
27.	A	28.	D	29.	A

DISCUSSION

Impetigo is a contagious skin infection that usually consists of discrete purulent lesions. Although most common among children in tropical or subtropical regions, the prevalence increases in northern climates during the summer months. Its peak incidence is among children 2 to 5 years old, although older children and adults can also be affected. There is no sex or racial predilection for the condition. Impetigo skin lesions are nearly always caused by group A streptococci or *Staphylococcus aureus* or both.

Impetigo usually occurs on exposed areas of the body; the infection most frequently affects the face and extremities. ♂ The lesions remain well localized, but are frequently multiple and can be either bullous or nonbullous. Bullous impetigo is usually caused by strains of *S. aureus* that produce a toxin causing cleavage in the superficial skin layer, with the causative pathogens usually present in the nose before the outbreak of the cutaneous disease. The bullous lesions usually appear initially as superficial vesicles that rapidly enlarge to form a bulla or blister that is often filled with a dark or purulent liquid and can take on a pustular appearance. The lesion ruptures, and a thin, lacquer-like crust typically forms quickly. The pattern of the lesion often reflects autoinoculation with the offending organism.

The lesions of nonbullous impetigo usually begin as papules that rapidly evolve into vesicles surrounded by an area of erythema. The pustules increase in size, breaking down in the next 4 to 6 days, forming characteristic thick crusts. About 70% of patients with impetigo have nonbullous lesions. In either form, the lesions heal slowly and leave depigmented areas.

Until more recently, nonbullous impetigo was usually caused by *Streptococcus* species. Now, most cases are caused by staphylococci alone or in combination with streptococci. Streptococci isolated from lesions are primarily group A organisms, but occasionally other serogroups (e.g., groups C and G) are responsible. Prospective studies of streptococcal impetigo have shown that the responsible microorganisms initially colonize the unbroken skin. As a result, personal hygiene has an influence on disease incidence in that colonization with a given streptococcal strain precedes the development of impetigo lesions by a mean duration of 10 days; inoculation of surface organisms into the skin by abrasions, minor trauma, or insect bites then ensues. Streptococcal strains can be transferred from the skin or impetigo lesions to the upper respiratory tract.

Rarely, an impetigo lesion can become deeply ulcerated, known as ecthyma. Although regional lymphadenitis occurs, systemic symptoms are usually absent.

When impetigo results in a few lesions, topical therapy is indicated with mupirocin (Bactroban) as the preferred agent. Mupirocin use is associated with higher cure rates compared with oral erythromycin, and both are noted to be superior to penicillin. Retapamulin (Altabax) ointment is a newer, effective, albeit expensive therapeutic option. Bacitracin and neomycin are less effective topical treatments; use of these products is not recommended for the treatment of impetigo.

Patients who have numerous lesions or who are not responding to topical agents should receive oral antimicrobials effective against *S. aureus* and *Streptococcus pyogenes*. In the past, penicillin was a common choice that was clinically effective because most cases were caused by *Streptococcus* species. Because *S. aureus* currently accounts for most cases of bullous impetigo and for a substantial portion of nonbullous infections, antimicrobials with a gram-positive spectrum of activity and stability in the presence of beta-lactamase, such as dicloxacillin, a first-generation or second-generation cephalosporin, azithromycin, or clarithromycin, is now often used as a first-line choice, particularly if methicillin-sensitive *S. aureus* (MSSA) is considered to be the likely causative pathogen. Impetigo caused by methicillin-resistant *S. aureus* (MRSA) is increasing in frequency, however. In addition, nearly one-half of MRSA strains show resistance to mupirocin.

Erythromycin-resistant strains of *S. aureus* and *S. pyogenes* are increasing in prevalence. The advent of infection by these resistant pathogens requires that other options also be considered, particularly if there is treatment failure with a first-line antimicrobial. These options include high-dose trimethoprim-sulfamethoxazole, and clindamycin. Minocycline and doxycycline, both tetracycline forms, can also be helpful, but should not be used in children younger than 11 years.

Even in these times of resistant pathogens, most episodes of impetigo resolve without complication or need for a second-line agent. In many areas of the world, cutaneous infections with nephritogenic strains of group A streptococci are the major antecedent of poststreptococcal glomerulonephritis, however. No conclusive data indicate that treatment of streptococcal pyoderma prevents nephritis. At the same time, treatment of impetigo is important to minimize risk of infectious transmission. Children with impetigo should be kept out of school or day care for 24 hours after initiation of antibiotic therapy, and family members should be checked for lesions.

Discussion Sources

Gilbert D, Moellering R, Eliopoulos G, Chambers H, Saag M. *The Sanford Guide to Antimicrobial Therapy*. 39th ed. Sperryville, VA: Antimicrobial Therapy, Inc; 2009:51.

Lewis L. www.emedicine.com/ped/topic1172.htm, eMedicine: Impetigo, accessed 9/4/09.

Stevens D, Bisno A, Chambers H, Everett ED, Patchen Dellinger E, Goldstein E, Gorbach S, Hirschmann J, Kaplan E, Montoya J, Wade J. Practice guidelines for the diagnosis and management of skin and soft-tissue infections. *Clin Infect Dis*. 2005; 41:1373–1406.

QUESTIONS

30. The use of which of the following medications contributes to the development of acne vulgaris?

    A. lithium
    B. propranolol
    C. tetracycline
    D. oral contraceptives

31. First-line therapy for acne vulgaris with closed comedones includes:

    A. oral antibiotics.
    B. isotretinoin.
    C. benzoyl peroxide.
    D. hydrocortisone cream.

32. When prescribing tretinoin (Retin-A), the NP advises the patient to:

    A. use it with benzoyl peroxide to minimize irritating effects.
    B. use a sunscreen because the drug is photosensitizing.
    C. add a sulfa-based cream to enhance antiacne effects.
    D. expect a significant improvement in acne lesions after approximately 1 week of use.

33. In the treatment of acne vulgaris, which lesions respond best to topical antibiotic therapy?

    A. open comedones
    B. cysts
    C. inflammatory lesions
    D. superficial lesions

34. Which of the following is indicated for the treatment of acne rosacea?

    A. metronidazole gel (MetroGel)
    B. benzyol peroxide
    C. erythromycin 2% solution (EryDerm 2% solution)
    D. azelaic acid 20% (Azelex cream)

35. You have initiated therapy for an 18-year-old man with acne vulgaris and have prescribed tetracycline. He returns in 3 weeks, complaining that his skin is "no better." Your next action is to:

    A. counsel him that 6 to 8 weeks of treatment is often needed before significant improvement is achieved.
    B. discontinue the tetracycline and initiate minocycline therapy.
    C. advise him that antibiotics are likely not an effective treatment for him and should not be continued.
    D. add a second antimicrobial agent.

36. Who is the best candidate for isotretinoin (Accutane) therapy?

    A. a 17-year-old patient with pustular lesions and poor response to benzoyl peroxide
    B. a 20-year-old patient with cystic lesions who has tried various therapies with minimal effect
    C. a 14-year-old patient with open and closed comedones and a family history of "ice pick" scars
    D. an 18-year-old patient with inflammatory lesions and improvement with tretinoin (Retin-A)

37. In a 22-year-old woman using isotretinoin (Accutane) therapy, the NP ensures follow-up to monitor for all of the following tests except:

    A. hepatic enzymes
    B. triglyceride measurements
    C. pregnancy test
    D. platelet count

38. Leonard is an 18-year-old man who has been taking isotretinoin (Accutane) for the treatment of acne for the past 2 months. Which of the following is the most important question for the clinician to ask at his follow-up office visit?

    A. Are you having any problems remembering to take your medication?
    B. Have you noticed any dry skin around your mouth since you started using Accutane?
    C. Do you notice any improvement in your skin?
    D. Have you noticed any recent changes in your mood?

ANSWERS

30.	A	31.	C	32.	B
33.	C	34.	A	35.	A
36.	B	37.	D	38.	D

DISCUSSION

Acne vulgaris is a common pustular disorder caused by a combination of factors. An increase in sebaceous activity causes plugging of follicles and retention of sebum, allowing an overgrowth of the organism, *Propionibacterium acnes*. This overgrowth allows an inflammatory reaction with the resulting wide variety of lesions, including open and closed comedones, cysts, and pustules. ☞

Topical and systemic antibiotics are used to treat acne and are particularly helpful as therapy for pustular lesions. The mechanism of action of antibiotics in acne therapy is probably not based solely on their antimicrobial action, but is likely in part a result of anti-inflammatory activity. Additional acne vulgaris agents include topical vitamin A derivatives such as tretinoin (Retin-A), synthetic retinoid (Accutane), and comedolytic (benzoyl peroxide) (Table 3–4).

Nearly all adolescents develop some acne vulgaris to some degree with milder cases resolving by early adulthood. Only 15% seek treatment for this problematic condition, which affects teenagers at a time in their lives when body image and social acceptance are usually of greater influence than they are at any other time of life. Numerous effective treatment options are available, however.

TABLE 3–4
Acne Medications

Acne Medication	Mechanism of Action and Considerations for Use
Benzoyl peroxide cream, lotion, various concentrations	• Antimicrobial against *P. acnes* and comedolytic effects • Lower strength formulation often as effective as higher strength and likely to cause less skin irritation • Often given in combination with topical antibiotics
Azelaic acid (Azelex) 20% cream	• Likely antimicrobial against *P. acnes,* keratolytic, possibly alters androgen metabolism • Expect ~6 weeks of therapy before noting improvement • Mild skin irritation with redness and dryness common with initial use, improves over time • Less potent, but less irritating than tretinoin preparations
Tretinoin (retinoic acid) gel, cream, various concentrations	• Decreases cohesion between epidermal cells, increases epidermal cell turnover, transforms closed to open comedones • Mild skin irritation with redness and dryness common with initial use, improves over time; expect ~6 weeks of therapy before noting improvement • Photosensitizing; advise patient to use sunscreen
Oral antibiotics (clindamycin, erythromycin, tetracycline, azithromycin, others)	• Antimicrobial against *P. acnes,* anti-inflammatory • Indicated for treatment of moderate papular inflammatory acne, usually when topical therapy has been inadequate • When skin is clear, taper off slowly over a few months while adding topical antibiotic agents; rapid discontinuation results in return of acne • Long-term therapy is often needed
Topical antibiotics (clindamycin, erythromycin, tetracycline, others)	• Antimicrobial against *P. acnes,* anti-inflammatory • Indicated in treatment of mild to moderate inflammatory acne vulgaris; less effective than oral antibiotics; often given in combination with benzoyl peroxide
Combined estrogen-progestin hormonal contraceptives such as birth control pills, ring, or patch	• Reduction in ovarian androgen production, decreased sebum production
Isotretinoin (Accutane) capsules, various strengths	• Likely inhibits sebaceous gland function • Indicated for treatment of cystic acne that does not respond to other therapies • Usual course of treatment is 4–6 months; discontinue when nodule count is reduced by 70%; repeat course only if needed after 2 months off drug • Prescriber and patient must be properly educated in use of drug and fully aware of adverse reactions profile, including cheilitis, conjunctivitis, hypertriglyceridemia, xerosis, photosensitivity, and potent teratogenicity. Women must use two types of highly effective contraception while on isotretinoin. Careful monitoring for mood destabilization and suicidal thoughts is an important part of patient care during isotretinoin use

Source: Gilbert D, Moellering R, Eliopoulos G, Chambers H, Saag M. *The Sanford Guide to Antimicrobial Therapy.* 39th ed. Sperryville, VA: Antimicrobial Therapy, Inc; 2009:47–48.

Acne-inducing drugs should be avoided, if possible. Certain medications, such as lithium and phenytoin (Dilantin), may need to be used, however. These medications can also cause acne in adults. In any event, drug-induced acne can be treated with conventional therapy (see Table 3–4).

Isotretinoin (Accutane) is effective in cystic acne that does not respond to conventional therapy. Although most patients who take it have adverse effects related only to dry skin, the prescriber and patient need to be well aware of potentially serious problems associated with its use, including pseudotumor cerebri (idiopathic intracranial hypertension), hypertriglyceridemia, elevated hepatic enzymes, and cheilitis. More recently, the U.S. Food and Drug Administration (FDA) ruled that labeling for the use of isotretinoin be changed to reflect a possible connection between its use and altered mood. During isotretinoin treatment, the patient should be observed closely for symptoms of depression, such as sad mood, irritability, impulsivity, altered sleep, loss of interest or pleasure in previously enjoyable activities, change in weight or appetite, and new problems with school or work performance. In addition, the patient should be asked about suicidal ideation and altered mood with every office visit. Patients should stop isotretinoin and they or their caregiver should contact their health-care professional right away if the patient has any of the previously mentioned symptoms. Simply discontinuing the offending medication might be insufficient, and further evaluation is likely needed. Isotretinoin is also a potent teratogen; women taking the medication should have two negative pregnancy tests, including one on the second day of their normal menstrual period, before beginning the medication. In addition, women using isotretinoin should use two forms of highly effective contraception and have a pregnancy test done monthly during therapy.

Discussion Sources

Gilbert D, Moellering R, Eliopoulos G, Chambers H, Saag M. *The Sanford Guide to Antimicrobial Therapy*. 39th ed. Sperryville, VA: Antimicrobial Therapy, Inc; 2009:47–48.

Robertson D, Mailbach H. Dermatologic pharmacology. In: Katzung B, *Katzung's Basic and Clinical Pharmacology*. 10th ed. New York, NY: McGraw-Hill Medical; 2006:991–1008.

United States Food and Drug Administration. http://www.fda.gov/cder/drug/infopage/accutane/default.htm, Center for Drug Evaluation and Research: isotretinoin (marketed as Accutane) capsule information, accessed 9/1/09.

QUESTIONS

39. A common infective agent in domestic pet cat bites is:
    A. viridans streptococcus species.
    B. *Pasteurella multocida.*
    C. *Bacteroides* species.
    D. *Haemophilus influenzae.*

40. Treatment of a cat bite wound should include prescribing:
    A. oral erythromycin.
    B. topical bacitracin.
    C. oral amoxicillin clavulanate.
    D. parenteral rifampin.

41. A 24-year-old man arrives at the walk-in center. He reports that he was bitten in the thigh by a raccoon while walking in the woods. The examination reveals a wound that is 1 cm deep on his right thigh. The wound is oozing bright red blood. Your next best action is to:
    A. administer high-dose parenteral penicillin.
    B. initiate antibacterial prophylaxis with amoxicillin.
    C. give rabies immune globulin and rabies vaccine.
    D. suture the wound after proper cleansing.

42. You see a 28-year-old man who was involved in a fight approximately 1 hour ago with another person, stating, "He bit me in the arm." Examination of the left forearm reveals an open wound consistent with this history. Your next best action is to:
    A. obtain a culture and sensitivity of the wound site.
    B. refer for rabies prophylaxis.
    C. irrigate the wound and débride as needed.
    D. close the wound with adhesive strips.

ANSWERS

39.	B	**40.**	C
41.	C	**42.**	C

DISCUSSION

Bite wounds should not be considered benign or inevitable. Intervention includes education to avoid further bites; a patient's history must include a complete documentation of events leading up to the bite.

All bites should be considered to carry significant infectious risk. This risk can vary from the relatively low rate of infection from dog bites (approximately 5%) to the very high rate from cat bites (approximately 80%). Initial therapy for all bite wounds should include vigorous wound cleansing with antimicrobial agents as appropriate and débridement if necessary. Starting short-term antimicrobial prophylactic therapy within 12 hours of the injury should be considered as directed by the location and origin of the bite wound, and tetanus immunization should be updated as needed (Table 3–5).

The clinician should check with local authorities for information on rabies when a bite involves domestic pets; because the rabies risk in this situation is usually negligible,

TABLE 3–5

Infectious Agents and Treatment in Bites

Type of Bite	Infective Agent	Prophylaxis or Treatment of Infection
Bat, raccoon, skunk	Uncertain; significant rabies risk	For bacterial infection Primary: amoxicillin with clavulanate, 875 mg/125 mg bid or 500 mg/125 mg tid Alternative: doxycycline, 100 mg bid Animal should be considered rabid, and patients should be given rabies immune globulin and vaccine
Cat	*Pasteurella multocida, Staphylococcus aureus*	Primary: amoxicillin with clavulanate, 875 mg/125 mg bid 500 mg/125 mg tid Alternative: cefuroxime, 0.5 g bid; doxycycline, 100 mg orally bid Switch to penicillin if *P. multocida* is cultured from wound Because 80% become infected, all wounds should be cultured and treated empirically
Dog	*P. multocida, S. aureus, Bacteroides* spp., others	Primary: amoxicillin with clavulanate, 875 mg/125 mg bid Alternative: clindamycin, 300 mg qid, plus a fluoro-quinolone; or clindamycin with TMP-SMX (children) Only 5% become infected. Treat only if bite is severe, or if significant comorbidity such as diabetes mellitus or immunosuppression
Human	*Streptococcus viridans, Staphylococcus epidermidis, Corynebacterium, Eikenella corrodens, S. aureus, Bacteroides* spp., *Peptostreptococcus*	Early, not yet infected: amoxicillin with clavulanate, 875 mg/125 mg bid for 5 days Later (3–24 hours, signs of infection): parenteral therapy with ampicillin with sulbactam, cefoxitin, others Penicillin allergy: Clindamycin with ciprofloxacin or TMP-SMX
Rat	*Streptobacillus moniliformis, Spirillum minus*	Primary: amoxicillin with clavulanate, 875 mg/125 mg bid Alternative: doxycycline Rabies prophylaxis not indicated
Pig or swine	Polymicrobial gram-positive cocci, gram-negative bacilli, anaerobes, *Pasteurella* spp.	Primary: amoxicillin with clavulanate, 875mg/125 mg bid Alternative: parenteral third-generation cephalosporin, others
Nonhuman primate	Herpesvirus simiae	Acyclovir

Source: Gilbert D, Moellering R, Eliopoulos G, Chambers H, Saag M. *The Sanford Guide to Antimicrobial Therapy*. 39th ed. Sperryville, VA: Antimicrobial Therapy, Inc; 2009:48–49.

rabies prophylaxis is not indicated. In recent years, there has been an increase in cases of rabies domestically, primarily from bites by usually docile, often nocturnal wild animals that attack without provocation. These include bats, foxes, woodchucks, squirrels, and skunks. Human bites carry no rabies risk.

Discussion Sources

Gilbert D, Moellering R, Eliopoulos G, Chambers H, Saag M. *The Sanford Guide to Antimicrobial Therapy*. 39th ed. Sperryville, VA: Antimicrobial Therapy, Inc; 2009:48–49.

Revis D, Seagle M. http://www.emedicine.com/ent/topic728.htm, eMedicine: Human bites, accessed 9/1/09.

QUESTIONS

43. A patient presents with a painful, blistering thermal burn involving the first, second, and third digits of his right hand. The most appropriate plan of care is to:

    A. apply an anesthetic cream to the area and open the blisters.

    B. apply silver sulfadiazine cream (Silvadene) to the area followed by a bulky dressing.

    C. refer the patient to burn specialty care.

    D. wrap the burn loosely with a nonadherent dressing and prescribe an analgesic agent.

44. You examine a patient with a red, tender thermal burn that has excellent capillary refill involving the entire surface of the anterior right thigh. The estimated involved body surface area (BSA) is appropriately:

    A. 5%.

    B. 9%.

    C. 13%.

    D. 18%.

45. A burn that is about twice as large as an adult's palmar surface of the hand encompasses a BSA of approximately ____%.

    A. 1

    B. 2

    C. 3

    D. 4

46. to 48. Match the following:

____ **46.** First-degree burn

____ **47.** Second-degree burn

____ **48.** Third-degree burn

    A. Affected skin blanches with ease.

    B. Surface is raw and moist.

    C. Affected area is white and leathery.

ANSWERS

43.	C	44.	B	45.	B
46.	A	47.	B	48.	C

DISCUSSION

As with bites, burn intervention includes asking for a complete history of the events leading up to the injury, to develop a plan for avoiding future events. In addition, education for burn avoidance for high-risk individuals for burn injury, such as children, elderly adults, and smokers, should be a routine part of primary care.

Generally, smaller (less than 10% of body surface area), minor (second-degree or lower) burns not involving a high-function area such as the hand or foot and of minimal cosmetic consequence can be treated in the outpatient setting. Treatment options include prevention of infection by the use of a topical antibiotic such as mafenide acetate (Sulfamylon) or silver sulfadiazine (Silvadene). An alternative is to use petroleum gauze dressing that provides protection to the affected area. Patients with any burn involving areas of high function such as the hands and feet or of significant cosmetic consequence such as the face should be referred promptly to specialty care.

First-degree and second-degree burns are characterized by erythema, hyperemia, and pain. With first-degree burns, the skin blanches with ease; skin with second-degree burns has blisters and a raw, moist surface. In third-degree burns, pain may be minimal, but the burns are usually surrounded by areas of painful first-degree and second-degree burns. The surface of third-degree burns is usually white and leathery. It is important to estimate the body surface area (BSA) affected by the burn (Fig. 3–1). A person's palmar surface represents a BSA of 1% throughout the life span and can provide a helpful guide in estimating the extent of a burn.

Discussion Sources

Gilbert D, Moellering R, Eliopoulos G, Chambers H, Saag M. *The Sanford Guide to Antimicrobial Therapy*. 39th ed. Sperryville, VA: Antimicrobial Therapy, Inc; 2009:48–49.

Narazady J, Alson R. http://www.emedicine.com/emerg/TOPIC72.HTM, eMedicine: Thermal burns, accessed 9/2/09.

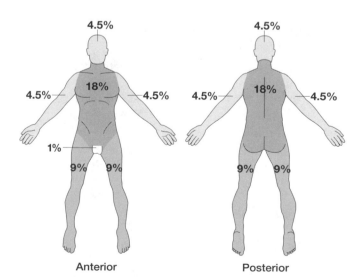

Figure 3–1 Rule of nines for calculating total burn surface area. *(Source: Adapted from Richard R, Staley M. Burn Care and Rehabilitation. Philadelphia, PA: FA Davis; 1994:109.)*

QUESTIONS

49. The most important aspect of skin care for individuals with atopic dermatitis is:
    A. frequent bathing with antibacterial soap.
    B. consistent use of medium-potency to high-potency topical steroids.
    C. application of lubricants.
    D. treatment of dermatophytes.

50. A common trigger agent for contact dermatitis is:
    A. exposure to nickel.
    B. use of fabric softener.
    C. washing with strong soap.
    D. eating spicy foods.

51. A common site for atopic dermatitis in an adult is on the:
    A. dorsum of the hand.
    B. face.
    C. neck.
    D. flexor surfaces.

52. A common site for atopic dermatitis in an infant is:
    A. the diaper area.
    B. the face.
    C. the neck.
    D. the posterior trunk.

53. The mechanism of action of pimecrolimus (Elidel) in the treatment of atopic dermatis is as a/an:
    A. immunomodulator.
    B. antimitotic.
    C. mast cell activator.
    D. exfoliant.

54. When counseling a patient about pimecrolimus (Elidel) use, you mention that:
    A. this is the preferred atopic dermatitis treatment in infants.
    B. there is a possibility of increased cancer risk with its use.
    C. the product is used interchangeably with topical corticosteroids.
    D. the product is a potent antihistamine.

ANSWERS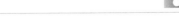

49.	C	50.	A	51.	D
52.	B	53.	A	54.	B

DISCUSSION

Atopic dermatitis, or eczema, is one manifestation of a type I hypersensitivity reaction. This type of reaction results from immunoglobulin E (IgE) antibodies occupying receptor sites on mast cells. This causes a degradation of the mast cell and subsequent release of histamine, resulting in vasodilation, mucous gland stimulation, and tissue swelling. Type I hypersensitivity reactions are usually divided into two subgroups: atopy and anaphylaxis.

The atopy subgroup includes many common clinical conditions, such as allergic rhinitis, atopic dermatitis, allergic gastroenteropathy, and allergy-based asthma. Atopic diseases have a strong familial component and tend to cause localized rather than systemic reactions. Individuals with atopic disease are often able to identify allergy-inducing agents. Allergic contact dermatitis is a form of eczematous dermatitis. Common causes of contact dermatitis include exposure to metals including nickel, rubber additives to shoes and gloves, some toiletries, and topical medications.

Criteria for the diagnosis of atopic dermatitis include the presence of itching and subsequent scratching, plus three or more of the following: red or inflamed rash, presence of excessive dryness/scaling, and location in skin folds of arms or legs. With severe outbreaks, vesicles are often present. Additional findings include early age at initial onset (0 to 5 years) and elevated serum IgE and peripheral blood eosinophil levels. In infants, the face is often involved, whereas the diaper area, owing to the occlusive, damp environment, is usually spared.

Treatment for atopic dermatitis includes avoiding offending agents, minimizing skin dryness by limiting soap and water exposure, and consistent use of lubricants. In general, the patient should be encouraged to treat the skin with care because it tends to be sensitive; the person with atopic dermatitis has an abnormal skin barrier that allows for loss of water and resulting dryness. When flares occur, the skin eruption is caused largely by histamine release. Antihistamines or topical and systemic corticosteroids or both are typically used to control flares. Cool, wet dressings made from a clean cloth with cool water or Burow's solution applied to the affected area for 30 minutes can provide significant symptom relief; application of an intermediate-potency topical corticosteroid is usually needed to control acute symptoms. After control of acute symptoms is achieved, the topical corticosteroid of lowest potency that yields the desired effect should be used (see Table 3–3).

Pimecrolimus (Elidel) and tacrolimus (Protopic) are immunomodulators that are helpful in the treatment of atopic dermatitis and offer an additional, noncorticosteroid option for atopic dermatitis. These products block T-cell stimulation by antigen-presenting cells and inhibit mast cell activation. Because of information from animal studies, case reports in a few patients, and knowledge of how drugs in this class work, an advisory about the potential for increased cancer risk with the use of these products has been released. Tacrolimus and pimecrolimus should be used only as labeled, and only if other prescription and supportive treatments have failed to work or cannot be tolerated. These products should not be used in children younger than 2 years.

Itch (pruritus) is a very distressing symptom; many patients say it is more distressing than pain. Pruritus is a cardinal symptom of many forms of dermatitis. Histamine contributes to the development of itching; the use of an antihistamine can provide relief. Pruritus tends to be worst at night, often causing disturbance in sleep. In particular, providing the patient with a bedtime dose of antihistamine can yield tremendous relief from itch and improve sleep. Hydroxyzine (Atarax) seems to provide better relief of itch than other antihistamines. Cetirizine (Zyrtec) is a less sedating antihistamine that is a metabolite of hydroxyzine.

Discussion Sources

Chamlin S. Atopic dermatitis. In: Rakel R, Bope E, eds. *Conn's Current Therapy 2008*. Philadelphia, PA: Saunders; 2008:848–850.

Food and Drug Administration Center for Drug Evaluation and Research. http://www.fda.gov/CDER/Drug/infopage/protopic/default.htm, Alert for healthcare professionals: tacrolimus (marketed as Protopic), accessed 9/2/09.

Robertson D, Mailbach H. Dermatologic pharmacology. In: Katzung, B, *Katzung's Basic and Clinical Pharmacology*. 10th ed. New York, NY: McGraw-Hill Medical; 2006:991–1008.

QUESTIONS

55. A 38-year-old woman with advanced human immunodeficiency virus (HIV) disease presents with a chief complaint of a painful, itchy rash over her trunk. Examination reveals linear vesicular lesions that do not cross the midline and are distributed over the posterior thorax. This is most consistent with:

    A. herpes zoster.
    B. dermatitis herpetiformis.
    C. molluscum contagiosum.
    D. impetigo.

56. A Tzanck smear that is positive for giant multinucleated cells was taken from a lesion caused by:

    A. herpesvirus.
    B. *S. aureus.*
    C. streptococci.
    D. allergic reaction.

57. When caring for an adult with an outbreak of shingles, you advise that:

    A. there is no known treatment for this condition.
    B. during outbreaks, the chickenpox virus is shed.
    C. although they are acutely painful, the lesions heal well without scarring or lingering discomfort.
    D. this condition commonly strikes young and old alike.

58. Risk factors for the development of postherpetic neuralgia include:

    A. age younger than 50 years at the time of the outbreak.
    B. severe prodromal symptoms.
    C. lumbar location of lesions.
    D. low volume of lesions.

59. Treatment options in postherpetic neuralgia include all of the following except:

    A. methylprednisolone.
    B. pregabalin.
    C. nortriptyline.
    D. topical lidocaine.

ANSWERS

| 55. | A | 56. | A | 57. | B |
| 58. | B | 59. | A | | |

DISCUSSION

Herpes zoster infection, commonly known as shingles, is an acutely painful condition caused by the varicella-zoster virus, the same agent that causes chickenpox. The virus lies dormant in the dorsal root ganglia of a dermatome. When activated, the characteristic blistering lesions occur along a dermatome, usually not crossing the midline. The resulting pain is burning, throbbing, or stabbing; intense itch is also occasionally described. The thoracic dermatomes are the most commonly involved sites, followed by the lumbar dermatomes.

Anyone who has had chickenpox is at risk for shingles, whereas recipients of varicella-zoster immunization have virtually no risk. Shingles is usually seen in elderly individuals, patients who are immunocompromised, and individuals with some other underlying health problem. When shingles is seen in younger adults, the possibility of HIV infection or other immunocompromised condition should be considered. During the acute attack, the chickenpox (varicella-zoster) virus is shed; patients can transmit this infection. Shingles is not communicable from person to person, however. Approximately 4% of patients with zoster develop a recurrent episode later in life.

Diagnosis of shingles is usually straightforward because of its characteristic lesions. If confirmation is needed, a Tzanck smear reveals giant multinucleated cells, a finding in all herpetic infections.

Scarring and postherpetic neuralgia are problematic sequelae of shingles. Initiating antiviral therapy with high-dose acyclovir (Zovirax), valacyclovir (Valtrex), or famciclovir

(Famvir), preferably within the first 72 hours of herpes zoster outbreak, helps limit the severity of the lesions and minimize the risk of postherpetic neuralgia and scarring. Systemic corticosteroids are often prescribed during the acute stage of shingles along with antivirals. This combination therapy usually results in more rapid resolution of pain, but not of zoster lesions.

Adequate analgesia should be offered to a person with shingles. Using a combination of topical agents such as Burow's solution with a high-potency nonsteroidal anti-inflammatory drug or opioid, or both, helps provide considerable relief. The patient should also be monitored for superinfection of lesions. Because of the risk of complication and possible compromise of vision, expert consultation should be sought if herpes zoster involves a facial dermatome. The rash usually resolves within 14 to 21 days.

Postherpetic neuralgia is defined as pain persisting at least 1 month after the rash has healed. Risk factors for the development of postherpetic neuralgia include the site of initial involvement, with greatest risk if outbreak involved the trigeminal or brachial plexus region; moderate risk with a thoracic outbreak; and lower risk with jaw, neck, sacral, and lumbar involvement. Additional risks include severe rash and intense prodromal pain. The incidence increases dramatically with age with only 4% of adults 30 to 50 years old reporting postherpetic neuralgia, and approximately 50% of adults older than 80 years reporting it. Tricyclic antidepressants (e.g., amitriptyline, nortriptyline, desipramine), gabapentin (Neurontin), pregabalin (Lyrica), opioids, and topical lidocaine patches are effective and are often used in the treatment of postherpetic neuralgia.

Zoster vaccine (Zostavax) is an immunization for protection against herpes zoster (or shingles) in adults 60 years old and older. The vaccine is prepared from a live, attenuated strain of varicella-zoster virus. Zostavax is designed to yield a more potent, higher titer than varicella virus live vaccine (Varivax), used in children for chickenpox. Because reactivation of the varicella virus seems to be related to a decline in varicella-zoster virus-specific immunity, the use of zoster vaccine significantly reduces shingles risk. This vaccine should be used even with a history of shingles.

Discussion Sources

Krause R. http://www.emedicine.com/emerg/TOPIC823.HTM, eMedicine: Herpes zoster, accessed 9/2/09.

McElveen WA, Gonzalez R, Sinclair D. http://www.emedicine.com/neuro/TOPIC317.HTM, eMedicine: Postherpetic neuralgia, accessed 9/2/09.

QUESTIONS

60. Characteristics of onychomycosis include all of the following except:
    A. it is readily diagnosed by clinical examination.
    B. nail hypertrophy.
    C. brittle nails.
    D. fingernails respond more readily to therapy than toenails.

61. When prescribing itraconazole (Sporanox), the NP considers that:
    A. the drug is a cytochrome P-450 3A4 inhibitor.
    B. one pulse cycle is recommended for fingernail treatment, and two cycles are needed for toenail therapy.
    C. continuous therapy is preferred in the presence of hepatic disease.
    D. taking the drug on an empty stomach enhances the efficacy of the product.

62. When prescribing pulse dosing with itraconazole for the treatment of fingernail fungus, the clinician realizes that:
    A. a transient increase in hepatic enzymes is commonly seen with its use.
    B. drug-induced leukopenia is a common problem.
    C. the patient needs to be warned about excessive bleeding because of the drug's antiplatelet effect.
    D. its use is contraindicated in the presence of iron-deficiency anemia.

63. In diagnosing onychomycosis, the NP considers that:
    A. nails often have a single midline groove.
    B. pitting is often seen.
    C. microscopic examination reveals hyphae.
    D. Beau lines are present.

ANSWERS

60.	A	61.	A
62.	A	63.	C

DISCUSSION

Onychomycosis, or dermatophytosis of the nail, is a chronic disfiguring disorder. The nails are dull, thickened, and lusterless with a pithy consistency. Parts of the nail often break off. Because trauma and other conditions can cause a similar appearance, confirmation of the diagnosis with microscopic examination for hyphae of the nail scrapings mixed with potassium hydroxide (KOH) is important, although it has a high rate of false-negative results. Fungal cultures should be obtained from pulverized nail scrapings or clippings.

Antifungals such as itraconazole (Sporanox), terbinafine (Lamisil), and fluconazole (Diflucan) offer well-tolerated effective treatment for fingernail and toenail fungal infections. These medications can be used in pulse cycles, with times of drug use alternating with abstinent periods. An example of pulse dosing is itraconazole, 400 mg daily for the first week of the month for 2 months to treat the fingernails and for 3 months to treat the toenails. The products are held within the nail matrix for months after therapy; this produces effective treatment at a considerably reduced cost compared with constant therapy. In addition, all oral antifungals have hepatotoxic potential and may cause an increase in hepatic enzyme levels. Pulse therapy lessens this risk considerably, however.

Caution is needed when itraconazole is prescribed because it inhibits cytochrome P-450 3A4, a pathway also used by drugs such as diazepam, digoxin, anticoagulants, and certain HIV protease inhibitors. In addition, fluconazole is a cytochrome P-450 2CP inhibitor, a pathway also used by drugs such as carbamazepine, some benzodiazepines, and calcium channel blockers. The concomitant use of these antifungals with the aforementioned medications can lead to significant drug interactions. Terbinafine has significantly less drug interaction potential.

Topical treatment has proved to be of little value because the fungal agent is held within the nail matrix. Oral agents such as griseofulvin require months of therapy with a high rate of relapse.

Discussion Sources

Blumberg M. http://www.emedicine.com/derm/topic300.htm, eMedicine: Onychomycosis, accessed 9/2/09.

Gilbert D, Moellering R, Eliopoulos G, Chambers H, Saag M. *The Sanford Guide to Antimicrobial Therapy.* 39th ed. Sperryville, VA: Antimicrobial Therapy, Inc; 2009:104–105.

Robertson D, Mailbach H. Dermatologic pharmacology. In: Katzung B, *Katzung's Basic and Clinical Pharmacology.* 10th ed. New York, NY: McGraw-Hill Medical; 2006:991–1008.

QUESTIONS

64. A 78-year-old resident of a long-term care facility complains of generalized itchiness at night that disturbs her sleep. Her examination is consistent with scabies. Which of the following do you expect to find on examination?

    A. excoriated papules on the interdigital area
    B. annular lesions over the buttocks
    C. vesicular lesions in a linear pattern
    D. honey-colored crusted lesions that began as vesicles

65. Which of the following represents the most accurate patient advice when using permethrin (Elimite) for treating scabies?

    A. To avoid systemic absorption, the medication should be applied over the body and rinsed off within 1 hour.
    B. The patient notices a marked reduction in pruritus within 48 hours of using the product.
    C. Itch often persists for a few weeks after successful treatment.
    D. It is a second-line product in the treatment of scabies.

66. When advising the patient about scabies contagion, you inform her that:

    A. mites can live for many weeks away from the host.
    B. close personal contact with an infected person is usually needed to contract this disease.
    C. casual contact with an infected person is likely to result in infestation.
    D. bedding used by an infected person must be destroyed.

ANSWERS

64. A   65. C   66. B

DISCUSSION

Scabies is a communicable skin disease caused by a host-specific mite, generally requiring close personal contact, such as sexual relations, to achieve contagion. Contact with used, unwashed bedding and clothing from an affected person can result in infection, however. Bedclothes and other items used by a person with scabies must be either washed in hot water or placed in the clothes dryer for a normal cycle. Alternatively, items can be placed in plastic storage bags for at least 1 week because mites do not survive for more than 3 to 4 days without contact with the host. The mites tend to burrow in areas of warmth, such as the finger webs, axillary folds, the belt line, areolae, scrotum, and penis, with lesions developing and clustering in these areas. The lesions often start with the characteristic burrows, but usually progress to a vesicular or papular form, usually with excoriation caused by scratching.

Permethrin (Elimite) lotion is the preferred method of treatment for scabies. The lotion must be left on for 8 to 14 hours to be effective. Despite effective therapy, individuals with scabies often have a significant problem with pruritus after permethrin treatment because of the presence of dead mites and their waste trapped in the skin, which causes an inflammatory reaction. This debris is eliminated from the body over a few weeks; the distress of itchiness passes at that time. Oral antihistamines, particularly for nighttime use, and low-potency to medium-potency topical corticosteroids should be offered to help with this problem (Table 3–6). In the past, lindane (Kwell) was used, but the use of this product presents potential problems with neurotoxicity and a resulting seizure risk and lower efficacy. In particular, lindane should not be used by pregnant women, children, and elderly patients.

Discussion Source

Cordoro E. http://www.emedicine.com/derm/TOPIC382.HTM, eMedicine: Scabies, accessed 9/2/09.

QUESTIONS

67. You examine a patient with psoriasis vulgaris and expect to find the following lesions:

    A. lichenified areas in flexor areas
    B. red, well-demarcated plaques on the knees
    C. greasy lesions throughout the scalp
    D. vesicular lesions over the upper thorax

68. Psoriatic lesions arise from:

    A. decreased skin exfoliation.
    B. rapid skin cell turnover, leading to decreased maturation and keratinization.
    C. inflammatory changes in the dermis.
    D. lichenification.

69. Anthralin (Drithocreme) is helpful in treating psoriasis because it has what kind of activity?

    A. antimitotic
    B. exfoliative
    C. vasoconstrictor
    D. humectant

70. Treatment options in generalized psoriasis vulgaris include all of the following except:

    A. psoralen with ultraviolet A light (PUVA) therapy.
    B. methotrexate.
    C. cyclosporine.
    D. systemic corticosteroids.

TABLE 3–6

Medications Used in the Treatment of Acute IgE-Mediated Hypersensitivity Reaction

Medications	Mechanism of Action	Comments
Antihistamines	Antagonize H_1-receptor sites. Prevent action of formed histamine, so helpful in treatment of acute allergic reaction	In acute reaction, give parenterally or in a quickly absorbed oral form such as chewable tablet or liquid First-generation products (diphenhydramine [Benadryl], chlorpheniramine [Chlor-Trimeton]) • Cross blood-brain barrier causing sedation • Anticholinergic activity can cause blurred vision, dry mucous membranes Second-generation products (loratadine [Claritin], cetirizine [Zyrtec], fexofenadine [Allegra]) • Little transfer across blood-brain barrier. Low rates of sedation • Less anticholinergic effect
Epinephrine	Alpha-1, beta-1, beta-2 agonists. Potent vasoconstrictor, cardiac stimulant, bronchodilator	• Initial therapy for anaphylaxis because of its multiple modes of reversing airway and circulatory dysfunction • Anaphylaxis usually responds quickly to epinephrine given parenterally
Oral corticosteroids	Inhibit eosinophilic action and other inflammatory mediators	• In higher dose and with longer therapy (>2 weeks), adrenal suppression may occur • Taper usually not needed if use is short-term (<10 days) and at lower dose (prednisone, 40–60 mg/day) • Potential for causing gastropathy

Source: www.anaphylaxis.com, www.aaaai.org/professionals/resources/pdf/anaphylaxis_2005.pdf, accessed 9/3/09.

71. Which of the following is not a potential adverse effect with long-term high-potency topical corticosteroid use?

- **A.** lichenification
- **B.** telangiectasia
- **C.** skin atrophy
- **D.** adrenal suppression

ANSWERS

67.	B	**68.**	B	**69.**	A
70.	D	**71.**	A		

DISCUSSION

Psoriasis vulgaris is a chronic skin disorder caused by accelerated mitosis and rapid cell turnover, which lead to decreased maturation and keratinization. This process prevents the dermal cells from "sticking" together, allowing for a shedding of cells in the form of characteristic silvery scales and leaving an underlying red plaque. Psoriasis is typically found in extensor surfaces; the lesions are most often found in plaques over the elbows and knees. The scalp and other surfaces are occasionally involved.

Topical corticosteroids have anti-inflammatory and mild antimitotic activity, which allows for regression of psoriatic plaques. A common treatment plan is to use a medium-potency to high-potency drug for short periods until the plaques resolve, and then to use a lower potency product three to four times a week to maintain remission. As with all dermatoses, consistent use of high-potency topical steroids is discouraged because of potential risk of skin atrophy, telangiectasia formation, corticosteroid-induced acne, and striae. In addition, the extensive use of topical corticosteroids leads to significant systemic absorption and potential subclinical adrenal function suppression. Tar preparations can be very helpful, but these products have a low level of patient acceptance because of the messiness and odor associated with these preparations.

Additional treatment options include use of anthralin (Drithocreme), a topical antimitotic, and calcipotriene, a topical vitamin D_3 derivative. Although offering effective psoriasis therapy, these products are significantly more expensive than topical corticosteroids and tars. Use should be reserved for corticosteroid-resistant conditions.

If psoriasis is generalized, covering more than 30% of body surface area, treatment with topical products is difficult and expensive. Ultraviolet A light exposure three times weekly is highly effective, but is associated with an increase in skin cancer risk and photoaging. For severe, recalcitrant psoriasis, cyclosporine, methotrexate, systemic retinoids and newer biological agents such as the tumor necrois factor antagonist infliximab (Remicade) are also used. Referral to a clinician with expertise in prescribing these agents is indicated.

Discussion Sources

Park R. http://www.emedicine.com/emerg/TOPIC489.HTM, eMedicine: Psoriasis vulgaris, accessed 9/3/09.

Robertson D, Mailbach H. Dermatologic pharmacology. In: Katzung, B, *Katzung's Basic and Clinical Pharmacology*. 10th ed. New York, NY: McGraw-Hill Medical; 2006:991–1008.

QUESTIONS

72. Which of the following best describes seborrheic dermatitis lesions?

- **A.** flaking lesions in the antecubital and popliteal spaces
- **B.** greasy, scaling lesions in the nasolabial folds
- **C.** intensely itchy lesions in the groin folds
- **D.** silvery lesions on the elbows and knees

73. In counseling a patient with seborrheic dermatitis on the scalp about efforts to clear lesions, you advise her to:

- **A.** use ketoconazole shampoo.
- **B.** apply petroleum jelly nightly to the affected area.
- **C.** coat the area with high-potency corticosteroid cream three times a week.
- **D.** expose the lesions periodically to sunlight.

74. A 64-year-old man with seborrhea mentions that his skin condition is "better in the summer when I get outside more and much worse in the winter." You respond:

- **A.** sun exposure is a recommended therapy for the treatment of this condition.
- **B.** although sun exposure is noted to improve the skin lesions associated with seborrhea, its use as a therapy is potentially associated with an increased rate of skin cancer.
- **C.** the lower humidity in the summer months noted in many areas of North America contributes to the improvement in seborrheic lesions.
- **D.** he should use high-potency topical corticosteroids during the winter months, tapering these off for the summer months.

ANSWERS

72.	B	**73.**	A	**74.**	B

DISCUSSION

Seborrheic dermatitis ♂ is a chronic, recurrent skin condition found in areas with a high concentration of sebaceous glands, such as the scalp, eyelid margins, nasolabial folds, ears, and upper trunk. Numerous theories are proposed for its cause. Because of the lesions' response to antifungal agents, the backbone of therapy for the condition, seborrheic dermatitis is most likely caused by an inflammatory reaction to *Malassezia* species (formerly *Pityrosporum* species), a yeast form present on the scalp of all humans. Further supporting this hypothesis is the fact that seborrhea is often found in immunocompromised patients and in chronically ill individuals (e.g., elderly adults and people with Parkinson disease). *Malassezia* organisms are likely a cofactor linked to T-cell depression, increased sebum levels, and an activation of the alternative complement pathway.

Skin lesions associated with seborrhea usually respond to topical antifungals such as ketoconazole. Class IV or lower corticosteroid creams, lotions, or solutions are also helpful during a flare (see Table 3–3); immune modulators such as pimecrolimus and tacrolimus, sulfur or sulfonamide combinations, and propylene glycol offer additional treatment options. The use of lubricants such as petroleum jelly can help remove stubborn lesions so that the lesions can be exposed to antifungal therapy (e.g., selenium sulfide or ketoconazole shampoo). Systemic ketoconazole or fluconazole is occasionally used if seborrheic dermatitis is severe or unresponsive.

As with any skin condition, high-potency topical corticosteroid use is discouraged because of the risk of subcutaneous atrophy, telangiectatic vessels, and other problems. Although seborrhea usually worsens in the winter and improves in the summer, exposing lesions to sunlight is not recommended because of the potential increase in skin cancer risk and photoaging.

Discussion Source

Selden S. http://www.emedicine.com/derm/topic396.htm, eMedicine: Seborrhea, accessed 9/3/09.

QUESTIONS

75. A 49-year-old man presents with a skin lesion suspicious for malignant melanoma. You describe the lesion as having:
    A. deep black-brown coloring throughout.
    B. sharp borders.
    C. a diameter of 3 mm or less.
    D. variable pigmentation.

76. A 72-year-old woman presents with a newly formed, painless, pearly, ulcerated nodule with an overlying telangiectasis on the upper lip. This most likely represents:
    A. an actinic keratosis.
    B. a basal cell carcinoma.
    C. a squamous cell carcinoma.
    D. molluscum contagiosum.

77. Which of the following represents the most effective method of cancer screening?
    A. skin examination
    B. stool for occult blood
    C. pelvic examination
    D. chest radiography

78. Risk factors for malignant melanoma include:
    A. Asian ancestry.
    B. history of blistering sunburn.
    C. family history of psoriasis vulgaris.
    D. presence of atopic dermatitis.

79. Skin lesions associated with actinic keratoses can be described as:
    A. a slightly rough, pink or flesh-colored lesion in a sun-exposed area.
    B. a well-defined, slightly raised, red, scaly plaque in a skinfold.
    C. a blistering lesion along a dermatome.
    D. a crusting lesion along flexor aspects of the fingers.

80. Treatment options for actinic keratoses include topical:
    A. hydrocortisone.
    B. 5-fluorouracil.
    C. acyclovir.
    D. doxepin.

ANSWERS

75.	D	76.	B	77.	A
78.	B	79.	A	80.	B

DISCUSSION

As with any area of dermatology, accurate diagnosis of a condition depends on knowledge of the description of the lesion and its most likely site of occurrence. The most potent risk factor for any skin cancer is sun exposure; patients should be instructed on sun avoidance. The consistent use of high–sun protection factor (SPF) sunscreen is critical and helps reduce, but not eliminate, the risk of squamous or basal cell carcinoma. Sunscreen use likely does little to minimize malignant melanoma risk.

Skin examination has the benefit of enabling the examiner to detect premalignant lesions (e.g., actinic keratoses and other precursor lesions to squamous cell carcinoma including keratoacanthoma) and malignant lesions.

Malignant melanoma is a malignancy that arises from melanocytes, cells that make the pigment melanin, and is the most common fatal dermatologic malignancy. "ABCDE" is a mnemonic for assessing malignant melanoma:

A = asymmetric with nonmatching sides

B = borders are irregular

C = color is not uniform; brown, black, red, white, blue

D = diameter usually larger than 6 mm, or the size of a pencil eraser

E = evolving lesions, either new or changing (most melanomas manifest as new lesions) ♂

Similar memory aids for squamous and basal cell carcinoma are as follows:

The characteristics of basal cell carcinoma (BCC) include a long latency period and low metastatic risk. Depending on lesion location, untreated BCC can lead to significant deformity and possibly altered function. As a result, early recognition and intervention is recommended. To help with BCC, remember this mnemonic; "PUT ON S'unscreen":

P = pearly papule

U = ulcerating

T = telangiectasia

O = on the face, scalp, pinnae

N = nodules = slow growing ♂

Compared with BCC, squamous cell carcinoma (SCC) tends to grow more rapidly and has a low but significant metastatic risk. Although difficult to distinguish from BCC by skin examination alone, the mnemonic "NO SUN" can help with the identification of early SCC lesions:

N = nodular

O = opaque

S = sun-exposed areas

U = ulcerating

N = nondistinct borders

Later lesions may also include scale and firm margins. ♂

Although the above-mentioned mnemonics are helpful in identifying these lesions, diagnosis of cutaneous malignancy requires a biopsy. Intervention depends on biopsy results and final diagnosis. Therapy is usually surgical, involving removal of the lesion with a reasonable "clean" or disease-free margin. Mohs micrographic surgery is recommended in the presence of skin tumors with aggressive histologic patterns or with invasive features. Nonsurgical options in BCC and SCC include destruction of the lesion with cryotherapy, electrodesiccation with curettage, focal radiation, and topical cancer chemotherapy. Intervention in malignant melanoma is based on additional factors including staging and sentinel node biopsy results; this requires expert opinion consultation.

Actinic keratoses are UV-induced skin lesions that can evolve into squamous cell carcinoma. Actinic keratoses begin as small rough spots that are easier felt than seen; the lesions are often best identified by rubbing the examining finger over the affected area and appreciating the sandpaper-like quality. Over time, the lesions enlarge, typically 3 to 10 mm in diameter, usually becoming scaly and red, although color can vary. Treatment of actinic keratoses, also known as solar keratoses, includes cryotherapy with liquid nitrogen. This causes destruction of the lesions with resulting crust for about 2 weeks, revealing healed tissue and usually an excellent cosmetic outcome. Alternatives include the use of 1% to 5% fluorouracil creams once a day for 2 to 3 weeks until the lesions become crusted over. As another alternative, 5% fluorouracil cream can be used once a day for 1 to 2 days weekly for 7 to 10 weeks. This regimen yields a similar therapeutic outcome without crusting or discomfort. Additional options include 5% imiquimod cream, topical diclofenac gel, and photodynamic therapy (PDT) with topical delta-aminolevulinic acid. Resurfacing with chemical peels and laser are additional destructive treatment options for actinic keratoses. ♂

Discussion Sources

Jacobs A, Orengo I. Cancers of the skin. In: Rakel R, Bope E, eds. *Conn's Current Therapy 2008*. Philadelphia, PA: Saunders; 2008:781–784.

Spencer J, Fulton J. http://www.emedicine.com/derm/topic9.htm, eMedicine: Actinic keratosis, accessed 9/3/09.

QUESTIONS

81. Which of the following is the most frequent cause of stasis ulcers?

    A. arterial insufficiency
    B. venous insufficiency
    C. diabetes mellitus
    D. fungal dermatitis

82. You examine the left lower extremity of a patient and find an ulcerated lesion with irregular borders and edema with brown discoloration of the surrounding tissue. The best treatment option at this time is:

    A. compression therapy.
    B. referral for surgical débridement.
    C. daily use of a topical antibiotic cream.
    D. application of a dry, sterile dressing.

83. A 70-year-old man presents with absent popliteal pulses and a cool, hairless foot with a 2-cm ulcer that has a "punched-out" appearance on the dorsum of the second toe. The appropriate next measure is to:

   A. arrange for evaluation for arterial insufficiency.

   B. apply wet to dry dressings.

   C. start the patient on a peripheral vasodilator.

   D. advise the patient to elevate his feet for 15 minutes three times a day.

ANSWERS

81. B   **82.** A   **83.** A

DISCUSSION

Stasis ulcers are most commonly caused by venous insufficiency, and far less commonly caused by arterial insufficiency, diabetes mellitus, and fungal infections. Poor venous return causes lower extremity edema, which leads to decreased tissue perfusion and the resulting risk of ulcer; a common patient complaint is a feeling of lower extremity heaviness and ache. Although the clinical presentation is relatively straightforward, the diagnosis of venous insufficiency is supported by the presence of venous reflux with color duplex ultrasound scanning.

Given that poor venous return is one of the core defects of the condition, compression therapy to 30 to 40 mm Hg at the ankle is optimal with wraps, graduated compression stockings, or compression pump and key to successful therapy. Venous stasis ulcers usually respond well to occlusive hydroactive dressings such as hydrocolloid gel (DuoDerm). An Unna boot also can help, but it requires weekly changing. If the wound does not respond, treatment with becaplermin (Regranex) or skin grafting is occasionally necessary; biopsy of the nonhealing lesion should be considered to rule out malignancy.

Regardless of the treatment chosen, venous stasis ulcers require long-term care, including good nutrition and expert wound management. Involving home help care and wound care management nursing experts greatly enhances success. Wound débridement is needed only when necrotic tissue is present, and antimicrobial therapy is needed when there are signs of infection.

The description of the lesion in Question 83 is consistent not with peripheral venous disease, but rather with peripheral arterial disease. The treatment of choice is revascularization of the limb to enhance circulation. This is the only treatment option that results in resolution of the lesion (see Chapter 9 for additional information). Arterial disease often coexists with venous disease, and the diagnosis can be supported by the presence of abnormal arterial brachial pressure index.

Discussion Source

Phillips T, Etufugh C. Venous stasis ulcers. In: Rakel R, Bope E, eds. *Conn's Current Therapy 2008*. Philadelphia, PA: Saunders; 2008:844–847.

QUESTIONS

84. Which of the following do you expect to find in the assessment of the person with urticaria?

   A. eosinophilia

   B. low erythrocyte sedimentation rate

   C. elevated thyroid-stimulating hormone level

   D. leukopenia

85. A 24-year-old woman presents with hive-form linear lesions that form over areas where she has scratched. These resolve within a few minutes. This most likely represent:

   A. dermographism.

   B. contact dermatitis.

   C. angioedema.

   D. allergic reaction.

86. An urticarial lesion is usually described as a:

   A. wheal.

   B. plaque.

   C. patch.

   D. papule.

ANSWERS

84. A   **85.** A   **86.** A

DISCUSSION

Urticaria is a condition in which eruptions of wheals or hives occur most often in response to allergen exposure. The most common cause is a type I hypersensitivity reaction. This type of reaction is caused when IgE antibodies occupy receptor sites on mast cells, causing degradation of the mast cell and subsequent release of histamine, vasodilation, mucous gland stimulation, and tissue swelling. As with most allergen-based conditions, eosinophilia, an increase in the number of circulating eosinophils, is usually present. Type I hypersensitivity reactions consist of two subgroups: atopy and anaphylaxis.

Urticarial lesions often develop as groups of intensely itchy wheals or hives. The lesions usually last less than 24 hours and often only 2 to 4 hours. New lesions can form, however, extending the outbreak to 1 to 2 weeks. ♂

Many common clinical conditions are included in the atopy subgroup, such as allergic rhinitis, atopic dermatitis, allergic gastroenteropathy, and allergy-based asthma. Atopic diseases have a strong familial component and tend to cause localized rather than systemic reactions. The person with atopic disease is often able to identify allergy-inducing agents. In addition to avoidance of offending agents, treatment for systemic atopic disease includes antihistamines, topical corticosteroids, and leukotriene modifiers (zafirlukast [Accolate], montelukast [Singulair]); systemic corticosteroids are often needed for severe flares.

Anaphylaxis typically causes a systemic IgE-mediated reaction to exposure to an allergen, often a drug (e.g., penicillin), insect venom (e.g., bee sting), or food (e.g., peanuts). Anaphylaxis is characterized by a wide variation in presentation, ranging from an urticarial reaction being noted in its mildest form to the presence of widespread vasodilation, urticaria, angioedema, and bronchospasm creating a life-threatening condition of airway obstruction coupled with circulatory collapse. First-line treatment includes avoiding or discontinuing use of the offending agent. Additional therapy is based on the clinical presentation. Simultaneously, maintaining airway patency and adequate circulation is critical.

TABLE 3–7

Clinical Manifestations of Anaphylaxis

Urticaria	Angioedema
Upper airway edema	Flush
Dyspnea and wheezing	Dizziness and syncope
Hypotension	GI symptoms
Headache	Substernal pain
Itch without rash	Seizure

Note: Although urticaria and angioedema are most consistently reported, the clinical presentation of anaphylaxis can be quite variable.

Angioedema and urticaria are subcutaneous anaphylactic reactions, but are not life-threatening unless tissue swelling impinges on the airway (Tables 3–7 and 3–8).

Discussion Sources

Linscott MS. http://www.emedicine.com/emerg/TOPIC628.HTM, eMedicine: Urticaria, accessed 9/2/09.

TABLE 3–8

Treatment of Anaphylaxis in Patient With Currently Patent Airway

Intervention	Comment
Immediate SC or IM administration of epinephrine	No contraindications to epinephrine use in anaphylaxis
	Failure to or delay in use associated with fatalities
Administer antihistamine such as diphenhydramine (Benadryl)	An important part of anaphylaxis treatment, but should be used only with, not instead of, epinephrine
Additional measures as dictated by patient response	Airway maintenance including supplemental oxygen
	IV fluids, vasopressor therapy corticosteroids
	Repeat epinephrine every 5 minutes if symptoms persist or increase
	Repeat antihistamine with or without H$_2$ blocker if symptoms persist
	Observe as dictated by patient response, keeping in mind that anaphylaxis reactions often have a protracted or biphasic response
Arrange follow-up care	Provide instruction on avoidance of provoking agent
	Give epinephrine autoinjector (EpiPen or Twinject) prescription with appropriate education about indications and safety of use

IM, intramuscular; IV, intravenous; SC, subcutaneous.

Source: www.anaphylaxis.com, www.aaaai.org/professionals/resources/pdf/anaphylaxis_2005.pdf, accessed 9/3/09.

QUESTIONS

87. When counseling a person who has a 2-mm verruca-form lesion on the hand, you advise that:

    A. bacteria are the most common cause of these lesions.
    B. lesions usually resolve without therapy in 12 to 24 months.
    C. there is a significant risk for future dermatologic malignancy.
    D. surgical excision is the treatment of choice.

88. The mechanism of action of imiquimod is as a/an:

    A. immunomodulator.
    B. antimitotic.
    C. keratolytic.
    D. irritant.

89. The most common human papillomavirus types associated with cutaneous, nongenital warts include:

    A. 1, 2, and 4.
    B. 6 and 11.
    C. 16 and 18.
    D. 32 and 36.

ANSWERS

| 87. | B | 88. | A | 89. | A |

DISCUSSION

Verruca vulgaris lesions are also known as warts. Human papillomavirus types 1, 2, and 4 cause most nongenital warts; virus is passed through direct person-to-person contact. Over a 12- to 24-month period, nearly all lesions resolve without therapy. Surgical excision is rarely indicated. Intervention is warranted if warts interfere with function, such as with painful plantar warts on the soles of the feet, or if the lesions are cosmetically problematic (Table 3–9).

Discussion Source

Housman T, Williford P. Warts (verrucae). In: Rakel R, Bope E, eds. *Conn's Current Therapy 2008*. Philadelphia, PA: Saunders; 2008:811–815.

TABLE 3–9

Treatment Options for Warts

Treatment	Instructions for Use	Comments
Liquid nitrogen	Apply to achieve a thaw time of 20–45 seconds	Usually good cosmetic results
	Two freeze-thaw cycles may be administered every 2–4 weeks until lesion is gone	Can be painful, requires multiple treatments
Keratolytic agents (Occlusal, Duofilm, DuoPlant, others)	Apply as directed until lesions resolve	Often needs long-term therapy before resolution
		Well tolerated
		With plantar warts, pare down lesion; then apply 40% salicylic acid plaster, changing every 5 days
Podophyllum resin (podofilox)	Patient applies three times a week for 4–6 weeks	Multiple cycles often needed
		Skin irritation common
Tretinoin	Apply bid to flat warts for 4–6 weeks	Needs consistent treatment for optimal results
Imiquimod (Aldara)	Frequency and duration of use depend on wart location	Immunomodulator
		Low rate of wart recurrence
Laser therapy	Used to dissect lesions	Needs 4–6 weeks to granulate tissue
		Best reserved for treatment-resistant warts

Source: Housman T, Williford P. Warts (verrucae). In: Rakel R, Bope E, eds. *Conn's Current Therapy 2008*. Philadelphia, PA: Saunders; 2008:811–815.

QUESTIONS

90. The most common causative organisms in cellulitis are:

A. *Escherichia coli* and *Haemophilus influenzae.*
B. *Bacteroides* species and other anaerobes.
C. group A beta-hemolytic streptococci and *S. aureus.*
D. pathogenic viruses.

91. Which of the following is the best treatment option for cellulitis when risk of infection with a methicillin-resistant pathogen is considered low?

A. dicloxacillin
B. amoxicillin
C. metronidazole
D. daptomycin

ANSWERS

91. C   92. A

DISCUSSION

Cellulitis is an acute infection of the subcutaneous tissue and skin, typically as part of a skin wound, such as an insect bite, surgical incision, abrasion, or other cutaneous trauma. The clinical presentation includes a warm, red, edematous area with sharply demarcated borders; lymphangitis, lymphadenitis, and, rarely, necrosis can also occur. Cellulitis is most commonly found in the extremities. The causative pathogen is usually a gram-positive organism such as group A beta-hemolytic streptococci and *S. aureus.* Rarely, particularly in immunocompromised individuals, certain gram-negative organisms are the causative agent.

Treatment for cellulitis involves the choice of an antimicrobial agent with strong gram-positive coverage (in streptococcal and staphylococcal infection); resistant pathogens, including methicillin-resistant *S. aureus* (MRSA), must be considered. Treatment options for cellulitis when MRSA risk is considered low include dicloxacillin or a macrolide such as azithromycin or clarithromycin. With significant MRSA risk, or when cellulitis surrounds an area of furunculosis or abscess, treatment should be aimed at treating MRSA and streptococcal infection (see next section on MRSA). Local therapy with warm soaks helps facilitate resolution.

Discussion Sources

Gilbert D, Moellering R, Eliopoulos G, Chambers H, Saag M. *The Sanford Guide to Antimicrobial Therapy.* 39th ed. Sperryville, VA: Antimicrobial Therapy, Inc; 2009:50–51.

Nichols R. Bacterial diseases of the skin. In: Rakel R, Bope E, eds. *Conn's Current Therapy 2008*. Philadelphia, PA: Saunders; 2008:824–825.

QUESTIONS

92. You see a 36-year-old man with no chronic health problems who presents with two furuncles, each around 4 cm in diameter, on the right anterior thigh. These lesions have been present for 3 days, slightly increasing in size during this time. He has no fever or other systemic symptoms. You advise the following:

A. incision and drainage of the lesion
B. a systemic antibiotic empirically
C. a topical antibiotic
D. aspiration of the lesion contents and prescription of a systemic antibiotic based on culture results

93. A woman was treated as an inpatient for a serious soft tissue infection with parenteral linezolid and now is being seen on day 3 of her illness and is being discharged to home. She is feeling better and appears by examination to be clinically improved. Culture results reveal MRSA, sensitive to trimethoprim-sulfamethoxazole, linezolid, daptomycin, vancomycin, and clindamycin, and resistant to cephalothin and erythromycin. Her antimicrobial therapy should be completed with:

A. oral cephalexin.
B. oral trimethoprim-sulfamethoxazole.
C. parenteral linezolid.
D. oral linezolid.

Answer the following questions true or false

____ 94. Skin lesions infected by community-acquired MRSA (CA-MRSA) often occur spontaneously on intact skin.

____ 95. CA-MRSA is most commonly spread from one person to another via air-borne pathogen transmission.

____ 96. All CA-MRSA strains are capable of causing necrotizing infection.

____ 97. The mechanism of resistance of MRSA is via the production of beta-lactamase.

____ 98. If a skin and soft tissue infection does not improve in 48 to 72 hours with antimicrobial therapy, infection with a resistant pathogen is likely the only cause.

____ 99. Most acute-onset necrotic skin lesions reported in North America are caused by spider bites.

____ 100. Rifampin must be prescribed with caution because this medication is a cytochrome P-450 isoenzyme inducer.

ANSWERS

92.	A	93.	B	94.	F
95.	F	96.	F	97.	F
98.	F	99.	F	100.	T

DISCUSSION

Staphylococcus aureus is a ubiquitous gram-positive organism that normally grows on the skin and mucous membranes and is a common cause of skin and soft tissue infections. Strains of *S. aureus* that produce beta-lactamase, which is an enzyme capable of neutralizing penicillins, were first noted in the 1940s and became the dominant community and hospital pathogenic forms of the organism from the 1950s through the early 2000s. During that time, *S. aureus* skin and soft tissue infections were treated with antimicrobials possessing activity against gram-positive organisms and had stability in the presence of beta-lactamase, such as the macrolides (erythromycin, azithromycin, clarithromycin), certain cephalosporins (e.g., cephalexin, cefadroxil), and semisynthetic penicillin forms that possess beta-lactamase stability (dicloxacillin, methicillin, oxacillin, nafcillin). As a result, these strains are known as methicillin-sensitive *S. aureus* (MSSA). An additional treatment option was an antimicrobial with a beta-lactamase inhibitor, such as amoxicillin-clavulanate. In the past 25 years, strains of *S. aureus* resistant to methicillin (MRSA) evolved into an important pathogen in hospital-associated and long-term care facility–associated infection. Until the early 2000s, however, MRSA was seldom noted in the community.

Across the United States, disease caused by MRSA acquired in the community (known as community-acquired or community-associated MRSA [CA-MRSA]) has been reported with increasing frequency. CA-MRSA is not simply an organism that has escaped the health-care facility and taken up residence in the community; in contrast to health-care–associated MRSA (HC-MRSA), in which numerous clones have been identified, two major clones are responsible for most CA-MRSA. One of these clones was implicated in a worldwide infectious disease outbreak more than 50 years ago. CA-MRSA infections usually involve the skin and soft tissues in the form of cellulitis, bullous impetigo, folliculitis, abscess, or an infected laceration. Less common is CA-MRSA–associated disease in the form of blood, bone, or joint infection or pneumonia. The Panton-Valentine leukocidin (PVL) toxin is present in approximately 77% of CA-MRSA strains and is rare in hospital-associated MRSA strains. The PVL toxin promotes lysis of human leukocytes, and it is associated with severe necrotizing skin infections and hemorrhagic pneumonia.

CA-MRSA is usually acquired during person-to-person, skin-to-skin contact, but inanimate objects such as countertops or other surfaces also contribute to CA-MRSA transmission. Although MRSA acquired in health-care facilities usually affects frail individuals, CA-MRSA is found predominately in otherwise healthy children and adults. Bearing this in mind, CA-MRSA infection does seem more common in impoverished populations and in certain ethnic groups, including African Americans and Native Americans. Additional risks include living in crowded conditions such as jails or prisons, participating in occupational or recreational activities with regular skin-to-skin contact such as wrestling, exposure to a person with CA-MRSA, and recent use of an antibiotic or recurrent skin infection (or both). Prevention of CA-MRSA includes appropriate hand hygiene, reduction of unnecessary skin-to-skin contact, and thorough cleaning of surfaces with a disinfectant solution.

The choice of therapy for skin and soft tissue infection must take into consideration issues of antimicrobial resistance and minimizing unnecessary antimicrobial use. According to the recommendations found in the *Sanford Guide,* in an afebrile patient with an abscess less than 5 cm in diameter, the first-line treatment of community-acquired skin and soft tissue infection is incision, drainage, and localized care such as warm soaks. A wound culture and sensitivity should be obtained to help guide treatment. If the abscess is equal to or greater than 5 cm in diameter, antimicrobial therapy should be added to the aforementioned localized treatment.

Given that the antimicrobials effective against MSSA (certain cephalosporins, penicillins, penicillin with beta-lactamase inhibitor combinations, and select macrolides) are ineffective in CA-MRSA, documentation of the organism's pattern of resistance can help direct therapy. Most strains of CA-MRSA remain sensitive to trimethoprim-sulfamethoxazole (TMP-SMX, Bactrim), and this is the primary antimicrobial therapy recommended, particularly in a person who is immunocompetent and without fever. Because successful therapy depends on achieving adequate concentration of the antimicrobial at the site of the infection, the recommended TMP-SMX dose is 2 double-strength tablets, and therapy should be continued for 5 to 10 days. When large, multiple lesions or fever or both are present, adding rifampin, 300 mg bid, to the aforementioned therapy is an option; however, few objective data exist to support this practice.

Rifampin must be prescribed with caution because this medication is a cytochrome P450 isoenzyme inducer. Its concomitant use with other medications causes a reduction in levels of numerous drugs, including methadone, cyclosporine, oral contraceptives, and many antiretrovirals. Rifampin should not be used alone to treat CA-MRSA because of the risk of developing resistance. In patients who are intolerant of sulfa drugs, alternatives to TMP-SMX therapy include doxycycline or minocycline. Linezolid (Zyvox) is another effective, albeit expensive, oral treatment option, which is usually reserved for use when the aforementioned medications are not tolerated or ineffective. When parenteral treatment is needed, commonly used management options include linezolid, vancomycin, and daptomycin. The last-mentioned is not indicated in the treatment of pneumonia.

Although TMP-SMX is usually active against CA-MRSA, its coverage against streptococcus is uncertain. If the causative pathogen of the skin and soft tissue infection is unclear, and streptococcal infection is considered a possibility, such as is seen in cellulitis or erysipelas, the antimicrobial choice should be aimed at choices that provide coverage against staphylococci and streptococci. In this situation, the *Sanford Guide* recommends using TMP-SMX with a beta-lactam such as a cephalosporin.

A person with CA-MRSA infection requires careful follow-up to ensure clinical resolution. Post-treatment cultures are unnecessary. Serious disease such as pneumonia or death resulting from CA-MRSA is, in many locations, a reportable disease.

As mentioned, the clinical presentation of CA-MRSA is usually as a cutaneous and soft tissue lesion in the form of boils and abscesses. Because a CA-MRSA lesion often has a dark or black center, the condition has often been attributed to a spider bite. In reality, spider bites are uncommon, usually occurring only when the arachnid is trapped in clothing or a shoe. In addition, few spider species have the capability of causing a significant bite. In particular, the brown recluse spider, or *Loxosceles reclusa,* can cause a necrotizing bite and is often blamed for lesions that are actually caused by CA-MRSA. Found primarily in the U.S. Midwest and Southeast, this arachnid hibernates during the winter, so bites, which are generally painless, occur between March and October. The term *recluse* depicts a shy creature that typically hides in shoes, boxes, and other small enclosed spaces. A single spider is occasionally spotted outside of its native region, having traveled in a suitcase or box. Only a small proportion of brown recluse spider bites become necrotic. When this occurs, a characteristic pattern known as the "red, white, and blue" sign follows, with a central purple-to-gray discoloration surrounded by a white ring of blanched skin and a large red halo. If necrosis occurs, a black eschar forms.

Discussion Sources

Gilbert D, Moellering R, Eliopoulos G, Chambers H, Saag M. *The Sanford Guide to Antimicrobial Therapy.* 39th ed. Sperryville, VA: Antimicrobial Therapy, Inc; 2009:48–49.

Roy H. http://www.emedicine.com/oph/topic652.htm, eMedicine: Spider bites, accessed 9/4/09.

Tolan R. http://www.emedicine.com/ped/topic2704.htm, eMedicine: *Staphylococcus aureus* infection, 2008, accessed 9/4/09.

www.cdc.gov/ncidod/dhqp/ar_mrsa_ca_posters.html, Consumer-oriented information from the CDC about infectious disease and spider bites, accessed 8/30/09.

4

Eye, Ear, Nose, and Throat Problems

QUESTIONS

1. A 74-year-old woman with well-controlled hypertension who is taking hydrochlorothiazide presents with a 3-day history of unilateral throbbing headache with difficulty chewing because of pain. On physical examination, you find a tender, noncompressible temporal artery. Blood pressure (BP) is 160/88 mm Hg, apical pulse is 98 bpm, and respiratory rate is 22/min; the patient is visibly uncomfortable. The most likely diagnosis is:

   A. giant cell arteritis.
   B. impending transient ischemic attack.
   C. complicated migraine.
   D. temporal mandibular joint dysfunction.

2. Therapeutic interventions for the patient in Question 1 should include:

   A. systemic corticosteroid therapy for many months.
   B. addition of an angiotensin-converting enzyme inhibitor (ACEI) to her antihypertensive regimen.
   C. warfarin therapy.
   D. initiation of topiramate (Topamax) therapy.

3. Concomitant disease seen with giant cell arteritis includes:

   A. polymyalgia rheumatica.
   B. acute pancreatitis.
   C. psoriatic arthritis.
   D. Reiter syndrome.

4. One of the most serious complications of giant cell arteritis is:

   A. hemiparesis.
   B. arthritis.
   C. blindness.
   D. uveitis.

ANSWERS

1.	A	2.	A
3.	A	4.	C

DISCUSSION

Giant cell or temporal arteritis is an autoimmune vasculitis that is most common in patients 50 to 85 years old; average age at onset is 70 years. A systemic disease affecting medium-sized and large-sized vessels, giant cell arteritis also causes inflammation of the temporal artery. Extracranial branches of the carotid artery are often involved; this often results in a tender or nodular, pulseless vessel, usually the temporal artery, accompanied by a severe unilateral headache. The temporal artery is occasionally normal, however. Giant cell arteritis and polymyalgia rheumatica are thought to represent two parts of a spectrum of disease and are often found together.

In an older adult, these clinical syndromes are often accompanied by respiratory tract symptoms (cough, sore throat, hoarseness) or mental status changes, rather than by the classically reported findings of headache, jaw claudication, and acute reduction or change in vision. The headache that is usually part of the presentation is occasionally reported as being located in the frontal, vertex, or occipital area, rather than in the temporal area.

Apart from relieving pain, treatment of giant cell arteritis helps minimize the risk of blindness, which is one of the most serious complications of the disease. Approximately 50% of patients with giant cell arteritis experience visual symptoms, including transient visual blurring, diplopia, eye pain, or sudden loss of vision; transient repeated episodes of blurred vision are usually reversible, but sudden loss of vision is an ominous sign and is almost always permanent. As soon as the diagnosis is made, high-dose systemic corticosteroid therapy should be initiated; this therapy typically involves

See full color images of this topic on DavisPlus at http://davisplus.fadavis.com | Keyword: Fitzgerald

prednisone, 1 to 2 mg/kg per day, until the disease seems to be under control, followed by a careful dose reduction until the lowest dose that can maintain clinical response can be determined. This dose is continued for 6 months to 2 years. When symptoms have been stable, and the corticosteroid therapy is going to be discontinued, a slow taper with close monitoring is warranted because of the risk of adrenal suppression and disease resurgence. Gastrointestinal cytoprotection with misoprostol or a proton pump inhibitor and bone protection with a bisphosphonate should also be provided to minimize these corticosteroid-related adverse effects. A cyclosporine-azathioprine or cyclosporine-methotrexate combination can be used as a corticosteroid-sparing treatment option or as an alternative in corticosteroid-resistant cases.

Diagnosis of giant cell arteritis should include a confirmatory arterial biopsy. Color duplex ultrasonography of the temporal arteries has been used as an alternative or complement to superficial temporal artery biopsy. Because the disease frequently skips portions of the vessel, biopsy specimens of multiple vessel sites should be obtained. C-reactive protein (CRP) and erythrocyte sedimentation rate (ESR), although nonspecific tests of inflammation, are usually markedly elevated.

The BP of the patient in Question 1 is probably elevated because of pain response. Analgesia should be given, and then BP should be measured again. Adding a second antihypertensive agent to this patient's treatment ignores the most likely underlying cause of her BP elevation.

Discussion Sources

Nesher G. Polymyalgia rheumatica and giant-cell arteritis. In: Rakel R, Bope E, eds. *Conn's Current Therapy 2009.* Philadelphia, PA: Saunders Elsevier; 2009:979–981.

Roque M. http://www.emedicine.com/OPH/topic254.htm, eMedicine: Giant cell arteritis, accessed 9/4/09.

QUESTIONS

5. An 88-year-old, community-dwelling man who lives alone has limited mobility because of osteoarthritis. Since his last office visit 2 months ago, he has lost 5% of his body weight and has developed angular cheilitis. You expect to find the following on examination:

   A. fissuring and cracking at the corners of the mouth
   B. marked erythema of the hard and soft palates
   C. white plaques on the lateral borders of the buccal mucosa
   D. raised, painless lesions on the gingiva

6. First-line therapy for angular cheilitis therapy includes the use of:

   A. metronidazole gel.
   B. hydrocortisone cream.
   C. topical nystatin.
   D. oral ketoconazole.

ANSWERS

5. A   6. C

DISCUSSION

Various oral and perioral infections are caused by *Candida* species, including angular cheilitis, ♂ also known as angular stomatitis, perlèche, or cheilosis. A major candidiasis risk factor is an immunocompromised state, whether resulting from advanced age, malnutrition, or HIV infection. In addition, physical characteristics can increase the risk for angular cheilitis, such as in an older adult who has a loss of vertical facial dimension because of loss of teeth, allowing for overclosure of the mouth; the resulting skin folds create a suitable environment for *Candida* growth.

Topical antifungals such as nystatin offer a reasonable first-line treatment for perioral and oral candidiasis. With particularly recalcitrant conditions and failure of topical therapy, systemic antifungals are occasionally needed. Treatment of the underlying condition is critical, as is maintenance of skin integrity through hygienic practices and skin lubrication.

Discussion Source

http://www.merck.com/mmpe/sec08/ch086/ch086f.html, Merck Manual online: Ear, nose, throat, and dental disorders, accessed 9/4/09.

QUESTIONS

7. A 19-year-old man presents with a chief complaint of a red, irritated right eye for the past 48 hours with eyelids that were "stuck together" this morning when he awoke. Examination reveals injected palpebral and bulbar conjunctiva; reactive pupils; vision screen with the Snellen chart of 20/30 in the right eye (OD), left eye (OS), and both eyes (OU); and purulent eye discharge on the right. This presentation is most consistent with:

   A. suppurative conjunctivitis.
   B. viral conjunctivitis.
   C. allergic conjunctivitis.
   D. mechanical injury.

8. A 19-year-old woman presents with a complaint of bilaterally itchy, red eyes with tearing that occurs intermittently throughout the year and is often accompanied by a ropelike eye discharge and clear nasal discharge. This is most consistent with conjunctival inflammation caused by a(n):

   A. bacterium.
   B. virus.
   C. allergen.
   D. injury.

9. Common causative organisms of acute suppurative conjunctivitis include all of the following except:

   A. *Staphylococcus aureus*.
   B. *Haemophilus influenzae*.
   C. *Streptococcus pneumoniae*.
   D. *Pseudomonas aeruginosa*.

10. Treatment options in suppurative conjunctivitis include all of the following ophthalmic preparations except:

    A. bacitracin–polymyxin B.
    B. ciprofloxacin.
    C. erythromycin.
    D. penicillin.

11. Treatment options in acute and recurrent allergic conjunctivitis include all of the following except:

    A. cromolyn ophthalmic drops.
    B. oral antihistamines.
    C. ophthalmological antihistamines.
    D. corticosteroid ophthalmic drops.

ANSWERS

7.	A	8.	C	9.	D
10.	D	11.	D		

DISCUSSION

Because therapy in conjunctivitis is in part aimed at eradicating or eliminating the underlying causes, accurate diagnosis is critical. A patient with a presumptive diagnosis of suppurative conjunctivitis requires antimicrobial therapy, whereas a person with allergic conjunctivitis 𝄐 benefits from therapy focused on identifying and limiting exposure to specific allergens and the appropriate use of antiallergic agents (Tables 4–1 and 4–2).

Discussion Source

Gilbert D, Moellering R, Eliopoulos G, Chambers H, Saag M. *The Sanford Guide to Antimicrobial Therapy*. 39th ed. Sperryville, VA: Antimicrobial Therapy, Inc; 2009:12–13.
World Allergy Organization. http://www.worldallergy.org/educational_programs/gloria/us/materials.php, Allergic conjunctivitis 2007, accessed 9/4/09.

QUESTIONS

12. Anterior epistaxis is usually caused by:

    A. hypertension.
    B. bleeding disorders.
    C. localized nasal mucosa trauma.
    D. a foreign body.

13. First-line intervention for anterior epistaxis includes:

    A. nasal packing.
    B. application of topical thrombin.
    C. firm pressure to the area superior to the nasal alar cartilage.
    D. chemical cauterization.

ANSWERS

12.	C	13.	C

TABLE 4–1

Allergic Conjunctivitis: Defining Terms

Intermittent (seasonal) allergic conjunctivitis	IgE-mediated diseases related to seasonal allergens Common triggers—depend on time of year and geographic location (April/May, tree pollens; June/July, grass pollens; July/August, mold spores and weed pollens; others dependent on local environmental factors)
Persistent (perennial) allergic conjunctivitis	IgE-mediated diseases are related to perennial allergens Common trigger—house dust mites (present in all geographic areas)

Source: http://www.worldallergy.org/educational_programs/gloria/guidelines.pdf, GLORIA guidelines for the treatment of allergic rhinitis and allergic conjunctivitis, accessed 9/5/09.

TABLE 4–2

Treatment of Common Bacterial Eye, Ear, Nose, and Throat Infection

Site of Infection	Common Pathogens	Recommended Antimicrobial	Comments
Suppurative conjunctivitis (nongonococcal, nonchlamydial)	*S. aureus,* *S. pneumoniae,* *H. influenzae* Outbreaks due to atypical *S. pneumoniae*	Primary: Ophthalmic treatment with FQ ocular solution (gatifloxacin, levofloxacin, moxifloxacin) Alternative: Ophthalmic treatment with bacitracin–polymyxin B with trimethoprim solution	Bacterial and viral conjunctivitis ("pink eye", usually caused by adenovirus) often self-limiting. Relieve irritative symptoms with use of cold artificial tear solution Most *S. pneumoniae* is resistant to tobramycin, gentamicin
Otitis externa (swimmer's ear)	*Pseudomonas* spp., *Proteus* spp., Enterobacteriaceae Acute infection often *S. aureus* Fungi rare etiology	Otic drops with ofloxacin or ciprofloxacin with hydrocortisone or polymyxin B with neomycin and hydrocortisone	Ear canal cleansing important. Decrease risk of reinfection by use of eardrops of 1:2 mixture or white vinegar and rubbing alcohol after swimming Do not use neomycin if tympanic membrane punctured
Malignant otitis externa in a person with diabetes mellitus, HIV/AIDS, on chemotherapy	*Pseudomonas* spp. in >90%	Oral ciprofloxacin for early disease suitable for outpatient therapy Other options available if inpatient therapy warranted in severe disease	Surgical débridement usually needed. MRI or CT to evaluate for osteomyelitis may be indicated Parenteral antimicrobial therapy may be warranted for severe disease
Acute otitis media	*S. pneumoniae,* *H. influenzae,* *M. catarrhalis,* viral or no pathogen (approximately 55% bacterial, *S. pneumoniae* most common)	If no antimicrobial therapy in the past month: amoxicillin at high dose (HD) (3-4 g/day in adults) or usual doses (1.75–3 g/day in adults) If antimicrobial therapy in past month: HD amoxicillin with or without clavulanate, cefdinir, cefpodoxime, cefprozil, cefuroxime If treatment failure >72 hours of therapy and no antimicrobial therapy in past month: HD amoxicillin with clavulanate, cefdinir, cefpodoxime, cefprozil, cefuroxime, or IM ceftriaxone (ceftriaxone daily × 3 days) If treatment failure >72 hours of therapy and antimicrobial therapy in past month: IM ceftriaxone qd × 3 days, clindamycin or tympanocentesis	Consider drug-resistant *S. pneumoniae* (DRSP) risk: antimicrobial therapy in past 3 months, age <2 years, day-care attendance. HD amoxicillin usually effective in DRSP Length of therapy: <2 years, 10 days; >2 years, 5–7 days If allergy to beta-lactam drugs: TMP-SMX, clarithromycin, azithromycin; all less effective against DRSP compared with other options. If penicillin allergy history is unclear or rash (no hive-form lesions), cephalosporins likely okay Clindamycin effective against DRSP, ineffective against *H. influenzae, M. catarrhalis* See Chapter 15, Pediatrics, for additional information
Exudative pharyngitis	Group A, C, G streptococcus, viral, HHV-6, *M. pneumoniae*	First-line: penicillin V PO × 10 days or benzathine penicillin IM × 1 dose if adherence an issue Alternative: erythromycin × 10 days, second generation cephalosporin × 4-6 d, azithromycin × 5 days, clarithromycin × 10 days Up to 35% *S. pyogenes* isolates resistant to macrolides	Vesicular, ulcerative pharyngitis usually viral. Only 10% of adult pharyngitis due to group A streptococcus No treatment recommended for asymptomatic group A streptococcus carrier For recurrent, culture-proven group A streptococcus, consider coinfection with beta-lactamase–producing organism, treat with amoxicillin with clavulanate or clindamycin

Source: Gilbert D, Moellering R, Eliopoulos G, Chambers H, Saag M. *The Sanford Guide to Antimicrobial Therapy.* 39th ed. Sperryville, VA: Antimicrobial Therapy, Inc; 2009.

DISCUSSION

Anterior epistaxis is usually the result of localized nasal mucosa dryness and trauma and is rarely a result of other causes such as hypertension or coagulation disorder. Most episodes can be easily managed with simple pressure—with firm pressure to the area superior to the nasal alar cartilage or an "entire nose pinched closed" position by the patient for a minimum of 10 minutes. If this action is ineffective, second-line therapies include nasal packing and cautery. If epistaxis is seen in the presence of a bleeding disorder, topical thrombin should be used.

Discussion Source

http://www.merck.com/mmpe/sec08/ch086/ch086f.html, Merck Manual online. Ear, nose, throat, and dental disorders, accessed 9/3/09.

QUESTIONS

14. A 58-year-old woman presents with a sudden left-sided headache that is most painful in her left eye. Her vision is blurred, and the left pupil is slightly dilated and poorly reactive. The left conjunctiva is markedly injected, and the eyeball is firm. Vision screen with the Snellen chart is 20/30 OD and 20/90 OS. The most likely diagnosis is:

    A. unilateral herpetic conjunctivitis.
    B. open-angle glaucoma.
    C. angle-closure glaucoma.
    D. anterior uveitis.

15. In caring for the patient in Question 14, the most appropriate next action is:

    A. prompt referral to an ophthalmologist.
    B. to provide analgesia and repeat the evaluation when the patient is more comfortable.
    C. to instill a corticosteroid ophthalmic solution.
    D. to patch the eye and arrange for follow-up in 24 hours.

16. A 48-year-old man presents with a new-onset right eye vision change accompanied by dull pain, tearing, and photophobia. The right pupil is small, irregular, and poorly reactive. Vision testing obtained by using the Snellen chart is 20/30 OS and 20/80 OD. The most likely diagnosis is:

    A. unilateral herpetic conjunctivitis.
    B. open-angle glaucoma.
    C. angle-closure glaucoma.
    D. anterior uveitis.

ANSWERS

| 14. | C | 15. | A | 16. | D |

DISCUSSION

The components of an ophthalmological emergency are a painful, red eye with a visual disturbance. In the case of angle-closure glaucoma, the patient usually presents with all of these findings, and, without intervention, blindness ensues in 3 to 5 days. Prompt referral to expert ophthalmological care focused on relieving acute intraocular pressure is needed; laser peripheral iridectomy after reduction of intraocular pressure with appropriate medications is usually curative. In contrast, open-angle glaucoma is a slowly progressive disease that seldom produces symptoms. In anterior uveitis, another cause of an occasionally dully painful red eye with visual change, the pupil is usually constricted, nonreactive, and irregularly shaped. Treatment includes medications to assist in pupillary dilation and corticosteroids, administered topically, by periocular injection, or systemically. Evaluation for the underlying cause, including autoimmune and inflammatory diseases and ocular trauma, of this uncommon condition should also be done.

Discussion Sources

Kilborne G. http://emedicine.medscape.com/article/798323, eMedicine: Iritis and uveitis, accessed 9/4/09.

Syed M, Bell N. Glaucoma. In: Rakel R, Bope E, eds. *Conn's Current Therapy 2008*. Philadelphia, PA: Saunders; 2008:194–196.

QUESTIONS

17. Which of the following is a common vision problem in the person with untreated primary open-angle glaucoma (POAG)?

    A. peripheral vision loss
    B. blurring of near vision
    C. difficulty with distant vision
    D. need for increased illumination

18. Which of the following is most likely to be found on the funduscopic examination in a patient with untreated POAG?

    A. excessive cupping of the optic disk
    B. arteriovenous nicking
    C. papilledema
    D. flame-shaped hemorrhages

19. Risk factors for POAG include all of the following except:

    A. African ancestry.
    B. type 2 diabetes mellitus.
    C. advanced age.
    D. blue eye color.

20. Treatment options for POAG include all of the following topical agents except:

    A. beta-adrenergic antagonists.
    B. alpha$_2$-agonists.
    C. prostaglandin analogues.
    D. mast cell stabilizers.

ANSWERS

17.	A		**18.**	A
19.	D		**20.**	D

DISCUSSION

Although the etiology of POAG is not completely understood, the result is elevated intraocular pressure caused by abnormal drainage of aqueous humor through the trabecular meshwork. POAG risk factors include African ancestry, diabetes mellitus, a family history of POAG, history of certain eye trauma and uveitis, and advancing age. A gradual-onset peripheral vision loss is most specific for open-angle glaucoma; this disease is the second most common cause of irreversible blindness in North America. Although all of these changes may be seen in patients with advanced open-angle glaucoma, changes in near vision are common as part of the aging process because of hardening of the lens (i.e., presbyopia) and the need for increased illumination. New onset of difficulty with distance vision can be found in patients with cataracts.

Glaucoma, whether open-angle or angle-closure, is primarily a problem with excessive intraocular pressure. Tonometry reveals intraocular pressure greater than 25 mm Hg; in angle-closure glaucoma, the abnormal measurement is usually documented on more than one occasion. As a result, the optic disk and cup are "pushed in," creating the classic finding often called glaucomatous cupping. This creates a cup-to-disk ratio of greater than 0.3 or asymmetry of cup-to-disk ratio of 0.2 or more. Papilledema, in which the optic disk bulges and the margins are blurred, is seen when there is excessive pressure behind the eye, as in increased intracranial pressure (Fig. 4–1).

Medical treatment options for primary open angle or angle-closure glaucoma include topical beta-adrenergic antagonists such as timolol, alpha$_2$ agonists such as brimonidine, carbonic anhydrase inhibitors such as dorzolamide, and prostaglandin analogues such as latanoprost. Because of their

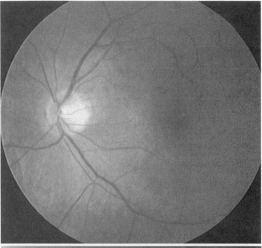
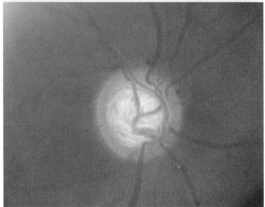
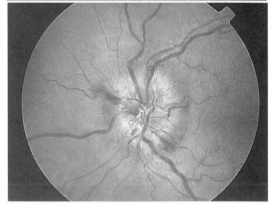

Figure 4–1 (A) Normal optic disk. (B) Glaucomatous cupping. (C) Bulging optic disk in papilledema.

ability to cause pupillary constriction, pilocarpine and similar medications are now seldom used. Laser trabeculoplasty and other surgical interventions are additional treatment options (Table 4–3).

Discussion Sources

http://www.merck.com/mmpe/sec09.html, Merck Manual online: Eye disorders, accessed 8/30/09.

Syed M, Bell N. Glaucoma. In: Rakel R, Bope E, eds. *Conn's Current Therapy 2008*. Philadelphia, PA: Saunders Elsevier; 2008:194–196.

TABLE 4–3

Treatment Options in Glaucoma

Chronic, Open-Angle Intervention	Acute, Angle-Closure Intervention

• Reduce production of intraocular fluid
  Topical beta-adrenergic antagonists
  Topical alpha$_2$-agonist
  Topical carbonic anhydrase inhibitors
  Surgical intervention if needed to attain
  normal pressures
    Photocoagulation
• Increase fluid outflow
  – Prostaglandin analogues
  – Surgical intervention if needed to attain
    normal pressures
    • Trabeculoplasty
    • Iridotomy
	• Prompt ophthalmological referral
	• Relieve acute intraocular pressure
	  – Reduce production of intraocular fluid
	    • Topical beta-adrenergic antagonists
	    • Topical alpha$_2$-agonist
	    • Topical carbonic anhydrase inhibitors
	  – Increase fluid outflow
	    • Prostaglandin analogues
	• Surgical intervention when pressure
	  normalized
	    Laser peripheral iridectomy

Source: Syed M, Bell N. Glaucoma. In: Rakel R, Bope E, eds. *Conn's Current Therapy 2008*. Philadelphia, PA: Saunders; 2008:194–196.

QUESTIONS

21. A 22-year-old woman presents with a "pimple" on her right eyelid. Examination reveals a 2-mm pustule on the lateral border of the right eyelid margin. This is most consistent with:

   A. a chalazion.
   B. a hordeolum.
   C. blepharitis.
   D. cellulitis.

22. A 22-year-old woman presents with a "bump" on her right eyelid. Examination reveals a 2-mm hard, non-tender swelling on the lateral border of the right eyelid margin. This is most consistent with:

   A. a chalazion.
   B. a hordeolum.
   C. blepharitis.
   D. cellulitis.

23. Treatment options for uncomplicated hordeolum include all of the following except:

   A. erythromycin ophthalmic ointment.
   B. warm compresses to the affected area.
   C. incision and drainage.
   D. oral antimicrobial therapy.

ANSWERS

21.   B   22.   A   23.   D

DISCUSSION

A hordeolum is often called a stye and is usually caused by a staphylococcal infection of a hair follicle on the eyelid. An internal hordeolum points toward the conjunctival eye surface, whereas an external hordeolum is found on the lid margin. A chalazion is an inflammatory eyelid condition that may not involve infection but can follow hordeolum and is characterized by a hard, nontender swelling of the upper or lower lid. Because treatment regimens for each of these differ significantly, accurate diagnosis is critical. Cellulitis is a serious complication of a hordeolum and is evidenced by widespread redness and edema over the eyelid.

Treatment for a simple hordeolum, or stye, includes warm compresses to the affected eye for 10 minutes three to four times a day. Local antimicrobial therapy with erythromycin or bacitracin ophthalmic ointment along the lid margin may accelerate resolution. Rarely, incision and drainage are needed. Oral antimicrobial therapy for an uncomplicated hordeolum is not warranted. An infrequently encountered complication of a hordeolum is cellulitis of the eyelid. If this occurs, ophthalmic consultation should be obtained, and appropriate systemic antimicrobial therapy should be promptly initiated. Because *S. aureus* is the most common pathogen, treatment options include the use of an antibiotic with gram-positive coverage and beta-lactamase stability with the possibility of methicillin-resistant strains. As a result, knowledge of local patterns of *S. aureus* is important.

Because this is an inflammatory, but not infectious disease, antimicrobial therapy for chalazion is not warranted. Treatment includes warm soaks of the area. If this is not helpful, referral to an ophthalmologist for intralesion corticosteroid injection or excision is recommended, particularly if the chalazion impairs lid closure or presses on the cornea.

Discussion Sources

Gilbert D, Moellering R, Eliopoulos G, Chambers H, Saag M. *The Sanford Guide to Antimicrobial Therapy*. 39th ed. Sperryville, VA: Antimicrobial Therapy, Inc; 2009:12–14.

http://www.merck.com/mmpe/sec08/ch086/ch086f.html, Merck Manual online: Ear, nose, throat, and dental disorders, accessed 9/4/09.

http://www.merck.com/mmpe/sec09.html, Merck Manual online: Eye disorders, accessed 9/4/09.

QUESTIONS

24. Which of the following is true concerning Ménière disease?

    A. Neuroimaging helps locate the offending cochlear lesion.
    B. Associated high-frequency hearing loss is common.
    C. It is largely a diagnosis of exclusion.
    D. Tinnitus is rarely reported.

25. Prevention and prophylaxis in Ménière's disease include all of the following except:

    A. avoiding ototoxic drugs.
    B. protecting the ears from loud noise.
    C. limiting sodium intake.
    D. restricting fluid intake.

26. to 29. Match the following to the lettered descriptions:

    ____ 26. dizziness
    ____ 27. vertigo
    ____ 28. nystagmus
    ____ 29. tinnitus

    A. perception that the person or the environment is moving
    B. subjective perception of altered equilibrium
    C. rhythmic oscillations of the eyes
    D. perception of abnormal hearing or head noises

ANSWERS

| 24. | C | 25. | D | 26. | B |
| 27. | A | 28. | C | 29. | D |

DISCUSSION

Ménière's disease, an idiopathic condition, and Ménière's syndrome, a condition with symptoms identical to those of Ménière's disease but in which an underlying cause has been identified, are believed to result from increased pressure within the endolymphatic system. In health, two fluids, one potassium-rich and the other potassium-poor, separated by a thin membrane, fill the chambers of the inner ear: endolymph and perilymph. Housed within the separating membrane is the nervous tissue of hearing and balance. Normally, the pressure exerted on these fluids is constant, allowing for normal balance and hearing. If the pressure of these fluids varies, the nerve-rich membranes are stressed, which causes disturbance in hearing, ringing in the ears, imbalance, a pressure sensation in the ear, and vertigo. The reason for the pressure changes varies, but most often they are caused by an increase in endolymphatic pressure that causes a break in the membrane separating the two fluids. When these fluids mix, the vestibular nerve receptors are bathed in the new, abnormal chemical mix, which leads to depolarization blockade and sudden change in the vestibular nerve firing rate. This creates an acute vestibular imbalance and the resulting sense of vertigo. Symptoms improve after the membrane is repaired, and normal sodium and potassium concentrations are restored.

A distinction needs to be made between Ménière's disease, usually idiopathic in origin, and Ménière's syndrome, usually secondary to various processes that interfere with normal production or resorption of endolymph, such as endocrine abnormalities, trauma, electrolyte imbalance, autoimmune dysfunction, medications, parasitic infections, and hyperlipidemia. Ménière's disease is largely a diagnosis of exclusion; diagnosis is made after other possible causes for the recurrent and often debilitating symptoms of dizziness, tinnitus, and low-frequency hearing loss have been ruled out. A distinct causative lesion cannot be identified. This condition is common and is characterized by repeat attacks; risk factors include use of ototoxic drugs such as aminoglycosides, long-term high-dose salicylate use, certain cancer chemotherapeutics, and exposure to loud noise.

Clinical presentation of Ménière's disease and Ménière's syndrome usually involves a history of episodes of vertigo with a sensation that the room is whirling about, often preceded by decreased hearing, low-tone roaring tinnitus, and a feeling of increased ear pressure. Particularly severe episodes are accompanied by nausea and vomiting. Attacks can last minutes to hours, with exhaustion often reported after the most severe symptoms have passed. Duration and frequency of attacks can vary, although common triggers include certain foods and drinks, mental and physical stress, and variations in the menstrual cycle.

Examination of a person with Ménière's disease typically reveals significant nystagmus or rhythmic oscillations of the eyes and slow movement toward one side, usually the side of the affected ear, with a rapid correction to the midline. The Weber tuning test result usually lateralizes to the unaffected ear, whereas the Rinne test shows that air exceeds bone conduction, a normal finding. Performing pneumatic otoscopy in the affected ear can elicit symptoms or cause nystagmus, whereas the same maneuver to the unaffected ear yields little response. Objective measures of hearing often reveal diminished hearing. The Romberg test is positive, with the patient showing increased swaying and difficulty staying balanced when standing with the eyes closed. Additional findings include a positive Fukuda marching step test, in which a directional drift, usually toward the affected ear, is noted when the patient is asked to perform a march step with the eyes closed. This latter maneuver may be impossible for a patient with severe symptoms. The result of the Dix-Hallpike test (i.e., observation of nystagmus while moving a patient from sitting to supine with the head angled 45 degrees to one side and then to the other) is occasionally also positive, indicating coexisting benign positional vertigo. Neuroimaging is usually not warranted, unless the examination reveals additional findings, or the diagnosis is unclear.

Treatment of Ménière disease is aimed at minimizing or preventing symptoms. Antihistamines such as meclizine (Antivert, Bonine) or antiemetics can minimize symptoms. Benzodiazepines can be used to help reinforce rest and minimize anxiety associated with severe symptoms; these options do not treat the underlying condition. Diuretics decrease fluid pressure load in the inner ear and can be used to prevent, but not treat, attacks; these medications do not help after the attack has been triggered. Corticosteroids also have been shown to be helpful, likely because of their anti-inflammatory properties, causing a reduction in endolymph pressure and potentially ameliorating vertigo, tinnitus, and hearing loss.

When standard therapy is ineffective and severe symptoms persist, chemical labyrinthectomy with intratympanic gentamicin is a treatment option. Surgery is reserved for patients with frequent, severely debilitating episodes that are unresponsive to other, less radical therapies; options include endolymphatic sac decompression, vestibular neurectomy, and surgical labyrinthectomy. The possible risk of permanent hearing loss with these interventions must be reviewed with the patient. In Ménière's syndrome, symptomatic treatment and intervention for the underlying cause are warranted.

Discussion Sources

http://www.merck.com/mmpe/sec08/ch086/ch086f.html, Merck Manual online: Ear, nose, throat, and dental disorders, accessed 9/4/09.
Li J. http://www.emedicine.com/ent/TOPIC232.HTM, eMedicine: Inner ear, Meniere disease, medical treatment, accessed 9/4/09.

QUESTIONS

30. You inspect the oral cavity of a 69-year-old man who has a 100–pack-year cigarette smoking history. You find a lesion suspicious for malignancy and describe it as:
    A. raised, red, and painful.
    B. a denuded patch with a removable white coating.
    C. an ulcerated lesion with indurated margins.
    D. a vesicular-form lesion with macerated margins.

31. A firm, painless, relatively fixed submandibular node would most likely be seen in the diagnosis of:
    A. herpes simplex.
    B. acute otitis media (AOM).
    C. bacterial pharyngitis.
    D. oral cancer.

ANSWERS

30. C   31. D

DISCUSSION

Risk factors for oral cancer include advancing age and tobacco and alcohol abuse. More recently, chronic infection with human papillomavirus type 16 has been appreciated as an oral cancer risk factor. Most commonly squamous cell carcinoma, an oral cancer is usually characterized by a relatively painless, firm ulceration or raised lesion. The lymphadenopathy associated with oral cancer consists of immobile nodes that are nontender when palpated. Self-limiting oral lesions, such as herpes simplex, oral candidiasis, and aphthous stomatitis, usually cause discomfort. With infection, the associated lymphadenopathy that follows drainage tracts is characterized by tenderness and mobility.

Discussion Sources

http://www.merck.com/mmpe/sec08/ch086/ch086f.html, Merck Manual online: Ear, nose, throat, and dental disorders, accessed 9/5/09.
http://www.oralcancerfoundation.org/facts, The Oral Cancer Foundation: Oral cancer facts, accessed 9/5/09.

QUESTIONS

32. A 45-year-old man presents with otitis externa. Likely causative pathogens include all of the following except:
    A. fungal agents.
    B. *P. aeruginosa.*
    C. *S. aureus.*
    D. *M. catarrhalis.*

33. Appropriate oral antimicrobial therapy for otitis externa with an accompanying facial cellulitis suitable for outpatient therapy includes a course of a:
    A. macrolide.
    B. cephalosporin.
    C. fluoroquinolone.
    D. penicillin.

34. Physical examination findings in otitis externa include:

   A. tympanic membrane immobility.
   B. increased ear pain with tragus palpation.
   C. tympanic membrane erythema.
   D. tympanic membrane bullae.

35. A risk factor for malignant external otitis includes:

   A. the presence of an immunocompromised condition.
   B. age younger than 21 years.
   C. a history of a recent upper respiratory tract infection (URI).
   D. a complicated course of otitis media with effusion.

ANSWERS

32.	D	**33.**	C
34.	B	**35.**	A

DISCUSSION

Risk factors for otitis externa include a history of recent ear canal trauma, usually after vigorous use of a cotton swab or other item to clean the canal, and conditions in which moisture is frequently held in the ear canal, such as with cerumen impaction and frequent swimming. Otitis externa can be caused by numerous pathogens, including various gram-positive organisms and fungi such as *Candida* or *Aspergillus* species. *P. aeruginosa* is the most common causative agent and the most likely organism in refractory otitis externa or accompanying cellulitis; cellulitis is a frequent complication of otitis externa, particularly in the presence of protracted infection or comorbidity, such as diabetes mellitus or immunosuppression.

Clinical presentation includes redness and edema of the ear canal accompanied by purulent or serous discharge and the hallmark finding of pain on tragus palpation or with the application of traction to the pinna. Facial, neck, or auricular cellulitis and unilateral neck lymphadenopathy are noted with complicated infection. When otitis externa is fungal in origin, usually the clinical presentation includes a report of less pain but more itch; ear discharge is usually described as being thicker and white to gray in color.

Malignant or necrosing otitis externa, in which infection invades the deeper soft tissue, is a complication that occurs in patients who are immunocompromised or in those who have received radiotherapy to the skull base; osteomyelitis of the temporal bone is often seen in this rare condition. Presentation includes the usual features of otitis externa and pain disproportionate to clinical findings. MRI or CT to evaluate for osteomyelitis is usually indicated, and surgical débridement is typically needed. Antipseudomonal antimicrobial therapy is usually reserved for severe cases. Parenteral antimicrobial therapy is often warranted for severe disease (see Table 4–2).

Effective topical therapies for otitis externa include otic suspension of an antimicrobial, such as an aminoglycoside, fluoroquinolone, or neomycin, with or without hydrocortisone solution and the combination of 2% nonaqueous acetic acid and hydrocortisone (VoSol HC Otic 2%). When the ear canal is edematous to the point where topical antimicrobial drops cannot be well distributed, an ear wick is usually inserted and left in place for 2 to 3 days. Aural hygiene using gentle suction to remove debris can be helpful; irrigation in the presence of acute infection is usually not advocated. Oral antibiotics should be prescribed in individuals with cellulitis of the face or neck skin, in persons in whom severe edema of the ear canal limits penetration of topical agents, and in immunocompromised persons. If this therapy proves ineffective or in the presence of severe disease, inpatient hospital admission and parenteral antimicrobial therapy is likely indicated.

Discussion Sources

Gilbert D, Moellering R, Eliopoulos G, Chambers H, Saag M. *The Sanford Guide to Antimicrobial Therapy*. 39th ed. Sperryville, VA: Antimicrobial Therapy, Inc; 2009:10.

Waitsman A. http://www.emedicine.com/ped/TOPIC1688.HTM, eMedicine: Otitis externa, accessed 9/5/09.

QUESTIONS

36. Likely causative organisms in AOM include:

   A. certain gram-positive and gram-negative bacteria.
   B. gram-negative bacteria and pathogenic viruses.
   C. rhinovirus and *S. aureus*.
   D. predominantly beta-lactamase–producing organisms.

37. Expected findings in AOM include:

   A. prominent bony landmarks.
   B. tympanic membrane immobility.
   C. itchiness and crackling in the affected ear.
   D. submental lymphadenopathy.

38. A 25-year-old woman has a 3-day history of left ear pain that began after 1 week of URI symptoms. On physical examination, you find that she has AOM. She is allergic to penicillin (use results in a hive-form reaction). The most appropriate antimicrobial option for this patient is:

   A. ciprofloxacin.
   B. clarithromycin.
   C. amoxicillin.
   D. cephalexin.

39. A reasonable treatment option for AOM that is not improved after 3-day therapy with an appropriate dosage of amoxicillin therapy is:

   A. cefuroxime.
   B. erythromycin.
   C. cephalexin.
   D. sulfamethoxazole.

40. Characteristics of *M. catarrhalis* include:

   A. high rate of beta-lactamase production.
   B. antimicrobial resistance resulting from altered protein-binding sites.
   C. often being found in middle ear exudate in recurrent otitis media.
   D. gram-positive organisms.

41. Which of the following is a characteristic of *H. influenzae*?

   A. Newer macrolides are ineffective against the organism.
   B. Its antimicrobial resistance results from altered protein-binding sites within the wall of the bacteria.
   C. Some isolates exhibit antimicrobial resistance via production of beta-lactamase.
   D. This is a gram-positive organism.

42. Which of the following is a characteristic of *S. pneumoniae*?

   A. mechanism of antimicrobial resistance primarily due to the production of beta-lactamase
   B. mechanism of antimicrobial resistance usually via altered protein-binding sites held within the microbe's cell
   C. organisms most commonly isolated from mucoid middle ear effusion
   D. gram-negative organisms

43. Clindamycin is most effective against which of the following organisms?

   A. *S. pneumoniae*
   B. *H. influenzae*
   C. *M. catarrhalis*
   D. Adenovirus

44. Which of the following is absent in otitis media with effusion?

   A. fluid in the middle ear
   B. otalgia
   C. fever
   D. itch

45. Treatment of otitis media with effusion usually includes:

   A. symptomatic treatment.
   B. antimicrobial therapy.
   C. an antihistamine.
   D. a mucolytic.

ANSWERS

36.	A	**37.**	B	**38.**	B
39.	A	**40.**	A	**41.**	C
42.	B	**43.**	A	**44.**	C
45.	A				

DISCUSSION

Although often considered a disease limited to childhood, AOM ♂ still ranks among the most frequent diagnoses noted in adult office visits. *S. pneumoniae, H. influenzae, M. catarrhalis,* and various viruses contribute to the infectious and inflammatory process of the middle ear. Eustachian tube dysfunction usually precedes the development of AOM, allowing negative pressure to be generated in the middle ear; this negative pressure enables pharyngeal pathogens to be aspirated into the middle ear, and the infection takes hold. Avoiding conditions that can cause eustachian tube dysfunction, such as upper respiratory infection, untreated or undertreated allergic rhinitis, tobacco use, and exposure to air pollution, can lead to a reduction in the occurrence of AOM.

S. pneumoniae causes 40% to 50% of AOM. It is the least likely of the three major causative bacteria to resolve without antimicrobial intervention, and infection with this organism usually causes the most significant otitis media symptoms. Numerous isolates of this organism exhibit resistance to many standard, well-tolerated, inexpensive antibiotic agents, including amoxicillin, certain cephalosporins, and the macrolides (azithromycin, clarithromycin, erythromycin). The mechanism of resistance is an alteration of intracellular protein-binding sites, which can typically be overcome by using higher doses of amoxicillin and select cephalosporins. A major risk factor for infection with drug-resistant *S. pneumoniae* is recent systemic antimicrobial use.

H. influenzae and *M. catarrhalis* are gram-negative organisms capable of producing beta-lactamase, an enzyme that cleaves the beta-lactam ring found in the penicillin, amoxicillin, and ampicillin molecule, rendering these antibiotics ineffective against the pathogen. These two organisms have high rates of spontaneous resolution in AOM (50% and 90%); however, *H. influenzae* is the organism most commonly isolated from mucoid and serous middle ear effusion. Beta-lactamase–producing organisms likely contribute less to AOM treatment failure than does prescribing inadequate dosages of amoxicillin needed to eradicate drug-resistant *S. pneumoniae*. Common viral agents that cause AOM include human rhinovirus, respiratory syncytial virus, and coronavirus. AOM caused by these viral agents usually resolves in 7 to 10 days with supportive care alone.

Appropriate assessment is critical for arriving at the diagnosis of AOM. The tympanic membrane may be retracted or bulging and is typically reddened with loss of translucency and mobility on insufflation. With recovery, tympanic membrane mobility returns in about 1 to 2 weeks, but middle ear effusion usually persists for 4 to 6 weeks. Itching and crackling in the ear is common in patients with AOM and in patients with serous otitis, also known as otitis media with effusion. The bony landmarks usually appear prominent when the tympanic membrane is retracted, a condition usually seen with eustachian tube dysfunction, which may not be present in patients with AOM. The submental node is not in the drainage tract of the middle ear and is not enlarged in patients with AOM. Rather, the nodes within the anterior cervical chain on the ipsilateral side of the infection are often enlarged and painful.

Otalgia, fever, and other symptoms that persist beyond 3 days of therapy usually indicate treatment failure. Repeat evaluation is in order. The organisms that cause recurrent otitis media are the same ones that cause acute disease. If amoxicillin fails to eradicate the infection, a drug-resistant pathogen, such as drug-resistant *S. pneumoniae,* might be the cause. In addition, the contribution of a beta-lactamase–producing organism, such as *H. influenzae* or *M. catarrhalis,* should be considered. If treatment failure occurs, the choice of a new antimicrobial depends on the initial medication that failed to eradicate the infection and patterns of recent antimicrobial use.

Discussion Sources

Cook K. http://www.emedicine.com/emerg/TOPIC351.HTM, eMedicine: Otitis media, accessed 9/5/09.

Gilbert D, Moellering R, Eliopoulos G, Chambers H, Saag M. *The Sanford Guide to Antimicrobial Therapy.* 39th ed. Sperryville, VA: Antimicrobial Therapy, Inc; 2009:10.

QUESTIONS

46. An 18-year-old woman has a chief complaint of a "sore throat and swollen glands" for the past 3 days. Her physical examination includes a temperature of 101°F (38.3°C), exudative pharyngitis, and tender anterior cervical lymphadenopathy. Right and left upper quadrant abdominal tenderness is absent. The most likely diagnosis is:

   A. *Streptococcus pyogenes* pharyngitis.
   B. infectious mononucleosis.
   C. viral pharyngitis.
   D. Vincent angina.

47. Treatment options for streptococcal pharyngitis for a patient with penicillin allergy include all of the following except:

   A. azithromycin.
   B. trimethoprim-sulfamethoxazole.
   C. clarithromycin.
   D. erythromycin.

48. You are seeing a 25-year-old man with *S. pyogenes* pharyngitis. He asks if he can get a "shot of penicillin" for therapy. You consider the following when counseling about the use of intramuscular penicillin:

   A. There is nearly a 100% cure rate in streptococcal pharyngitis when it is used.
   B. Treatment failure rates approach 20%.
   C. It is the preferred agent in treating group G streptococcal infection.
   D. Injectable penicillin has a superior spectrum of antimicrobial coverage compared with the oral version of the drug.

49. With regard to pharyngitis caused by group C streptococci, the NP considers that:

   A. potential complications include glomerulonephritis.
   B. appropriate antimicrobial therapy helps to facilitate more rapid resolution of symptoms.
   C. infection with these organisms carries a significant risk of subsequent rheumatic fever.
   D. acute infectious hepatitis can occur if not treated with an appropriate antimicrobial.

50. Clinical presentation of peritonsillar abscess includes:

   A. occipital lymphadenopathy.
   B. congested cough.
   C. muffled "hot potato" voice.
   D. abdominal pain.

51. Patients with strep throat can be cleared to return to work or school after ___ hours of antimicrobial therapy.

   A. 12
   B. 24
   C. 36
   D. 48

52. When advising a patient with scarlet fever, the NP considers that:

   A. there is increased risk for poststreptococcal glomerulonephritis.
   B. the rash often peels during recovery.
   C. an injectable cephalosporin is the preferred treatment option.
   D. throat culture is usually negative for group A streptococci.

53. The incubation period for *S. pyogenes* is usually:

   A. 1 to 3 days.
   B. 3 to 5 days.
   C. 6 to 9 days.
   D. 10 to 13 days.

54. The incubation period for *M. pneumoniae* is usually:

    A. less than 1 week.

    B. 1 week.

    C. 2 weeks.

    D. 3 weeks.

55. All of the following are common causes of penicillin treatment failure in streptococcal pharyngitis except:

    A. infection with a beta-lactamase–producing *Streptococcus* strain.

    B. failure to initiate or complete the antimicrobial course.

    C. concomitant infection or carriage with a beta-lactamase–producing organism.

    D. inadequate penicillin dosage.

ANSWERS

46.	A	**47.**	B	**48.**	B
49.	B	**50.**	C	**51.**	B
52.	B	**53.**	B	**54.**	D
55.	A				

DISCUSSION

S. pyogenes, also known as group A beta-hemolytic streptococcus, is the causative pathogen in 15% to 40% of sore throats in school-aged children, but is less common in children younger than 3 years and in teenagers and adults. The organism is transmitted primarily via saliva and droplet contact. The incubation period lasts an average of 3 to 5 days, but can be up to 3 months. Clinical presentation of exudative pharyngitis caused by *S. pyogenes* includes complaints of sore throat and fever, and evidence of large, beefy tonsils, usually covered with exudate; palatial petechiae; and anterior cervical lymphadenopathy. Communicability gradually decreases over several weeks in untreated patients. Patients are no longer contagious within 24 hours of initiation of appropriate antimicrobial therapy. Asymptomatic nasopharyngeal carriage is common.

S. pyogenes is not the sole cause of bacterial exudative pharyngitis. Another causative pathogen implicated is *Mycoplasma pneumoniae.* Infection with this organism is uncommon in children 5 years or younger and is most often seen in teenagers and younger adults. Clinical presentation includes inflammatory exudate, pharyngeal edema and erythema, cervical lymphadenopathy, and tonsillar enlargement. Because this organism is also a cause of acute bronchitis, the person with *M. pneumoniae* pharyngitis often has a bothersome dry cough; rapid streptococcal screen and standard throat culture fail to reveal the presence of this organism and yield negative results. The incubation period

for *M. pneumoniae* is approximately 3 weeks, and it is usually contracted via cough and respiratory droplet. Clinical findings most often associated with viral pharyngitis include cough, nasal discharge, hoarseness, pharyngeal ulcerations, conjunctival inflammation, and diarrhea. Groups C and G streptococci cause pharyngitis, but infection with these organisms carries minimal risk for rheumatic fever or glomerulonephritis. The infection and its resulting symptoms clear without antimicrobial therapy, but taking an appropriate antimicrobial helps minimize symptoms.

Complications of bacterial pharyngitis include peritonsillar abscess, rheumatic fever, and acute glomerulonephritis. Clinical presentation of peritonsillar abscess includes progressively worsening sore throat, often worse on one side; trismus (inability or difficulty in opening the mouth); drooling; a muffled, "hot potato" voice with an erythematous, swollen tonsil with contralateral uvular deviation; and cervical lymphadenopathy. Because airway compromise is a potentially life-threatening consequence of peritonsillar abscess, ultrasonography or CT of the affected region should be promptly obtained to confirm the diagnosis. Treatment with appropriate antimicrobial therapy, needle aspiration, and airway maintenance must be initiated promptly. Antimicrobial therapy initiated early in the course of acute pharyngitis minimizes peritonsillar abscess risk.

Rheumatic fever is usually caused by *S. pyogenes* serotypes 1, 3, 5, 6, 14, 18, 19, and 24; on average, onset of symptoms of carditis and arthritis begins about 19 days (range 7 to 35 days) after the onset of sore throat symptoms. Antimicrobial treatment is helpful in minimizing rheumatic fever risk. Acute glomerulonephritis is also a complication of *S. pyogenes,* usually serotypes 1, 3, 4, 12, and 25 when associated with pharyngitis and serotypes 2, 4, 9, 55, 57, 59, and 60 when associated with skin infection. Onset of glomerulonephritis symptoms is usually 1 to 3 weeks after pharyngeal or skin infection. Although poststreptococcal glomerulonephritis is usually a self-limiting condition, patients can develop renal scarring with chronic proteinuria or hematuria. Antimicrobial therapy does not minimize glomerulonephritis risk. Infrequently seen but potentially purulent complications of streptococcal pharyngitis include otitis media, sinusitis, peritonsillar and retropharyngeal abscess, and suppurative cervical adenitis.

Scarlet fever is the clinical condition seen when a scarlatiniform rash with a fine sandpaper-like texture erupts during streptococcal pharyngitis, usually on the second day of illness. The rash starts on the trunk and spreads widely, usually sparing the palms and soles, and usually peels during recovery. Treatment of scarlet fever is identical to treatment of streptococcal pharyngitis and carries no increased risk of complications or sequelae.

A positive throat culture for *Streptococcus pyogenes* is considered the diagnostic standard in streptococcal pharyngitis. A potential drawback is that a positive result does not distinguish between acute viral pharyngitis with group A streptococcus carriage and acute streptococcal pharyngitis. Despite this, all patients with a positive throat culture should be treated with an appropriate antimicrobial. Rapid antigen detection tests detect the presence of the group A streptococcus carbohydrate antigen and can be completed in minutes, but with lower sensitivity and specificity than standard throat culture. As a result, many authorities advocate treating in the presence of a positive rapid streptococcal screen and following up negative studies with a throat culture in a patient in whom there is a high index of suspicion. If a rapid streptococcal test result is positive, antimicrobial treatment should be initiated immediately.

If a throat culture is performed, the question is raised as to whether treatment should be initiated while results are awaited or when a positive throat culture is noted. In the former, some patients need to be notified of the need to discontinue antimicrobial therapy if the culture results are negative; some unneeded antibiotic would have been consumed, potentially contributing to the development of resistant pathogens. In the latter case, treatment for patients with positive cultures is delayed by 2 days. This delay poses little risk in an otherwise well person.

In the treatment of bacterial pharyngitis caused by *S. pyogenes,* penicillin remains highly effective. When the total daily dosage is given in equally divided twice-daily doses, treatment outcomes are equivalent to regimens of three or four times daily with significantly improved adherence. A single dose of injectable penicillin given intramuscularly offers a one-time treatment option. Limitations include increased risk of serious reaction with penicillin allergy and a treatment failure rate similar to that of a completed course of oral therapy. Of group A beta-hemolytic streptococcus isolates, 35% are resistant to macrolides or clindamycin, so these drugs should be used only when a patient has a penicillin allergy. Advice on the use of symptomatic treatment with salt-water gargles, throat lozenges, and analgesics should also be given.

When penicillin therapy fails, it is seldom because of a resistant *S. pyogenes* strain. Rather, oropharyngeal carriage with a beta-lactamase–producing organism, such as *H. influenzae,* is often the problem; the presence of beta-lactamase renders the penicillin ineffective. Treatment with an antimicrobial stable in the presence of beta-lactamase, such as amoxicillin-clavulanate, a cephalosporin, or macrolide, is likely to be effective. If the streptococcal test result is negative, and the patient continues to have symptoms, infection with *M. pneumoniae* or *Chlamydophila* (*Chlamydia*) *pneumoniae* should be considered, particularly if cough is present. A macrolide or fluoroquinolone should be prescribed because beta-lactams (penicillins, cephalosporins) are less effective.

The treatment of *S. pyogenes* carriage, defined as a positive throat culture in an individual who has no symptoms, warrants mention. Antimicrobial therapy for *S. pyogenes* carriage is indicated only when an outbreak of rheumatic fever or glomerulonephritis is in process, or when there is an outbreak of streptococcal pharyngitis in a closed or semiclosed environment, such as a correctional facility or college dormitory. First-line therapy includes treatment with clindamycin or amoxicillin with clavulanate; rifampin with penicillin can also be used.

Discussion Sources

Fitzgerald MA. Pharyngitis: evaluation and treatment issues. *Nurse Pract.* 2008.

Gilbert D, Moellering R, Eliopoulos G, Chambers H, Saag M. *The Sanford Guide to Antimicrobial Therapy.* 39th ed. Sperryville, VA: Antimicrobial Therapy, Inc; 2009:45–46.

University of Michigan Health System: Pharyngitis. Ann Arbor, MI: University of Michigan Health System; 2006. http://www.guideline.gov/summary/summary.aspx?doc_id=10630&nbr=5567, accessed 9/4/09.

QUESTIONS

56. A 25-year-old woman who has seasonal allergic rhinitis likes to spend time outdoors. She asks you when the pollen count is likely to be the lowest. You respond:

    A. "Early in the morning."
    B. "During breezy times of the day."
    C. "After a rain shower."
    D. "When the sky is overcast."

57. You prescribe nasal corticosteroid spray for a patient with allergic rhinitis. What is the anticipated onset of symptom relief with its use?

    A. immediately with the first spray
    B. 1 to 2 days
    C. a few days to a week
    D. 2 or more weeks

58. Which of the following medications is most appropriate for allergic rhinitis therapy in an acutely symptomatic 24-year-old machine operator?

    A. nasal cromolyn
    B. diphenhydramine
    C. flunisolide nasal spray
    D. loratadine

59. Antihistamines work primarily through:

    A. vasoconstriction.
    B. action on the histamine-1 (H_1) receptor sites.
    C. inflammatory mediation.
    D. peripheral vasodilation.

60. Decongestants work primarily through:

    A. vasoconstriction.
    B. action on the H_1 receptor sites.
    C. inflammatory mediation.
    D. peripheral vasodilation.

61. Which of the following medications affords the best relief of acute nasal itch?

   A. anticholinergic nasal spray
   B. oral decongestant
   C. corticosteroid nasal spray
   D. oral antihistamine

62. According to the Allergic Rhinitis and Its Effects on Asthma (ARIA) treatment guidelines, which of the following medications affords the best relief of acute nasal congestion?

   A. anticholinergic nasal spray
   B. decongestant nasal spray
   C. corticosteroid nasal spray
   D. oral antihistamine

63. According to the ARIA treatment guidelines, which of the following medications affords the least control of rhinorrhea associated with allergic rhinitis?

   A. anticholinergic nasal spray
   B. antihistamine nasal spray
   C. corticosteroid nasal spray
   D. cromolyn nasal spray

64. Ipratropium bromide (Atrovent) helps control nasal secretions through:

   A. antihistaminic action.
   B. anticholinergic effect.
   C. vasodilation.
   D. vasoconstriction.

65. Oral decongestant use should be discouraged in patients with:

   A. allergic rhinitis.
   B. migraine headache.
   C. cardiovascular disease.
   D. chronic bronchitis.

66. Cromolyn's mechanism of action is as a/an:

   A. anti–immunoglobulin E antibody.
   B. vasoconstrictor.
   C. mast cell stabilizer.
   D. leukotriene modifier.

67. In the treatment of allergic rhinitis, leukotriene modifiers should be used as:

   A. an agent to relieve nasal itch.
   B. an inflammatory inhibitor.
   C. a rescue drug.
   D. an intervention in acute inflammation.

68. According to the Global Resources in Allergy (GLORIA) guidelines, which of the following is recommended for intervention in persistent allergic conjunctivitis?

   A. topical mast cell stabilizer with a topical antihistamine
   B. ocular decongestant
   C. topical nonsteroidal anti-inflammatory drug
   D. topical corticosteroid

69. Allergy immunotherapy is most successful in controlling allergies caused by:

   A. dust mites.
   B. molds.
   C. animal dander.
   D. air pollution.

ANSWERS

56.	C	57.	C	58.	D
59.	B	60.	A	61.	D
62.	B	63.	D	64.	B
65.	C	66.	C	67.	B
68.	A	69.	A		

DISCUSSION

The most important component of allergic rhinitis and allergic conjunctivitis ♂ therapy is avoidance of the allergen. In seasonal allergic rhinitis, pollens are often triggers. Pollen counts are generally the highest early in the morning because these substances are released during the night. After a rain shower, the air is relatively cleansed of the offending agent.

Because the mechanism of action of corticosteroid nasal spray in allergic rhinitis therapy is prevention of production of inflammatory substances, corticosteroid and mast cell stabilizer nasal sprays are effective at preventing, but not acutely controlling, symptoms of allergic rhinitis. At least a few days to 1 week of use is needed before symptom relief is achieved. Antihistamines prevent action of formed histamine, a potent inflammatory mediator, and can be used to control acute allergic symptoms. A nonsedating second-generation antihistamine such as loratadine (Claritin) is the best choice for active adults. Diphenhydramine (Benadryl) is an example of a rapidly acting, sedating, first-generation antihistamine. All antihistamines work by blocking H_1 receptor sites. Decongestants act as vasoconstrictors, opening edematous nasal passages and relieving congestion.

The person with allergic rhinitis should also be evaluated for allergic conjunctivitis. Often, the nasal symptoms are more distressing, and the patient simply fails to mention that the eyes often itch and tear. The inflammatory mediator–filled tears from allergic conjunctivitis drain into the nose, making allergic rhinitis symptoms significantly worse. Treatment of allergic conjunctivitis includes allergen avoidance and use of products that help prevent the formation of inflammatory mediators, such as ophthalmic mast cell stabilizers and antihistamines. Oral antihistamines can help with symptom management (Tables 4–4 and 4–5 and Figs. 4–2 and 4–3).

Discussion Sources

Allergic Rhinitis and Its Impact on Asthma (ARIA) At-a-glance Pocket Guidelines. 1st ed. http://www.ga2len.net//files_new/filesPublic/Educ_ARIA_Glance_2007FINALVERSION.pdf, accessed 9/5/09.

World Allergy Organization: http://www.worldallergy.org/educational_programs/gloria/us/materials.php, Allergic conjunctivitis 2007, accessed 9/5/09.

World Allergy Organization: http://www.worldallergy.org/educational_programs/gloria/us/materials.php, Allergic rhinitis 2007, 9/5/09.

QUESTIONS

70. Which of the following findings is most consistent with the diagnosis of acute bacterial rhinosinusitis (ABRS)?

    A. upper respiratory tract infections persisting beyond 7 to 10 days or worsening after 5 to 7 days
    B. mild midfacial fullness and tenderness
    C. preauricular lymphadenopathy
    D. marked eyelid edema

71. The most common causative bacterial pathogen in ABRS is:

    A. *M. pneumoniae.*
    B. *S. pneumoniae.*
    C. *M. catarrhalis.*
    D. *H. influenzae.*

TABLE 4–4
Allergic Conjunctivitis Treatment

Nondrug therapies for all classifications	• Nondrug therapies • Avoidance of allergen • Cool compresses • Preservative-free artificial tears • Sunglasses to ameliorate photosensitivity, and possibly provide a degree of barrier protection against air-borne allergens

For intermittent, seasonal allergic conjunctivitis	• Controller therapy with
	  • Topical antihistamine or topical cromolyn *or*
	  • Topical antihistamine with mast cell stabilizer *or*
	  • Topical antihistamine with vasoconstrictor *or*
	  • Topical NSAID
	• If inadequate control for intermittent, seasonal
	  • Oral antihistamine

Specific allergen immunotherapy (allergen vaccination)	• Helpful in managing persistent allergic rhinitis and conjunctivitis • Of value in patients with multiorgan symptoms of IgE-mediated allergic sensitization • Risk-to-benefit ratio must be considered in all cases • Highly effective in selected patients • Evaluation and treatment must be made by a clinician with background in allergen immunotherapy with facilities to treat anaphylaxis

OTC and older pharmacotherapies	• Can be helpful, but should not be overused or abused. These products generally treat the presenting problem (eye redness or itch), but do not fully address the underlying problem (allergy)
	  • Ocular vasoconstrictors, helpful at reducing eye redness, but not recommended for regular use. OTC products are often combined with an antihistamine
	  • Topical NSAID such as ketorolac helpful in reducing ocular itch and redness

Topical ocular corticosteroids	• Topical ocular corticosteroids should be prescribed and monitored only by a suitably qualified clinician such as specialist in allergy or ophthalmology, and only in the presence of severe allergic ocular disease for short-term use • Prolonged use can lead to secondary bacterial infection, glaucoma, and cataracts. With short-term use, increased risk for ocular viral or fungal infection

Source: www.worldallergy.org/gloria, GLORIA guidelines for the treatment of allergic rhinitis and allergic conjunctivitis (2007 Update), accessed 9/5/09.

TABLE 4–5

Medications Used in the Treatment of Allergic Rhinitis

Therapeutic Goal	Intervention	Comment
Controller therapy to prevent formation of inflammatory mediators	• Corticosteroid nasal spray (beclomethasone [Beconase], fluticasone [Flonase], others) • Leukotriene modifiers (montelukast [Singulair], zafirlukast [Accolate]) • Mast cell stabilizer (intranasal and optic cromolyn [NasalCrom])	• Controller therapy usually needs to be used for a few days to 2 weeks before maximum effect noted. Little effect on acute symptoms
Rescue therapy by inactivating formed inflammatory mediators	• Oral antihistamines (first-generation [chlorpheniramine, diphenhydramine, others], second-generation (loratadine, cetirizine, fexofenadine, levocetirizine, others) • Antihistamine nasal spray (azelastine [Astelin] nasal spray) • Antihistamine optic drops (ketotifen [Zaditor] optic drops) • Short-term oral corticosteroids if needed for severe allergic symptoms	• Using only antihistamine rescue therapy usually not as effective on overall disease control as consistent use of controller therapy with rescue therapy as an adjunct
Rescue therapy and symptom relief by minimizing nasal discharge	• Anticholinergic nasal spray (Ipratropium bromide [Atrovent]) • Antihistamine nasal spray (Astelin, others)	• Helpful adjuncts as part of rescue therapy for patient with bothersome profuse nasal discharge
Rescue therapy and symptom relief by minimizing nasal congestion	Oral and nasal decongestants (alpha-adrenergic agonists such as pseudoephedrine [Sudafed])	• Potential for vasoconstriction and increased blood pressure and heart rate. Avoid or use with caution in hypertension, cardiovascular disease

ARIA Classification

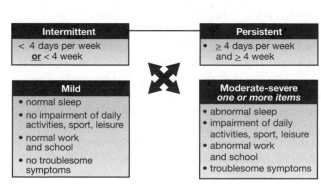

symptoms reported prior to treament

Figure 4–2 ARIA classification. *(Source: Bousquet J, Van Cauwenberge P, Khaltaev N. Allergic rhinitis and its impact on asthma. J Allergy Clin Immunol. 2001;108 [Suppl]:S147–S334.)*

Treatment of allergic rhinitis: ARIA Guidelines

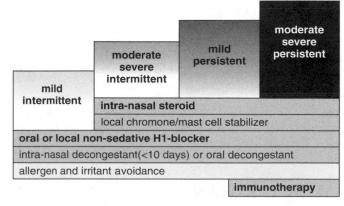

Figure 4–3 Treatment of allergic rhinitis according to ARIA guidelines. *(Source:http://www.whiar.org/docs/ARIA_PG_08_View_WM.pdf, ARIA Workshop Report: management of allergic rhinitis and its impact on asthma: global primary care education, accessed 9/5/09.)*

72. Which of the following is inconsistent with the clinical presentation of ABRS?

A. nasal congestion responsive to decongestant use
B. maxillary toothache
C. colored nasal discharge
D. antecedent event such as acute upper respiratory tract infection or allergic rhinitis

73. Which of the following is a first-line therapy for the treatment of ABRS in an adult with no recent antimicrobial use?

A. amoxicillin
B. trimethoprim-sulfamethoxazole
C. clarithromycin
D. levofloxacin

74. Which of the following represents a therapeutic option for ABRS in a patient with no recent antimicrobial care with treatment failure after 72 hours of appropriate-dose first-line antimicrobial therapy?

A. clindamycin
B. clarithromycin
C. ofloxacin
D. high-dose amoxicillin with clavulanate

75. A 34-year-old man with penicillin allergy presents with ABRS. Three weeks ago, he was treated with doxycycline for "bronchitis." You now prescribe:

A. clarithromycin.
B. levofloxacin.
C. cephalexin.
D. amoxicillin.

76. The most appropriate pharmacologic intervention for treating ABRS in a 45-year-old person who is moderately ill with the condition is:

A. erythromycin.
B. high-dose amoxicillin with clavulanate.
C. cephalexin.
D. ciprofloxacin.

ANSWERS

70.	A	71.	B	72.	A
73.	A	74.	D	75.	B
76.	B				

DISCUSSION

ABRS is a clinical condition resulting from inflammation of the lining of the membranes of the paranasal sinuses caused by bacterial infection. Risk factors include any condition that alters the normal cleansing mechanism of the sinuses, including viral infection, allergies, tobacco use, and abnormalities in sinus structure. Inhaled tobacco use disturbs normal sinus mucociliary action and drainage, causing secretions to pool, and increases the risk of superimposed bacterial infection. In addition, viral URI and poorly controlled allergic rhinitis cause similar dysfunction, increasing ABRS risk. The observation of purulent discharge from one of the nasal turbinates is a highly sensitive finding in ABRS. Midfacial fullness is common in patients with uncomplicated URI, and anterior cervical lymphadenopathy is often found in many infectious and inflammatory conditions involving the head and pharynx. Marked eyelid edema is found only when the infection has extended beyond the sinuses and an orbital cellulitis has formed, a potentially life-threatening complication of ABRS.

Because ABRS is a clinical diagnosis based on patient presentation, with findings also reported in patients with a viral URI, the problem arises as to how to differentiate these two common conditions. The Sinus and Allergy Health Partnership (SAHP) guidelines recommend that the diagnosis of ABRS be considered only in patients in whom the URI-like symptoms, such as facial fullness, cough, and nasal discharge, either persist for at least 10 days or worsen after 5 to 7 days because viral infection is usually resolved or significantly improved before these time parameters.

S. pneumoniae is the causative organism in most ABRS; this pathogen is also the least likely of the three major causative bacteria to resolve without antimicrobial intervention, and it causes the most significant symptoms. This organism exhibits resistance to numerous antibiotic agents, including lower dose amoxicillin, certain cephalosporins, and macrolides. The mechanism of resistance is alterations of intracellular protein-binding sites, which can typically be overcome by using higher doses of amoxicillin, certain cephalosporins, and respiratory fluoroquinolones (levofloxacin [Levaquin] or moxifloxacin [Avelox]). Recent antimicrobial use is the major risk for infection with drug-resistant *S. pneumoniae*.

H. influenzae and *M. catarrhalis* are gram-negative organisms capable of producing beta-lactamase; the presence of this enzyme renders the penicillins ineffective. Although these two organisms have relatively high rates of spontaneous resolution without antimicrobial intervention in AOM, infections caused by these pathogens seldom resolve without antimicrobial therapy in ABRS. Empirical antimicrobial therapy in ABRS should be aimed at choosing an agent with significant activity against gram-positive (*S. pneumoniae*) and gram-negative organisms (*H. influenzae, M. catarrhalis*), with consideration for drug-resistant *S. pneumoniae* risk and possible need for stability in the presence of beta-lactamase. If there is treatment failure, the choice of a new antimicrobial depends on the initial medication that failed to eradicate the infection and patterns of recent antimicrobial use (Table 4–6). Intervention in underlying contributory causes, such as treating allergic rhinitis and encouraging the cessation of tobacco use, is crucial to treatment success.

TABLE 4–6

Sinus and Allergy Health Partnership Treatment Guidelines for Empiric Antimicrobial Therapy in ABRS

Patient Characteristics	Initial Therapy	No Improvement or Worsening After 72 Hours
Adults with mild disease and no prior antimicrobial use in the past 4–6 weeks • Need antimicrobial activity against *S. pneumoniae* (likely low risk DRSP), *H. influenzae*, *M. catarrhalis* (consider beta-lactamase production	• Amoxicillin (1.5–4 g/day) *or* • Amoxicillin/clavulanate (Augmentin) (1.75–4 g/ 250 mg/day) *or* • Cefpodoxime (Vantin), cefuroxime (Ceftin), or cefdinir (Omnicef)	• HD amoxicillin/clavulanate (4 g/day) *or* • Respiratory fluoro-quinolone such as lev-ofloxacin (Levaquin) or moxifloxacin (Avelox)
Adults with mild disease and beta-lactam allergy and no prior antimicrobial use in the past 4–6 weeks) • Avoid beta-lactams (penicillins, cephalosporins) • Need antimicrobial activity against *S. pneumoniae* (likely low-risk DRSP), *H. influenzae*, *M. catarrhalis* (consider beta-lactamase production)	• TMP/SMX (Bactrim) *or* • Doxycycline *or* • Azithromycin (Zithromax), clar-ithromycin (Biaxin), erythromycin	• Levofloxacin or moxi-floxacin *or* • Clindamycin with rifampin
Adults with mild disease with a history of prior antimi-crobial use in the past 4–6 weeks *or* Adults with moderate disease with or without prior antimicrobial use • Need antimicrobial activity against *S. pneumoniae* with significant DRSP risk, *H. influenzae*, *M. catarrhalis* (consider beta-lactamase production) • With moderate disease, need antimicrobial with low risk of treatment failure	• Levofloxacin or moxifloxacin *or* • HD amoxicillin/ clavulanate *or* • Ceftriaxone (Rocephin) *or* • Clindamycin with rifampin	Re-evaluate patient • Consider alternate diagno-sis, complication
Adults with mild disease with prior antimicrobial use in past 4–6 weeks and beta-lactam allergy *or* Adults with moderate disease with or without prior antibiotic use and beta-lactam allergy • Avoid beta-lactams (penicillins, cephalosporins) • Need antimicrobial activity against *S. pneumoniae* with significant DRSP risk, *H. influenzae*, *M. catarrhalis* (consider beta-lactamase production) • With moderate disease, need antimicrobial with low risk of treatment failure	• Levofloxacin or moxifloxacin *or* • Clindamycin plus rifampin	Re-evaluate patient • Consider alternate diagno-sis, complication

Sources: Sinus and Allergy Health Partnership Treatment Guidelines. *Otolaryngol Head Neck Surg.* 2004;130:1–45, Gilbert D, Moellering R, Eliopoulos G, Chambers H, Saag M. *The Sanford Guide to Antimicrobial Therapy.* 39th ed. Sperryville, VA: Antimicrobial Therapy, Inc; 2009: 46–47.

Discussion Sources

Antimicrobial treatment guidelines for acute bacterial rhinosinusitis. Sinus and Allergy Health Partnership. *Otolaryngol Head Neck Surg.* 2004;123(1 Pt 2):1–31.

Gilbert D, Moellering R, Eliopoulos G, Chambers H, Saag M. *The Sanford Guide to Antimicrobial Therapy.* 39th ed. Sperryville, VA: Antimicrobial Therapy, Inc; 2009:46–47.

QUESTIONS

77. Which of the following best describes hearing loss associated with presbycusis?

    A. rapidly progressive, often asymmetric, and in all frequencies
    B. slowly progressive, usually symmetric, and predominantly high frequency
    C. variable in progression, usually unilateral, and in the midrange frequencies
    D. primarily conductive and bilateral with slow progress

78. A 78-year-old woman has early bilateral senile cataracts. Which of the following situations would likely pose the greatest difficulty?

    A. reading the newspaper
    B. distinguishing between the primary colors
    C. following extraocular movements
    D. reading road signs while driving

79. Which of the following is consistent with the visual problems associated with presbyopia?

    A. bilateral peripheral vision loss
    B. blurring of near vision
    C. difficulty with distant vision
    D. loss of the central vision field

80. Which of the following is consistent with the visual problems associated with macular degeneration?

    A. peripheral vision loss
    B. blurring of near vision
    C. difficulty with distant vision
    D. loss of the central vision field

81. All of the following are consistent with normal age-related vision changes except:

    A. need for increased illumination.
    B. increasing sensitivity to glare.
    C. washing out of colors.
    D. gradual loss of peripheral vision.

ANSWERS

77.	B	**78.**	D	**79.**	B
80.	D	**81.**	D		

DISCUSSION

Aging is associated with many changes in the senses. Presbycusis is a progressive, symmetric, high-frequency, age-related sensory hearing loss that is likely caused by cochlear deterioration. Speech discrimination is usually the primary problem; an individual with presbycusis often reports the ability to hear another person talking, but has limited ability to understand the content of the speech.

Distance vision poses the greatest problem for individuals with senile cataracts. As the lens becomes more opaque, near vision also deteriorates. Other visual changes of age-related cataracts include loss of ability to distinguish contrasts and progressive dimming of vision. Close vision is usually retained, and there are occasional improvements in reading ability.

Presbyopia refers to age-related vision changes caused by a progressive hardening of the lens. Patients most often complain of close vision problems, usually first manifested by difficulty with reading smaller print. Other normal age-related vision changes include a progressive yellowing of the lens and decreased flexibility of the sclera, in part leading to the perception of washing out of colors, difficulty seeing under low illumination, and increased sensitivity to glare.

Macular degeneration is the most common cause of blindness and vision loss in elderly adults. Vision changes seen in macular degeneration include loss of the central vision field. This disease is seen more often in women of European descent. A history of cigarette smoking and a family history of the disease are often found as well; excessive sun exposure has also been implicated as a risk factor for macular degeneration. The ophthalmological examination reveals hard drusen or yellow deposits in the macular area. Soft drusen can also be seen. These appear larger, paler, and less distinct.

Discussion Source

Kennedy-Malone L, Fletcher K, Plank L. *Management Guidelines for Nurse Practitioners Working with Older Adults.* 2nd ed. Philadelphia, PA: FA Davis; 2004.

5 Chest Disorders

QUESTIONS

1. Which of the following best describes asthma?

    A. intermittent airway inflammation with occasional bronchospasm

    B. a disease of bronchospasm that leads to airway inflammation

    C. chronic airway inflammation with superimposed bronchospasm

    D. relatively fixed airway constriction

2. The patient you are evaluating is having an asthma flare. You have assessed that his condition is appropriate for office treatment. You expect to find the following on physical examination:

    A. tripod posture

    B. inspiratory crackles

    C. increased vocal fremitus

    D. hyperresonance on thoracic percussion

3. A 44-year-old man has a long-standing history of moderate persistent asthma that is normally well controlled by fluticasone with salmeterol (Advair) via metered-dose inhaler, 1 puff twice a day, and the use of albuterol one to two times a week as needed for wheezing. Three days ago, he developed a sore throat, clear nasal discharge, body aches, and a dry cough. In the past 24 hours, he has had intermittent wheezing that necessitated the use of albuterol, 2 puffs every 3 hours, which produced partial relief. Your next most appropriate action is to obtain a:

    A. chest radiograph.

    B. measurement of oxygen saturation (SaO_2).

    C. peak expiratory flow (PEF) measurement.

    D. sputum smear for white blood cells (WBCs).

4. You examine a 24-year-old woman who has an acute asthma flare. She is using budesonide (Pulmicort) and albuterol as directed and continues to have difficulty with coughing and wheezing. Her PEF is 55% of personal best. Her medication regimen should be adjusted to include:

    A. theophylline.

    B. salmeterol (Serevent).

    C. prednisone.

    D. montelukast (Singulair).

5. Which of the following is most likely to appear on a chest radiograph of a person during an acute asthma attack?

    A. hyperinflation

    B. atelectasis

    C. consolidation

    D. Kerley B signs

6. A 36-year-old man with asthma also needs antihypertensive therapy. Which of the following products should you avoid prescribing?

    A. hydrochlorothiazide

    B. propranolol

    C. nicardipine

    D. enalapril

7. Which of the following is inconsistent with the clinical presentation of poorly controlled asthma?

    A. a troublesome nocturnal cough at least 2 nights per week

    B. need for albuterol to relieve shortness of breath at least twice a week

    C. morning sputum production

    D. patient report that asthma is somewhat controlled

8. The cornerstone of moderate persistent asthma drug therapy is the use of:
   A. oral theophylline.
   B. mast cell stabilizers.
   C. short-acting beta$_2$-agonists.
   D. inhaled corticosteroids.

9. Sharon is a 29-year-old woman with moderate intermittent asthma. She is not using prescribed inhaled corticosteroids, but is using albuterol prn to relieve her cough and wheeze with reported satisfactory clinical effect. Currently she uses about 2 albuterol metered-dose inhalers per month and is requesting a prescription refill. You consider that:
   A. albuterol use can continue at this level.
   B. excessive albuterol use is a risk factor for asthma death.
   C. she should also use salmeterol (Serevent) to reduce her albuterol use.
   D. theophylline should be added to her treatment plan.

10. In the treatment of asthma, leukotriene receptor antagonists should be used as:
    A. long-acting bronchodilators.
    B. inflammatory inhibitors.
    C. rescue drugs.
    D. intervention in acute inflammation.

11. According to the National Asthma Education and Prevention Program Expert Panel Report-3 (NAEPP EPR-3) guidelines, which of the following is not a risk for asthma death?
    A. hospitalization or an emergency department visit for asthma in the past month
    B. current use of systemic corticosteroids or recent withdrawal from systemic corticosteroids
    C. difficulty perceiving airflow obstruction or its severity
    D. rural residence

12. An 18-year-old high school senior presents, asking for a letter stating that he should not participate in gym class because he has asthma. The most appropriate response is to:
    A. write the note because gym class participation could trigger asthma symptoms.
    B. excuse him from outdoor activities only to avoid pollen exposure.
    C. remind him that with appropriate asthma care, he should be capable of participating in gym class.
    D. write a note to excuse him from indoor activities only to avoid dust mite exposure.

13. After inhaled corticosteroid or leukotriene modifier therapy is initiated, clinical effects are usually seen:
    A. on the first day of use.
    B. within 1 to 2 weeks.
    C. in about 3 to 4 weeks.
    D. in about 1 to 2 months.

14. Compared with albuterol, levalbuterol (Xopenex) has:
    A. a different mechanism of action.
    B. the ability potentially to provide greater bronchodilation with a lower dose.
    C. an anti-inflammatory effect similar to that of an inhaled corticosteroid.
    D. a contraindication to use in elderly patients.

15. Which of the following is consistent with the NAEPP comment on the use of inhaled corticosteroids (ICS) for a child with asthma?
    A. The potential but small risk of delayed growth with ICS is well balanced by their effectiveness.
    B. ICS should be used only if leukotriene modifiers fail to control asthma.
    C. Permanent growth stunting is consistently noted in children using ICS.
    D. Leukotriene modifiers are equal in therapeutic effect to the use of a long-acting beta$_2$-agonist.

16. A potential adverse effect from ICS use is:
    A. oral candidiasis.
    B. tachycardia.
    C. weight loss.
    D. insomnia.

17. Clinical findings characteristic of asthma include all of the following except:
    A. a recurrent spasmodic cough that is worse at night.
    B. recurrent shortness of breath and chest tightness with exercise.
    C. a congested cough that is worse during the day.
    D. wheezing with and without associated respiratory infections.

18. Which of the following best describes the mechanism of action of short-acting beta$_2$-agonists?
    A. reducer of inflammation
    B. inhibition of secretions
    C. modification of leukotrienes
    D. smooth muscle relaxation

19. Regarding the use of long-acting beta$_2$-agonists (LABAs), which of the following is true?

    A. LABAs enhance the anti-inflammatory action of corticosteroids.
    B. Use of LABAs is associated with a small increase in risk of asthma death.
    C. LABAs reduce asthma exacerbations.
    D. LABAs can be tried before ICS to relieve bronchospasm.

20. Which of the following is the therapeutic objective of using inhaled ipratropium bromide in the treatment of acute asthma exacerbation?

    A. a recommendation for use with short-acting beta$_2$ agonists in the hospital
    B. an increase in vagal tone in the airway
    C. inhibition of muscarinic cholinergic receptors
    D. an increase in salivary and mucous secretions

21. Which of the following is true regarding the use of systemic corticosteroids?

    A. Parenteral therapy is preferred over the oral route.
    B. Tapering down the dosage is required if used for 5 to 7 days as is typical in an asthma flare.
    C. These medications provide action against the formation of various inflammatory mediators.
    D. The adult dose to treat an asthma flare should not exceed the equivalent of prednisone 40 mg daily.

22. Compared with short-acting beta$_2$ agonists, long-acting beta$_2$ agonists:

    A. are recommended as a first-line therapy in mild persistent asthma.
    B. have a significantly different pharmacodynamic profile.
    C. have a rapid onset of action across the drug class.
    D. should be added to therapy only when ICS use does not provide adequate asthma control.

Answer the following questions true or false.

____ 23. Most prescribers are well versed in the relative potency of ICS and prescribe an appropriate dose for the patient's clinical presentation.

____ 24. Approximately 80% of the dose of an ICS is systemically absorbed.

____ 25. Leukotriene modifiers and ICS are interchangeable clinically because both groups of medications have equivalent anti-inflammatory effect.

____ 26. Little systemic absorption of mast cell stabilizers occurs with inhaled or intranasal use.

____ 27. Mast cell stabilizers need to be used generally three or more times per day for approximately 3 weeks before a significant clinical effect is seen.

ANSWERS

1.	C	2.	D	3.	C
4.	C	5.	A	6.	B
7.	C	8.	D	9.	B
10.	B	11.	D	12.	C
13.	B	14.	B	15.	A
16.	A	17.	C.	18.	D
19.	B	20.	C	21.	C
22.	D	23.	F	24.	F
25.	F	26.	T	27.	T

DISCUSSION

Asthma is a common chronic disorder of the airways that is complex and characterized by variable and recurring symptoms, airflow obstruction, bronchial hyperresponsiveness, and underlying inflammation. Although the condition ranks second after allergic rhinitis as the most common chronic respiratory disease in North America, many persons with asthma continue to be undiagnosed and untreated (Table 5–1).

Asthma is a lower airway obstructive disease with clinical findings that are consistent with air trapping (Table 5–2). Wheeze is often considered to be the hallmark of the disease. A decrease in forced expiratory volume at 1 second (FEV$_1$) or peak expiratory flow rate (PEFR) is usually noted before

---

TABLE 5–1

Making the Diagnosis: Is It Asthma?

Is there a history of:
- Recurrent wheezing?
- Recurrent chest tightness?
- Recurrent cough?
- Recurrent difficulty breathing?
- Troublesome cough at night?
- Cough or wheeze after exercise?
- Symptoms worse after exposure to airborne allergens, viral infections, smoke, pollutants, or other irritants?
- Symptoms influenced by menstrual cycle, strong emotions (especially laughing, crying)?

Consider the diagnosis of asthma and perform spirometry if any of these indicators are present. These indicators are not diagnostic by themselves, but the presence of multiple key indicators increases the probability of the diagnosis of asthma. Spirometry is needed to make the diagnosis of asthma

Source: Report of the Expert Panel: http://www.nhlbi.nih.gov/guidelines/asthma/, Guidelines for the diagnosis and management of asthma (EPR-3), accessed 9/12/09.

TABLE 5–2
Clinical Findings in Asthma or Chronic Obstructive Pulmonary Disease Flare

Condition	Physical Examination Findings
Lower airway disease with resulting air trapping as found in asthma or chronic obstructive pulmonary disease flare or poor disease control	Hyperresonance on thoracic percussion
	Decreased tactile fremitus
	Wheeze (expiratory first, inspiratory later)
	Prolonged expiratory phase of forced exhalation
	Low diaphragms
	Increased anterior-posterior diameter
	Reduction in forced expiratory volume at 1 second (FEV_1) or peak expiratory flow rate (early finding)
	Reduction in arterial oxygen saturation (SaO_2) (later finding)

Source: Mangione S. *Physical Diagnosis Secrets*. 2nd ed. St. Louis, MO: Elsevier Health Sciences; 2007.

the onset of other obstructive airway findings, however, such as wheeze; for many individuals with asthma, cough is present as a lower airway obstructive sign, and wheeze is absent or rarely present.

According to the NAEPP EPR-3, the goals of asthma care, with a brief explanation of the rationale for each objective, are as follows:

- *Minimal or, ideally, no chronic symptoms such as cough and wheeze, including nocturnal symptoms*
  - Asthma symptoms typically follow a circadian rhythm, in which bronchospasm is worse during the night sleep hours. A marker of effective airway inflammation control is minimal nocturnal symptoms.
- *Few to no emergency department visits or emergency physician visits, and no hospitalizations for asthma-related problems*
  - When airway inflammatory control is poor, patients with asthma typically use emergency services for treatment of frequent acute flares. With appropriate asthma instruction to help the patient manage acute and chronic airway inflammation and its resulting symptoms, emergency visits and hospitalizations can be minimized or eliminated.
- *Minimize airway remodeling*
  - In the past, the airway restriction noted in asthma, no matter how severe, was believed to be fully reversible.

The current concept is that chronic and recurrent airway inflammation can lead to progressive loss of lung function.

- *Minimal (ideally, no) use of prn short-acting beta₂ agonist (two or fewer days per week with beta₂ agonist use aside from use before sports participation)*
  - Asthma is a disease with a core problem of airway inflammation with subsequent superimposed bronchospasm. The need for short-acting beta₂ agonist use as a rescue drug should be viewed as failure to provide adequate airway inflammatory control. Excessive beta₂ agonist use is a risk factor for asthma death (see Table 5–1).
- *No limitations on activities, including exercise*
  - When airway inflammation control is inadequate, asthma symptoms such as cough or wheeze can accompany or immediately follow physical activity. An individual with well-controlled asthma should be able and encouraged to participate in fitness and leisure activities.

Because of the wide range of asthma medications currently available, the NP, patient, and family can work together to find a lifestyle and treatment regimen that provide optimal care with minimal to few adverse medication effects.

The backbone of mild persistent, moderate persistent, or severe persistent asthma therapy is the use of an inflammatory controller drug (Table 5–3). Numerous medications are approved and used for this purpose, including inhaled corticosteroids (ICS) (e.g., budesonide [Pulmicort], fluticasone [Flovent]), mast cell stabilizers (e.g., nedocromil [Tilade], cromolyn [Intal]), and leukotriene modifiers (e.g., montelukast [Singulair], zafirlukast [Accolate]). Although all these products have anti-inflammatory capability, ICS have proved to be the most effective in preventing airway inflammation and are recognized as the preferred controller drug for all classifications of asthma (Table 5–4; see Table 5–3).

ICS use is also recommended in children with asthma as the preferred anti-inflammatory agent; the potential but small risk of delayed growth with their use is well balanced by the effectiveness of these medications. Use of mast cell stabilizers, although quite safe, is limited by the need for consistent use for many weeks before clinical effectiveness is seen. The clinical effects of an ICS is usually seen within the first 1 to 2 weeks of use; approximately 10% to 15% of the dose of ICS delivered via metered dose inhaler (MDI) is systemically absorbed. Primary care providers are often poorly informed as to the relative potency of a given ICS and prescribe too low a dose for the asthma severity; this is a major issue that potentially limits the effectiveness of ICS (see Table 5–4). Leukotriene modifiers, also known as leukotriene receptor antagonists (e.g., montelukast [Singulair], zafirlukast [Accolate]) are helpful as "add-on" anti-inflammatory medications in patients with moderate persistent or severe persistent asthma when disease control is inadequate with the use of an ICS or as an alternative to ICS use in mild persistent asthma.

The EPR-3 guidelines mention medications that are seldom used in the management of asthma. Zileuton (Zyflo)

TABLE 5–3

Asthma Stages and Treatment for Children ≥12 Years and Adults

Intermittent	Mild Persistent	Moderate Persistent		Severe Persistent	
Step 1	Step 2	Step 3	Step 4	Step 5	Step 6
Preferred SABA prn	*Preferred* Low-dose ICS	*Preferred* Medium-dose ICS	*Preferred* Medium-dose ICS + LABA	*Preferred* High-dose ICS + LABA	*Preferred* High-dose ICS + LABA + oral corticosteroid
	Alternative Mast cell stabilizer (cromolyn, nedrocromil), LTRA, or theophylline	*or* Low-dose ICS + LABA	*Alternative* Medium-dose ICS	*and* Omalizumab use can be considered for patients who have allergies	*and* Consider omalizumab for patients who have allergies
		Alternative Low-dose ICS and LTRA, theophylline, *or* zileuton	*and* LTRA, theophylline, *or* zileuton		

ICS, inhaled corticosteroid; LABA, long-acting beta₂ agonist; LTRA, leukotriene receptor antagonist; SABA, short-acting beta₂ agonist.
Source: NAEPP. http://www.nhlbi.nih.gov/guidelines/asthma/epr3/resource.pdf, accessed 9/10/09..

TABLE 5–4

Estimated Comparative Daily Doses for Inhaled Corticosteroid (ICS) Therapy in Patients 12 Years and Older

	Low Daily Dose	Medium Daily Dose	High Daily Dose
Beclomethasone HFA 40 or 80 mcg/puff	80–240 mcg	>240–480 mcg	>480 mcg
Budesonide DPI 180 mcg/inhalation	180–540 mcg	>540–1080 mcg	>1080 mcg
Flunisolide 250 mcg/puff	500–1000 mcg	1000–2000 mcg	>2000 mcg
Flunisolide HFA 80 mcg/puff	320 mcg	320–640 mcg	>640 mcg
Fluticasone HFA MDI 44, 110, or 220 mcg/puff	88–264 mcg	264–440 mcg	>440 mcg
Fluticasone DPI 50, 100, or 250 mcg/puff	100–300 mcg	300–500 mcg	>500 mcg
Mometasone DPI 200 mcg/puff	200 mcg	400 mcg	>400 mcg

Source: NAEPP. http://www.nhlbi.nih.gov/guidelines/asthma/epr3/resource.pdf, accessed 9/10/09.

is also a leukotriene modifier; periodic hepatic enzyme monitoring is required during use. Theophylline is a mild bronchodilator with significant drug-drug interaction potential, a narrow therapeutic index, and requirement for periodic serological drug level monitoring. Rescue medications that relieve acute superimposed bronchospasm include short-acting beta₂ agonists (SABA), such as albuterol (Proventil, Ventolin), levalbuterol (Xopenex), and pirbuterol (Maxair). Compared with albuterol and pirbuterol, levalbuterol, a single isomer of the racemate albuterol, is often better tolerated with potentially better bronchodilation than the other short-acting beta₂ agonists, owing to its lower recommended dose. Long-acting beta₂ agonists (LABA), including salmeterol (Serevent) and formoterol (Foradil), have a pharmacodynamic profile identical to SABA, but with a significantly different pharmacokinetic profile. In addition, the LABA class received a boxed warning from the U.S. Food and Drug Administration (FDA) because LABA use is associated with increased risk of asthma death in certain patient groups and should not be used in patients with asthma that is well controlled with an ICS alone.

In the event of an asthma flare, treatment should be intensified. This includes removing or minimizing contributing factors to the flare, such as exposure to allergens. The most common reason for a protracted asthma exacerbation is a viral respiratory tract infection.

The patient should have an individualized asthma action plan to guide care during an exacerbation, outlining use of inhaled bronchodilators and other therapies, including when to seek urgent care at the physician's office or emergency department care. A systemic corticosteroid such as prednisone usually is added, providing an additional anti-inflammatory intervention. In the absence of severe gastrointestinal upset, the oral route should be used for corticosteroid administration. A recommended systemic prednisone dose for an adult is 40 to 60 mg total daily dose, given in a twice-daily divided dose if desired, for 3 to 10 days, with 5 to 7 days average use. Other corticosteroids are also used; knowledge of the relative potency of systemic corticosteroids is important to ensure safe and effective practice (Table 5–5). Severe exacerbations can occur at all asthma severity levels.

Discussion Sources

Chrousos G. Adrenal corticosteroids and adrenocorticosteroid antagonists. In: Katzung BG, ed. *Basic and Clinical Pharmacology*. 10th ed. New York, NY: Lange Medical Books/McGraw-Hill; 2007:635–652.

Report of the Expert Panel. http://www.nhlbi.nih.gov/guidelines/asthma, Guidelines for the diagnosis and management of asthma (EPR-3), accessed 9/10/09.

Schatz M. Asthma in adolescents and adults. In: Rakel R, Bope E, eds. *Conn's Current Therapy 2009*. Philadelphia, PA: Saunders Elsevier; 2009:763–770.

Stringer J. Receptor theory. In: Stringer J, ed. *Basic Concepts in Pharmacology*. 3rd ed. New York, NY: McGraw-Hill; 2006:7–12.

QUESTIONS

28. When discussing immunizations with a 64-year-old woman with chronic obstructive pulmonary disease (COPD), you advise that she:
    A. receive live attenuated influenza virus vaccine.
    B. avoid immunization against influenza because of the risk associated with the vaccine.
    C. receive inactivated influenza virus vaccine.
    D. take an antiviral for the duration of the influenza season.

29. When used in treating COPD, ipratropium bromide (Atrovent) is prescribed to achieve which of the following therapeutic effects?
    A. increase mucociliary clearance
    B. reduce alveolar volume
    C. bronchodilation
    D. mucolytic action

30. What is the desired therapeutic action of inhaled corticosteroids when used to treat COPD?
    A. reversal of fixed airway obstruction
    B. improvement of central respiratory drive
    C. reduction of airway inflammation
    D. mucolytic activity

31. Which is most consistent with the diagnosis of COPD?
    A. FEV₁/FVC ratio equal to or less than 0.70
    B. dyspnea on exhalation
    C. elevated diaphragms noted on x-ray
    D. polycythemia noted on complete blood cell count

TABLE 5–5
Relative Potency of Systemic Corticosteroids

Higher potency corticosteroids (equipotent doses)	Betamethasone, 0.6–0.75 mg	Half-life 36–54 hr
	Dexamethasone, 0.75 mg	
Medium potency corticosteroids (equipotent doses)	Methylprednisolone, 4 mg	Half-life 18–36 hr
	Triamcinolone, 4 mg	
	Prednisolone, 5 mg	
	Prednisone, 5 mg	
Lower potency (equipotent doses)	Hydrocortisone, 20 mg	Half-life 8–12 hr
	Cortisone, 25 mg	

Source: *Drug Facts and Comparisons*. Philadelphia, PA: Wolters Kluwer Health; 2009.

32. Which of the following characteristics is found in the early stages of chronic bronchitis?

   A. enlargement of air spaces distal to the terminal bronchiole
   B. excessive mucus production
   C. alveolar fibrosis
   D. dyspnea at rest

33. Which of the following characteristics is most often found in patients with emphysema?

   A. alpha₁ antiprotease deficiency
   B. enlargement of air spaces distal to the terminal bronchiole
   C. alveolar fibrosis
   D. hypertrophy of the larger airways

34. According to the Global Initiative for Chronic Obstructive Lung Disease (GOLD) COPD guidelines, which of the following medications is indicated for all COPD stages?

   A. short-acting inhaled bronchodilator
   B. inhaled corticosteroid
   C. mucolytic agent
   D. theophylline

35. According to the GOLD COPD guidelines, the goal of inhaled corticosteroid use in stage III or severe COPD is to:

   A. minimize the risk of repeated exacerbations.
   B. improve cough function.
   C. reverse alveolar hypertrophy.
   D. help mobilize secretions.

36. Which of the following corticosteroid doses is most potent?

   A. methylprednisolone 8 mg
   B. triamcinolone 10 mg
   C. prednisone 15 mg
   D. hydrocortisone 18 mg

37. Which of the following pathogens is often implicated in a COPD exacerbation caused by bacterial respiratory tract infection?

   A. *Legionella* species
   B. *Streptococcus pyogenes*
   C. *Haemophilus influenzae*
   D. *Staphylococcus aureus*

38. Which is the most appropriate choice for therapy of mild acute COPD exacerbation in a 42-year-old man?

   A. levofloxacin
   B. daptomycin
   C. linezolid
   D. Antimicrobial therapy is usually not indicated.

39. Which is the most appropriate choice of antimicrobial therapy for a severe COPD exacerbation in a 52-year-old man?

   A. azithromycin
   B. amoxicillin
   C. trimethoprim-sulfamethoxazole
   D. fosfomycin

40. An organism often associated with COPD exacerbation in a person with advanced disease and repeated exacerbations is:

   A. *Pseudomonas aeruginosa.*
   B. *Chlamydophila (Chlamydia) pneumoniae.*
   C. *Streptococcus pneumoniae.*
   D. *Haemophilus influenzae.*

41. You see a 67-year-old man with stage IV (very severe) COPD who asks, "When should I use my home oxygen?" You respond:

   A. as needed when short of breath.
   B. primarily during sleep hours.
   C. preferably during waking hours.
   D. for at least 15 hours a day.

42. With a COPD exacerbation, a chest x-ray should be obtained:

   A. routinely in all patients
   B. when attempting to rule out a concomitant pneumonia.
   C. if sputum volume is increased.
   D. when work of breathing is increased.

43. Which of the following best describes the role of theophylline in COPD treatment?

   A. indicated in moderate to very severe COPD
   B. use limited by narrow therapeutic profile and drug-drug interaction potential
   C. a potent bronchodilator
   D. available only in parenteral form

44. All of the following are consistent with the GOLD COPD recommendation for pulmonary rehabilitation except:

   A. indicated in all COPD stages
   B. goals include improvement in overall well-being
   C. an underused therapeutic option
   D. components aimed at reducing the deconditioning common in COPD

ANSWERS

28. C	29. C	30. C
31. A	32. B	33. B
34. A	35. A	36. C
37. C	38. D	39. A
40. A	41. D	42. B
43. B	44. A	

DISCUSSION

Chronic obstructive pulmonary disease (COPD) is a preventable and treatable disease with significant extrapulmonary effects that may contribute to the severity in individual patients. The pulmonary component is characterized by airflow limitation that is not fully reversible. The airflow limitation is usually progressive and associated with an abnormal inflammatory response of the lung to noxious particles or gases. This response results in a decrease in the ratio of forced expiratory volume at 1 second (FEV_1) to forced vital capacity (FVC).

Chronic bronchitis and emphysema are two conditions that are also chronic lung disorders. The diagnosis of chronic bronchitis is made clinically, with the patient reporting the presence of excessive mucus production for 3 or more months per year for at least 2 consecutive years in the absence of other causes. Emphysema is characterized by permanent enlargement of the air spaces distal to the terminal bronchiole without fibrosis. These terms are not used as part of the Global Obstructive Lung Disease (GOLD) guidelines for the diagnosis and management of COPD.

Because 80% of all cases of COPD can be attributed directly to tobacco use, encouraging the patient to stop smoking is an important clinical goal. Despite symptoms, many patients continue to smoke. Raising the issue of smoking cessation at every visit and offering assistance with this is an important part of the ongoing care of the person with COPD. Counseling about general respiratory hygiene should also be provided, including information on minimizing exposure to passive smoking, allergens, and air pollution, and advice on hydration, nutrition, and avoiding respiratory tract infection. Immunization against influenza via inactive virus vaccine should be encouraged and should be given annually. Cigarette smokers, people with asthma, and anyone with COPD should also be encouraged to receive antipneumococcal vaccine.

Symptoms associated with COPD are usually classified as symptoms associated with airway irritation, such as cough and sputum production, and symptoms associated with altered lung mechanics, such as dyspnea and wheezing. Patients with COPD typically present for care in the fifth and sixth decades of life, usually after having some symptoms, particularly sputum production and cough, for more than a decade. As the disease progresses, dyspnea with exertion is often reported. A person with COPD does not need to report symptoms to meet diagnostic criteria for the disease (Table 5–6). Later in the course of COPD, dyspnea at rest is occasionally noted.

Tiotropium bromide (Spiriva) and ipratropium bromide (Atrovent) are anticholinergic agents considered to be part of the backbone drugs in treatment of patients with moderate, severe, and very severe COPD (Table 5–7; see Table 5–6). Atropine analogues act as muscarinic antagonists.

TABLE 5–6

GOLD Chronic Obstructive Pulmonary Disease (COPD) Therapy at Each Stage of COPD

I—Mild	II—Moderate	III—Severe	IV—Very Severe
• FEV_1/FVC <70% • FEV_1 ≥80% predicted	• FEV_1/FVC <70% • 50% ≤ FEV_1 <80% predicted	• FEV_1/FVC <70% • 30% ≤ FEV_1 <50% predicted	• FEV_1/FVC <70% • FEV_1 <30% predicted or FEV_1 <50% predicted plus chronic respiratory failure

Active reduction of risk factor(s); influenza vaccination ⟶

Add short-acting bronchodilator such as albuterol (when needed)

Add regular treatment with one or more long-acting bronchodilators such as tiotropium (Spiriva) or ipratroprium bromide (Atrovent), salmeterol (Serevent), formoterol (Foradil), or arformoterol (Brovana) (when needed); *Add* rehabilitation

Add inhaled corticosteroids if repeated exacerbations

Add long-term oxygen if chronic respiratory failure

Consider surgical treatments

FEV_1, force expiratory volume in 1 second; FVC, forced vital capacity.

TABLE 5–7

Medications Used for Treating Patients With Asthma and Chronic Obstructive Pulmonary Disease (COPD)

Medication	Mechanism of Action	Indication	Comment
Inhaled corticosteroids mometasone (Asmanex) fluticasone (Flovent) budesonide (Pulmicort) beclomethasone (Qvar)	Block late-phase activation to allergen, inhibit inflammatory cell migration and activation	Controller drug, prevention of inflammation	Need consistent use to be helpful. Cornerstone medication of most asthma levels
Mast cell stabilizer Cromolyn sodium (Intal) nedocromil (Tilade)	Halts degradation of mast cells and release of histamine and other inflammatory mediators (mast cell stabilizer)	Controller drug, prevention of inflammation	Need consistent use to be helpful Less clinical effect compared with inhaled corticosteroids
Leukotriene receptor antagonist, also known as leukotriene modifier (montelukast [Singulair], zafirlukast [Accolate]) leukotriene inhibitor (zileuton [Zyflo])	Inhibit action of inflammatory mediator (leukotriene) by blocking select receptor sites	Controller drug, prevention of inflammation	Likely less effective than inhaled corticosteroids Particularly effective add-on medication when disease control is inadequate with inhaled corticosteroid, when asthma is complicated by allergic rhinitis. In mild persistent asthma, an alternative, although not preferred, therapeutic option for controller therapy
Systemic corticosteroids (oral or parenteral)	Inhibit eosinophilic action and other inflammatory mediators	Treatment of acute inflammation such as in asthma flare or COPD exacerbation	Oral route preferred whenever possible. Indicated in treatment of acute asthma flare to reduce inflammation In higher dose and with longer therapy (>2 weeks), adrenal suppression may occur No taper needed if use is short-term (<10 days) and at lower dose (prednisone, 40–60 mg/d or less) Potential for causing gastropathy, particularly gastric ulcer and gastritis
Albuterol (Ventolin, Proventil) pirbuterol (Maxair)	Beta$_2$ agonists; bronchodilation via stimulation of beta$_2$ receptor site	Rescue drugs for treatment of acute bronchospasm	Albuterol and pirbuterol • Onset of action 15 min • Duration of action 4–6 hr

Continued

TABLE 5–7

Medications Used for Treating Patients With Asthma and Chronic Obstructive Pulmonary Disease (COPD)—cont'd

Medication	Mechanism of Action	Indication	Comment
Levalbuterol (Xopenex) Long-acting beta₂ agonists (salmeterol [Serevent] formoterol [Foradil]) arformoterol [Brovana])	Long-acting beta₂ agonists; bronchodilation through stimulation of receptor site beta₂	Prevention of bronchospasm	Salmeterol • Onset of action 1 hr • Duration of action 12 hr • Indicated for prevention rather than treatment of bronchospasm • Patient should also have short-acting beta₂ agonist as rescue drug Formoterol • Onset of action 15–30 min • Duration of action 12 hr • Indicated for prevention rather than treatment of bronchospasm • Patient should also have short-acting beta₂ agonist as rescue drug Although long-acting beta₂ agonist use decreases number of asthma episodes, the use of these medicines may increase the chances of a severe asthma episode and rarely increase risk of asthma death. FDA-mandated box warning about this risk
Ipratropium bromide (Atrovent) Tiotropium bromide (Spiriva)	Anticholinergic and muscarinic antagonist, yielding bronchodilation	Treatment and prevention of bronchospasm	Onset of action ≥30 min Best used to avoid rather than treat bronchospasm associated with COPD and asthma Well tolerated
Theophylline	Mild bronchodilator via nonphosphodiesterase inhibitor. Possible mild anti-inflammatory effect	Prevention of bronchospasm, mild anti-inflammatory	Narrow therapeutic index drug with numerous potential drug interactions Monitor carefully for toxicity by checking drug levels and clinical presentation

Source: Report of the Expert Panel. http://www.nhlbi.nih.gov/guidelines/asthma/, Guidelines for the diagnosis and management of asthma (EPR-3), accessed 9/12/09.

Muscarinic receptor sites are located in organs innervated by the parasympathetic nervous system. When these sites are stimulated, bronchoconstriction occurs; blocking these receptor sites leads to bronchodilation. Ipratropium and tiotropium act as bronchodilators, but have no sympathomimetic effects or action at beta₂ receptor sites, such as with albuterol. In contrast to albuterol, muscarinic antagonists have a longer onset of action (usually longer than ½ hour), and are best used to avoid, rather than treat, the bronchospasm associated with COPD. Use of these medications also can help reduce the volume of secretions produced in COPD. If a patient with COPD continues to have symptoms despite consistent use of a full therapeutic dose of ipratropium or tiotropium, a beta₂ agonist should be added to provide additional bronchodilation through another mechanism of action.

Theophylline, which has mild bronchodilation and anti inflammatory action, is used less commonly than in the past partly because of its narrow therapeutic index, need for ongoing drug level monitoring, and marginal therapeutic effect. Inhaled corticosteroids are also used to minimize airway inflammation and possibly to limit the frequency and severity of COPD exacerbations.

Pulmonary rehabilitation should be encouraged for all patients with moderate, severe, or very severe COPD (stages 2– 4). The goal of this intervention is to improve quality of life, decrease symptoms, and increase physical participation in activities of daily living. Components of a pulmonary rehabilitation program include reversing the effects of physical deconditioning, social isolation, weight loss, muscle wasting, and altered mood often noted with COPD. Because of issues of funding, access, and lack of provider and patient knowledge of this helpful intervention, pulmonary rehabilitation is an underused, yet helpful intervention.

Long-term oxygen therapy for patients with COPD should be considered, particularly as the disease progresses, or when a patient presents with advanced disease (Table 5–8). The goal of therapy is to ensure adequate oxygen delivery to the vital organs by increasing the baseline PaO₂ at rest to 60 mm Hg or greater at sea level or producing SaO₂ equal to or greater than 90%, or both. When indicated, oxygen therapy should be used for more than 15 hours per day. Many patients wait until they are breathless, then attempt to correct this with as-needed oxygen use and fail to achieve maximum benefit; these benefits include not only improved overall well-being, but also increased survival.

Exacerbations of respiratory symptoms that necessitate treatment are important clinical events in COPD. The most common causes of an exacerbation are infection of the tracheobronchial tree and air pollution, but the cause of about one third of severe exacerbations cannot be identified. Inhaled bronchodilators (beta₂ agonists or anticholinergics or both) are effective for the treatment of COPD exacerbation. If baseline FEV₁ is less than 50% of predicted, a systemic corticosteroid, with oral route preferred, such as prednisone 40 mg daily for 10 days, should be added; knowledge of the

TABLE 5–8

Long-term Oxygen Therapy in Chronic Obstructive Pulmonary Disease

GOAL	To ensure adequate oxygen delivery to vital organs by increasing baseline PaO₂ at rest to ≥60 mm Hg at sea level or producing SaO₂ ≥90%, or both
INDICATIONS TO INITIATE LONG-TERM (>15 HOURS/DAY) OXYGEN THERAPY	PaO₂ <55 mm Hg *or* SaO₂ <88% with or without hypercapnia PaO₂ 55–69 mm Hg *or* SaO₂ 89% in the presence of cor pulmonale, right heart failure, or polycythemia (hematocrit >56%)

Source: www.goldcopd.org/Guidelineitem.asp?l1=2&l2=1&intId =1116, accessed 9/9/09.

relative potency of these drugs is important to safe and effective clinical practice (see Table 5–5). An inhaled corticosteroid such as nebulized budesonide (Pulmicort) is a helpful treatment option during nonacidotic exacerbations. Theophylline is occasionally used, with consideration for the previously identified cautions and limitations.

Antimicrobial therapy is not always needed as part of treatment of a COPD exacerbation because the cause can be nonbacterial in origin, such as an environmental problem or viral infection. Use of an antibiotic is likely indicated, however, when symptoms of breathlessness and cough are accompanied by altered sputum characteristics that suggest bacterial infection, such as increased purulence or change in volume. The therapeutic choice should be dictated by antimicrobial coverage for the major bacterial pathogens involved in COPD exacerbation, while taking into account local patterns of bacterial resistance (Tables 5–9 and 5–10). Because of the possibility of a concomitant pneumonia, a chest x-ray should be obtained when the patient presents with fever or unusually low SaO₂ or both; in the absence of these findings, a chest x-ray is not usually needed.

Noninvasive intermittent positive-pressure ventilation during a particularly severe acute exacerbation can improve blood gas values and pH, reduce in-hospital mortality, decrease the need for invasive mechanical ventilation and intubation, and decrease the length of hospital stay. As with the care of all patients with airway disease, the provider should assist the patient in developing a plan for smoking cessation and avoidance of second-hand smoke.

TABLE 5-9

Pathogens Associated With Chronic Obstructive Pulmonary Disease Exacerbation

Respiratory Bacteria	Viral (20%–50%)	Less Common Respiratory Bacteria (Usually in Presence of Advanced Disease and Repeated Exacerbations)
Gram-positive • S. pneumoniae Gram-negative • H. influenzae • M. catarrhalis Atypical pathogens • M. pneumoniae • C. pneumoniae • Legionella spp.	Rhinovirus Influenza virus	Enterobacteriaceae spp. Pseudomonas spp.

Source: Balter MS, La Forge J, Low DE, Mandell L, Grossman RF; Canadian Thoracic Society; Canadian Infectious Disease Society. Canadian guidelines for the management of acute exacerbations of chronic bronchitis. *Can Respir J.* 2003;10(Suppl B):3B-32B.

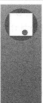

TABLE 5-10

Recommendations for Antimicrobial Therapy in Chronic Obstructive Pulmonary Disease (COPD) Exacerbations

Mild to moderate COPD exacerbation/ acute exacerbation of chronic bronchitis	Antimicrobial therapy usually not indicated. If prescribed, consider using the following agents: • Amoxicillin • Cephalosporin • Trimethoprim-sulfamethoxazole • Doxycycline
More severe COPD exacerbation/acute exacerbation of chronic bronchitis	Use one of the following agents: • Amoxicillin-clavulanate • Cephalosporin • Azithromycin • Clarithromycin • Fluoroquinolone with activity against drug-resistant S. pneumoniae

Source: Gilbert D, Moellering R, Eliopoulos G, Chambers H, Saag M. *The Sanford Guide to Antimicrobial Therapy.* 39th ed. Sperryville, VA: Antimicrobial Therapy, Inc; 2009:33—34.

Discussion Sources

Gilbert D, Moellering R, Eliopoulos G, Chambers H, Saag M. *The Sanford Guide to Antimicrobial Therapy.* 39th ed. Sperryville, VA: Antimicrobial Therapy, Inc; 2009:33–34.

Global Strategy for Diagnosis, Management, and Prevention of COPD. http://www.goldcopd.com/GuidelinesResources.asp, accessed 9/9/09.

Simpson T, Garcia JA, Jenkinson S. Management of chronic obstructive pulmonary disease. In: Rakel R, Bope E, eds. *Conn's Current Therapy 2009.* Philadelphia, PA: Saunders Elsevier; 2009:231–236.

QUESTIONS

45. You examine a 28-year-old woman who has emigrated from a country where tuberculosis (TB) is endemic. She has documentation of receiving bacille Calmette-Guérin (BCG) vaccine as a child. With this information, you consider that:

    A. she will always have a positive tuberculin skin test (TST) result.
    B. biannual chest radiographs are needed to assess her health status accurately.
    C. a TST finding of 10 mm or more induration should be considered a positive result.
    D. isoniazid therapy should be given for 6 months before TST is undertaken.

46. A 33-year-old woman works in a small office with a man recently diagnosed with active pulmonary TB. Which of the following would be the best plan of care for this woman?

    A. She should receive TB chemoprophylaxis if her TST result is 5 mm or more in induration.
    B. Because of her age, TB chemoprophylaxis is contraindicated even in the presence of a positive TST result.
    C. If the TST result is positive, but the chest radiograph is normal, no further evaluation or treatment is needed.
    D. Further evaluation is needed only if the TST result is 15 mm or more in induration.

47. Compared with TST, potential advantages of the QuantiFERON-TB Gold test (QTF-G) include all of the following except:

    A. ability to have entire testing process complete with one clinical visit.
    B. results are available within 24 hours.
    C. interpretation of test is not subject to reader bias.
    D. provides a prediction as to who is at greatest risk for disease development.

For the following questions, answer "yes" or "no" in response to the question, "Does this patient have a reactive TST?"

_____ **48.** A 45-year-old woman with type 2 diabetes mellitus and chest radiograph finding consistent with previous TB and a 7-mm induration

_____ **49.** A 21-year-old man with no identifiable TB risk factors and a 10-mm induration

_____ **50.** A 31-year-old man with HIV and a 6-mm induration

_____ **51.** A 45-year-old woman from a country where TB is endemic who has an 11-mm induration

_____ **52.** A 42-year-old woman with rheumatoid arthritis who is taking etanercept (Enbrel) who has a 7-mm induration

53. Risk factors for development of infection reactivation in patients with latent TB infection include all of the following except:

A. diabetes mellitus.
B. immunocompromise.
C. long-term oral corticosteroid therapy.
D. male gender.

54. Clinical presentation of progressive primary TB most commonly includes all of the following except:

A. malaise.
B. fever.
C. dry cough.
D. frank hemoptysis.

ANSWERS

45.	C	**46.**	A	**47.**	D
48.	Yes	**49.**	No	**50.**	Yes
51.	Yes	**52.**	Yes	**53.**	D
54.	D				

DISCUSSION

Pulmonary tuberculosis (TB) is a chronic bacterial infection, caused by *Mycobacterium tuberculosis* and transmitted through aerosolized droplets. With an estimated 20% to 43% of the world's population infected, the disease occurs disproportionately in disadvantaged populations, such as the homeless, the malnourished, and people living in overcrowded and substandard housing. About 30% of individuals exposed to the causative organism become infected. In an immunocompetent host, when the organism is acquired, an immune reaction ensues to help contain the infection within granulomas. This stage, known as primary TB, is usually symptom-free. Viable organisms can lie dormant within the granulomas for years, however; this stage is known as latent TB infection (LTBI). A person with LTBI does not have active disease and is not contagious.

Without treatment, individuals with LTBI have a 10% lifetime risk of reactivation of the disease, known as postprimary TB, with 50% of the reactivations occurring within the first 2 years of primary infection. This increases to a risk of 10% per year in the presence of HIV infection; increased rates of reactivation are also noted with other forms of immunocompromise (systemic corticosteroid or other immunosuppressive drug use, many chronic illnesses) or diabetes mellitus. After primary infection, about 5% of patients do not mount a containing immune response and develop progressive primary TB.

Public health measures to ensure adequate shelter, hygiene, and nutrition for the vulnerable public is an important primary prevention measure against the spread of TB infection. TST is an effective method of identifying individuals infected with *M. tuberculosis*. This test, when performed on an asymptomatic patient, is an example of secondary prevention or health screening. The test is performed by injecting 0.1 mL of purified protein derivative transdermally. The results should be checked within 48 to 72 hours, with the transverse measurement of any change in the test site measured in millimeters of induration, not simply redness. A positive TST result is usually noted within 2 to 10 weeks of acquiring the organism. Thresholds for a positive TST result vary in different clinical conditions (Table 5–11). The interpretation of the test is the same in the presence or absence of bacille Calmette-Guérin (BCG) vaccination history. In certain circumstances, two-step testing and anergy testing should be considered.

The TST has limitations, including the need for multiple visits, one to inject the PPD then a return visit to read or interpret the test, and a low sensitivity in the people with immunosuppression, a group at high risk for reactivation. In addition, test results can be compromised by poor injection technique or the use of an inferior purified protein derivative product. As a result, alternative testing has been developed and is gaining increased acceptance. A blood test, known by its trade name QuantiFERON-TB, detects interferon-γ, which is released by T lymphocytes in response to *M. tuberculosis*–specific antigens. This test can be performed from a blood sample obtained on a single provider visit, with results available within 24 hours. In addition, its sensitivity is greater in patients with immunocompromise or with a history of receiving BCG vaccine.

Any patient with a positive TST or QuantiFERON-TB test result should have a chest x-ray to help exclude the diagnosis of active pulmonary tuberculosis. In addition, a careful evaluation for clinical evidence of active disease, including malaise, weight loss, fever, night sweats, and chronic cough, should be carried out; these findings often evolve over 4 to 6 weeks in a person with active TB, and atypical presentation is common in immunocompromised individuals. Although

TABLE 5–11

Classification of Tuberculin Skin Test Reaction

An **induration of ≥5 mm** is considered positive in:	An **induration of ≥10 mm** is considered positive in:	An **induration of ≥15 mm** is considered positive in any person, including persons with no known risk factors for TB. Targeted skin testing programs should be conducted only in high-risk groups, however
• HIV-infected persons • A recent contact of a person with tuberculosis (TB) disease • Persons with fibrotic changes on chest radiograph consistent with prior TB • Patients with organ transplants • Persons who are immunosuppressed for other reasons (e.g., taking the equivalent of >15 mg/d of prednisone for ≥1 mo, taking TNF-α antagonists)	• Recent immigrants (<5 yr) from high-prevalence countries • Injection drug users • Residents and employees of high-risk congregate settings • Mycobacteriology laboratory personnel • Persons with clinical conditions that place them at high risk • Children <4 y.o. • Infants, children, and adolescents exposed to adults in high-risk categories	

Source: Centers for Disease Prevention and Control. http://www.cdc.gov/tb/publications/factsheets/testing/skintesting.htm, Tuberculin skin testing, accessed 9/10/09.

blood-tinged sputum is occasionally reported, the cough associated with TB is often dry; frank hemoptysis is rarely reported. The chest examination is usually normal, with dyspnea seldom reported unless disease is extensive.

Chemoprophylaxis therapy with isoniazid and other agents to prevent the development of active pulmonary TB should be considered for patients with latent tuberculosis—that is, positive tuberculin test results, but negative chest radiograph results and no suspicion of disease revealed by health history or physical examination. The duration of isoniazid therapy is 6 to 9 months, depending on the dosing regimen. Rifampin is an alternative choice if isoniazid cannot be taken or is poorly tolerated. Although the risk of liver toxicity with anti-TB drug use increases with age, age alone is not a contraindication to its use, particularly in individuals at higher risk.

In the presence of active pulmonary TB, multiple antimicrobial therapies are administered that are aimed not only at eradicating the infection, but also at minimizing the risk of developing a resistant pathogen. In this era of multidrug-resistant TB, it is prudent to consult with local TB experts to ascertain the local patterns of susceptibility. With latent and active disease, public health involvement is critical to maximize the patient outcome and minimize risk to the general population.

Discussion Sources

National Center for HIV/AIDS, Viral Hepatitis, STD and TB Prevention, Division of Tuberculosis Elimination. http://www.cdc.gov/tb/, accessed 9/10/09.

Sharma S, Mohan A. Tuberculosis and other mycobacterial diseases. In: Rakel R, Bope E, eds. *Conn's Current Therapy 2009.* Philadelphia, PA: Saunders Elsevier; 2009:282–290.

QUESTIONS

55. to 59. According to the American Thoracic Society/ Infectious Disease Society of American (ATS/IDSA) Consensus Guidelines on the Management of Community-Acquired Pneumonia in Adults, which of the following is the most appropriate antimicrobial for treatment of community-acquired pneumonia (CAP) in:

55. A 42-year-old man with no comorbidity and no recent antimicrobial use?

    A. azithromycin

    B. cefpodoxime

    C. trimethoprim-sulfamethoxazole

    D. ciprofloxacin

56. A 46-year-old well woman who cannot take a macrolide?

    A. clarithromycin

    B. amoxicillin

    C. doxycycline

    D. fosfomycin

57. A 78-year-old woman with COPD?

    A. clindamycin

    B. high-dose amoxicillin with a macrolide

    C. nitrofurantoin

    D. ceftriaxone

58. A 69-year-old man with heart failure and type 2 diabetes?

   A. respiratory fluoroquinolone
   B. amoxicillin with a beta-lactamase inhibitor
   C. cephalosporin
   D. a macrolide

59. A 58-year-old woman who has a dry cough, headache, malaise, no recent antimicrobial use, and no comorbidity who takes no medication?

   A. clarithromycin
   B. amoxicillin
   C. levofloxacin
   D. trimethoprim-sulfamethoxazole

60. Which of the following is a quality of respiratory fluoroquinolones?

   A. activity against drug-resistant *S. pneumoniae* (DRSP)
   B. poor activity against atypical pathogens
   C. predominantly hepatic route of elimination
   D. absence of photosensitizing action

61. The mechanism of resistance of DRSP is through the cell's:

   A. beta-lactamase production.
   B. hypertrophy of cell membrane.
   C. alteration in protein-binding sites.
   D. failure of DNA gyrase reversal.

62. The primary mechanism of antimicrobial resistance of *H. influenzae* is through the organism's:

   A. beta-lactamase production.
   B. hypertrophy of cell membrane.
   C. alteration in protein-binding sites.
   D. failure of DNA gyrase reversal.

63. Which of the following characteristics applies to macrolides?

   A. consistent activity against DRSP
   B. contraindicated in pregnancy
   C. effective against atypical pathogens
   D. unstable in the presence of beta-lactamase

64. According to the ATS/IDSA guidelines, what is the usual length of antimicrobial therapy for the treatment of CAP for outpatients?

   A. less than 5 days
   B. 5 to 7 days
   C. 7 to 10 days
   D. 10 to 14 days

65. Modifying factors for increased *P. aeruginosa* risk include all of the following except:

   A. corticosteroid use.
   B. structural lung disease.
   C. malnutrition.
   D. day-care attendance.

66. Which of the following best describes the mechanism of transmission in an atypical pneumonia?

   A. microaspiration
   B. respiratory droplet
   C. surface contamination
   D. aerosolized contaminated water

67. Risk factors for death resulting from pneumonia include:

   A. viral origin.
   B. history of allergy.
   C. renal insufficiency.
   D. polycythemia.

68. All of the following antimicrobial strategies help facilitate the development of resistant pathogens except:

   A. longer course of therapy.
   B. lower antimicrobial dosage.
   C. higher antimicrobial dosage.
   D. prescribing a broader spectrum agent.

69. Findings of increased tactile fremitus and dullness to percussion at the right lung base in the person with CAP likely indicate an area of:

   A. atelectasis.
   B. pneumothorax.
   C. consolidation.
   D. cavitation.

70. Which of the following represents findings in an acceptable sputum specimen for Gram staining?

   A. many squamous epithelial cells and few WBCs
   B. three or more stained organisms
   C. few squamous epithelial cells and many WBCs
   D. motile bacteria with monocytes

71. You are caring for a 52-year-old man who is currently smoking 1.5 PPD and has a 40-pack-year cigarette smoking history and has CAP. It is the third day of his antimicrobial therapy, and he is without fever, is well hydrated, and is feeling less short of breath. His initial chest x-ray revealed a right lower lobe infiltrate. Physical examination today reveals peak inspiratory crackles with increased tactile fremitus in the right posterior thorax. Which of the following represents the most appropriate next step in this patient's care?

   A. His current plan of care should continue because he is improving by clinical assessment.
   B. A chest radiograph should be taken today to confirm resolution of pneumonia.
   C. Given the persistence of abnormal thoracic findings, his antimicrobial therapy should be changed.
   D. A computed tomography scan of the thorax is needed today to image better any potential thoracic abnormalities.

72. While seeing a 62-year-old who is hospitalized with CAP, the NP considers that:

   A. antipneumococcal vaccine should be given when antimicrobial therapy has been completed.
   B. antipneumococcal vaccine can be given today, and influenza vaccine can be given in 2 weeks.
   C. influenza vaccine can be given today, and antipneumococcal vaccine can be given in 2 weeks.
   D. influenza and antipneumococcal vaccines should be given today.

73. Risk factors for infection with DRSP include all of the following except:

   A. systemic antimicrobial therapy in the previous 3 months.
   B. exposure to children in day care.
   C. age older than 65 years.
   D. use of inhaled corticosteroids.

74. The mechanism of transmission of *Legionella* species is primarily via:

   A. respiratory droplet.
   B. inhalation of contaminated water.
   C. contact with a contaminated surface.
   D. hematogenous spread.

Identify the following organisms as a gram positive, gram negative, or atypical pathogen.

___ **75.** *Streptococcus pneumoniae*

___ **76.** *Haemophilus influenzae*

___ **77.** *Legionella* species

___ **78.** *Chlamydophila pneumoniae*

___ **79.** *Mycoplasma pneumoniae*

ANSWERS

55.	A	**56.**	C	**57.**	B
58.	A	**59.**	A	**60.**	A
61.	C	**62.**	A	**63.**	C
64.	B	**65.**	D	**66.**	B
67.	C	**68.**	C	**69.**	C
70.	C	**71.**	A	**72.**	D
73.	D	**74.**	B	**75.**	Gram positive
76.	Gram negative	**77.**	Atypical		
78.	Atypical	**79.**	Atypical		

DISCUSSION

Pneumonia is the most common cause of death from infectious disease and is the eighth leading cause of overall mortality in the United States. Although pneumonia is often considered a disease primarily of older adults and persons with chronic illness, most episodes occur in immunocompetent community-dwelling individuals; about 20% of children develop pneumonia by age 5 years. Most often caused by bacteria or virus, pneumonia is an acute lower respiratory tract infection involving lung parenchyma, interstitial tissues, and alveolar spaces. The term *community-acquired pneumonia* (CAP) is used to describe the onset of disease in a person who resides within the community, not in a nursing home or other care facility, with no recent (<2 weeks') hospitalization.

Patients with pneumonia usually present with cough (>90%), dyspnea (66%), sputum production (66%), and pleuritic chest pain (50%), although nonrespiratory symptoms, including fatigue and gastrointestinal upset, are also commonly reported. As with other infectious diseases, elderly patients may report fewer symptoms and often present with an elevated resting respiratory rate and generally feeling ill. Chest x-ray is helpful in the assessment of the person with CAP. Characteristic infiltrate patterns are typically seen with certain pathogens, such as interstitial infiltrates with atypical pathogens or viruses and areas of consolidation with *Streptococcus pneumoniae*. Therapy should be based on patient characteristics and risk factors, however, rather than the pattern of the radiographic abnormality. According to the recommendations of the IDSA/ATS Consensus Guidelines, an abnormal chest radiograph and clinical findings are required to confirm the diagnosis of pneumonia.

Although numerous organisms are capable of causing pneumonia, relatively few are seen with frequency. *S. pneumoniae*, also known as the pneumococcal organism, is a gram-positive diplococcus, is the most common CAP pathogen in adults, and is found in most deaths caused by CAP. Pneumonia caused by *H. influenzae* is predominantly a disease of tobacco users. After many years of smoking, the tracheobronchial tree becomes colonized with this gram-negative coccobacillus. *Mycoplasma pneumoniae* and *Chlamydophila* (formerly *Chlamydia*) *pneumoniae* are common causative pathogens of CAP. These organisms are transmitted by coughing and are often found among people living in closed communities, such as households, college dormitories, military barracks, and residential centers, including long-term care facilities. *M. pneumoniae, C. pneumoniae, Legionella* species and respiratory viruses are often referred to as atypical pathogens (causing atypical pneumonia) because these organisms are not detectable via Gram stain and cannot be cultured on standard bacterial media.

Usually contracted by inhaling mist or aspirating liquid that comes from a water source contaminated with the organisms, pulmonary infection with *Legionella* species can result in pneumonia ranging from mild to severe disease; there is no evidence for person-to-person spread of the disease. Risk factors for severe disease with *Legionella* species, capable of causing the most serious illness of the atypical pathogens, include tobacco use, airway disease, and diabetes mellitus. With airway impairment, pneumonia is often caused by anaerobic gram-negative bacilli or mixed gram-negative organisms (Table 5–12).

TABLE 5–12

Community-acquired Pneumonia: Likely Causative Pathogens

OUTPATIENT	S. pneumoniae
	M. pneumoniae
	C. pneumoniae
	Respiratory viruses including influenza A/B, RSV, adenovirus, parainfluenza
INPATIENT, NOT TREATED IN THE INTENSIVE CARE UNIT	S. pneumoniae
	M. pneumoniae
	C. pneumoniae
	Legionella spp.
	H. influenzae
	Respiratory viruses including influenza A/B, RSV, adenovirus, parainfluenza

RSV, respiratory syncytial virus.
Source: Mandell L, Wunderink RG, Anzueto A, Bartlett JG, Campbell GD, Dean NC, Dowell SF, File TM Jr, Musher DM, Niederman MS, Torres A, Whitney CG; Infectious Diseases Society of America; American Thoracic Society. Infectious Disease Society of America/American Thoracic Society consensus guidelines on the management of community-acquired pneumonia in adults. *Clin Infect Dis.* 2007;44 (Suppl 2):S27-S72. Available at www.journals.uchicago.edu/ CID/journal/issues/v44nS2/41620/41620.html, accessed 9/20/09.

Successful community-based care of a person with pneumonia depends on many factors. The patient must have intact gastrointestinal function and be able to take and tolerate oral medications and adequate amounts of fluids. A competent caregiver must be available. Also, the patient should be able to return for follow-up examination and evaluation.

Certain patient characteristics increase the likelihood of death from pneumonia and should alert the NP to consider hospitalization and aggressive therapy. These include age older than 65 years and severe electrolyte or hematological disorder, such as serum sodium concentration of less than 130 mEq/L, hematocrit less than 30%, or absolute neutrophil count of less than 1000/mm³. The presence of a comorbid disease, such as impaired renal function, diabetes mellitus, heart failure, immunosuppression, and airway dysfunction, poses increased risk, as do abnormalities in vital signs, such as fever, tachycardia, tachypnea, and hypotension. The pathogen responsible for pneumonia also needs to be considered because pneumonia death risk is increased when *S. aureus*, often seen in postinfluenza pneumonia, or gram-negative rods such as *Klebsiella pneumoniae*, found frequently in pneumonia in alcohol abusers, cause infection. Risks for CAP by *Pseudomonas aeruginosa* include structural lung disease, long-term corticosteroid therapy (prednisone use of ≥10 mg/day, or its equivalent) and broad-spectrum antibiotic therapy in the previous month, and malnutrition.

Sputum Gram staining and culture are helpful in ascertaining the pathogen in less than 50% of persons with CAP. Most often, the sputum specimen is inadequate, coming from the oropharynx rather than the chest. Clues to an inadequate specimen are the presence of numerous epithelial cells with few WBCs. Conversely, if numerous WBCs and few epithelial cells are found, the specimen is from the chest.

Because definitive identification of the organism is unlikely, the choice of antimicrobial agent to treat pneumonia is largely empirical, directed at the most likely causative organism in view of patient characteristics, such as age and comorbidity. Because pneumococcal pneumonia, caused by *S. pneumoniae*, carries a significant risk for mortality, the chosen antimicrobial should always be effective against this pathogen, regardless of patient presentation. Choosing an antimicrobial with activity against atypical organisms (*M. pneumoniae, C. pneumoniae, Legionella* species) and gram-positive and gram-negative organisms (*S. pneumoniae, H. influenzae*) helps ensure optimal outcome.

An additional consideration is antimicrobial resistance. Factors that facilitate the development of resistant microbes include repeated exposure to a given agent, underdosing (eradicating more sensitive organisms, leaving more resistant pathogens untouched), and an unnecessarily prolonged period of treatment. Shorter course high-dose therapy maximizes and exploits concentration-dependent killing by achieving higher maximum concentration and area under the curve/minimal inhibitory concentration values; allowing treatment of difficult pathogens, increased tissue penetration, and improved patient adherence to the regimen; and minimizing the development of resistance.

S. pneumoniae has shown increasing resistance to beta-lactams (antimicrobials containing the beta-lactam ring, including penicillins and cephalosporins), macrolides (an antimicrobial class including erythromycin, clarithromycin, and azithromycin), and tetracyclines (an antimicrobial class including tetracycline, doxycycline, and minocycline); strains with these resistance characteristics are known as drug-resistant *S. pneumoniae* (DRSP) or multidrug-resistant *S. pneumoniae*. The mechanism of resistance of DRSP is a result of an alteration in intracellular protein-binding sites, rendering formerly effective antimicrobials incapable of destroying the pathogen. Risk factors for DRSP include systemic antimicrobial therapy in the previous 3 months, exposure to children in day care, age older than 65 years, alcohol abuse, multiple comorbidities (e.g., COPD, coronary heart disease, diabetes mellitus), and immunosuppressive state including use of corticosteroids and other immunosuppressing medications and chronic illness.

Respiratory fluoroquinolones (e.g., levofloxacin [Levaquin], gemifloxacin [Factive], moxifloxacin [Avelox]) provide enhanced activity against DRSP and atypical organism coverage and stability in the presence of beta-lactamase. High-dose amoxicillin ($\geq$3 g/d) and certain cephalosporins, such as cefuroxime, are additional treatment options. Macrolides (erythromycin, azithromycin [Zithromax, Zmax], clarithromycin [Biaxin]) and tetracyclines (tetracycline, minocycline [Minocin], doxycycline) do not consistently exhibit activity against DRSP; use of these products could result in treatment failure in the presence of DRSP risk.

H. influenzae has the capacity to produce beta-lactamase, rendering penicillins ineffective; this varies regionally, but averages approximately 25% to 40% nationwide. Antimicrobials stable in the presence of beta-lactamase include macrolides, respiratory fluoroquinolones, and cephalosporins; adding clavulanate to amoxicillin (Augmentin) inactivates beta-lactamase and provides effective activity against *H. influenzae*. Because atypical pathogens do not have a true cell wall, beta-lactams are ineffective against these organisms. Macrolides, tetracyclines, and respiratory fluoroquinolones provide activity against these pathogens.

The American Thoracic Society and the Infectious Disease Society of America offer guidelines for CAP assessment and intervention. Factors influencing the choice of antimicrobial agent include patient comorbidity and risk if treatment fails. All treatment options offer activity against *S. pneumoniae, H. influenzae,* and atypical pathogens, the most common organisms implicated in CAP; consideration also needs to be given for DRSP risk (Tables 5–13 and 5–14).

NPs are ideally positioned to help minimize risk for pneumonia through immunization and hygienic measures. Nearly two-thirds of all fatal cases of pneumonia are caused by *S. pneumoniae,* the pneumococcal organism. Although available for nearly 30 years, antipneumococcal vaccine (e.g., Pneumovax) continues to be underused. The use of influenza vaccine can help minimize the risk of postinfluenza pneumonia, an often debilitating and potentially fatal condition. Both vaccines can be given together and in the presence of moderately severe illness. Ensuring adequate ventilation, reinforcing cough hygiene, and proper hand washing can help minimize pneumonia risk.

Discussion Sources

Gilbert D, Moellering R, Eliopoulos G, Chambers H, Saag M. *The Sanford Guide to Antimicrobial Therapy*. 39th ed. Sperryville, VA: Antimicrobial Therapy, Inc.; 2009:35–37.

Mandell L, Wunderink RG, Anzueto A, Bartlett JG, Campbell GD, Dean NC, Dowell SF, File TM Jr, Musher DM, Niederman MS, Torres A, Whitney CG; Infectious Diseases Society of America; American Thoracic Society. Infectious Disease Society of America/American Thoracic Society consensus guidelines on the management of community-acquired pneumonia in adults. *Clin Infect Dis*. 2007;44(Suppl 2):S27-S72. www.journals.uchicago.edu/CID/journal/issues/v44nS2/41620/41620.html, accessed 9/12/09.

QUESTIONS

80. You examine a 38-year-old woman who has presented for an initial examination and Papanicolaou test. She has no complaint. Her blood pressure (BP) is 144/98 mm Hg bilaterally and her body mass index (BMI) is 31. The rest of her physical examination is unremarkable. Your next best action is to:

    A. initiate antihypertensive therapy.
    B. arrange for at least two additional BP measurements during the next 2 weeks.
    C. order blood urea nitrogen, creatinine, and potassium ion measurements and urinalysis.
    D. advise her to reduce her sodium intake.

81. You see a 68-year-old woman as a patient who is transferring care into your practice. She has a 10-year history of hypertension, diabetes mellitus, and hyperlipidemia. Current medications include hydrochlorothiazide, glipizide, metformin, simvastatin, and daily low-dose aspirin. Today's BP reading is 138/88 mm Hg, and the rest of her history and examination is unremarkable. Your next best action is to:

    A. prescribe an angiotensin-converting enzyme inhibitor (ACEI).
    B. have her return for a BP check in 1 week.
    C. advise that her current therapy is adequate.
    D. start therapy with a alpha-adrenergic antagonist.

TABLE 5–13

Community-acquired Pneumonia: Likely Causative Pathogens, Characteristics, and Effective Antimicrobials

Pathogen	Description	Antimicrobial Resistance	Comment
S. pneumoniae	Gram-positive diplococci	Via altered protein binding sites in bacterial cell (~25% nationwide) DRSP risk: Recent antimicrobial use (within past 3 mo), age ≥65 yr, exposure to a child in day care, alcohol abuse, medical comorbidities, immunosuppressive therapy or illness Effective antimicrobials for nonresistant *S. pneumoniae*: Macrolides (azithromycin, clarithromycin, erythromycin), standard-dose amoxicillin (1.5–2.5 g/d), select cephalosporins, tetracyclines including doxycycline Preferred antimicrobials for DRSP: High-dose (3–4 g/d) amoxicillin, telithromycin* (Ketek), respiratory fluoroquinolones (moxifloxacin, levofloxacin, gemifloxacin)	Most common cause of fatal community-acquired pneumonia
M. pneumoniae *C. pneumoniae*	Not revealed by Gram stain	Effective antimicrobials: Macrolides, respiratory fluoroquinolones, tetracyclines including doxycycline Ineffective antimicrobials: Beta-lactams (cephalosporins, penicillins)	Largely transmitted by cough, often seen in people who have recently spent extended time in close proximity (closed communities such as correctional facilities, college dormitories, long-term care facilities)
H. influenzae	Gram-negative bacillus	Beta-lactamase production (~40% nationwide) Effective antimicrobials: Agents with activity against gram-negative organisms and stable in presence of or active against beta-lactamase—macrolides, cephalosporins, amoxicillin-clavulanate, respiratory fluoroquinolones, tetracyclines including doxycycline	Common respiratory pathogen with tobacco-related lung disease
Legionella spp.	Not revealed by Gram stain	Effective antimicrobials: Macrolides, respiratory fluoroquinolones, tetracyclines, including doxycycline Ineffective antimicrobials: Beta-lactams (cephalosporins, penicillins)	Usually contracted by inhaling mist or aspirating liquid that comes from a water source contaminated with *Legionella*. No evidence for person-to-person spread of the disease

DRSP, drug-resistant *S. pneumoniae*.
Source: Gilbert D, Moellering R, Eliopoulos G, Chambers H, Saag M. *The Sanford Guide to Antimicrobial Therapy*. 39th ed. Sperryville, VA: Antimicrobial Therapy, Inc.; 2009.
*Per FDA Advisory, health-care providers should monitor patients taking telithromycin for signs or symptoms of liver problems and the drug promptly discontinued if this occurs. Visit www.fda.gov for the latest FDA telithromycin advisory information.

82. You examine a 78-year-old woman with long-standing, poorly controlled hypertension. When evaluating her for hypertensive target organ damage, you look for evidence of:

A. lipid abnormalities.
B. hyperinsulinemia and insulin resistance.
C. left ventricular hypertrophy.
D. clotting disorders.

83. Diagnostic testing for a patient with new stage 1 primary hypertension diagnosis should include all of the following except:

A. hematocrit.
B. uric acid.
C. creatinine.
D. potassium.

TABLE 5–14

Infectious Disease Society of America/American Thoracic Society (IDSA/ATS) Community-acquired Pneumonia Classification and Recommended Treatment

IDSA/ATS Classification	Likely Causative Pathogens	Recommended Treatment	Comment
Previously healthy No recent (within 3 mo) antimicrobial use	*S. pneumoniae* (gram-positive) with low DRSP risk Atypical pathogens (*M. pneumoniae, C. pneumoniae, Legionella*) Respiratory virus	Strong recommendation • Macrolide such as azithromycin, clarithromycin, or erythromycin **Or** Weak recommendation • Doxycycline	Erythromycin: Limited gram-negative coverage Erythromycin, clarithromycin: CYP3A4 inhibitors
Comorbidities including COPD, diabetes, renal or congestive heart failure, asplenia, alcoholism, immunosuppressing conditions or use of immunosuppressing medications, malignancy, or use of an antimicrobial in past 3 mo	*S. pneumoniae* (gram-positive) with DRSP risk *H. influenzae* (gram-negative) Atypical pathogens (*M. pneumoniae, C. pneumoniae*) Respiratory virus	Respiratory fluoroquinolone (levofloxacin,* moxifloxacin or gemifloxacin) **Or** Advanced macrolide plus beta-lactam such as high-dose amoxicillin (3–4 g/d), high-dose amoxicillin-clavulanate (4 g/d), ceftriaxone (Rocephin), cefpodoxime (Vantin), cefuroxime (Ceftin) Alternative to macrolide: Doxycycline	Recent antimicrobial use increases risk of infection with DRSP. Given comorbidity, risk of poor outcome if treatment failure Recent use of fluoroquinolone should dictate selection of a nonfluoroquinolone regimen, and vice versa

*With levofloxacin use, the 750 mg dose × 5 days regimen is recommended.
COPD, chronic obstructive pulmonary disease; DRSP, drug-resistant *S. pneumoniae*.
Source: Mandell L, Wunderink RG, Anzueto A, Bartlett JG, Campbell GD, Dean NC, Dowell SF, File TM Jr, Musher DM, Niederman MS, Torres A, Whitney CG; Infectious Diseases Society of America; American Thoracic Society. Infectious Disease Society of America/American Thoracic Society consensus guidelines on the management of community-acquired pneumonia in adults. *Clin Infect Dis*. 2007;44(Suppl 2):S27-S72. Available at www.journals.uchicago.edu/CID/journal/issues/v44nS2/41620/41620.html, accessed 9/12/09.

84. In the person with hypertension, which of the following would likely yield the greatest potential reduction in BP in a patient with a BMI of 30?

    A. 10-kg weight loss
    B. dietary sodium restriction to 2.4 g (6 g NaCl) per day
    C. regular aerobic physical activity, such as 30 minutes of brisk walking most days of the week
    D. moderate alcohol consumption

85. Which of the following medications is a dihydropyridine calcium channel blocker?
    A. lisinopril
    B. verapamil
    C. amlodipine
    D. doxazosin

86. Which of the following medications is a nondihydropyridine calcium channel blocker?

    A. lisinopril
    B. diltiazem
    C. amlodipine
    D. prazosin

87. Which of the following medications is an alpha-adrenergic antagonist?

    A. enalapril
    B. diltiazem
    C. felodipine
    D. doxazosin

88. Which of the following medications is an ACEI?

    A. trandolapril
    B. clonidine
    C. felodipine
    D. doxazosin

89. Which of the following medications is an angiotensin receptor antagonist?

    A. trandolapril
    B. methyldopa
    C. telmisartan
    D. atenolol

90. Which of the following medications is a beta-adrenergic receptor antagonist?

    A. clonidine
    B. spironolactone
    C. hydrochlorothiazide
    D. pindolol

91. The mechanism of action of aliskiren (Tekturna) is as a/an:

    A. ACEI
    B. beta-adrenergic antagonist
    C. centrally acting agent
    D. direct renin inhibitor

92. In obtaining an office BP measurement, which of the following is most reflective of the Seventh Report of the National High Blood Pressure Education Program for the Prevention, Detection, Evaluation, and Treatment of High Blood Pressure (JNC-7) recommendations?

    A. Patient should sit in chair with feet flat on floor for at least 5 minutes before obtaining the reading.
    B. The BP cuff should not cover more than 50% of the upper arm.
    C. The patient should sit on the edge of the examination table without arm support to enhance reading accuracy.
    D. Obtaining the BP reading immediately after the patient walks into the examination room is recommended.

93. A BP elevation noted only at an office visit is commonly known as _____ hypertension.

    A. provider-induced
    B. clinical
    C. white coat
    D. pseudo

94. The most important goal of treating hypertension is to:

    A. strive to reach recommended numeric BP measurement.
    B. avoid disease-related target organ damage.
    C. develop a plan of care with minimal adverse effects.
    D. treat concomitant health problems often noted in the person with this condition.

95. You start a patient with hypertension who is already receiving an ACEI on spironolactone. You advise the patient to return in 4 weeks to check which of the following laboratory parameters?

    A. sodium
    B. calcium
    C. potassium
    D. chloride

96. A 68-year-old woman presents with hypertension and BP of 145–155/92–96 mm Hg documented over 2 months on three different occasions. ECG and creatinine are normal, and she has no proteinuria. Clinical findings include the following: BMI 26.4; no S_3, S_4, or murmur; and point of maximal impulse at fifth intercostal space, mid-clavicular line. Which of the following represents the best intervention?

    A. Initiate therapy with atenolol.
    B. Initiate therapy with hydrochlorothiazide.
    C. Initiate therapy with methyldopa.
    D. Continue to monitor BP, and start drug therapy if evidence of target organ damage.

97. Which of the following can have a favorable effect on a comorbid condition in a person with hypertension?

    A. chlorthalidone in gout
    B. propranolol with airway disease
    C. verapamil in migraine headache
    D. methyldopa in an older adult

98. According to recommendations found in JNC-7, all of the following medications are designated as having a compelling indication for use in the person with high cardiovascular disease risk except:

    A. doxazosin.
    B. hydrochlorothiazide.
    C. atenolol.
    D. trandolapril.

99. You see a 59-year-old man with poorly controlled hypertension. On physical examination, you note grade 1 hypertensive retinopathy. You anticipate all of the following will be present except:

    A. patient report of acute visual change.
    B. narrowing of the terminal arterioles.
    C. sharp optic disc borders.
    D. absence of retinal hemorrhage.

100. A 52-year-old woman whose blood pressure is consistently 130–135/82–86 mm Hg who is otherwise well is considered to have:

    A. normal blood pressure.
    B. prehypertension.
    C. stage 1 hypertension.
    D. stage 2 hypertension.

101 to 106. According to information found in the Seventh Report of the Joint National Committee on the Prevention, Detection, Evaluation, and Treatment of Hypertension (JNC-7), which of the following medications has a compelling indication for use in the following patient conditions? (The medications listed can be used more than once. A given condition may have more than one medication indicated.)

____	**101.** Heart failure	**A.**	thiazide diuretic
____	**102.** Diabetes mellitus	**B.**	beta blocker
____	**103.** Chronic renal disease	**C.**	ACEI
____	**104.** High risk for coronary artery disease	**D.**	angiotensin receptor blocker (ARB)
____	**105.** After myocardial infarction (MI)	**E.**	aldosterone antagonist
____	**106.** Recurrent stroke	**F.**	calcium channel blocker

ANSWERS

80.	B	81.	A	82.	C
83.	B	84.	A	85.	C
86.	B	87.	D	88.	A
89.	C	90.	D	91.	D
92.	A	93.	C	94.	B
95.	C	96.	B	97.	C
98.	A	99.	A	100.	B
101.	A, B, C, D, E		102.	A, B, C, D, F	
103.	C, D		104.	A, B, C, F	
105.	B, C, E		106.	A, C	

DISCUSSION

Hypertension (HTN) is a complex disease with a core defect of vascular dysfunction that leads to select target organ damage (TOD); the target organs include the brain, eye, heart, and kidneys (Table 5–15). Appropriate HTN treatment significantly reduces TOD risk. When a BP reading of 115/75 mm Hg is used as a starting point, cardiovascular disease risk doubles with each increment of 20/10 mm Hg. HTN control leads to a reduction of stroke incidence by 35% to 40%, reduction of MI by 20% to 25%, and reduction of heart failure by 50%. Long-standing poorly controlled HTN is the leading cause of new-onset heart failure.

The JNC-7 report provides evidence-based guidance for the diagnosis, prevention, and treatment of HTN. Following are some JNC-7 highlights:

- Accurate clinical assessment depends on proper measurement of BP. The patient should be seated in a chair with feet flat on floor, without crossed legs, with arm supported at heart level, for at least 5 minutes before taking the BP measurement, not on an examination table with feet dangling. Failure to perform these measures can lead to an artificially elevated reading and lack of standardization from visit to visit. The BP cuff should be wide enough to cover more than 80% of the upper arm, and the cuff's bladder should be approximately 40% of the arm circumference. The use of a cuff that does not meet these qualifications can lead to a falsely elevated BP reading.

- People with systolic BP of 120 to 139 mm Hg or diastolic BP of 80 to 89 mm Hg should be considered to have prehypertension. Lifestyle modification to prevent cardiovascular disease is indicated. In individuals older than 50, systolic BP greater than 140 mm Hg is a more important risk factor for cardiovascular disease than diastolic BP; the wider the pulse pressure (difference between systolic and diastolic BPs), the greater the cardiovascular risk.

- In stage 1 HTN (140–159/90–99 mm Hg), a thiazide diuretic is indicated for most individuals with uncomplicated HTN, alone or in combination with an ACEI, an ARB, a beta-blocker, or a calcium channel blocker. In stage 2 HTN (≥160/≥100 mm Hg), a combination of two or more drugs, one usually a thiazide diuretic, is needed by most patients. Most patients need multidrug therapy to meet BP goals. Lifestyle modification yields significant improvement in BP measurements (Table 5–16).

TABLE 5–15

Hypertension: A Complex Disease With a Core Defect of Vascular Dysfunction That Leads to Select Target Organ Damage

Target Organ	Potential Damage Outcome With Known Moderation as a Result of Effective Antihypertension Therapy
Brain	Stroke, vascular (multi-infarct) dementia
Cardiovascular system	Atherosclerosis, myocardial infarction, left ventricular hypertrophy, heart failure
Kidney	Hypertensive nephropathy, renal failure
Eye	Hypertensive retinopathy with risk for blindness

TABLE 5–16

Lifestyle Modification in Hypertension According to JNC-7

Modification	Recommendation	Average Systolic Blood Pressure Reduction Rate
Weight reduction	Maintain normal body weight (body mass index 18.5–24.9 kg/m²)	5–20 mm Hg/10 kg
DASH eating plan	Adopt a diet rich in fruits, vegetables, and low-fat dairy products with reduced content of saturated and total fat	8–14 mm Hg
Dietary sodium reduction	Reduce dietary sodium intake to <100 mmol/d (2.4 g sodium or 6 g sodium chloride)	2–8 mm Hg
Aerobic physical activity	Regular aerobic physical activity (e.g., brisk walking) at least 30 min per day, most days of the week	4–9 mm Hg
Moderation of alcohol consumption	Men: limit to <2 drinks* per day Women and lighter weight persons: limit to <1 drink* per day	2–4 mm Hg

*1 drink = ½ oz or 15 mL ethanol (e.g., 12 oz beer, 5 oz wine, 1.5 oz 80-proof whiskey).
Source: National Heart, Blood and Lung Institute: The Seventh Report of the Joint National Committee on Prevention, Detection, Evaluation, and Treatment of High Blood Pressure (JNC7), available at www.nhlbi.nih.gov/guidelines/hypertension/, accessed 10/12/09.

- The most important goal of HTN treatment is the avoidance of TOD. JNC-7 recommendations for BP goals include less than 130/80 mm Hg in the presence of renal impairment or diabetes mellitus or both, and less than 140/90 mm Hg in the absence of compelling indications for a lower level and more stringent control.
- In more than two-thirds of hypertensive individuals, their HTN cannot be controlled on one drug, and they require two or more antihypertensive agents selected from different drug classes. Many conditions provide compelling indications to use certain drugs (Table 5–17).
- Along with the traditional risks, microalbuminuria (MA) or glomerular filtration rate of less than 60 mL/min is identified in the JNC-7 report as a cardiovascular risk factor. When adjusted for other risk factors, the relative risk of ischemic heart disease associated with MA is increased twofold. An interaction between MA and cigarette smoking has been noted, and the presence of MA more than doubled the predictive effect of the conventional atherosclerotic risk factors for development of ischemic heart disease. MA not only is an independent predictor of ischemic heart disease, but also substantially increases the risk associated with other established risk factors. Because the person with MA has significant cardiovascular disease risk, JNC-7 recommendations for HTN treatment include thiazide diuretics, beta blockers, ACEIs, and calcium channel blockers, particularly nondihydropyridines; in the presence of chronic renal disease, as manifested by MA, recommendations also include the use of an ACEI and an ARB.
- People of African ancestry show reduced BP responses to monotherapy with ACEIs, ARBs, and beta blockers compared with diuretics or calcium channel blockers. Although complete explanations for these racial differences are unknown, what is known is that HTN is the most common cause of renal failure in African Americans. An ACEI or an ARB should be prescribed to minimize renal disease risk. Using an ACEI or an ARB as part of multidrug therapy, including a calcium channel blocker and thiazide diuretic, is likely to be needed. Nondihydropyridine calcium channel blockers (verapamil, diltiazem) are particularly helpful for BP control and renal protection.

Discussion Sources

National Heart, Blood and Lung Institute. http://www.nhlbi.nih.gov/guidelines/hypertension/, The Seventh Report of the Joint National Committee on Prevention, Detection, Evaluation, and Treatment of High Blood Pressure (JNC7), accessed 9/12/09.

Prisant M. Hypertension. In: Rakel R, Bope E, eds. *Conn's Current Therapy 2009*. Philadelphia, PA: Saunders Elsevier; 2009:349–360.

TABLE 5–17

JNC-7 Compelling Indications for Individual Drug Classes

	Thiazide Diuretic	Beta-adrenergic Receptor Antagonist (Beta Blocker)	Angiotensin-converting Enzyme Inhibitor (ACEI)	Angiotensin Receptor Blocker (ARB)	Calcium Antagonist (Calcium Channel Blocker)	Aldosterone Antagonist: Compelling Indications Post Myocardial Infarction
Heart failure	✓	✓	✓	✓		✓
Post myocardial infarction		✓	✓			✓
High coronary disease risk	✓	✓	✓		✓	
Diabetes	✓	✓	✓	✓	✓	
Chronic renal disease			✓	✓		
Recurrent stroke prevention	✓		✓			

QUESTIONS

107. You examine a 24-year-old woman with mitral valve prolapse (MVP). Her physical examination findings may also include:

  A. pectus excavatum.
  B. obesity.
  C. petite stature.
  D. hyperextensible joints.

108. In performing a cardiac examination in a person with MVP, you expect to find:

  A. an early to mid systolic, crescendo-decrescendo murmur.
  B. a pansystolic murmur.
  C. a low-pitched, diastolic rumble.
  D. a mid to late systolic murmur.

109. Additional findings in MVP include:

  A. an opening snap.
  B. a mid-systolic click.
  C. a paradoxical splitting of the second heart sound (S_2).
  D. a fourth heart sound (S_4).

110. Intervention for patients with MVP may include:

  A. restricted activity because of low cardiac output.
  B. control of fluid intake to minimize risk of volume overload.
  C. routine use of beta-adrenergic antagonists to control palpitations.
  D. encouragement of a regular program of aerobic activity.

111. When a heart valve fails to open to its normal orifice size, it is said to be:

  A. stenotic.
  B. incompetent.
  C. sclerotic.
  D. regurgitant.

112. When a heart valve fails to close properly, it is said to be:

  A. stenotic.
  B. incompetent.
  C. sclerotic.
  D. regurgitant.

113. You are evaluating a patient who has rheumatic heart disease. When assessing her for mitral stenosis, you auscultate the heart, anticipating finding the following murmur:

  A. systolic with wide radiation over the precordium
  B. localized diastolic with little radiation
  C. diastolic with radiation to the neck
  D. systolic with radiation to the axilla

114. In evaluating mitral valve incompetency, you expect to find the following murmur:

  A. systolic with radiation to the axilla
  B. diastolic with little radiation
  C. diastolic with radiation to the axilla
  D. localized systolic

115. In evaluating the person with aortic stenosis, the NP anticipates finding 12-lead ECG changes consistent with:

A. right bundle branch block.

B. extreme axis deviation.

C. right atrial enlargement.

D. left ventricular hypertrophy.

116. Of the following patients, who is in greatest need of endocarditis prophylaxis when planning dental work?

A. a 22-year-old woman with MVP with trace mitral regurgitation noted on echocardiogram

B. a 54-year-old woman with a prosthetic aortic valve

C. a 66-year-old man with cardiomyopathy

D. a 58-year-old woman who had a three-vessel coronary artery bypass graft with drug-eluting stents 1 year ago

117. Of the following people, who has no significant increased risk for developing bacterial endocarditis?

A. a 43-year-old woman with a bicuspid aortic valve

B. a 55-year-old man who was diagnosed with a Still's murmur during childhood

C. a 45-year-old woman with a history of endocarditis

D. a 75-year-old man with dilated cardiomyopathy

118. You are examining an elderly woman and find a grade 3/6 crescendo-decrescendo systolic murmur with radiation to the neck. This is most likely caused by:

A. aortic stenosis

B. aortic regurgitation.

C. anemia.

D. mitral stenosis.

119. Aortic stenosis in a 15-year-old is most likely:

A. a sequela of rheumatic fever.

B. a result of a congenital defect.

C. calcific in nature.

D. found with atrial septal defect.

120. A physiological murmur has which of the following characteristics?

A. occurs late in systole

B. is noted in a localized area of auscultation

C. becomes softer when the patient moves from supine to standing

D. frequently obliterates S_2

121. You are examining an 18-year-old man who is seeking a sports clearance physical examination. You note a mid-systolic murmur that gets louder when he stands. This may represent:

A. aortic stenosis.

B. hypertrophic cardiomyopathy.

C. a physiologic murmur.

D. a Still's murmur.

122. According to recommendations of the American Heart Association (AHA), which of the following antibiotics should be used for endocarditis prophylaxis in patients who are allergic to penicillin?

A. erythromycin

B. dicloxacillin

C. azithromycin

D. ofloxacin

123. A grade III systolic heart murmur is usually:

A. softer than the S_2 heart sound.

B. about as loud as the S_1 heart sound.

C. accompanied by a thrill.

D. heard across the precordium but without radiation.

124. The S_3 heart sound has all of the following characteristics except:

A. heard in early diastole

B. a presystolic sound

C. noted in the presence of ventricular overload

D. heard best with the bell of the stethoscope

125. The S_4 heart sound has which of the following characteristics?

A. After it is initially noted, it is a permanent finding.

B. It is noted in presence of poorly controlled hypertension.

C. It is heard best in early diastole.

D. It is a high-pitched sound best heard with the diaphragm of the stethoscope.

126. Of the following individuals, who is most likely to have a physiological split S_2 heart sound?

A. a 19-year-old healthy athlete

B. a 49-year-old with well-controlled hypertension

C. a 68-year-old with stable heart failure

D. a 78-year-old with cardiomyopathy

ANSWERS

107.	A	108.	D	109.	B
110.	D	111.	A	112.	B
113.	B	114.	A	115.	D
116.	B	117.	B	118.	A
119.	B	120.	C	121.	B
122.	C	123.	B	124.	B
125.	B	126.	A			

DISCUSSION

Heart murmurs are caused by the sounds produced from turbulent blood flow. Blood traveling through the chambers and great vessels is usually silent. When the flow is sufficient to generate turbulence in the wall of the heart or great vessel, a murmur occurs.

Murmurs are often benign; the examiner simply hears the blood flowing through the heart, but no cardiac structural abnormality exists. Certain cardiac structural problems, such as valvular and myocardial disorders, can contribute to the development of a murmur, however (Table 5–18).

Normal heart valves allow one-way, unimpeded, forward blood flow through the heart. The entire stroke output is able to pass freely during one phase of the cardiac cycle (diastole with the atrioventricular valves, systole with the others), and there is no backflow of blood. When a heart valve fails to open to its normal orifice, it is stenotic. When it fails to close appropriately, the valve is incompetent, causing regurgitation of blood to the previous chamber or vessel. Both of these events place a patient at significant risk for embolic disease.

Physiologic murmurs are heard in the absence of cardiac pathology. The term *physiologic* implies that the reason for murmur is something other than obstruction to flow, and that the murmur is present with a normal gradient across the valve. This murmur is heard in 80% of thin adults or children if the cardiac examination is performed in a sound-proof booth, and it is best heard at the left sternal border. The physiological murmur occurs in early to mid systole, leaving the S_1 and S_2 heart sounds intact. In addition, an individual with a benign systolic ejection murmur denies having cardiac symptoms and has an otherwise normal cardiac examination, including an appropriately located point of maximum impulse and full pulses. Because no cardiac pathology is present with a physiologic murmur, no endocarditis prophylaxis is needed.

Aortic stenosis (AS) is the inability of the aortic valves to open to an optimal orifice. The aortic valve normally opens to 3 cm²; AS usually does not cause significant symptoms until the valvular orifice is limited to 0.8 cm². The disease is characterized by a long symptom-free period with rapid clinical deterioration at the onset of symptoms, including dyspnea, syncope, chest pain, and heart failure (HF). Low pulse pressure, the difference between the systolic and diastolic blood pressure, is a characteristic of severe AS.

When AS is present in adults who are middle-aged and older, it is most often the acquired form. In an older adult, the problem is usually calcification, leading to the inability of the valve to open to its normal orifice. Valvular changes in middle-aged adults without congenital AS are usually the sequelae of rheumatic fever and represent about 30% of valvular dysfunction seen in rheumatic heart disease.

AS may be present in children and younger adults and is usually caused by a congenital bicuspid (rather than tricuspid) valve or by a three-cusp valve with leaflet fusion. This defect is most often found in boys and young men, and is commonly accompanied by a long-standing history of becoming excessively short of breath with increased activity such as running. The physical examination is usually normal except for the associated cardiac findings.

The heart murmur of mitral regurgitation (MR) arises from mitral valve incompetency or the inability of the mitral valve to close properly. This incompetency allows a retrograde flow from a high-pressure area (left ventricle) to an area of lower pressure (left atrium). MR is most often caused by the degeneration of the mitral valve, commonly by rheumatic fever, endocarditis, calcific annulus, rheumatic heart disease, ruptured chordae, or papillary muscle dysfunction. In MR resulting from rheumatic heart disease, there is usually some degree of mitral stenosis. After the person becomes symptomatic, the disease progresses in a downhill course leading to HF over the next 10 years.

Mitral valve prolapse (MVP) is likely the most common valvular heart problem; it is present in perhaps 10% of the population. The degree of distress (chest pain, dyspnea) may depend in part on the degree of MR, although some studies have failed to reveal any difference in the rates of chest pain in patients with or without MVP. Potentially the greatest threat is the rupture of chordae, usually seen only in those with connective tissue disease, especially Marfan syndrome. Most patients with MVP have a benign condition in which one of the valve leaflets is unusually long and buckles or prolapses into the left atrium, usually in mid-systole. At that time, a click occurs that is followed by a short murmur caused by regurgitation of blood into the atrium. Cardiac output is usually uncompromised, and the event goes unnoticed by the patient. The clinician may detect this on examination, however. Echocardiography fails to reveal any abnormality, simply noting the valve buckling followed by a small-volume MR. If there are no cardiac complaints and the rest of the cardiac examination, including the ECG, is normal, no further evaluation is needed.

One way of describing this variation from the norm is to inform the patient that one leaflet of the mitral valve is a bit longer than usual. The "holder" (valve orifice) is of average size, however. This discrepancy causes the valve to buckle a bit, just as a person's foot would if forced into a shoe that is

TABLE 5–18

Assessment of Common Cardiac Murmurs in Adults

WHEN EVALUATING AN ADULT WITH CARDIAC MURMUR

Ask about major symptoms of heart disease: chest pain, heart failure symptoms, palpitations, syncope, activity intolerance

The bell of the stethoscope is most helpful for auscultating lower pitched sounds, whereas the diaphragm is most helpful for higher pitched sounds

Systolic murmurs are graded on a 1–6 scale, from barely audible to audible with stethoscope off the chest. Grade 3 murmur is about as loud as S_1 or S_2, whereas grade 2 murmur is slightly softer; grade 1 murmur is difficult to hear. Grade ≥ 4 murmurs are usually accompanied by a thrill, or the feel of turbulent blood flow. Diastolic murmurs are usually graded on the same scale, but abbreviated to grades 1–4 because these murmurs are not loud enough to reach grades 5 and 6

A critical part of the evaluation of a person with a heart murmur is to decide to offer antimicrobial prophylaxis. No prophylaxis is needed with benign murmurs. Please refer to the American Heart Association's Guideline for the latest advice

Murmur	Important Cardiac Examination Findings	Additional Findings	Comments
Physiological (also known as innocent, functional)	Grade 1–3/6 early to mid systolic murmur heard best at left sternal border, but usually audible over precordium	No radiation beyond precordium. Softens or disappears with standing, increases in intensity with activity, fever, anemia. S_1, S_2 intact, normal PMI	Etiology probably flows over aortic valve. May be heard in ~80% of thin adults if examined in soundproof room. Asymptomatic with no report of chest pain, heart failure symptoms, palpitations, syncope, activity intolerance
Aortic stenosis	Grade 1–4/6 harsh systolic murmur, usually crescendo-decrescendo pattern, heard best at second right intercostal space, apex, softens with standing	Radiates to carotids, may have diminished S_2, slow filling carotid pulse, narrow pulse pressure, loud S_4, heaving PMI. The greater the degree of stenosis, the later the peak of murmur	In younger adults, usually congenital bicuspid valve. In older adults, usually calcific, rheumatic in nature. Dizziness and syncope ominous signs, pointing to severely decreased cardiac output
Aortic sclerosis	Grade 2–3/6 systolic ejection murmur heard best at second right intercostal space	Carotid upstroke full, not delayed, no S_4, absence of symptoms	Benign thickening or calcification, or both, of aortic valve leaflets. No change in valve pressure gradient. Also known as "50 over 50" murmur as found in >50% adults >50 y.o.
Aortic regurgitation	Grade 1–3/4 high-pitched blowing diastolic murmur heard best at third left intercostal space	May be enhanced by forced expiration, leaning forward. Usually with S_3, wide pulse pressure, sustained thrusting apical impulse	More common in men, usually from rheumatic heart disease, but occasionally due to latent syphilis
Mitral stenosis	Grade 1–3/4 low-pitched late diastolic murmur heard best at the apex, localized. Short crescendo-decrescendo rumble, similar to a bowling ball rolling down an alley or distant thunder	Often with opening snap, accentuated S_1 in the mitral area. Enhanced by left lateral decubitus position, squat, cough, immediately after Valsalva	Nearly all rheumatic in origin. Protracted latency period, then gradual decrease in exercise tolerance leading to rapid downhill course owing to low cardiac output. Atrial fibrillation common

Continued

TABLE 5–18

Assessment of Common Cardiac Murmurs in Adults—cont'd

Murmur	Important Cardiac Examination Findings	Additional Findings	Comments
Atrial septal defect (uncorrected)	Grade 1–3/6 systolic ejection murmur at the pulmonic area	Widely split S_2, right ventricular heave	Typically without symptoms until middle age, then present with congestive heart failure. Persistent ostium secundum in mid septum
Pulmonary hypertension	Narrow splitting S_2, murmur of tricuspid regurgitation	Report of shortness of breath nearly universal	Seen with right ventricular hypertrophy, right atrial hypertrophy as identified by ECG, echocardiogram. Secondary pulmonary hypertension may be a consequence of dexfenfluramine (Redux), "phen/fen" (phentermine with fenfluramine) use (Dexfenfluramine and fenfluramine no longer available on the North American market due to safety issues.)
Mitral regurgitation	Grade 1–4/6 high-pitched blowing systolic murmur, often extending beyond S_2. Sounds like long "haaa," "hooo." Heard best at right lower scapular border	Radiates to axilla, often with laterally displaced PMI. Decreased with standing, Valsalva maneuver. Increased by squat, hand grip	Found in ischemic heart disease, endocarditis, RHD. With RHD, often with other valve abnormalities (aortic stenosis, mitral stenosis, aortic regurgitation)
Mitral valve prolapse	Grade 1–3/6 late systolic crescendo murmur with honking quality heard best at apex. Murmur follows mid-systolic click	With Valsalva or standing, click moves forward into earlier systole, resulting in a longer sounding murmur. With hand grasp, squat, click moves back further into systole, resulting in a shorter murmur	Often seen with minor thoracic deformities such as pectus excavatum, straight back, and shallow anterior-posterior diameter. Chest pain is sometimes present, but there is a question as to whether mitral valve prolapse itself is cause

PMI, point of maximal impulse; RHD, rheumatic heart disease.
Source: Goolsby MJ. *Advanced Assessment: Interpreting Findings and Formulating Differential Diagnoses*. Philadelphia, PA: Davis; 2005.
Mangione S. *Physical Diagnosis Secrets*. 2nd ed. St. Louis, MO: Elsevier Health Sciences; 2007.

one or two sizes too small. As a result, the heart makes an extra set of sounds (click and murmur), but is not diseased or damaged. MVP is often found in patients with minor thoracic deformities such as pectus excavatum, a dish-shaped concave area at T1, and scoliosis. The exact nature of this correlation of findings is not understood.

The second and much smaller group of patients with MVP has systolic displacement of one or both of the mitral leaflets into the left atrium alone with valve thickening and redundancy, usually accompanied by mild to moderate MR. This group typically has additional health problems, such as Marfan syndrome or other connective tissue disease. There is a risk of bacterial endocarditis in this group because structural cardiac abnormality is present.

Barring other health problems, patients with MVP usually have normal cardiac output and tolerate a program of aerobic activity. This activity should be encouraged to pro-mote health and well-being. The degree of MVP is increased, however, which increases intensity of the murmur, when cir-culating volume is low. Maintaining a high level of fluid intake should be encouraged for patients with MVP. Treatment with a beta-adrenergic antagonist (beta blocker) is indicated only when symptomatic recurrent tachycardia or palpitations is an issue.

Hypertrophic cardiomyopathy is a disease of the cardiac muscle. The ventricular septum is thick and asymmetrical, leading to potential blockage of the outflow tract. Patients often exhibit symptoms of cardiac outflow tract blockage with activity because the hypertrophic ventricular walls better approximate with the increased force of myocardial contraction associated with exercise. The presentation of hypertrophic cardiomyopathy can be sudden cardiac death. Idiopathic hypertrophic subaortic stenosis is a type of car-diomyopathy. Because it is an autosomal dominant disorder, a strong family history is often present. Patients with this disorder are usually young adults with a history of dyspnea with activity, but they may also be asymptomatic.

The American Heart Association (AHA) has developed guidelines for the evaluation of infectious endocarditis risk. Although in the past, infectious endocarditis prophylaxis was used liberally for most individuals with a past or current history of heart murmur or structural cardiac abnormality, the AHA has long advocated for restraint in this practice, recognizing that infectious endocarditis is much more likely to result from frequent exposure to random bacteremias associated with daily activities than from bacteremia caused by a dental, gastrointestinal tract, or genitourinary tract pro-cedure; maintenance of optimal oral health and hygiene is likely more important than prophylactic antibiotics for a dental procedure in reducing infectious endocarditis risk. Infectious endocarditis prophylaxis is considered a reason-able option, however, for people at highest risk, including individuals with an infectious endocarditis history or a pros-thetic heart valve (Table 5–19).

Heart sound abnormalities are commonly noted in poorly controlled hypertension (S_4) and heart failure (S_3). Knowledge of the timing and qualities of these sounds is an important component of safe and effective practice (Table 5–20).

Discussion Sources

Goolsby MJ, Grubbs L. *Advanced Assessment: Interpreting Findings and Formulating Differential Diagnoses.* Philadelphia, PA: FA Davis; 2007.

http://www.americanheart.org/presenter.jhtml?identifier =3004539, Prevention of Endocarditis: Guidelines from the American Heart Association, accessed 9/12/09.

QUESTIONS

127. Causes of unstable angina include all of the following except:
    A. ventricular hypertrophy.
    B. vasoconstriction.
    C. nonocclusive thrombus.
    D. inflammation or infection.

128. Which of the following is most consistent with a per-son presenting with unstable angina?
    A. a 5-minute episode of chest tightness brought on by stair climbing and relieved by rest
    B. a severe, searing pain that penetrates the chest and lasts about 30 seconds
    C. chest pressure lasting 20 minutes that occurs at rest
    D. "heartburn" relieved by position change

129. In assessing a woman with or at risk for acute coronary syndrome (ACS), the NP considers that the patient will likely present:
    A. in a manner similar to that of a man with equiva-lent disease.
    B. at the same age as a man with similar health problems.
    C. more commonly with angina and less commonly with acute MI.
    D. less commonly with HF.

130. The cardiac finding most commonly associated with unstable angina is:
    A. physiological split S_2.
    B. S_4.
    C. opening snap.
    D. summation gallop.

131. Which of the following changes on the 12-lead ECG do you expect to find in a patient with acute coronary syndrome (ACS)?
    A. flattened T wave
    B. R wave larger than 25 mm
    C. ST segment deviation (>0.05 mV)
    D. fixed Q wave

132. Beta-adrenergic antagonists are used in ACS therapy because of their ability to:
    A. reverse obstruction-fixed vessel lesions.
    B. reduce myocardial oxygen demand.
    C. enhance myocardial vessel tone.
    D. stabilize atriol volume.

TABLE 5–19

Prevention of Endocarditis: Guidelines From the American Heart Association

PRIMARY REASONS FOR REVISIONS OF INFECTIOUS ENDOCARDITIS (IE) PROPHYLAXIS GUIDELINES

IE is much more likely to result from frequent exposure to random bacteremias associated with daily activities than from bacteremia caused by a dental, gastrointestinal (GI) tract, or genitourinary (GU) tract procedure

Prophylaxis may prevent very few, if any, cases of IE in individuals who undergo a dental, GI tract, or GU tract procedure

The risk of antibiotic-associated adverse events exceeds the benefit, if any, from prophylactic antibiotic therapy

Maintenance of optimal oral health and hygiene may reduce incidence of bacteremia from daily activities and is more important than prophylactic antibiotics for a dental procedure to reduce the risk of IE

CARDIAC CONDITIONS ASSOCIATED WITH HIGHEST RISK OF ADVERSE OUTCOME FROM ENDOCARDITIS FOR WHICH PROPHYLAXIS WITH DENTAL PROCEDURES IS REASONABLE

Prosthetic cardiac valve or prosthetic material used for cardiac valve repair

Previous IE

Congenital heart disease (CHD)*

- Unrepaired cyanotic CHD, including palliative shunts and conduits
- Completely repaired congenital heart defect with prosthetic material or device, whether placed by surgery or by catheter intervention, during the first 6 mo after the procedure†
- Repaired CHD with residual defects at the site or adjacent to the site of a prosthetic patch or prosthetic device (which inhibit endothelialization)

   Cardiac transplantation recipients who develop cardiac valvulopathy

DENTAL, ORAL, OR RESPIRATORY TRACT OR ESOPHAGEAL PROCEDURES: GIVE 30–60 MINUTES BEFORE PROCEDURE

Adults	Children
Amoxicillin 2 g PO	Amoxicillin 50 mg/kg PO
IF UNABLE TO TAKE ORAL MEDICATION	
Ampicillin 2 g IM or IV	Ampicillin 50 mg/kg IM or IV
Cefazolin or ceftriaxone 1 g IM or IV	Cefazolin or ceftriaxone 50 mg/kg IM or IV
ORAL, IF PENICILLIN OR AMPICILLIN ALLERGIC	
Clindamycin 600 mg	Clindamycin 20 mg/kg
Cephalexin‡§ 2 g	Cephalexin §50 mg/kg
Azithromycin or clarithromycin 500 mg	Azithromycin or clarithromycin 15 mg/kg
IF PENICILLIN OR AMPICILLIN ALLERGIC AND UNABLE TO TAKE ORAL MEDICATION	
Cefazolin§ or ceftriaxone§ 1 g IM or IV	Cefazolin§ or ceftriaxone §50 mg/kg IM or IV
Clindamycin 600 mg IM or IV	Clindamycin 20 mg/kg IM or IV

*Except for the conditions listed, antibiotic prophylaxis is no longer recommended for any other form of CHD.

†Prophylaxis is reasonable because endothelialization of prosthetic material occurs within 6 mo after the procedure.

‡Or other first-generation or second-generation oral cephalosporin in equivalent adult or pediatric dosage.

§Cephalosporins should not be used in an individual with a history of anaphylaxis, angioedema, or urticaria with penicillins or ampicillin.

Source: Prevention of Endocarditis. Available at http://www.americanheart.org/presenter.jhtml?identifier=3004539, Guidelines from the American Heart Association, accessed 9/12/09.

TABLE 5–20

Heart Sounds

Heart Sound	Significance	Heard Best	Comment
S_1	Marks beginning of systole. Produced by events surrounding closure of mitral and tricuspid valve.	Best heard at apex with the diaphragm	"**Lub** dub" Heard nearly simultaneous with carotid upstroke
S_2	Marks end of systole. Produced by events surrounding closure of aortic and pulmonic valves	Best heard at base with diaphragm	"Lub **dub**"
Physiological split S_2	Widening of normal interval between aortic and pulmonic components of S_2. Caused by delay in pulmonic component	Heard best in pulmonic region	The split *increases* on patient *in*spiration. Found in most adults <30 y.o., fewer beyond this age. Benign finding
Pathological split S_2	Fixed split—no change with inspiration Paradoxical split—narrows or closes with inspiration	Heard best in pulmonic region	Fixed split often found in uncorrected septal defect Paradoxical split often found in conditions that delay aortic closure, such as left bundle branch block Finding can resolve with treatment of underlying condition
Pathological S_3	Marker of ventricular overload or systolic dysfunction or both	Heard in early diastole, can sound like it is "hooked on" to the back of S_2 Low pitch, best heard with bell, might miss with diaphragm	For diagnosis of heart failure, correlate with additional findings such as dyspnea, tachycardia, crackles Finding can resolve with treatment of underlying condition
S_4	Marker of poor diastolic function, most often found in poorly controlled hypertension or recurrent myocardial ischemia	Heard late in diastole, can sound like it is "hooked on" to the front of S_1 Sometimes called a presystolic sound Soft, low pitch (higher pitch than S_3), best heard with bell	Finding can resolve with treatment of underlying condition

133. Nitrates are used in ACS therapy because of their ability to:

   A. reverse fixed vessel obstruction.
   B. reduce myocardial oxygen demand.
   C. cause vasodilation.
   D. stabilize cardiac rhythm.

134. Which of the following is most consistent with a patient presenting with acute MI?

   A. a 5-minute episode of chest tightness brought on by stair climbing
   B. a severe, localized pain that penetrates the chest and lasts about 3 hours
   C. chest pressure lasting 20 minutes that occurs at rest
   D. retrosternal diffuse pain for 30 minutes accompanied by diaphoresis

135. Which of the following changes on the 12-lead ECG would you expect to find in a patient with history of acute transmural MI 6 months ago?

   A. 2-mm ST segment elevation
   B. R wave larger than 25 mm
   C. T wave inversion
   D. deep Q waves

136. Which of the following changes on the 12-lead ECG would you expect to find in a patient with myocardial ischemia?

   A. 2-mm ST segment elevation
   B. S wave larger than 10 mm
   C. T wave inversion
   D. deep Q waves

137. Thrombolytic therapy is indicated in patients with chest pain and ECG changes such as:

   A. 1-mm ST segment depression in leads V1 and V3.
   B. physiologic Q waves in leads aVF, V5, and V6.
   C. 3-mm ST segment elevation in leads V1 to V4.
   D. T wave inversion in leads aVL and aVR.

138. An abnormality of which of the following is the most sensitive marker for myocardial damage?

   A. aspartate aminotransferase
   B. creatine phosphokinase (CPK)
   C. troponin I (cTnI)
   D. lactate dehydrogenase

139. All of the following should be prescribed as part of therapy in ACS except:

   A. aspirin.
   B. metoprolol.
   C. lisinopril.
   D. nisoldipine.

140. Which of the following is an absolute contraindication to the use of thrombolytic therapy?

   A. history of hemorrhagic stroke
   B. BP of 160/100 mm Hg or greater at presentation
   C. current use of warfarin
   D. active peptic ulcer disease

141. The recommended low-density lipoprotein goal for a 64-year-old man with diabetes mellitus who had an MI 2 years ago should be less than:

   A. 70 mg/dL (<1.8 mmol/L).
   B. 100 mg/dL (< 2.6 mmol/L).
   C. 130 mg/dL (< 3.4 mmol/L).
   D. 160 mg/dL (< 4.1 mmol/L).

142. Which of the following is least likely to be reported in ACS?

   A. newly noted pulmonary crackles
   B. transient MR murmur
   C. hypotension
   D. pain reproduced with palpation

ANSWERS

127.	A	**128.**	C	**129.**	C
130.	B	**131.**	C	**132.**	B
133.	C	**134.**	D	**135.**	D
136.	C	**137.**	C	**138.**	C
139.	D	**140.**	A	**141.**	A
142.	D				

DISCUSSION

ACS (acute MI, unstable angina) and angina pectoris, most often caused by atherosclerosis, result from an imbalance in the ability to supply the myocardium with sufficient oxygen to meet its metabolic demands. In stable angina, patterns of symptom provocation are usually predictable, with exertion often causing discomfort that is promptly relieved with rest, use of nitroglycerin via sublingual tablet or spray, or both. The discomfort associated with an anginal episode is described by many terms—*pressure, pain, tightness, heaviness,* and *suffocation.* Testing to support the angina diagnosis includes a resting 12-lead ECG (though this is normal in about 50% of individuals with the disease) and exercise ECG or other form of stress testing, often with myocardial nuclear imaging. Computed tomography to document coronary artery calcification is another noninvasive test.

Treatment includes beta blockers because these agents reduce myocardial workload through lowering heart rate, lowering stroke volume, and blunting of catecholamine response and aspirin therapy; most patients with angina also have an indication for ACEI use. A calcium channel blocker is often added if anginal symptoms occur two or more times per week, and no contraindications to calcium channel blocker use exist. Sustained-effect nitroglycerin via the oral or topical route (patch or ointment) can be added if nocturnal symptoms are present. Nitroglycerin via sublingual tablet or spray should be prescribed with advice on its use for acute symptoms and education to monitor frequency of use to detect patterns of anginal triggers and disease instability. Use of nitrates enhances myocardial perfusion through peripheral and central vasodilation. Overall cardiovascular risk reduction is also important, with the use of appropriate dyslipidemia agents, with HMG-CoA reductase inhibitor therapy (statin) therapy nearly always indicated. Coronary angiography should be considered if exercise tolerance is poor, significant abnormality is noted on resting or exercise ECG or myocardial imaging, or symptoms become less stable.

Unstable angina is defined as a new onset of symptoms at rest or worsening symptoms with activities that did not previously provoke symptoms. Certain characteristics increase or decrease the likelihood of ACS (Tables 5–21 and 5–22).

TABLE 5–21

Chest Pain, Typical of Myocardial Ischemia or Myocardial Infarction

- Substernal compression or crush
- Pressure, tightness, heaviness, cramping, aching sensation
- Unexplained indigestion, belching, epigastric pain
- Radiating pain to neck, jaw, shoulders, back, or one or both arms
- Dyspnea, nausea/vomiting, diaphoresis

Source: American College of Cardiology/American Heart Association 2007 Guidelines for the Management of Patients with Unstable Angina/Non–ST-Elevation Myocardial Infarction. http://circ.ahajournals.org/cgi/content/short/CIRCULATIONAHA.107.185752v1, Executive summary: a report of the American College of Cardiology/American Heart Association Task Force on Practice Guidelines (Writing Committee to Revise the 2002 Guidelines for the Management of Patients with Unstable Angina/Non–ST-Elevation Myocardial Infarction), accessed 9/12/09.

TABLE 5–22

Likelihood That Signs and Symptoms Represent Acute Coronary Syndrome Secondary to Coronary Artery Disease

Feature	High Likelihood Any of the Following Present	Intermediate Likelihood: Absence of High-likelihood Features and Presence of Any of the Following	Low Likelihood Absence of High- or Intermediate-likelihood Features but Many Have the Following
History	Chest or left arm pain or discomfort as chief symptom producing documented angina	Chest or left arm pain or discomfort as chief symptom Age >70 yr Male sex Diabetes mellitus	Probable ischemic symptoms in absence of any intermediate-likelihood characteristics Recent cocaine use
Examination	Pulmonary edema New rales Transient mitral regurgitation murmur Hypotension	Extracardiac vascular disease	Chest discomfort reproduced by palpation
ECG findings	New or presumably new transient ST segment deviation (≥0.05 mV) or T wave inversion (≥0.2 mV) with symptoms	Fixed Q waves Abnormal ST segments or E waves not documented as new	T wave flattening or inversion in leads with dominant R waves ECG
Cardiac markers	Elevated cTnT, cTnI, or CPK-MB	Normal	Normal

Source: American College of Cardiology/American Heart Association 2007 Guidelines for the Management of Patients with Unstable Angina/Non–ST-Elevation Myocardial Infarction. http://circ.ahajournals.org/cgi/content/short/CIRCULATIONAHA.107.185752v1, Executive summary: a report of the American College of Cardiology/American Heart Association Task Force on Practice Guidelines (Writing Committee to Revise the 2002 Guidelines for the Management of Patients with Unstable Angina/Non–ST-Elevation Myocardial Infarction), accessed 9/12/09.

The clinical presentation of unstable angina (ACS) represents an emergency and should be handled accordingly.

S_4 is often heard with myocardial ischemia and poorly controlled angina pectoris. This sound of poor myocardial relaxation (compliance) and diastolic dysfunction may potentially cause decreased cardiac output. The third heart sound (S_3) is the sound of poor myocardial contractility and systolic dysfunction, and usually leads to decreased cardiac output; this abnormal heart sound is often heard in the presence of heart failure.

Women usually have onset of coronary heart disease at significantly older ages and are likely to present differently than men. Dyspnea is often an anginal equivalent in older women. In a study of 515 women with ACS, 95% reported new or different symptoms in weeks before the event, including unusual fatigue (70%), sleep disturbance (48%), shortness of breath (42%), indigestion (39%), and anxiety (35%). Symptoms experienced by the women during ACS included shortness of breath (58%), weakness (55%), unusual fatigue (43%), diaphoresis (39%), dizziness (39%), and chest pain or pressure (30%); 43% of the woman had no chest discomfort during the event.

Men often have their first manifestation of coronary heart disease in the form of MI, whereas women initially present first with angina pectoris, which may lead to MI. Women younger than 60 years often have a presentation similar to that of men, however. Atypical MI presentation is often noted in both sexes when patients are older than 80 years.

MI/ACS most commonly occurs when an atherosclerotic plaque ruptures, leading to the formation of an occlusive thrombus. Coronary artery spasm can also occur, adding to the vessel obstruction. A patient with suspected ACS needs to be assessed promptly and accurately because therapy to reinstitute vessel patency (e.g., thrombolysis, percutaneous angioplasty, coronary artery bypass grafting) should be initiated early in the process to limit myocardial damage. The 12-lead ECG should be assessed for changes consistent with myocardial ischemia, myocardial injury, and MI.

In approximately 75% of patients admitted to the hospital for MI, this condition is ruled out. At least 25% of all MIs are clinically silent, however. To reduce unneeded hospitalization and to detect asymptomatic MI/ACS, diagnostic tests that are highly sensitive and specific for myocardial damage are needed.

Creatine phosphokinase (CK) isoenzyme MB (CK-MB) has long been used as a serum marker of myocardial damage. CK-MB level increases within 6 to 12 hours of MI, begins to decrease within 24 to 48 hours, and usually returns to normal in about 60 hours. Because CK-MB clears quickly, its use in late detection of MI is limited. In addition, false-positive and false-negative results are noted.

Troponin is a regulatory protein of the myofibril with three major subtypes: C, I, and T. Subtypes I (cTnI) and T (cTnT) are released in the presence of myocardial damage. Both increase rapidly within the first 12 hours after MI; cTnT typically remains elevated for about 168 hours, and cTnI remains elevated for about 192 hours. cTnI is the more cardiac-specific measure and is sensitive for small-volume myocardial damage. cTnT levels can be elevated in chronic renal failure, muscle trauma, and rhabdomyolysis. cTnI is more sensitive and specific than ECG and CK-MB in diagnosing unstable angina and non–Q wave MI. In addition, cTnI results are available quickly through a rapid assay. Protracted elevation of cTnI after MI or unstable angina may be a predictor of increased mortality. People with angina without documented MI have a significantly higher risk of death within 42 days if cTnI is persistently elevated.

The AHA periodically publishes guidelines for the management of patients with ST segment elevation MI, unstable angina, and non–ST segment elevation MI developed from consensus of nursing and medical experts and evidence-based health care. The AHA recommends the following therapy:

- Nitroglycerin via spray or sublingual tablet should be given, followed by parenteral nitroglycerin.
- Supplemental oxygen should be administered to patients with cyanosis or respiratory distress, and pulse oximetry or arterial blood gas determination should be done to confirm adequate arterial SaO_2 (>90%).
- Adequate analgesia should be provided with intravenous morphine sulfate when symptoms are not immediately relieved by nitroglycerin, or when pulmonary congestion or severe agitation or both are present.
- A beta blocker should be given if there are no contraindications. The first dose should be administered intravenously. An ACEI should be given if no contraindications exist.
- Aspirin should be given, 160 to 325 mg orally in a chewable nonenteric form. Other antiplatelet agents, such as clopidogrel (Plavix), may be used if aspirin allergy or intolerance is present or as adjunctive therapy.
- A history, physical examination, 12-lead ECG, and cardiac marker tests should be performed promptly.

With a diagnosis of ACS and ST segment elevation, the patient should be evaluated for reperfusion; the examiner should look for ST segment elevation greater than 1 mm in contiguous leads. The presence of these changes usually indicates acute coronary artery occlusion, usually from thrombosis. In addition, clinically significant ST segment elevation largely dictates reperfusion therapy with the use of thrombolytic therapy, primary percutaneous transluminal coronary angioplasty, or other revascularization options. These therapies have the best effect on clinical outcomes if used within 6 hours after onset of chest pain, but may be helpful 7 to 12 hours or more after MI symptoms begin. When thrombolysis is used, heparin is usually given for at least 48 hours to ensure continued vessel patency. Before giving a thrombolytic agent such as tissue plasminogen activator or streptokinase, the prescriber must be aware of absolute and relative contraindications to thrombolytic therapy (Table 5–23).

If left bundle branch block is evident on ECG, and the clinical scenario is consistent with acute MI, standard acute MI care should be offered. Patients with a presentation

TABLE 5–23

Contraindications and Cautions for Fibrinolysis in ST Segment Elevation Myocardial Infarction*

ABSOLUTE CONTRAINDICATIONS	Any prior intracranial hemorrhage
	Known structural cerebral vascular lesion (e.g., arteriovenous malformation)
	Known malignant intracranial neoplasm (primary or metastatic)
	Ischemic stroke within 3 mo *except* acute ischemic stroke within 3 hr
	Suspected aortic dissection
	Active bleeding or bleeding diathesis (excluding menses)
	Significant closed-head or facial trauma within 3 mo
RELATIVE CONTRAINDICATIONS	History of chronic, severe, poorly controlled hypertension
	Severe uncontrolled hypertension on presentation (systolic blood pressure >180 mm Hg or diastolic blood pressure >110 mm Hg)†
	History of prior ischemic stroke >3 mo, dementia, or known intracranial pathology not covered in contraindications
	Traumatic or prolonged (>10 min) CPR or major surgery (within <3 weeks)
	Recent (within 2–4 weeks) internal bleeding
	Noncompressible vascular punctures
	For streptokinase/anistreplase: prior exposure (>5 days ago) or prior allergic reaction to these agents
	Pregnancy
	Active peptic ulcer
	Current use of anticoagulants: the higher the INR, the higher the risk of bleeding

*Viewed as advisory for clinical decision making and may not be all-inclusive or definitive.
†Could be an absolute contraindication in low-risk patients with ST segment elevation myocardial infarction.
INR, international normalized ratio.
Source: American College of Cardiology/American Heart Association 2007 Guidelines for the Management of Patients with Unstable Angina/Non–ST-Elevation Myocardial Infarction. http://circ.ahajournals.org/cgi/content/short/CIRCULATIONAHA.107.185752v1, Executive Summary. A Report of the American College of Cardiology/American Heart Association Task Force on Practice Guidelines (Writing Committee to Revise the 2002 Guidelines for the Management of Patients with Unstable Angina/Non–ST-Elevation Myocardial Infarction), accessed 4/8/09.

suggestive of MI but without ST segment changes should not receive thrombolysis. These patients should be hospitalized and placed on continuous ECG monitoring for rhythm disturbances; disturbances that are noted should be appropriately treated. Serial 12-lead ECGs should be obtained, and results should be correlated with clinical measures of myocardial necrosis, such as CPK or CK isoenzymes and troponin. Aspirin therapy should be continued, and heparin use should be considered, particularly in the presence of a large anterior MI or left ventricular mural thrombus because of increased risk of embolic stroke.

If no contraindications are present, beta blocker and ACEI therapy should be initiated promptly because the use of these products is associated with reduced mortality and morbidity after MI. Beta blocker and ACEI therapy should be continued indefinitely. Before hospital discharge, patients should undergo standard exercise testing to assess functional capacity, efficacy of current medical regimen, and risk stratification for subsequent cardiac events.

Ongoing care includes a goal of reducing low-density lipoprotein cholesterol to less than 100 mg/dL (<2.6 mmol/L) and in some very high-risk patients, including individuals with diabetes mellitus and established coronary artery disease, to less than 70 mg/dL (<1.8 mmol/L), using diet, exercise, and, as is typically needed, drug therapy. This ongoing care is in keeping with an overall plan to reduce or eliminate all cardiac risk factors, including inactivity, smoking, and obesity.

Discussion Sources

American College of Cardiology/American Heart Association 2007 Guidelines for the Management of Patients with Unstable Angina/Non–ST-Elevation Myocardial Infarction: Executive Summary. http://circ.ahajournals.org/cgi/content/short/CIRCULATIONAHA.107.185752v1, A Report of the American College of Cardiology/American Heart Association Task Force on Practice Guidelines (Writing Committee to Revise the 2002 Guidelines for the Management of Patients with Unstable Angina/Non–ST-Elevation Myocardial Infarction), accessed 9/12/09.

American College of Cardiology/American Heart Association (ACC/AHA) Task Force on Practice Guidelines. http://circ.ahajournals.org/cgi/content/full/116/23/2762, 2007 Chronic Angina Focused Update of the ACC/AHA 2002 Guidelines for the Management of Patients with Chronic Stable Angina, accessed 9/12/09.

McSweeney J, Cody M, O'Sullivan P, Elberson K, Moser D, Garvin B. Women's early warning symptoms of acute myocardial infarction. *Circulation.* 2003;108:2619–2623.

National Heart, Lung, and Blood Institute. http://www.nhlbi.nih.gov/guidelines/cholesterol/index.htm, National Cholesterol Education Program Adult Treatment Panel III Guidelines for Lipid Goals, accessed 4/8/09.

QUESTIONS

143. You examine an 82-year-old woman who has a history of heart failure (HF). She is in the office because of increasing shortness of breath. When auscultating her heart, you note a tachycardia with a rate of 104 bpm and an extra heart sound early in diastole. This sound most likely represents:

    A. summation gallop.
    B. S$_3$.
    C. opening snap.
    D. S$_4$.

144. You examine a 65-year-old man with dilated cardiomyopathy and HF. On examination, you expect to find all of the following except:

    A. jugular venous distention.
    B. tenderness on right upper abdominal quadrant palpation.
    C. point of maximal impulse at the fifth intercostal space, mid-clavicular line.
    D. peripheral edema.

145. One of the most underused classes of drugs in the treatment of heart failure is:

    A. beta blockers.
    B. ACEIs.
    C. calcium channel blockers.
    D. loop diuretics.

146. The rationale for using beta blocker therapy in treating a patient with HF is to:

    A. increase myocardial contractility.
    B. reduce the effects of circulating catecholamines.
    C. relieve concomitant angina.
    D. stabilize cardiac rhythm.

147. An ECG finding in a patient who is taking digoxin in a therapeutic dose typically includes:

    A. shortened P-R interval.
    B. slightly depressed, cupped ST segments.
    C. widened QRS complex.
    D. tall T waves.

148. A potential adverse effect of ACEI when used with spironolactone therapy is:

    A. hypertension.
    B. hyperkalemia.
    C. renal insufficiency.
    D. proteinuria.

149. ECG findings in a patient with digoxin toxicity would most likely include:

    A. atrioventricular heart block.
    B. T wave inversion.
    C. sinus tachycardia.
    D. pointed P waves.

150. Patients reporting symptoms of digoxin toxicity are most likely to include:

    A. anorexia.
    B. disturbance in color perception.
    C. blurred vision.
    D. diarrhea.

151. Which of the following is among the most common causes of HF?

    A. dietary indiscretion
    B. COPD
    C. hypertensive heart disease
    D. anemia

152. Which of the following medications is an aldosterone antagonist?

    A. clonidine
    B. spironolactone
    C. hydrochlorothiazide
    D. furosemide

153. Which of the following best describes orthopnea?

    A. shortness of breath with exercise
    B. dyspnea that develops when the individual is recumbent and is relieved with elevation of the head
    C. shortness of breath that occurs at night, characterized by a sudden awakening after a couple of hours of sleep, with a feeling of severe anxiety, breathlessness, and suffocation
    D. dyspnea at rest

154. Which of the following is unlikely to be noted in the person experiencing HF?

    A. elevated serum B-type natriuretic peptide (BNP)
    B. Kerley B lines noted on chest x-ray
    C. left ventricular hypertrophy on ECG
    D. evidence of hemoconcentration on hemogram

155. Which of the following medications is an alpha/beta-adrenergic antagonist?

   A. atenolol
   B. metoprolol
   C. propranolol
   D. carvedilol

156. Which of the following best describes the patient presentation of New York Heart Association stage III heart disease?

   A. Ordinary physical activity does not cause undue fatigue, dyspnea, or palpitations.
   B. Ordinary physical activity results in fatigue, palpitations, dyspnea, or angina.
   C. Less-than-ordinary activity leads to fatigue, dyspnea, palpitations, or angina.
   D. Discomfort increases with any physical activity.

ANSWERS

143.	B	144.	C	145.	A
146.	B	147.	B	148.	B
149.	A	150.	A	151.	C
152.	B	153.	B	154.	D
155.	D	156.	C			

DISCUSSION

Heart failure (HF) occurs as a result of altered cardiac function that leads to inadequate cardiac output and a resulting inability to meet the oxygen and metabolic demands of the body. Hypertensive heart disease and atherosclerosis are the leading causes of HF. Less common causes include pneumonia (as a result of increased right-sided heart workload), anemia (because of the resulting decreased oxygen-carrying capability of the blood), and increased sodium intake (because of the resultant increase in circulating volume).

Clinical presentation of an acute exacerbation of HF includes dyspnea, or shortness of breath (SOB), that increases in severity, seen in a spectrum from exertional dyspnea (SOB with exercise), orthopnea (SOB that typically develops quickly when the individual is recumbent and is relieved with elevation of the head), paroxysmal nocturnal dyspnea (SOB that occurs at night, characterized by a sudden awakening after a couple hours of sleep, with a feeling of severe anxiety, breathlessness, and suffocation), and dyspnea at rest to acute pulmonary edema. Additional reported history often includes nocturia, fatigue, and weakness. Except for the mildest cases, crackles heard over the lung bases are characteristic; in severe cases, there is wheezing and expectoration of frothy, blood-tinged sputum. S_3 is usually noted, typically disappearing on resolution of the acute event.

Additional findings usually include tachycardia, diaphoresis, pallor, and peripheral cyanosis with pallor. Although edema is considered a classic finding in HF, a substantial gain of extracellular fluid volume (i.e., a minimum of 5 L in adults) must occur before peripheral edema is manifested. As a result of liver engorgement from elevated right-sided heart pressures, hepatojugular reflux, hepatic engorgement, and tenderness are typically noted. The point of maximal impulse is normally at the fifth intercostal space, mid-clavicular line. This shifts laterally and perhaps over more than one intercostal space in the presence of dilated cardiomyopathy and its resultant increase in cardiac size.

Patients with HF are often assigned a classification of heart disease from the New York Heart Association (NYHA), where a relationship between symptoms and the amount of effort required for provocation is assessed. In treating an acute HF exacerbation, a patient often is initially consistent with a higher classification category (NYHA III or IV). After treatment, the assignment of lower category (NYHA I or II) is likely noted and should be a clinical goal.

ECG helps to identify the presence of left atrial enlargement, left ventricular hypertrophy, and dysrhythmias often noted in HF but not specific to the diagnosis. ECG changes consistent with acute myocardial ischemia or MI as the cause of HF may also be revealed.

Laboratory testing in HF usually includes evaluation to rule in or rule out potential underlying causes (e.g., anemia, infection, renal insufficiency). B-type natriuretic peptide (BNP) is an amino acid structure common to all natriuretic peptides. The cardiac ventricles are the major source of plasma BNP; the amount in circulation is in proportion to ventricular volume expansion and pressure overload. As part of the evaluation of a patient with dyspnea and suspected HF, an elevated BNP level helps to support the diagnosis. The increased circulating volume found in HF can occasionally lead to evidence of hemodilution on hemogram; this corrects as circulating volume is normalized.

Findings on chest radiograph in HF include cardiomegaly and alveolar edema with pleural effusions and bilateral infiltrates in a butterfly pattern. Additional findings are loss of sharp definition of pulmonary vasculature, haziness of hilar shadows, and thickening of interlobular septa, also known as Kerley B lines. As part of the evaluation of heart valve function and competency, an echocardiogram is usually obtained. Radionuclide evaluation of left ventricular function provides helpful information on global heart function. Angiography and further studies should be directed by clinical presentation and other health risks.

The goal of HF therapy is threefold: reduction of preload, reduction of systemic vascular resistance (afterload reduction), and inhibition of the renin and sympathetic nervous system. Because ACEIs and angiotensin receptor blockers (ARBs) cause central and peripheral vasodilation, these medications result in a reduction in cardiac workload and improvement in cardiac output. Although ACEIs and ARBs are the cornerstone of HF therapy, their use can be associated with adverse effects. Most common is hypotension, particularly when one of these agents is prescribed for a person who is currently taking a diuretic or vasodilator. To avoid hypotension, ACEI or ARB therapy should be started at low dosages and increased slowly to achieve a therapeutic response. Renal insufficiency can be precipitated by ACEI or ARB therapy; this usually occurs only in the presence of renal artery stenosis or underlying renal disease. Hyperkalemia with ACEI or ARB use is usually seen only with concurrent use of a potassium-sparing diuretic/aldosterone antagonist, such as spironolactone (Aldactone); in advancing renal disease; or in a poor hydration state, including overly aggressive diuretic use.

Diuretics assist with circulating volume and preload reduction. Unless contraindicated, a potassium-sparing diuretic such as spironolactone should be used because of its neurohumoral effects, allowing sodium excretion and enhanced vasodilation. These effects are achieved by the drug's ability to bind competitively at receptors found in aldosterone-dependent sodium-potassium exchange sites in the renal tubule.

Beta-adrenergic blockers are used to inhibit chronotropic and inotropic responses to beta-adrenergic stimulation; the use of an alpha/beta blocker such as carvedilol (Coreg) can provide the additional benefit of a vasodilating effect through its action blockade at the alpha receptors. Long-term beta-adrenergic antagonist (beta blocker) use has been shown to improve cardiac function, to reduce myocardial ischemia, to decrease myocardial oxygen consumption, and possibly to reduce the incidence of sudden cardiac death. This drug class is underused in HF therapy.

Digoxin has a positive inotropic effect and slows conduction through the atrioventricular node. A prolongation of the P-R interval and cupping of the ST segment are typically seen in ECGs of patients taking a therapeutic dose of digoxin. Because it is a medication with narrow therapeutic index and with significant drug-drug interactions and a potential proarrhythmic effect, clinical vigilance is needed with digoxin use. In digoxin toxicity, numerous cardiac effects can be seen; atrioventricular block is the most common, whereas anorexia is the most commonly reported by patients. Visual changes are rarely reported. Digoxin use does not prolong survival in patients with systolic HF, but its use is associated with reduced hospital admissions, improved functional class, reduced symptoms of HF, and improved quality of life.

Discussion Sources

A Report of the American College of Cardiology Foundation/ American Heart Association Task Force on Practice Guidelines. http://circ.ahajournals.org/cgi/content/full/119/14/1977, 2009 Focused update: ACCF/AHA guidelines for the diagnosis and management of heart failure in adults, accessed 9/12/09.

Zevitz M. eMedicine. http://www.emedicine.com/MED/ topic3552.htm, Heart failure, accessed 9/12/09.

QUESTIONS

157. Pertussis (whooping cough) is most often transmitted via:
    A. contact with an item contaminated by a person with the infection.
    B. respiratory droplet.
    C. contaminated food.
    D. inhalation of contaminated water that has been vaporized.

158. The person with pertussis is most likely to transmit the infection to another person during the _____ stage.
    A. prodromal
    B. catarrhal
    C. paroxysmal
    D. convalescent

159. Which of the following is an appropriate antimicrobial therapy for the person with pertussis?
    A. amoxicillin
    B. cefprozil
    C. clarithromycin
    D. ofloxacin

Pertussis: True or false?

____ 160. The incubation period of the causative organism is usually 7 to 10 days.

____ 161. The causative bacterium, *Bordetella pertussis*, is a gram-negative organism.

____ 162. Because of low contagion risk, household members of a person with pertussis should be treated only if symptoms occur.

ANSWERS

157.	B	158.	B	159.	C
160.	T	161.	T	162.	F

DISCUSSION

Pertussis, or whooping cough, is an acute infectious disease caused by the bacterium *Bordetella pertussis*, an aerobic gram-negative rod. Before widespread use of the vaccine, available since the 1940s, more than 200,000 cases of this infection were reported annually in the United States. The incidence of pertussis infection has decreased dramatically in the postvaccine era, yet pertussis remains a significant public health threat with a steadily increasing number of cases during the past two decades. In developing countries with low levels of immunization against pertussis, this illness causes at least 250,000 deaths per year.

B. pertussis transmission most commonly occurs through contact with respiratory droplets and less commonly through contact with a recently contaminated item from an infected individual. The incubation period is usually 7 to 10 days (range 4 to 21 days, rarely 42 days). Pertussis is highly communicable, as evidenced by secondary attack rates of 80% among susceptible household contacts.

The clinical course of pertussis is divided into three stages:

- *Catarrhal stage*: The illness is similar to the common cold and is characterized by complaints related to upper respiratory tract infection, including nasal discharge, sneezing, low-grade fever, and an intermittent cough. This stage usually lasts 1 to 2 weeks. The person with pertussis is highly infectious during this stage.
- *Paroxysmal stage*: At the onset of this stage, the person with pertussis seems to have a lingering cold. Although the nasal symptoms are usually resolved, the cough worsens, however, because the pathogen has attached to the respiratory cilia and produced toxins that paralyze the cilia and induce inflammation of the respiratory tract. The result is an inability to clear the airways normally and a resulting stagnation of pulmonary secretions. The characteristic paroxysms occur, with numerous, rapid coughs as the airways attempt to mobilize and expel thick sputum. An episode of paroxysmal cough is followed by a long inspiration with a characteristic whooping sound. Although this is a distressing symptom for adults, infants and young children with pertussis often vomit in response to the cough episode and quickly become exhausted. Younger children often lack the respiratory effort needed for the rapid intake of air needed to induce a whoop; the absence of this characteristic sound should not cause the clinician to eliminate pertussis as a possible cause of persistent cough. During the first week of this stage, the number of daily cough attacks increases to an average of 15 per day, most often occurring at night. This level of cough remains unchanged for 2 to 3 weeks, then gradually becomes less frequent. The paroxysmal stage usually lasts 1 to 10 weeks with an average duration of 5 to 6 weeks. The person with pertussis is highly infectious for the first 2 weeks of the catarrhal stage.
- *Convalescent stage:* Gradual recovery occurs in this stage. The cough is less paroxysmal and disappears over 2 to 3 weeks. Cough can return, however, if the person with recent pertussis develops a respiratory tract infection over the next 6 to 12 months after the illness. The mechanism of this cough is likely residual airway inflammation and does not signify a recurrence of the original illness.

Although adolescents and younger adults account for most cases of pertussis reported more recently, often the first person in the household with the infection is an older adult. Infants are at highest risk, however, for having pertussis-associated complications. The most common complication, and the cause of most pertussis-related deaths, is secondary bacterial pneumonia. Neurological complications are also most common in infants and include seizures and encephalopathy, often resulting from the hypoxia induced by coughing or pathogen-related toxins. Older children and adults can develop pertussis-associated pneumonia and encephalopathy; rib fracture, pneumothorax, and subdural hematomas have also been reported in these age groups as complications directly related to cough paroxysms.

The diagnosis of pertussis is usually based on health history and physical examination with confirming laboratory tests. Specimens for analysis should be obtained from the posterior nasopharynx. Testing options include polymerase chain reaction (PCR), direct fluorescent antibody (DFA) testing, and standard bacterial culture. Serological testing is also available and gaining in utility. Because of the challenges of obtaining a clinically useful specimen, consultation with the local or regional public health department is advised at the time of testing. Guidelines on pertussis surveillance and outbreak control are available on the National Immunization Program website and from the local or regional public health department.

Treatment of the person with pertussis is largely supportive. Antimicrobial therapy helps eliminate the organisms from secretions, limiting the likelihood of communicating the disease to another person; however, this treatment does not shorten the length of the illness. Pertussis treatment options for infants and children include azithromycin, erythromycin, and clarithromycin. Options for adults include azithromycin, erythromycin, clarithromycin, and trimethoprim-sulfamethoxazole; azithromycin provides the most rapid elimination of pathogen nasal carriage. In addition to treating the person with pertussis, equally important is the provision of prophylactic antimicrobial therapy to close contacts regardless of age and immunization status with erythromycin, azithromycin, or clarithromycin.

Given the ease of communication and severity and duration of pertussis, primary prevention of the disease via immunization is important. More recent recommendations include expanded use of pertussis vaccine in the form of Tdap (tetanus, diphtheria, acellular pertussis vaccine) in the preteen to adult age group.

Discussion Sources

Centers for Disease Control and Prevention. http://www.cdc.gov/ncidod/dbmd/diseaseinfo/pertussis_t.htm, Pertussis, accessed 9/12/09.

Recommended antimicrobial agents for the treatment and postexposure prophylaxis of pertussis. 2005 CDC Guidelines. *MMWR Morb Mortal Wkly Rep*. 2005;54(No. RR-14):1–16.

6

Abdominal Disorders

QUESTIONS

1. You examine a 59-year-old man with a chief complaint of new onset of rectal pain after a bout of constipation. On examination, you note an ulcerated lesion on the posterior midline of the anus. This presentation is most consistent with:

   A. perianal fistula.
   B. anal fissure.
   C. external hemorrhoid.
   D. Crohn proctitis.

2. Rectal bleeding associated with hemorrhoids is usually described as:

   A. streaks of bright red blood on the stool.
   B. dark brown to black in color and mixed in with normal-appearing stool.
   C. a large amount of brisk red bleeding.
   D. significant blood clots and mucus mixed with stool.

3. Therapy for hemorrhoids includes all of the following except:

   A. weight control.
   B. low-fat diet.
   C. topical corticosteroids.
   D. the use of a stool softener.

ANSWERS

1. B   2. A   3. B

DISCUSSION

In anal fissure, there is an ulcer or tear of the margin of the anus. Most fissures occur posteriorly. Risk factors include constipation, diarrhea, recent childbirth, and anal intercourse or other anal insertion practices. The best treatment for anal fissure is avoidance of the condition through adequate fiber and fluid intake, avoiding constipation, and minimizing or eliminating activity that triggers or contributes to the condition.

The superior hemorrhoidal veins form internal hemorrhoids, whereas the inferior hemorrhoidal veins form external hemorrhoids. Both forms are normal anatomical findings but cause discomfort when there is an increase in the venous pressure and resulting dilation and inflammation, such as in childbirth, obesity, constipation, and prolonged sitting. Over time, tissue and vessel redundancy develop, resulting in rectal protrusion and increased risk for bleeding. With chronically protruding or prolapsing hemorrhoids, the patient often reports itch, mucous leaking, and staining of undergarments with streaks of stool. Manual reduction of the protruding hemorrhoid after evacuation can be helpful.

As with anal fissure, prevention of hemorrhoidal engorgement and inflammation is the best treatment. Strategies include weight control, high-fiber diet, regular exercise, and increased fluid intake. Treatment for acute hemorrhoid flare-ups includes the use of astringents and topical corticosteroids, sitz baths, and analgesics. Surgical intervention is warranted when more conservative therapy fails to yield clinical improvement. These therapies are also used to treat patients with anal fissure.

Discussion Source

Hyman N. Hemorrhoids, anal fissure, and anorectal abscess and fistula. In: Rakel R, Bope E, eds. *Conn's Current Therapy.* Philadelphia, PA: Saunders Elsevier; 2009:525–527.

QUESTIONS

4. All of the following are typically noted in a young adult with the diagnosis of acute appendicitis except:

   A. epigastric pain.
   B. positive obturator sign.
   C. rebound tenderness.
   D. marked febrile response.

 See full color images of this topic on DavisPlus at http://davisplus.fadavis.com | Keyword: Fitzgerald

5. A 26-year-old man presents with acute abdominal pain. As part of the evaluation for acute appendicitis, you order a white blood cell (WBC) count with differential and anticipate the following results:

   A. total WBCs, 4500 mm³; neutrophils, 35%; bands, 2%; lymphocytes, 45%
   B. total WBCs, 14,000 mm³; neutrophils, 55%; bands, 3%; lymphocytes, 38%
   C. total WBCs, 16,500 mm³; neutrophils, 66%; bands, 8%; lymphocytes, 22%
   D. total WBCs, 18,100 mm³; neutrophils, 55%; bands, 3%; lymphocytes, 28%

6. In evaluating a patient with suspected appendicitis, the clinician considers that:

   A. the presentation may differ according to the anatomical location of the appendix.
   B. this is a common reason for acute abdominal pain in elderly patients.
   C. vomiting before onset of abdominal pain is often seen.
   D. the presentation is markedly different from the presentation of pelvic inflammatory disease.

7. The psoas sign can be best described as abdominal pain elicited by:

   A. passive extension of the hip.
   B. passive flexion and internal rotation of the hip.
   C. deep palpation.
   D. asking the patient to cough.

8. The obturator sign can be best described as abdominal pain elicited by:

   A. passive extension of the hip.
   B. passive flexion and internal rotation of the hip.
   C. deep palpation.
   D. asking the patient to cough.

9. To support the diagnosis of acute appendicitis with suspected appendiceal rupture, you consider obtaining the following abdominal imaging study:

   A. magnetic resonance image
   B. computed tomography (CT) scan
   C. ultrasound
   D. flat plate

10. Which of the following WBC forms is an ominous finding in the presence of severe bacterial infection?

    A. neutrophil
    B. lymphocyte
    C. basophil
    D. metamyelocyte

11. Which of the following best represents the peak ages for occurrence of acute appendicitis?

    A. 1 to 20 years
    B. 20 to 40 years
    C. 10 to 30 years
    D. 30 to 50 years

12. Clinical findings most consistent with appendiceal rupture include all of the following except:

    A. abdominal discomfort less than 24 hours in duration.
    B. fever greater than 102°F (>38°C).
    C. palpable abdominal mass.
    D. marked leukocytosis with total WBC greater than 20,000/mm³.

ANSWERS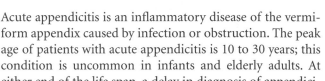

4.	D	5.	C	6.	A
7.	A	8.	B	9.	B
10.	D	11.	C	12.	A

DISCUSSION

Acute appendicitis is an inflammatory disease of the vermiform appendix caused by infection or obstruction. The peak age of patients with acute appendicitis is 10 to 30 years; this condition is uncommon in infants and elderly adults. At either end of the life span, a delay in diagnosis of appendicitis commonly occurs because providers do not consider appendicitis a possibility.

There is no true classic presentation of acute appendicitis. Vague epigastric or periumbilical pain often heralds its beginning, with the discomfort shifting to the right lower quadrant over the next 12 hours. Pain is often aggravated by walking or coughing. Nausea and vomiting are late symptoms that invariably occur a number of hours after the onset of pain; this late onset helps to differentiate appendicitis from gastroenteritis, in which vomiting usually precedes abdominal cramping. The presentation of appendicitis also differs significantly according to the anatomical position of the appendix, with pain being reported in the epigastrium, flank, or groin. The obturator and psoas signs indicate inflammation of the respective muscles and strongly suggest peritoneal irritation and the diagnosis of appendicitis; these signs are also known as obturator muscle and iliopsoas muscle signs. Rebound tenderness indicates the likelihood of peritoneal irritation and helps with the diagnosis of acute appendicitis. ♂

A total WBC count and differential are obtained as part of the evaluation of patients with suspected appendicitis.

The most typical WBC count pattern found in this situation is the "left shift." A "left shift" is usually seen in the presence of severe bacterial infection, such as acute appendicitis, bacterial pneumonia, and pyelonephritis. The following are typically noted in the "left shift":

- Leukocytosis: An elevation in the total WBC.
- Neutrophilia: An elevation in the number of neutrophils in circulation. Neutrophilia is defined as an absolute neutrophil count (ANC) of greater than 7000 neutrophils/mm^3. The ANC is calculated by multiplying the percentage of neutrophils by the total WBC in mm^3. A total WBC (TWBC) of 12,000 mm^3 × 70% neutrophils yields an ANC of 8300 neutrophils/mm^3. Neutrophils are also known as "polys" or "segs," both referring to the polymorph shape of the segment nucleus of this WBC.
- Bandemia: An elevation in the number of bands or young neutrophils in circulation. Usually less than 4% of the total WBCs in circulation are bands. When this percentage is exceeded, and the absolute band count (ABC) is greater than 500 mm^3, bandemia is present. A TWBC of 12,000 mm^3 with 8% bands yields an ABC of 860/mm^3. The presence of bandemia indicates that the body has called up as many mature neutrophils as were available in the storage pool and is now accessing less mature forms. The presence of bandemia further reinforces the seriousness of the infection. An increase in circulating bands also occurs in pneumonia, meningitis, septicemia, pyelonephritis, and tonsillitis when caused by bacterial infection.

Although additional neutrophil forms exist, these do not belong in circulation even with severe infection. Myelocytes and metamyelocytes are immature neutrophil forms that are typically found in only the granulopoiesis pool. The presence of these cells is an ominous marker of life-threatening infection, and these are occasionally found in the presence of appendiceal rupture.

In addition to the WBC differential, abdominal or transvaginal ultrasound reveals the inflamed appendix, usually greater than 6 mm in diameter, with a diagnostic accuracy of greater than 85%. Ultrasound offers an option in women or children with an equivocal presentation. CT of the abdomen is more accurate, however, because of its ability to define better the anatomical abnormality associated with appendicitis. CT is the preferred diagnostic procedure when there is a suspicion of appendiceal perforation because this study reveals periappendiceal abscess formation or when an atypical presentation raises the issue of another possible diagnosis. Appendiceal perforation is usually associated with a marked leukocytosis with total WBC count often exceeding 20,000 mm^3 to 30,000 mm^3, fever greater than 102°F (>38°C), peritoneal inflammation findings, symptoms lasting longer than 24 hours, and an ill-defined right lower quadrant abdominal mass that is usually indicative of abscess formation.

Surgical removal of an inflamed appendix via laparoscopy or laparotomy is indicated. If there is evidence of rupture with localized abscess and peritonitis, CT-directed abscess aspiration may be indicated first, with an appendectomy performed after appropriate antimicrobial therapy.

Discussion Source

Ferri F. Appendicitis. In: *Ferri's Fast Facts*. Philadelphia, PA: Elsevier Mosby; 2005:67–68.

Ferri F. Appendicitis. In *Ferri's Best Test: A Practical Guide to Clinical Laboratory Medicine and Diagnostic Imaging*. 2nd ed. Philadelphia, PA: Elsevier Mosby; 2009:190.

QUESTIONS

13. Which of the following is not a risk factor for bladder cancer?

    A. occupational exposure to textile dyes
    B. cigarette smoking
    C. occupational exposure to heavy metals
    D. long-term aspirin use

14. A 68-year-old man presents with suspected bladder cancer. You consider that its most common presenting sign or symptom is:

    A. painful urination.
    B. fever and flank pain.
    C. painless frank hematuria.
    D. palpable abdominal mass.

15. In a person diagnosed with superficial bladder cancer without evidence of metastases, you realize that:

    A. the prognosis for 2-year survival is poor.
    B. a cystectomy is indicated.
    C. despite successful initial therapy, local recurrence is common.
    D. systemic chemotherapy is the treatment of choice.

16. Persistent microscopic hematuria would be the primary finding in about ___% of individuals with bladder cancer.

    A. 10
    B. 20
    C. 30
    D. 40

ANSWERS

| 13. | D | 14. | C |
| 15. | C | 16. | B |

DISCUSSION

Bladder cancer is the second most common urologic malignancy after prostate cancer. It is usually a disease that occurs later in life—the mean age at diagnosis is 65 years—and it is more common in men. Risk factors include cigarette smoking, which accounts for most cases, and exposure to industrial chemicals, including paints, dyes, and solvents. Primary prevention of bladder cancer through risk reduction is critical.

Gross painless hematuria is the most common presenting sign of bladder cancer; persistent microscopic hematuria is the only finding in about 20% of individuals presenting with the disease. Irritative voiding symptoms and urinary frequency without fever are reported occasionally. Abdominal mass is palpable only with advanced disease.

Most patients with newly diagnosed bladder cancer have superficial disease, which allows for effective treatment through bladder-sparing surgery and intravesical chemotherapy. Meticulous follow-up is critical because recurrence is often seen, necessitating repeat chemotherapy and other therapies. Long-term survival is the norm with this noninvasive form of the disease. With invasive disease, treatment is dictated by type of tumor, degree of invasion, and presence of metastatic disease; long-term survival is based on numerous factors.

Discussion Source

Cookson M, Chang S. Malignant tumors of the urogenital tract. In: Rakel R, Bope E, eds. *Conn's Current Therapy*. Philadelphia, PA: Saunders Elsevier; 2009:731–742.

QUESTIONS

17. A 43-year-old woman has a 12-hour history of sudden onset of right upper quadrant abdominal pain with radiation to the shoulder, fever, and chills. She has had similar, milder episodes in the past. Examination reveals marked tenderness to right upper quadrant abdominal palpation. Her most likely diagnosis is:

    A. hepatoma.
    B. acute cholecystitis.
    C. acute hepatitis.
    D. cholelithiasis.

18. Which of the following is usually not seen in the diagnosis of acute cholecystitis?

    A. elevated lactic dehydrogenase level
    B. increased alkaline phosphatase level
    C. leukocytosis
    D. elevated aspartate aminotransferase (AST) level

19. Murphy's sign can be best described as abdominal pain elicited by:

    A. right upper quadrant abdominal palpation.
    B. asking the patient to stand on tiptoes and then letting body weight fall quickly onto the heels.
    C. asking the patient to cough.
    D. percussion.

20. Risk factors for cholelithiasis include all of the following except:

    A. genetics.
    B. rapid weight loss.
    C. obesity.
    D. high-fiber diet.

21. Imaging in a patient with suspected symptomatic cholelithiasis usually includes obtaining an abdominal:

    A. magnetic resonance image.
    B. CT scan.
    C. ultrasound (right upper quadrant).
    D. flat plate.

22. Which of the following is most likely to be found in a person with acute cholecystitis?

    A. fever
    B. vomiting
    C. jaundice
    D. palpable gallbladder

ANSWERS

| 17. | B | 18. | A | 19. | A |
| 20. | D | 21. | C | 22. | B |

DISCUSSION

Cholelithiasis is defined as a condition in which there is the formation of calculi or gallstones, but without the presence of gallbladder or associated structure. The most common form of stones is cholesterol or cholesterol-dominant (80% to 85%). Major risk factors for this condition include age older than 50 years, female gender, obesity, hyperlipidemia, rapid weight loss (including patients who have undergone bariatric surgery), pregnancy, genetic factors, and ingestion of a diet with a high glycemic index. About 75% of all patients with cholelithiasis have no symptoms and become aware of the condition only when it is found during evaluation for another health problem. About 10% to 25% of individuals initially without symptoms become symptomatic over the next decade. In the absence of symptoms, prophylactic cholecystectomy is not usually indicated. Many patients with cholelithiasis have intermittent right upper quadrant abdominal pain, however; right upper quadrant abdominal ultrasound usually reveals the problem, and cholecystectomy is then indicated. Stone-dissolving medications such as ursodeoxycholic acid are available, but can take 2 years to dissolve stones. Approximately 50% of patients treated with stone-dissolving medications have a return of stones within 5 years; consequently, the use of this therapy has largely fallen out of favor.

Acute cholecystitis results from an acute inflammation of the gallbladder, nearly always caused by gallstones. Right upper quadrant or epigastric pain and tenderness are present along with vomiting (>70%) and occasional fever (33%); vomiting often affords temporary symptom relief. Tenderness on palpating the right upper quadrant of the abdomen significant enough to cause inspiratory arrest (Murphy's sign) is nearly always present. A palpable gallbladder is rarely noted.

Approximately 25% to 50% of those affected have some degree of jaundice. Leukocytosis is usually present with a typical total WBC count of 12,000 mm³ to 20,000 mm³, and levels of the hepatic enzymes, including gamma glutamyl transferase (GGT) and alkaline phosphatase (ALP), often increase (Table 6–1).

ALP is an enzyme found in rapidly dividing or metabolically active tissue, such as the liver, bone, and intestine, and, in women during pregnancy, placenta. Elevated levels can reflect damage or accelerated cellular division in any of these areas, but most circulating ALP is of hepatic origin. ALP level increases in response to any obstruction in the biliary systems; it is a sensitive indicator of intrahepatic or extrahepatic cholestasis. GGT, an enzyme involved in the transfer of amino acids across cell membranes, is found primarily in the liver and kidneys. In liver disease, increased level of GGT usually parallels changes in ALP, which makes it a useful marker of

TABLE 6–1
Hepatic Enzyme Elevations and Their Significance

Enzyme Elevation	Comment, Associated Conditions	Example
Alanine aminotransferase (ALT, formerly known as SGPT)	Measure of hepatic cellular enzymes found in circulation, elevated when hepatocellular damage is present. Highly liver specific. This enzyme has circulatory half-life of 37–57 hr; levels increase relatively slowly in response to hepatic damage and clear gradually after damage ceases. See AST for contrast in this rise and fall pattern In hepatitis A, B, C, D, or E, or drug-associated or industrial chemical–associated hepatitis, ALT usually increases higher than AST, with enzyme increases ≥10 times ULN In nonalcoholic fatty liver steatohepatitis (NASH, also known as nonalcoholic fatty liver disease [NAFLD]), ALT usually increases higher than AST, with enzyme increases usually within 3 times ULN	A 22 y.o. woman with acute hepatitis A AST 678 U/L (normal 0–31 U/L) ALT 828 U/L (normal 0–31 U/L) ALT:AST ratio >1 A 66 y.o. woman with obesity, type 2 diabetes mellitus and nonalcoholic fatty liver disease AST 44 U/L ALT 78 U/L ALT:AST ratio >1
Aspartate aminotransferase (AST, formerly known as SGOT)	Measure of hepatic cellular enzymes found in circulation, elevated when hepatocellular damage is present. Enzyme also present in lesser amounts in skeletal muscle and myocardium AST has circulatory half-life of ~12–24 hr; levels increase in response to hepatic damage and clear quickly after damage ceases In alcohol-related hepatic injury, with HMG-CoA reductase inhibitor ("statin") use (rare finding in <0.5% statin users), AST usually increases higher than ALT In acetaminophen overdose, massive increases in AST and ALT are often noted, >20 times ULN	A 38 y.o. man with a 10-yr history of increasingly heavy alcohol use AST 83 U/L (normal 0–31 U/L) ALT 50 U/L (normal 0–31 U/L) AST:ALT ratio >1 A 26 y.o. man with intentional acetaminophen overdose AST 15,083 U/L (normal 0–31 U/L) ALT 10,347 U/L (normal 0–31 U/L)

Continued

TABLE 6–1

Hepatic Enzyme Elevations and Their Significance—cont'd

Enzyme Elevation	Comment, Associated Conditions	Example
Alkaline phosphatase (ALP)	Enzyme found in rapidly dividing or metabolically active tissue, such as liver, bone, intestine, placenta. Elevated levels can reflect damage or accelerated cellular division in any of these areas. Most in circulation is of hepatic origin. Levels increase in response to biliary obstruction and are a sensitive indicator of intrahepatic or extrahepatic cholestasis	A 40 y.o. woman with acute cholecystitis AST 45 U/L (0–31) ALT 55 U/L (0–31) ALP 225 U/L (0–125)
Gamma glutamyl transferase (GGT)	Enzyme involved in the transfer of amino acids across cell membranes. Found primarily in the liver and kidney In liver disease, usually parallels changes in alkaline phosphatase Marked elevation often noted in obstructive jaundice, hepatic metastasis, intrahepatic cholestasis	A 40 y.o. woman with acute cholecystitis AST 45 U/L (0–31) ALT 55 U/L (0–31) ALP 225 U/L (0–125) GGT 245 U/L (0–45)

ULN, upper limits of normal.

Source: Ferri F. *Ferri's Best Test: A Practical Guide to Clinical Laboratory Medicine and Diagnostic Imaging,* 2nd ed. Philadelphia, PA: Elsevier Mosby; 2009.

hepatic disease in obstructive jaundice, metastasis to the liver, and intrahepatic cholestasis. In addition, GGT can serve as a backup marker with elevated ALP. If the ALP level is elevated and the GGT level is normal, ALP elevation is likely caused by its bone, not hepatic, fraction. Other laboratory abnormalities include mildly elevated total serum bilirubin and amylase levels; total bilirubin greater than 4 mg/dL is uncommon and suggests an alternative diagnosis such as choledocholithiasis.

Combined with the health history, physical examination findings, and laboratory testing, imaging results help to support the diagnosis of cholecystitis. Right upper quadrant abdominal ultrasound usually reveals stones; a hepatoiminodiacetic acid (HIDA) scan is more sensitive and specific at revealing an obstructed cystic duct.

Acute cholecystitis symptoms usually subside with conservative therapy, such as a low-fat diet of clear liquids and analgesics. Antimicrobial therapy may be indicated with evidence of infection. Cholecystectomy, usually performed via laparoscope, should be considered because of the likelihood of recurrence. In a person who is seriously ill with other health problems and considered too high a risk to undergo cholecystectomy, ultrasound-guided gallbladder aspiration or percutaneous cholecystostomy can delay or occasionally eliminate the need for further surgical intervention.

Discussion Source

Caddy G. Cholelithiasis and cholecystitis. In: Rakel R, Bope E, eds. *Conn's Current Therapy*. Philadelphia, PA: Saunders Elsevier; 2009:494–496.

Ferri F. Cholecystitis. In: *Ferri's Fast Facts*. Philadelphia, PA: Elsevier Mosby; 2005:117–118.

QUESTIONS

23. Which of the following is true concerning colorectal cancer?

    A. Most colorectal cancers are found during rectal examination.
    B. Rectal carcinoma is more common than cancers involving the colon.
    C. Early manifestations include abdominal pain and cramping.
    D. Later disease presentation often includes iron deficiency anemia.

24. According to the American Cancer Society recommendations, which of the following is the preferred method for annual colorectal cancer screening in a 51-year-old man?

    A. digital rectal examination
    B. fecal occult blood test
    C. colonoscopy
    D. barium enema study

25. Which of the following is most likely to be noted in a person with colorectal cancer?

    A. gross rectal bleeding
    B. weight loss
    C. few symptoms
    D. nausea and vomiting

26. Which of the following does not increase a patient's risk of developing colorectal cancer?

   A. family history of colorectal cancer
   B. familial polyposis
   C. personal history of neoplasm
   D. long-term aspirin therapy

ANSWERS

23.	D	24.	B
26.	D	25.	C̶ D̶

DISCUSSION

Colorectal cancer is the second leading cause of cancer death in the United States, with approximately 5% of the population developing the disease. Most colorectal malignancies prove to be adenocarcinomas, with about 70% found in the colon and 30% found in the rectum. Risk factors include a history of inflammatory bowel disease (ulcerative colitis [UC] and Crohn disease), personal history of neoplasia, age older than 50 years, a family history of colorectal cancer, and familial polyposis syndrome. In addition, an autosomal dominant condition known as hereditary nonpolyposis colorectal cancer (HNPCC) has been identified. Although this condition accounts for only about 3% of all colorectal cancers, persons with this risk factor tend to develop disease earlier and have a 70% likelihood of colon cancer by age 65 years. A thorough family history is important in assessing an individual's risk of colorectal cancer. A diet high in fat, high in red meat, and low in calcium has also been implicated as a contributing factor. The use of antioxidants, calcium supplements, and low-dose aspirin has been shown in limited study to reduce colorectal cancer rates.

A person presenting with colorectal cancer is usually asymptomatic until disease is quite advanced. At that time, vague abdominal complaints coupled with iron deficiency anemia (as a result of chronic low-volume blood loss) is often noted. The mass is most often beyond the examining digit. As a result, digital rectal examination is an ineffective method of colorectal cancer screening. In addition, the American Cancer Society colorectal cancer screening guidelines do not recommend the use of the fecal occult blood test (FOBT) obtained via the digital rectal examination in the provider's office, which is not an adequate substitute for the recommended at-home procedure of collecting two samples from three consecutive specimens. Toilet-bowl FOBT tests also are not recommended. Compared with guaiac-based tests for the detection of occult blood, immunochemical tests are more patient-friendly, and are likely to be equal or better in sensitivity and specificity. There is no justification for repeating FOBT in response to an initial positive finding. Colonoscopy should be done if test results are positive.

The most commonly recommended colorectal cancer screening method in adults is a colonoscopy at 10-year intervals, starting at age 50 years. Alterative testing methods and schedules include flexible sigmoidoscopy, double-contrast barium enema, and CT colonography (virtual colonoscopy) every 5 years starting at age 50 years. Stool DNA test, also starting at age 50 years, is an option being used more frequently.

Alternative screening schedules, usually including more frequent testing or earlier testing or both, are considered when colorectal cancer risk factors are increased. These risk factors include a personal history of colorectal cancer or adenomatous polyps, Crohn disease or UC, a strong family history (first-degree relative [parent, sibling, or child] younger than 60 years or two or more first-degree relatives of any age) of colorectal cancer or polyps, or a known family history of hereditary colorectal cancer syndromes such as familial adenomatous polyposis or HNPCC. These alternative schedules should be pursued in conjunction with expert consultation.

Treatment of colorectal cancer usually includes surgery combined with chemotherapy and radiation. Long-term survival depends on many factors, including the size and depth of the tumor, the presence of positive nodes, and the overall health of the patient.

Discussion Source

Albo D. Tumors of the colon and rectum. In: Rakel R, Bope E, eds. *Conn's Current Therapy*. Philadelphia, PA: Saunders Elsevier; 2009:558–563.

Rex D, Johnson D, Anderson J, Schoenfield P, Burke C, Inadomi J. http://www.gi.org/media/releases/ACG2009CRCGuideline.pdf, American College of Gastroenterology Guidelines for Colorectal Cancer 2008, 2009, accessed 9/12/09.

QUESTIONS

27. Which of the following is most consistent with the presentation of a patient with colonic diverticulosis?

   A. diarrhea and leukocytosis
   B. constipation and fever
   C. few or no symptoms
   D. frank blood in the stool with reduced stool caliber

28. Which of the following is most consistent with the presentation of a patient with acute colonic diverticulitis?

   A. cramping, diarrhea, and leukocytosis
   B. constipation and fever
   C. right-sided abdominal pain
   D. frank blood in the stool with reduced stool caliber

29. The location of discomfort with acute diverticulitis is usually in which of the following areas of the abdomen?

   A. epigastrium
   B. left lower quadrant
   C. right lower quadrant
   D. suprapubic

30. Prevention of acute colonic diverticulitis includes:

   A. use of antidiarrheal agents.
   B. avoiding gas-producing foods.
   C. high-fiber diet.
   D. low-dose antibiotic therapy.

31. You are seeing Mr. Lopez, a 68-year-old man with suspected acute colonic diverticulitis. In choosing an appropriate imaging study to support this diagnosis, which of the following abdominal imaging studies is most appropriate?

   A. flat plate
   B. ultrasound
   C. CT scan
   D. barium enema

32. Recommended antimicrobial therapy in acute diverticulitis includes:

   A. amoxicillin with clarithromycin.
   B. linezolid with daptomycin.
   C. ciprofloxacin with metronidazole.
   D. nitrofurantoin with doxycycline.

33. Lower gastrointestinal (GI) hemorrhage associated with diverticular disease usually manifests as:

   A. a painless event.
   B. a condition noted to be found with a marked febrile response.
   C. a condition accompanied by crampy abdominal pain.
   D. a common chronic condition.

ANSWERS

27.	C	28.	A	29.	B
30.	C	31.	C.	32.	C
33.	A				

DISCUSSION

In colonic diverticulosis, bulging pockets are present in the intestinal wall, most commonly in the wall of the sigmoid colon. Inflammation is not present, however, and the patient is usually asymptomatic; diverticulosis is often found during studies done for other reasons, such as colorectal cancer screening. A major risk factor for the condition is long-term low-fiber diet. When symptoms are present in diverticulosis, left-sided abdominal cramping, increased flatus, and a pattern of constipation alternating with diarrhea are often reported. Intervention includes a high-fiber diet; use of fiber supplements such as bran, psyllium, or methylcellulose; or both. The goal of treatment is to minimize the risk of complications such as diverticulitis. Although avoidance of seeds and other similar food products has been recommended in the past as a way to avoid acute diverticulitis, few studies exist to support this dietary change.

In acute colonic diverticulitis, the diverticula are inflamed, causing fever, leukocytosis, diarrhea, and left lower quadrant abdominal pain. Intestinal perforation is the likely origin of the condition, with the perforation ranging from pinpoint lesions that cause local infection and respond to conservative management to major tears, which necessitate surgical repair and are often complicated by intra-abdominal abscess or peritonitis. Imaging is often obtained to support the diagnosis and assess disease severity or complications. An abdominal CT scan is helpful in identifying findings consistent with the condition inducing bowel wall thickening; complications including abscess and fistulas can also be identified with this diagnostic modality. A plain abdominal film is often normal in milder disease, but can be helpful in identifying free air, indicated diverticular perforation, or altered bowel air patterns consistent with obstruction. Because of the potential risk of complication, a barium enema should not be obtained during an acute episode of diverticular disease. Abdominal ultrasound is not helpful in this condition. Occasionally, diverticular hemorrhage, caused by an erosion of a vessel by a fecalith held in a diverticular sac, can occur. The condition usually manifests with painless lower GI bleeding. The management is usually directed by the clinical presentation and usually includes fluid and blood replacement; surgical intervention is often required.

In mild cases of diverticulitis, conservative management is adequate, including increased fluid intake, rest, and a low-residue diet for the duration of the illness and antimicrobial therapy. Because of its strong activity against anaerobic organisms implicated in the conditions, metronidazole is an antibiotic of choice. A second agent with activity against the anaerobes implicated, such as ciprofloxacin, levofloxacin, or trimethoprim-sulfamethoxazole (TMP-SMX), should be added because the infection is often polymicrobial (Table 6–2). If the patient fails to respond within 2 to 3 days or becomes significantly worse during that time, particularly if peritoneal signs develop, an abdominal CT scan and specialty consultation should be obtained.

Measures to prevent colonic diverticulosis and diverticulitis include regular aerobic exercise, adequate hydration, and a high-fiber diet. All of these measures help increase bowel motility and tone.

TABLE 6–2

Antimicrobial Treatment Options in Acute Diverticulitis

Causative Organisms	Primary Oral Treatment Regimen When Suitable for Outpatient Therapy	Alternative Oral Treatment Regimen When Suitable for Outpatient Therapy
Enterobacteriaceae, *P. aeruginosa, Bacteroides* spp., enterococci	TMP-SMX-DS bid or ciprofloxacin 750 mg bid or levofloxacin 750 mg qd plus metronidazole 500 mg q 6 hr, all for 7–10 days	Amoxicillin-clavulanate ER 1000/62.5 mg 2 tabs bid × 7–10 days *or* Moxifloxacin 400 mg q 24 hr × 7–10 days

TMP-SMX, trimethoprim-sulfamethoxazole.
Source: Gilbert D, Moellering R, Eliopoulos G, Sande M. *The Sanford Guide to Antimicrobial Therapy*. 39th ed. Sperryville, VA: Antimicrobial Therapy, Inc; 2009:19.

Discussion Source

Ferri F. Diverticular disease. In; *Ferri's Fast Facts*. Philadelphia, PA: Elsevier Mosby; 2005:154–156.
Maxwell P, Chappuis C. Diverticula of the alimentary tract. In: Rakel R, Bope E, eds. *Conn's Current Therapy*. Philadelphia, PA: Saunders Elsevier; 2009:511–514.

QUESTIONS

34. The gastric parietal cells produce:

    A. hydrochloric acid.
    B. a protective mucosal layer.
    C. prostaglandins.
    D. prokinetic hormones.

35. Antiprostaglandin drugs cause stomach mucosal injury primarily by:

    A. a direct irritative effect.
    B. altering the thickness of the protective mucosal layer.
    C. decreasing peristalsis.
    D. modifying stomach pH level.

36. A 24-year-old man presents with a 3-month history of upper abdominal pain. He describes it as an intermittent, centrally located "burning" feeling in his upper abdomen, most often occurring 2 to 3 hours after meals. His presentation is most consistent with the clinical presentation of:

    A. acute gastritis.
    B. gastric ulcer.
    C. duodenal ulcer.
    D. cholecystitis.

37. When choosing pharmacologic intervention to prevent recurrence of duodenal ulcer in a middle-aged man, you prescribe:

    A. a proton pump inhibitor (PPI).
    B. timed antacid use.
    C. antimicrobial therapy.
    D. a histamine$_2$-receptor antagonist (H$_2$RA).

38. The H$_2$RA most likely to cause drug interactions with phenytoin and theophylline is:

    A. cimetidine.
    B. famotidine.
    C. nizatidine.
    D. ranitidine.

39. Which of the following is least likely to be found in a patient with gastric ulcer?

    A. history of long-term naproxen use
    B. age younger than 50 years
    C. previous use of H$_2$RA or antacids
    D. cigarette smoking

40. Nonsteroidal anti-inflammatory drug (NSAID)–induced peptic ulcer can be best limited by the use of:

    A. an antacid.
    B. an H$_2$RA.
    C. an appropriate antimicrobial.
    D. misoprostol.

41. Cyclooxygenase-1 (COX-1) contributes to:

    A. the inflammatory response.
    B. pain transmission.
    C. maintenance of gastric protective mucosal layer.
    D. renal arteriole constriction.

42. Cyclooxygenase-2 (COX-2) contributes to:
    A. the inflammatory response.
    B. pain transmission inhibition.
    C. maintenance of gastric protective mucosal layer.
    D. renal arteriole constriction.

43. A 64-year-old woman presents with a 3-month history of upper abdominal pain. She describes the discomfort as an intermittent, centrally located "burning" feeling in the upper abdomen, most often with meals and often accompanied by mild nausea. Use of an over-the-counter H₂RA affords partial symptom relief. She also uses naproxen sodium on a regular basis for the control of osteoarthritis pain. Her clinical presentation is most consistent with:
    A. acute gastroenteritis.
    B. gastric ulcer.
    C. duodenal ulcer.
    D. chronic cholecystitis.

44. The most sensitive and specific test for *Helicobacter pylori* infection from the following list is:
    A. stool Gram stain, looking for the offending organism.
    B. serological testing for antigen related to the infection.
    C. organism-specific stool antigen testing.
    D. fecal DNA testing.

45. Which of the following medications is a PPI?
    A. loperamide
    B. metoclopramide
    C. nizatidine
    D. lansoprazole

ANSWERS

34.	A	35.	B	36.	C
37.	C	38.	A	39.	B
40.	D	41.	C	42.	A
43.	B	44.	C	45.	D

DISCUSSION

GI irritation and ulcer occur when there is an imbalance between gastric protective mechanisms and irritating factors such as hydrochloric acid and other digestive juices. Gastric parietal cells secrete hydrochloric acid, mediated by histamine₂-receptor sites.

The normal stomach pH is about 2, which kills many swallowed bacteria and viruses. Gastric acid production is about 1 to 2 mEq/hr in a resting, empty stomach and increases to 30 to 50 mEq/hr after a meal. The stomach is protected by numerous mechanisms, including a mucus coat with a gel layer. This layer provides mechanical protection from shearing as a result of ingestion of rough substances. In addition, bicarbonate is held within the protective layer and helps maintain pH to protect the mucosa from stomach acidity. Endogenous prostaglandins stimulate and thicken the mucus layer, enhance bicarbonate secretion, and promote cell renewal and blood flow. Endogenous prostaglandin levels normally decrease with age, which places older adults at increased risk for gastric damage. As part of the stress response, there is an increase in endogenous gastric acid and pepsin production and the potential for gastric mucosa injury and gastritis. Exogenous reasons for damage to the stomach's protective mechanism include the use of standard NSAIDs such as ibuprofen and naproxen, corticosteroid use, tobacco use, and infection with *H. pylori*.

Peptic ulcer disease is located in areas, such as the duodenum, stomach, esophagus, and small intestine, that are exposed to peptic juices such as acid and pepsin. Peptic ulcer disease usually includes loss of mucosal surface, extending to muscularis mucosae, that is at least 5 mm in diameter, with most losses being two to five times this size. Although an upper GI series identifies more than 80% of all ulcers larger than 0.5 cm, upper GI endoscopy identifies nearly all such ulcers. Ulcers are capable of brisk bleeding, scarring, and perforation. GI erosion is usually seen in patients with gastritis. These are superficial mucosal lesions, usually less than 5 mm in diameter, that tend to ooze rather than bleed. With healing, there is no scarring (Table 6–3).

The clinical presentation of peptic ulcer disease differs according to the location of the lesion. Symptoms associated with acute gastritis and gastric ulcer often become worse with eating because of the increase in irritating stomach acid production on top of the lesion. The symptoms often lessen within an hour as food buffers the acid. In contrast, duodenal ulcer symptoms often worsen as the stomach pH decreases when emptying after a meal, resulting in a sensation of stomach burning about 2 hours after a meal.

Duodenal ulcer is more common than gastric ulcer. The most potent risk factor for this condition is most likely infection with *H. pylori*, a gram-negative, spiral-shaped organism with sheathed flagella found in at least 90% of patients with duodenal ulcer. The pathogen is also found in about 40% to 70% of individuals with gastric ulcer. Infection with *H. pylori* is transmitted via the oral-fecal and oral-oral route, and rates of infection approach 100% in developing nations with impure water supplies. In developed nations with pure water supplies, at least 75% of the population older than 50 years has been infected at some time. Eradication of the organism dramatically alters the risk of relapse. Numerous antimicrobial combinations are effective in treating symptomatic *H. pylori* infection (Table 6–4).

Stool antigen testing is the most cost-effective method of diagnosing *H. pylori* infection, particularly when coupled with

TABLE 6–3

Assessing a Patient With Peptic Ulcer Disease

Location and Type of Peptic Ulcer Disease	Risk and Contributing Factors	Presenting Signs and Symptoms	Diagnostic Testing
Duodenal ulcer	*Helicobacter pylori* infection (most common), NSAID use, corticosteroid use (much less common)	Epigastric burning, gnawing pain about 2–3 hr after meals; relief with foods, antacids Clusters of symptoms with periods of feeling well; awakening at 1–2 a.m. with symptoms common, morning waking pain rare Tender at the epigastrium, left upper quadrant abdomen; slightly hyperactive bowel sounds	Stool antigen testing >90% sensitive and specific If *H. pylori* stool antigen test is positive and PUD history, assume active infection and treat because cost of treatment less than that of confirmatory endoscopy. Repeat stool antigen test >8 wk post-treatment. *H. pylori* testing; serological testing for anti–*H. pylori* antibodies positive with acute infection but can take decades post infection to decline. A less sensitive and specific option compared with stool antigen testing Urea breath test establishes presence of acute infection Endoscopy with biopsy and urease testing of biopsy specimen or staining, looking for *H. pylori* organisms, is diagnostic gold standard
Gastric ulcer	NSAID and corticosteroid use (potent risk factor) Cigarette smoking Male:female ratio equal Peak incidence in fifth and sixth decades of life; nearly all found in patients without *H. pylori* infection are caused by NSAID use	Pain often reported with or immediately after meals Nausea, vomiting, weight loss common	Difficulty distinguishing gastric ulcer from stomach cancer through UGI imaging UGI endoscopy with biopsy vital Need confirmation of presence of *H. pylori* before treatment, as is present in some of cases
Nonerosive gastritis, chronic type B (antral) gastritis	Most likely caused by *H. pylori* infection	Nausea Burning and pain limited to upper abdomen without reflux symptoms	Upper endoscopy is helpful diagnostic test
Erosive gastritis	Usually secondary to alcohol and NSAID use, ASA use, stress *H. pylori* infection usually not a factor	Nausea Burning and pain limited to upper abdomen without reflux symptoms; bleeding common	Upper endoscopy is helpful diagnostic test

ASA, acetylsalicylic acid; NSAID, nonsteroidal anti-inflammatory drug; PUD, peptic ulcer disease; UGI, upper gastrointestinal.

TABLE 6–4

Treatment Options in *Helicobacter Pylori* Infection Associated With Peptic Ulcer Disease

Antimicrobials and Acid-Suppressing Medication	Usual duration of Therapy	Comments
Bismuth salicylate 2 tabs qid plus metronidazole 500 mg qid plus tetracycline 500 mg qid plus omeprazole 20 mg bid	14 days	Less effective if doxycycline is substituted for tetracycline. An older regimen that requires multiple medications carefully timed to avoid possible bismuth chelation effect. An alternative when clarithromycin therapy should be avoided or is less desirable. *H. pylori* resistance to amoxicillin and metronidazole uncommon
Amoxicillin 1 g bid plus clarithromycin 500 mg bid plus omeprazole 20 mg or rabeprazole 20 mg bid	14 days	Well tolerated 85%–95% effective if taken as directed. Consider possible drug-drug interactions with using a CYP 450 3A4 inhibitor such as clarithromycin. Rates of *H. pylori* resistance to clarithromycin increasing
Sequential therapy with rabeprazole 20 mg bid plus amoxicillin 1 g bid × 5 days then rabeprazole 20 mg bid plus clarithromycin 500 mg plus tinidazole 500 mg bid × additional 5 days	10 days total	Generally well tolerated. Helpful when a shorter course of therapy is desirable

Source: Gilbert D, Moerlling R, Eliopoulos G, Chambers H, Saag M. *The Sanford Guide to Antimicrobial Therapy*. 39th ed. Sperryville, VA: Antimicrobial Therapy, Inc; 2009:18.

a clinical presentation consistent with peptic ulcer disease. Serological testing is also available, with the limitation that titers can take years to decline after effective treatment; however, 50% of patients have undetectable titers 12 to 18 months after therapy. The organism produces urease, which breaks down urea into ammonia and CO_2; this allows the organism to control pH in its local environment in the stomach by neutralizing H^+ ions in gastric acid. As a result, urea breath testing is also a helpful diagnostic procedure when attempting to establish the presence of *H. pylori* infection, although it is usually more expensive than the stool antigen test.

In the past, the adage "no stress, no extra acid, no ulcer" was often quoted. Treatment for peptic ulcer disease often included the use of psychotropic medications for relief of stress, according to the hypothesis that this would reduce the acid production. In reality, only 30% to 40% of persons with duodenal ulcer have higher than average acid secretion rates. In addition, coffee drinking and occasional alcohol use are not risk factors for peptic ulcer disease. Alcohol abuse with cirrhosis remains a risk factor, however. *H. pylori* is also found in individuals with asymptomatic gastritis and dyspepsia without ulceration; eradication of the organism does not seem to make a difference in symptoms in patients with these conditions.

Suppression or neutralization of gastric acid is a critical part of peptic ulcer disease therapy. H_2RAs (whose names have the "-tidine" suffix, such as ranitidine [Zantac], famotidine

[Pepcid], and cimetidine [Tagamet]) competitively block the binding of histamine to the H_2-receptor site, reducing the secretion of gastric acid. In prescription dosages, these products suppress approximately 90% of hydrochloric acid production, whereas over-the-counter dosages suppress about 80%. These products are generally well tolerated. Cimetidine is the only H_2RA that significantly inhibits cytochrome P-450, slowing metabolism of many drugs. As a result, drug interactions between cimetidine and warfarin, diazepam, phenytoin, quinidine, carbamazepine, theophylline, imipramine, and other medications can occur; these interactions are not noted with the use of the other H_2RAs.

Proton pump inhibitors (PPIs) include omeprazole (Prilosec), esomeprazole (Nexium), and lansoprazole (Prevacid). These drugs inhibit gastric acid secretion by inhibiting the final step in acid secretion by altering the activity of the "proton pump" (H^+,K^+-ATPase). As a result, there is a virtual cessation of stomach hydrochloric acid production, particularly owing to its significant action against the postprandial acid surge. PPI use is indicated in the treatment of peptic ulcer disease and gastroesophageal reflux disease (GERD) when an H_2RA is ineffective, and in refractory erosive esophagitis and Zollinger-Ellison syndrome.

A significant amount of peptic ulcer disease, particularly gastric ulcer, acute gastritis, and NSAID-induced gastropathy, is caused by use of NSAIDs. This is partly because of the action of these products against cyclooxygenase.

Cyclooxygenase-1 (COX-1) is an enzyme found in gastric mucosa, small and large intestine mucosa, kidneys, platelets, and vascular epithelium. COX-1 contributes to the health of these organs through numerous mechanisms, including the maintenance of the protective gastric mucosal layer and proper renal perfusion. Cyclooxygenase-2 (COX-2) is an enzyme that produces prostaglandins important in the inflammatory cascade and pain transmission. The standard NSAIDs and systemic corticosteroids inhibit the synthesis of COX-1 and COX-2, controlling pain and inflammation, but producing gastric and renal complications. NSAIDs such as celecoxib (Celebrex) spare COX-1 and are more COX-2-selective and afford pain and inflammatory control. Although shorter-term studies supported lower rates of gastropathy with COX-2-selective NSAIDS (COX-2 inhibitors), this effect usually attenuates with longer term use and is absent with concomitant aspirin use. In addition, use of COX-2 inhibitors can be associated with increased risk for cardiovascular and cerebrovascular events.

Besides the use of a standard NSAID, major risk factors for gastric ulcer include age older than 60 years, history of peptic ulcer disease (especially gastric ulcer), and previous use of H_2RA or antacids for the treatment of GI symptoms. Additional, less potent risk factors include cigarette smoking, cardiac disease, and alcohol use; taking more than one NSAID; and the concurrent use of NSAIDs and anticoagulants.

H_2RAs likely offer protection against NSAID-induced duodenal ulcer and perhaps gastritis, but not against gastric ulcer. PPIs afford better protection against peptic ulcer disease. A prostaglandin analogue, misoprostol (Cytotec), is a drug specifically designed for gastric protection with NSAID; the use of this medication is possibly helpful in minimizing renal injury secondary to NSAID use.

Discussion Sources

Ferri F. Peptic ulcer disease. In: *Ferri's Fast Facts*. Philadelphia, PA: Elsevier Mosby; 2005:324–326.

Gilbert D, Moerlling R, Eliopoulos G, Chambers H, Saag M. *The Sanford Guide to Antimicrobial Therapy*. 39th ed. Sperryville, VA: Antimicrobial Therapy, Inc; 2009:18.

Kenthu S, Moss S. Gastritis and peptic ulcer disease. In: Rakel R, Bope E, eds. *Conn's Current Therapy*. Philadelphia, PA: Saunders Elsevier; 2009:527–533.

QUESTIONS

46. A 45-year-old woman complains of periodic "heartburn." Examination reveals a single altered finding of epigastric tenderness without rebound. As first-line therapy, you advise:
    A. avoiding trigger foods.
    B. the use of a prokinetic agent.
    C. a daily dose of a PPI.
    D. increased fluid intake with meals.

47. You see a 62-year-old man diagnosed with esophageal columnar epithelial metaplasia. You realize he is at increased risk for:
    A. esophageal stricture.
    B. adenocarcinoma.
    C. gastroesophageal reflux.
    D. *H. pylori* colonization.

48. In caring for a patient with symptomatic gastroesophageal reflux, you prescribe a PPI to:
    A. enhance motility.
    B. increase the pH of the stomach.
    C. reduce lower esophageal pressure.
    D. help limit *H. pylori* growth.

49. Which of the following represents the optimal dosing schedule for sucralfate (Carafate)?
    A. Each tablet should be taken with a snack.
    B. The medication should be taken with a full meal for buffering effect.
    C. To achieve maximal therapeutic effect, the drug must be taken on an empty stomach.
    D. Sucralfate should be taken with other prescribed medications to enhance compliance.

50. Which of the following is most likely to be found in a 50-year-old woman with new-onset reflux esophagitis?
    A. initiation of estrogen-progestin hormonal therapy
    B. recent weight loss
    C. report of melena
    D. evidence of *H. pylori* infection

51. Which of the following is likely to be reported in a patient with persistent GERD?
    A. hematemesis
    B. chronic sore throat
    C. diarrhea
    D. melena

52. A 58-year-old man recently began taking an antihypertensive medication and reports that his "heartburn" has become much worse. He is most likely taking:
    A. atenolol.
    B. trandolapril.
    C. amlodipine.
    D. losartan.

53. You prescribe a fluoroquinolone antibiotic to a 54-year-old woman who has occasional GERD symptoms that she treats with an antacid. When discussing appropriate medication use, you advise that she should take the antimicrobial:
    A. with the antacid.
    B. separated from the antacid use by 2 to 4 hours before or 4 to 6 hours after taking the fluoroquinolone.
    C. without regard to antacid use.
    D. apart from the antacid by about 1 hour on either side of the fluoroquinolone dose.

ANSWERS

46.	A	47.	B	48.	B
49.	C	50.	A	51.	B
52.	C	53.	B		

DISCUSSION

GERD is a common but troublesome condition. Reflux of stomach contents occurs regularly. Most reflux is asymptomatic with no resulting esophageal injury. GERD is present when there are symptoms or evidence of tissue damage. The most common GERD presentation includes dyspepsia, chest pain at rest, and postprandial fullness. In addition, non-GI symptoms, including chronic hoarseness, sore throat, nocturnal cough, and wheezing, are often reported, occasionally in the absence of more classic GERD symptoms, and particularly when the condition is chronic.

Reflux-induced esophageal injury, also known as reflux esophagitis, is present in 40% of patients with GERD. Erosions and ulcerations in squamous epithelium of esophagus are present and are most common in elderly patients. Complications of reflux esophagitis include esophageal stricture and columnar epithelial metaplasia, also known as Barrett esophagus. This is a risk factor for adenocarcinoma of the esophagus. Decreased lower esophageal sphincter tone and the resulting reflux of gastric contents cause GERD. Esophageal mucosal irritation results from exposure to hydrochloric acid and pepsin.

Certain medications can cause a decrease in lower esophageal sphincter pressure and worsen GERD, including estrogen, progesterone, theophylline, calcium channel blockers, and nicotine. Initial therapy for patients with GERD includes reducing intake of offending medications and of GERD-enhancing foods such alcohol, tomato-based products, chocolate, peppermint, colas, and citrus juices. Behavioral intervention includes avoiding or minimizing conditions or situations that encourage esophageal reflux and includes the following: remaining upright and avoiding assuming the supine position within 3 hours of a meal, eating smaller meals, eliminating occasions of overeating, and abstaining from high-fat meals. Because abdominal obesity contributes to GERD, weight loss can also be helpful. Elevation of the head of the bed on 4-inch blocks may also offer some relief; propping the head and upper thorax on pillows is not effective.

The use of antacids after meals and at bedtime is often sufficient to control milder, particularly intermittent, GERD symptoms. Antacids neutralize secreted acids and inactivate pepsin and bile salts. These medications are most effective when used 1 to 3 hours after meals and at bedtime. Antacids interact with many other medications and should be used at least 2 hours apart; with the use of a fluoroquinolone such as ciprofloxacin, antacid use should be 2 to 4 hours before or 4 to 6 hours after the fluoroquinolone.

If the use of antacids and lifestyle modification are inadequate to control milder, intermittent GERD symptoms, an H_2RA at full prescription strength bid should be added. If there is no improvement in 6 weeks, longer-term H_2RA therapy is unlikely to be helpful. With moderate to severe symptoms that do not respond to a prescription dosage of H_2RA, a PPI such as omeprazole (Prilosec) or lansoprazole (Prevacid) should be prescribed. Compared with H_2RAs, PPIs have superior postprandial and nocturnal acid suppression. Adding sucralfate, 1 g qid on an empty stomach, should be considered, particularly when nonsystemic medication use is preferred, such as during pregnancy. Sucralfate's mechanism of action is as a mucosal protective agent that acts by forming an adhesive gel that binds to the site of an ulcer or irritation. A small amount adheres to normal mucosa. It has no effect on acid formation, but inactivates pepsin, while stimulating the formation of prostaglandins. Because it can inactivate many other drugs, sucralfate should be taken at least 2 hours before or after any other medication. In addition, it should be taken on an empty stomach. Prokinetic agents, such as metoclopramide (Reglan), offer an additional treatment option. Concerns about extrapyramidal movements developing with use of metoclopramide coupled with relatively little evidence of clinical utility limit the usefulness of this product.

In patients with classic GI and extra-GI symptoms, the diagnosis of GERD is usually made clinically with no specific diagnostic testing performed, particularly when clinical response is noted with standard therapy. If a standard GERD treatment regimen is unsuccessful, expert consultation with a gastroenterology specialist should be sought. GI referral should also be considered if there are "alarm" findings, such as concurrent anemia or unexpected weight loss.

Upper GI endoscopy should be performed and appropriate biopsy specimens should be obtained in patients at risk for Barrett esophagus (BE), a premalignant metaplastic process that typically involves the distal esophagus. Risk factors for BE include GERD of long duration, certain ethnicity (i.e., white, Hispanic), male gender, advancing age, tobacco use, and obesity. Intervention in BE is based on aggressive acid suppression, with the anticipated end product of minimizing further esophageal damage. For patients with established BE of any length and with no dysplasia after two consecutive examinations within 1 year, an acceptable interval for additional surveillance is every 3 years. The clinician should remain aware of the latest recommendations on BE intervention and surveillance.

Surgical intervention in GERD is a treatment option usually limited to patients with the most severe symptoms that are not improved by the use of standard treatment. As additional endoscopic interventions become available, with evidence of the long-term efficacy and safety of the procedures, this option is likely to increase in utility.

Discussion Sources

DeVault K. Gastroesophageal reflux. In: Rakel R, Bope E, eds. *Conn's Current Therapy*. Philadelphia, PA: Saunders Elsevier; 2009:552–555.

Standards of Practice Committee, Lichtenstein DR, Cash BD, Davila R, Baron TH, Adler DG, Anderson MA, Dominitz JA, Gan SI, Harrison ME 3rd, Ikenberry SO, Qureshi WA, Rajan E, Shen B, Zuckerman MJ, Fanelli RD, Van Guilder T. Role of endoscopy in the management of GERD. *Gastrointest Endosc.* 2007;66:219–224.

QUESTIONS

54. You are caring for a 45-year-old woman from a developing country. She reports that she had "yellow jaundice" as a young child. Her physical examination is unremarkable. Her laboratory studies are as follows: AST, 22 U/L (normal, 0 to 31 U/L); alanine aminotransferase (ALT), 25 U/L (normal, 0 to 40 U/L); hepatitis A virus immunoglobulin G (HAV IgG) positive. Laboratory testing reveals:
    A. chronic hepatitis A.
    B. no evidence of prior or current hepatitis A infection.
    C. resolved hepatitis A infection.
    D. prodromal hepatitis A.

55. The most common source of hepatitis A infection is:
    A. sharing intravenous drug equipment.
    B. cooked seafood.
    C. contaminated water supplies.
    D. sexual contact.

56. In addition to the laboratory work described, results reveal the following for the above-mentioned patient: hepatitis B surface antigen (HBsAg) positive. These findings are most consistent with:
    A. no evidence of hepatitis B infection.
    B. resolved hepatitis B infection.
    C. chronic hepatitis B.
    D. evidence of effective hepatitis B immunization.

57. A 38-year-old man with a recent history of injection drug use presents with malaise, nausea, fatigue, and "yellow eyes" for the past week. After ordering diagnostic tests, you confirm the diagnosis of acute hepatitis B. Anticipated laboratory results include:
    A. hepatitis B surface antibody (HBsAb).
    B. neutrophilia.
    C. thrombocytosis.
    D. the presence of HBsAg.

58. Clinical findings in patients with acute hepatitis B likely include all of the following except:
    A. abdominal rebound tenderness.
    B. scleral icterus.
    C. a smooth, tender, palpable hepatic border.
    D. report of myalgia.

59. You see a woman who has been sexually involved with a man newly diagnosed with acute hepatitis B. She has not received hepatitis B immunization. You advise her to:
    A. start hepatitis B immunization series.
    B. limit the number of sexual partners.
    C. be tested for HBsAb.
    D. receive hepatitis B immune globulin and start hepatitis B immunization series.

60. Which of the following statements is true concerning hepatitis C infection?
    A. It usually manifests with jaundice, fever, and significant hepatomegaly.
    B. Among health-care workers, it is most commonly found in nurses.
    C. More than 50% of persons with acute hepatitis C go on to develop chronic infection.
    D. Interferon therapy is consistently curative.

61. Which of the following characteristics is predictive of severity of chronic liver disease in a patient with chronic hepatitis C?
    A. female gender, age younger than 30
    B. co-infection with hepatitis B, daily alcohol use
    C. acquisition of virus through intravenous drug use, history of hepatitis A infection
    D. frequent use of aspirin, nutritional status

62. When answering questions about hepatitis A vaccine, you consider that all of the following are true except:
    A. it does not contain live virus.
    B. it should be offered to individuals who frequently travel to developing countries.
    C. it is a recommended immunization for health-care workers.
    D. it is given as a single dose.

63. To prevent an outbreak of hepatitis D infection, a NP plans to:
    A. promote a campaign for clean food supplies.
    B. immunize the population against hepatitis B.
    C. offer antiviral prophylaxis against the agent.
    D. encourage frequent hand washing.

64. Which of the following is true concerning hepatitis B vaccine?

   A. The vaccine contains live hepatitis B virus.
   B. The NP should consider checking postvaccination HBsAb titers only for individuals at highest risk for infection.
   C. The vaccine is contraindicated in the presence of HIV infection.
   D. Postvaccination arthralgias are often reported.

65. Hyperbilirubinemia can cause all of the following except:

   A. potential displacement of highly protein-bound drugs.
   B. scleral icterus.
   C. cola-colored urine.
   D. reduction in urobilinogen.

66. Monitoring for hepatoma in a patient with chronic hepatitis B or C often includes periodic evaluation of:

   A. erythrocyte sedimentation rate.
   B. HBsAb.
   C. alpha-fetoprotein.
   D. urobilinogen.

67. Which of the following is an expected laboratory result in a patient with acute hepatitis A infection (normal values: AST, 0 to 31 U/L; ALT, 0 to 40 U/L)?

   A. AST, 55 U/L; ALT, 50 U/L
   B. AST, 320 U/L; ALT, 190 U/L
   C. AST, 320 U/L; ALT, 300 U/L
   D. AST, 640 U/L; ALT, 870 U/L

68. Which of the following is most likely to be reported in a patient taking a 3-hydroxy-3-methylglutaryl–coenzyme A (HMG-CoA) reductase inhibitor (statin)?

   A. AST, 41 U/L; ALT, 28 U/L
   B. AST, 320 U/L; ALT, 190 U/L
   C. AST, 32 U/L; ALT, 120 U/L
   D. AST, 440 U/L; ALT, 670 U/L

69. When discussing the use of immunoglobulin (IG) with a 60-year-old woman who was recently exposed to the hepatitis A virus, you consider that:

   A. IG is derived from pooled donated blood.
   B. the product must be used within 1 week of exposure to provide protection.
   C. its use in this situation constitutes an example of active immunization.
   D. a short, intense flu-like illness often occurs after its use.

70. You see a 48-year-old woman with nonalcoholic fatty liver disease. Evaluation of infectious hepatitis includes the following:

   Anti-HAV IgG—negative
   Anti-HBs—negative
   Anti-HCV—negative

   When considering her overall health status, you advise receiving which of the following vaccines?

   A. immunization against hepatitis A and B as based on her lifestyle risk factors
   B. immunization against hepatitis B and C
   C. immunization against hepatitis A and B
   D. immunization against hepatitis A, B, and C

71. Which of the following hepatitis forms is most effectively transmitted from the man to the woman via heterosexual vaginal intercourse?

   A. hepatitis A
   B. hepatitis B
   C. hepatitis C
   D. hepatitis D

ANSWERS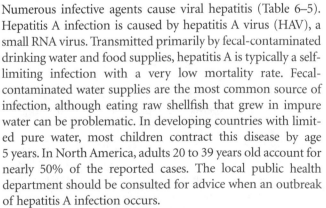

54.	C	55.	C	56.	C	57.	D
58.	A	59.	D	60.	C	61.	B
62.	D	63.	B	64.	B	65.	D
66.	C	67.	D	68.	A	69.	A
70.	C	71.	B				

DISCUSSION

Numerous infective agents cause viral hepatitis (Table 6–5). Hepatitis A infection is caused by hepatitis A virus (HAV), a small RNA virus. Transmitted primarily by fecal-contaminated drinking water and food supplies, hepatitis A is typically a self-limiting infection with a very low mortality rate. Fecal-contaminated water supplies are the most common source of infection, although eating raw shellfish that grew in impure water can be problematic. In developing countries with limited pure water, most children contract this disease by age 5 years. In North America, adults 20 to 39 years old account for nearly 50% of the reported cases. The local public health department should be consulted for advice when an outbreak of hepatitis A infection occurs.

All children and some other groups should be immunized against HAV. Candidates for immunization include individuals who reside in or travel to areas where the disease is endemic, food handlers, sewage workers, animal handlers, day-care attendees and workers, long-term care residents

TABLE 6–5

Infectious Hepatitis: Key Features to Transmission and Diagnosis

Type	Route of Transmission	Immunization Available? Postexposure Prophylaxis?	Sequelae	Disease Marker
Hepatitis A	Fecal-oral	Immunization: Yes Postexposure prophylaxis with IG for close contacts	None, survive or die	*Acute disease marker* • HAV IgM (M—miserable) • Elevated hepatic enzymes >10 × upper limits of normal *Chronic disease marker* • None, as chronic hepatitis A does not exist *Disease in past, history of immunization* • Anti-HAV (total of HAV IgM and HAV IgG) present • Hepatic enzymes normalize *Still susceptible to hepatitis A infection* • Anti-HAV negative

Hepatitis B	Blood, body fluids	Immunization: Yes Postexposure prophylaxis with HBIG for blood, body fluid contacts	Chronic hepatitis B, hepatocellular carcinoma, hepatic failure	*Acute disease markers*
				• HBsAg
				• HBeAg
				• Elevated hepatic enzymes >10 × upper limits of normal
				Chronic disease marker
				• Patient without symptoms
				• Normal or slightly elevated hepatic enzymes
				• HBsAg
				  • Only present if HBV on board
				  • Surrogate marker for HBV
				Hepatitis B in past, history of immunization
				• HBsAb (anti-HBs)
				  • A protective antibody, unable to get HBV in the future
				• Hepatic enzyme normalized
				Still susceptible to hepatitis B infection
				• HBsAg negative
				• Anti-HBc negative
				• HBsAb (anti-HBs) negative

Hepatitis C	Blood, body fluids	No No	Chronic hepatitis C, hepatocellular carcinoma, hepatic failure	*Acute disease marker* • Anti-HCV present • HCV viral RNA • Elevated hepatic enzymes *Chronic disease marker* • Anti-HCV present • HCV viral RNA • Normal to slightly elevated hepatic enzymes *Disease in the past* • Anti-HCV present (nonprotective antibody) • HCV RNA absent • Normalized hepatic enzymes
Hepatitis D	Blood, body fluids	No, but prevent hepatitis B and you can prevent hepatitis D	Severe infection, hepatic failure, death	*Acute or chronic* hepatitis B (HBsAg) markers plus hepatitis D IgM. Usually with markedly elevated hepatic enzymes.

Note: This is not intended as an exhaustive presentation of hepatitis markers.

and workers, military personnel, and health-care workers. Injection drug users also benefit from the vaccine. HAV is rarely transmitted sexually or from needle sharing; rather, injection drug users often live in conditions that facilitate the oral-fecal transmission of HAV. In addition, co-infection with hepatitis A and C, co-infection with hepatitis A and B, or acute hepatitis A in addition to chronic liver disease may lead to a rapid deterioration in hepatic function. Persons with chronic hepatitis B or C or both or any chronic liver disease should be immunized against hepatitis A. Persons who have clotting factor disorders and are receiving clotting factor concentrates who have not had hepatitis A should also be immunized. Updated hepatitis A vaccine guidelines have been expanded to include all individuals who would like to be immunized against the condition.

Two doses of HAV vaccine are usually given 6 to 12 months apart to ensure an enhanced immunological response; an alternative accelerated dosing schedule is also licensed for use with a combined hepatitis A and B vaccine. Hepatitis A vaccine, which does not contain live virus, is usually well tolerated without systemic reaction. Post-exposure prophylaxis against hepatitis A is also available; IG and HAV vaccine are used for this purpose. For healthy persons 12 months to 40 years old, a dose of hepatitis A vaccine at the age-appropriate dose is preferred to IG because of vaccine advantages that include long-term protection and ease of administration. For persons older than 40 years, IG is preferred because of the lack of information regarding vaccine performance and the more severe manifestations of hepatitis A in this age group; vaccine can be used if IG cannot be obtained. IG, a form of passive immunity, is highly effective in preventing HAV infection if given within 2 weeks of exposure. IG is a product derived from pooled blood that contains preformed antibodies against the virus and has an outstanding safety profile.

Hepatitis B is caused by a small double-stranded DNA virus that contains an inner core protein of hepatitis B core antigen and an outer surface of HBsAg. Hepatitis B virus (HBV) is usually transmitted through an exchange of blood and body fluids. Acute hepatitis B is a serious illness that can lead to hepatic failure. Approximately 5% of individuals with acute hepatitis B go on to develop chronic hepatitis B; chronic hepatitis B is a potent risk factor for hematoma or primary hepatocellular carcinoma and hepatic cirrhosis. A person with chronic hepatitis B continues to be able to transmit the virus, although the person appears clinically well.

Hepatitis B infection can be prevented by limiting exposure to blood and body fluids and through immunization. Recombinant hepatitis B vaccine, which does not contain live virus, is well tolerated; one contraindication to receiving the vaccine is a personal history of anaphylaxis to baker's yeast. In the United States, this vaccine has been routinely used in children since 1986; as a result, most of the population born during or after 1986 have been immunized. The vaccine should be offered to adults born before 1986 and to all who have not been immunized, particularly persons at

highest risk for contracting the virus. Nonimmunized individuals being treated for other sexually transmitted infections should be encouraged to receive protection against HBV. Refer to the latest immunization guidelines for further information on this important public health issue.

Infants who become infected perinatally with HBV have an estimated 25% lifetime chance of developing hepatocellular carcinoma or cirrhosis. As a result, all pregnant women should be screened for HBsAg at the first prenatal visit, regardless of HBV vaccine history. Because the HBV vaccine is not 100% effective, and perinatal transmission is possible, a woman could have carried HBV before becoming pregnant. About 90% to 95% of individuals who receive the vaccine develop HBsAb (anti-HBs) after three doses, implying protection from the virus. Routine testing for the presence of HBsAb after immunization is not recommended. HBsAb testing should be considered, however, to confirm the development of HBV protection in persons with high risk for infection (e.g., certain health-care workers who have risk for frequent and high-volume blood exposures, injection drug users, sex workers) and persons at risk for a poor immune response (e.g., dialysis patients, patients with immunosuppression).

Booster doses of hepatitis B vaccine are recommended only in certain circumstances. For hemodialysis patients, the need for booster doses should be assessed by annual testing for antibody to hepatitis B surface antigen (anti-HBs). A booster dose should be administered when anti-HBs levels decline to less than 10 mIU/mL. For other immunocompromised persons (e.g., HIV-infected persons, hematopoietic stem-cell transplant recipients, and persons receiving chemotherapy), the need for booster doses has not been determined. When anti-HBs levels decline to less than 10 mIU/mL, annual anti-HBs testing and booster doses should be considered for persons with an ongoing risk for exposure. Ongoing serological surveillance in immunocompetent persons is not recommended.

Post-exposure prophylaxis is effective in preventing HBV infection. In a person who has written documentation of a complete hepatitis B vaccine series and who did not receive post-vaccination testing, a single vaccine booster dose should be given with a nonoccupational known HBsAg-positive exposure source. A person who is in the process of being vaccinated, but who has not completed the vaccine series should receive the appropriate dose of hepatitis B immunoglobulin (HBIG) and should complete the vaccine series. Unvaccinated persons should receive HBIG and hepatitis B vaccine as soon as possible, preferably within 24 hours, after exposure. Testing for HIV, other sexually transmitted infections, and hepatitis A and C should also be offered, and post-exposure prophylaxis and immunization should be offered where applicable. Owing to the complexity of care, intervention for a person with occupational exposure should be done with expert consultation in this area.

Currently, treatment with pegylated interferon and an antiviral such as entecavir, adefovir, and lamivudine has shown clinical utility in inducing remission in some patients with chronic hepatitis B. Because of the rapid advances being made in this area, the NP and patient must be aware of the most up-to-date treatment options.

Hepatitis C infection is transmitted through the exchange of blood and body fluids. A single-strain RNA virus causes the infection. Although it is the most frequent cause of blood transfusion–associated hepatitis, less than 4% of all cases of hepatitis C can be attributed to this cause. Since the advent of screening of the blood supply for hepatitis C virus (HCV), the risk of transfusion-associated hepatitis C has decreased from 10% in the early 1980s to 0.1% today. More than 50% of cases of HCV infection are caused by injection drug use with needle sharing. Other risk behaviors include tattooing, branding, piercing, or other similar practices when shared or poorly sanitized equipment is used. Transmission through sexual contact is possible, but this risk seems to be relatively low. Maternal-fetal transmission is also uncommon and is usually limited to women with high circulating HCV levels. Transmission through breastfeeding has not been reported.

The HCV incubation period is about 6 to 7 weeks, and the infection rarely causes a serious acute illness. Diagnosis is made by the presence of anti-HCV, an antibody that persists in the presence of the virus and is not protective. At least 50% to 80% of individuals with hepatitis C go on to develop chronic infection and exhibit anti-HCV along with a positive hepatitis C viral load. Progression to cirrhosis occurs in about 20% of people infected with chronic hepatitis C after 20 years of disease. HCV-related cirrhosis risk is increased in men, with disease acquisition after age 40 years, and in people who drink the equivalent of 50 g or more of alcohol per day (15 g alcohol = 12 oz beer, 5 oz wine, 1.5 oz 80 proof whiskey). If anti-HCV persists in the absence of a positive hepatitis C viral load, this suggests that active infection is not present.

Because of the significant potential sequelae of chronic hepatitis C infection, expert consultation should be obtained so that the patient and primary care provider are well versed on the latest evaluation, monitoring, and treatment options. Currently, treatment with pegylated interferon and select antivirals has shown clinical utility in inducing remission in some patients with chronic hepatitis C; response depends on many factors, including other health problems, viral genotype, and viral load. Because of the rapid advances being made in this area, the clinician and patient must be aware of the most up-to-date treatment options.

Because the hepatitis D virus is an RNA virus that can occur only concurrently in the presence of HBV, it is found only in persons with acute or chronic hepatitis B. A patient with hepatitis B and D acute co-infection has a course of illness similar to that in a patient with only hepatitis B infection. If a patient with chronic hepatitis B becomes superinfected with hepatitis D virus, a fulminant or severe acute hepatitis often results. Prevention of hepatitis B through immunization also prevents hepatitis D.

The presentation of viral hepatitis, most commonly with acute HAV and HBV infection, usually includes malaise, myalgia, fatigue, nausea, and anorexia. Aversion to cigarette smoke exposure is often reported. Occasionally, arthritis-like symptoms and skin rash are also noted. Mild fever occasionally occurs. Hepatomegaly with usually mild right upper quadrant abdominal tenderness without rebound is found in about 50% of patients, with splenomegaly in about 15%. Jaundice typically occurs about 1 week after the onset of symptoms. Jaundice is not found in most cases, however. The course of the illness is typically 2 to 3 weeks. During this period, a gradual increase in energy, appetite, and well-being is reported.

Laboratory findings common to all forms of viral hepatitis include leukopenia with lymphocytosis. Atypical lymphocytes are often found. Bilirubin in the urine is usually found in the absence of icterus. Hepatic enzyme elevation is universal. Serological findings help with the diagnosis of the type of hepatitis. Knowledge of measures to prevent hepatitis or minimize its acquisition after exposure is important to safe, effective practice (see Table 6–5).

The test of liver enzymes is an evaluation of the degree of hepatic inflammation. Hepatic enzymes are found in the circulation because of hepatic growth and repair. The aspartate aminotransferase (AST) level increases in response to hepatocyte injury, as often occurs in alcohol abuse, acetaminophen misuse or overdose, and rarely the therapeutic use of HMG-CoA reductase inhibitors (lipid-lowering drugs whose names have the "-statin" suffix, such as simvastatin). This enzyme is also found in skeletal muscle, myocardium, brain, and kidneys in smaller amounts, and so damage to these areas may also cause an increase in AST.

AST (formerly known as serum glutamic oxaloacetic transaminase [SGOT]) is a hepatic enzyme with a circulatory half-life of approximately 12 to 24 hours; levels increase in response to hepatic damage and clear quickly after damage ceases. AST elevation is generally found in only about 10% of problem drinkers. If the AST level is elevated with normal alanine aminotransferase (ALT) level and mild macrocytosis (mean corpuscular volume >100 fL, seen in about 30% to 60% of men who drink five or more drinks per day and in women who drink three or more drinks per day), long-standing alcohol abuse is the likely cause.

ALT (formerly known as serum glutamate pyruvate transaminase [SGPT]) is more specific to the liver, having limited concentration in other organs. This enzyme has a longer half-life, 37 to 57 hours, than AST. Elevation of ALT levels persists longer after hepatic damage has ceased. The greatest elevation of this enzyme is likely seen in hepatitis caused by infection or inflammation, with a lesser degree of elevation noted in the presence of alcohol abuse. When evaluating a patient with suspected substance abuse causing hepatic dysfunction, the NP must note the degree of AST or ALT elevation.

An increase in bilirubin level is typically found in patients with viral hepatitis. Clinical jaundice is found when the total bilirubin level exceeds 2.5 mg. Bilirubin is the degradation product of heme, with 85% to 90% arising from hemoglobin and a smaller percentage arising from myoglobin.

Bilirubin is produced at a rate of about 4 mg/kg/d in healthy individuals. Because the rate of excretion usually matches the rate of production, the levels remain low and stable. Reticuloendothelial cells take in haptoglobin, a protein that binds with hemoglobin from aged red blood cells (RBCs). The reticuloendothelial cells remove the iron from hemoglobin for recycling. The remaining substances are degraded to bilirubin in its unconjugated, or indirect, form. This form is not water-soluble.

When unconjugated bilirubin is released into the circulation, it binds to albumin and is transported to the liver. When unconjugated bilirubin arrives at the liver, hepatocytes detach bilirubin from the albumin. It is then in a water-soluble form, also known as conjugated, or direct, bilirubin. Conjugated bilirubin loosely attaches to albumin and is easily detached in the kidney. The passing of small amounts of conjugated bilirubin through the kidney gives urine its characteristic yellow color. Conjugated bilirubin not excreted by the kidney is reabsorbed by the small intestine and converted to urobilinogen by bacterial action in the gut. This urobilinogen can be reabsorbed into the circulation, and excess amounts can appear in the urine. Small amounts of urobilinogen may also be found in a fecally contaminated urine sample because urobilinogen is normally found in the large intestine.

When there is an excess of urinary excretion of bilirubin, as found in patients with viral hepatitis, urine develops a characteristic brown color, often described by a patient as looking like cola or dark tea. Also, excess bilirubin could displace drugs with a high propensity for protein (albumin) binding, increasing free drug and possibly causing drug toxicity.

Treatment of acute viral hepatitis is largely supportive. Corticosteroids, antiviral agents, and interferon are used occasionally. Because of the seriousness of hepatitis B and C sequelae and risk of the development of chronic infection, considerable research is under way to develop effective, well-tolerated therapies. Chronic hepatitis B and C are potent risk factors for hematoma or primary hepatocellular carcinoma. Periodic monitoring for alpha-fetoprotein is often used to look for an increase in the level that indicates hepatic tumor growth, usually coupled with imaging such as abdominal ultrasound or CT. Consultation with a hepatitis specialist and awareness of the latest recommendations for ongoing monitoring are critical.

Discussion Sources

A comprehensive immunization strategy to eliminate transmission of hepatitis B virus infection in the United States: recommendations of the Advisory Committee on Immunization Practices, Part I: immunization of infants, children, and adolescents. *MMWR Morb Mortal Wkly Rep.* 2005;54(No. RR-16).

Centers for Disease Control and Prevention. http://www.cdc.gov/NCIDOD/DISEASES/hepatitis/a, National Center for HIV/AIDS, Viral Hepatitis, STD, and TB Prevention: viral hepatitis A, accessed 9/16/09.

Centers for Disease Control and Prevention. http://www.cdc.gov/hepatitis/HBV/HBVfaq.htm#general, Hepatitis B FAQs for health professionals, accessed 9/16/09.

Gilbert D, Moerlling R, Eliopoulos G, Chambers H, Saag M. *The Sanford Guide to Antimicrobial Therapy.* 39th ed. Sperryville, VA: Antimicrobial Therapy, Inc; 2009:138–140.

Jain M, Brailita D. Acute and chronic hepatitis. In: Rakel R, Bope E, eds. *Conn's Current Therapy.* Philadelphia, PA: Saunders Elsevier; 2009:533–539.

QUESTIONS

72. Which of the following is an expected finding in a patient with chronic renal failure?

    A. hypokalemia
    B. hypotension
    C. constipation
    D. anemia

73. The use of which of the following medications can precipitate acute renal failure in a patient with bilateral renal artery stenosis?

    A. corticosteroids
    B. angiotensin II receptor antagonists
    C. beta-adrenergic antagonists
    D. cephalosporins

74. A 78-year-old man presents with fatigue and difficulty with bladder emptying. Examination reveals a distended bladder, but is otherwise unremarkable. The blood urea nitrogen (BUN) level is 88 mg/dL (31.4 mmol/L); the creatinine level is 2.8 mg/dL (247.5 μmol/L). This clinical assessment is most consistent with:

    A. prerenal azotemia.
    B. acute glomerulonephritis.
    C. acute tubular necrosis.
    D. postrenal azotemia.

75. A 68-year-old woman with heart failure presents with tachycardia, S_3 heart sound, and basilar crackles bilaterally. Blood pressure is 90/68 mm Hg; BUN level is 58 mg/dL (20.7 mmol/L); creatinine level is 2.4 mg/dL (212.1 μmol/L). This clinical presentation is most consistent with:

    A. prerenal azotemia.
    B. acute glomerulonephritis.
    C. tubular necrosis.
    D. postrenal azotemia.

76. Which of the following is found early in the development of chronic renal failure?

    A. persistent proteinuria
    B. elevated creatinine level
    C. acute uremia
    D. hyperkalemia

77. Angiotensin-converting enzyme inhibitors can limit the progression of some forms of renal disease by:

   A. increasing intraglomerular pressure.
   B. reducing efferent arteriolar resistance.
   C. enhancing afferent arteriolar tone.
   D. increasing urinary protein excretion.

78. Objective findings in patients with glomerulonephritis include all of the following except:

   A. edema.
   B. urinary RBC casts.
   C. proteinuria.
   D. hypotension.

79. An increase in creatinine from 1 to 2 mg/dL is typically seen with a _____ loss in renal function.

   A. 25%
   B. 50%
   C. 75%
   D. 100%

80. Creatinine clearance usually:

   A. approximates glomerular filtration rate.
   B. does not change as part of normative aging.
   C. is greater in women compared with men.
   D. increases with hypotension.

81. Creatinine is best described as:

   A. a substance produced by the kidney.
   B. a product related to skeletal muscle metabolism.
   C. produced by the liver and filtered by the kidney.
   D. a by-product of protein metabolism.

ANSWERS

72.	D	73.	B	74.	D
75.	A	76.	A	77.	B
78.	D	79.	B	80.	A
81.	B				

DISCUSSION

Renal failure can be either acute or chronic. In acute renal failure, a precipitating event or cause is often easily identifiable. With prerenal azotemia, the most common cause of acute renal failure, the kidneys are hypoperfused, which often leads to acute tubular necrosis. Reasons for this hypoperfusion include decreased circulating volume, as seen in patients with dehydration and acute blood loss; decreased cardiac output, as seen in patients with heart failure; or excessive sequestering of fluid, as seen in patients with burns. Postrenal azotemia is caused by obstruction to urine flow and is an uncommon cause of renal failure. In intrinsic renal failure, there is disease within the kidney at the levels of the renal tubules, glomeruli, interstitium, or vessels. Etiologies include glomerulonephritis and acute interstitial nephritis. Laboratory findings in these more common forms of acute renal failure vary (Table 6–6).

Typical findings in renal failure include increased serum creatinine and blood urea nitrogen (BUN) levels. Creatinine is the end product of creatine metabolism, which arises from skeletal muscle. Because creatinine excretion by a healthy kidney is very efficient, measurement of creatinine is used as a surrogate marker of kidney function; creatinine production equals creatinine excretion. As the kidney fails, the creatinine level increases. BUN is derived from the breakdown of protein from dietary or other sources. BUN level typically increases (uremia) more rapidly than creatinine level in response to decreased renal perfusion and can increase from prerenal, renal, and postrenal causes of kidney failure. In particular, elevated BUN level with a normal creatinine level is occasionally found in patients with healthy kidneys but with severe dehydration. In addition, GI bleeding usually causes a marked increase in BUN level without corresponding increase in creatinine as the gut digests and absorbs proteins found in the blood.

Anemia is typically seen in patients with chronic renal failure. Erythropoietin, a glycoprotein growth factor produced primarily by the kidneys, influences the undifferentiated stem

TABLE 6–6

Etiology of and Findings in Acute Renal Failure

Disease Causing Acute Renal Failure	Typical Etiology	Laboratory Findings
Acute glomerulonephritis	Poststreptococcal infection, autoimmune diseases	BUN:Cr ratio >20:1 Urinalysis: renal casts, RBCs
Acute interstitial nephritis	Allergic reaction, drug reaction	BUN:Cr ratio <20:1 Urinalysis: WBC casts, eosinophils
Acute tubular necrosis	Hypotension, nephrotoxins	BUN:Cr ratio <20:1 Urinalysis: granular casts, renal tubular cells

BUN, blood urea nitrogen; Cr, creatinine; RBCs, red blood cells; WBC, white blood cell.

cell to form the RBC precursor. With end-stage renal disease, erythropoietin response is reduced because of limited supply; that is, as the kidney fails, erythropoietin production declines. In addition, as is common in chronic illness, RBC life span is shortened. These factors result in a normocytic, normochromic anemia in the presence of a low reticulocyte count, the characteristics of anemia of chronic disease. This problem is treated with recombinant erythropoietin, transfusion, and correction of additional anemia risk factors.

Discussion Sources

Ferri F. *Ferri's Best Test: A Practical Guide to Clinical Laboratory Medicine and Diagnostic Imaging.* 2nd ed. Philadelphia, PA: Saunders Elsevier; 2009.

Fitzgerald M. Hematologic disorders. In: Youngkin E, Sawin K, Kissinger J, Israel D, eds. *Pharmacotherapeutics: A Primary Care Clinical Guideline.* 2nd ed. Saddle River, NJ: Prentice-Hall; 2005.

Kraut J. Chronic renal failure. In: Rakel R, Bope E, eds. *Conn's Current Therapy.* Philadelphia, PA: Saunders Elsevier; 2009:725–731.

National Kidney Foundation Kidney Disease Outcomes Quality Initiative. http://www.kidney.org/professionals/KDOQI/, accessed 9/16/09.

Schroeder K. Acute renal failure. In: Rakel R, Bope E, eds. *Conn's Current Therapy.* Philadelphia, PA: Saunders Elsevier; 2009:721–725.

QUESTIONS

82. Which of the following is most likely to be part of the clinical presentation of an otherwise healthy woman with uncomplicated lower urinary tract infection (UTI)?
    A. urinary frequency
    B. fever
    C. suprapubic tenderness
    D. lower GI upset

83. A 36-year-old afebrile woman with no health problems presents with dysuria and frequency of urination. Her urinalysis findings include results positive for nitrites and leukocyte esterase. You evaluate these results and consider that she likely has:
    A. purulent vulvovaginitis.
    B. a gram-negative UTI.
    C. cystitis caused by *Staphylococcus saprophyticus*.
    D. urethral syndrome.

84. The most likely causative organism in community-acquired UTI is:
    A. *Klebsiella* species.
    B. *Proteus mirabilis*.
    C. *Escherichia coli*.
    D. *Staphylococcus saprophyticus*.

85. Preferred therapy for an uncomplicated UTI in an otherwise healthy woman includes:
    A. TMP-SMX.
    B. amoxicillin.
    C. azithromycin.
    D. cephalexin.

86. The notation of alkaline urine in a patient with a UTI may point to infection caused by:
    A. *Klebsiella* species.
    B. *P. mirabilis*.
    C. *E. coli*.
    D. *S. saprophyticus*.

87. Which of the following is the most accurate information in caring for a 40-year-old man with cystitis?
    A. This is a common condition in men of this age.
    B. A gram-positive organism is the likely causative pathogen.
    C. A urological evaluation should be considered.
    D. Pyuria is rarely found.

88. A 44-year-old woman presents with pyelonephritis. The report of her urinalysis is least likely to include:
    A. WBC casts.
    B. positive nitrites.
    C. 3+ protein.
    D. rare RBCs.

89. An example of a first-line therapeutic agent for the treatment of pyelonephritis is:
    A. amoxicillin with clavulanate.
    B. trimethoprim-sulfamethoxazole.
    C. ciprofloxacin.
    D. nitrofurantoin.

90. With fluoroquinolone use, length of antimicrobial therapy during uncomplicated pyelonephritis is typically:
    A. 5 days.
    B. 1 week.
    C. 2 weeks.
    D. 3 weeks.

91. Risk factors for UTI in women include:
    A. postvoid wiping back to front.
    B. low lactobacilli colonization.
    C. hot tub use.
    D. wearing pantyhose.

92. Which of the following is not a gram-negative organism?
    A. *E. coli*
    B. *K. pneumoniae*
    C. *P. mirabilis*
    D. *S. saprophyticus*

93. You see a 70-year-old woman in a walk-in center with a chief complaint of increased urinary frequency and dysuria. Urinalysis reveals pyuria and positive nitrites. She mentions she has a "bit of kidney trouble, not too bad." Recent evaluation of renal status is unavailable. In considering antimicrobial therapy for this patient, you prescribe:

   A. nitrofurantoin.
   B. fosfomycin.
   C. ciprofloxacin.
   D. tetracycline.

ANSWERS

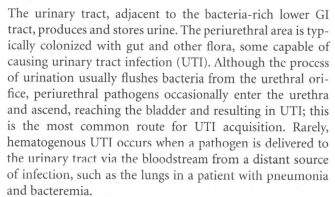

82.	A	83.	B	84.	C
85.	A	86.	B	87.	C
88.	C	89.	C	90.	B
91.	B	92.	D	93.	C

DISCUSSION

The urinary tract, adjacent to the bacteria-rich lower GI tract, produces and stores urine. The periurethral area is typically colonized with gut and other flora, some capable of causing urinary tract infection (UTI). Although the process of urination usually flushes bacteria from the urethral orifice, periurethral pathogens occasionally enter the urethra and ascend, reaching the bladder and resulting in UTI; this is the most common route for UTI acquisition. Rarely, hematogenous UTI occurs when a pathogen is delivered to the urinary tract via the bloodstream from a distant source of infection, such as the lungs in a patient with pneumonia and bacteremia.

UTIs can involve mucosal tissue (cystitis) or soft tissue (pyelonephritis, prostatitis). Anatomically, the infection can be limited to the lower urinary tract (cystitis involving the bladder and urethra) or the upper tract (pyelonephritis). Complicated UTI can occur in either the upper or the lower urinary tract, but is accompanied by an underlying condition that increases the risk for failing therapy, such as obstruction, urological dysfunction, or resistant pathogens. Most UTIs occur via an ascending route.

UTI is typically diagnosed by clinical presentation and a few physical examination and laboratory findings. In an otherwise healthy woman, history of the present illness usually reveals a complaint of dysuria, often reported as an internal discomfort, with urinary frequency and urgency, but without fever or constitutional symptoms. Although suprapubic tenderness and pain are often considered part of the clinical presentation, this is found in only about 20% of women with an uncomplicated UTI. Back pain, fever, nausea, and vomiting are more often associated with pyelonephritis and, in

rare cases, with cystitis; many patients with pyelonephritis also report lower UTI symptoms. Although vaginal infection and irritation can cause dysuria, most women who have dysuria without vaginal discharge have a UTI, not vaginitis.

Hemorrhagic cystitis is characterized by large quantities of visible blood in the urine. Its etiology can be bacterial infection or infection with adenovirus types 7, 11, 21, and 35, papovirus, and influenza A, or it can be a result of radiation, cancer chemotherapy, or certain immunosuppressive medications. The clinical presentation usually depends on its origin; with all causes, irritative voiding symptoms are typically reported. When the disease is infectious in origin, signs and symptoms of infection may also be encountered. Adenovirus is a common cause and is self-limiting in nature. Hemorrhagic cystitis is often confused with glomerulonephritis, but hypertension and abnormal renal function are absent in the former.

Acute pyelonephritis is an infection of the renal parenchyma and renal pelvis, caused by ascending cystitis; most episodes are uncomplicated and not accompanied by risk of treatment failure such as obstruction, urological dysfunction, or a multidrug-resistant uropathogen. Irritative voiding symptoms similar to symptoms of cystitis, fever, flank pain, an acutely ill appearance, costovertebral tenderness, and pyuria are usually reported; GI upset including vomiting is often noted. WBC with differential usually reveals leukocytosis, neutrophilia, and bandemia.

Urine dipstick testing is commonly done in the outpatient setting when UTI is suspected because it is simple and convenient and yields immediate results. Leukocyte esterase, nitrites, protein, and blood are the important features in evaluating for UTI. The presence of leukocyte esterase on a urine dipstick is equivalent to 4 WBCs or more per high-power field (HPF). Nearly all (≥96%) patients with UTI have pyuria equivalent to more than 10 WBCs/HPF. Some uropathogens are capable of reducing dietary nitrates in the urine to nitrite; this is an indirect test for bacteriuria. When this finding is coupled with a leukocyte esterase response, the likely offending organism is a gram-negative pathogen (*E. coli*, *Proteus* species, *Klebsiella pneumoniae*). The nitrite test result is occasionally falsely negative in UTI with a low colony count or with recently voided or dilute urine. In addition, this test does not detect organisms unable to reduce nitrate to nitrite, such as enterococci, staphylococci, or adenovirus. Small amounts of protein and RBCs may also be positive on dipstick testing in cases of UTI (Table 6–7).

Urine culture is important when diagnosis is unclear, or UTI is recurrent. The presence of more than one organism often indicates a contaminated urine specimen, and collection and testing should be repeated. The presence of 10^5 or more colony-forming units (CFUs) per milliliter of bacteria is the traditional diagnostic indicator for UTI. In the presence of dysuria and other symptoms for UTI, 10^2 CFU/mL confirms the diagnosis.

Certain factors protect against or increase the risk for UTI. Male sex is recognized as a potent protective factor, in part because of the longer urethral length than in women;

TABLE 6–7
Common Urinalysis Dipstick Findings in Urinary Tract Infection

Finding	Significance	Comment
Color	Typically pale yellow to colorless	Change in urine color is not synonymous with UTI or disease
Clarity	Typically clear	Pyuria causes urinary turbidity
Odor	Mild characteristic odor	Rancid or ammonia odor in urea-splitting organism
Specific gravity (SG)	Dilute urine: SG ≤1.008 Concentrated urine: SG >1.020	Dilute or concentrated urine may influence results of urine chemical test strip testing
Leukocyte esterase	Test for enzyme present in WBCs	Positive results indicate presence of neutrophils >5 WBCs/HPF, an indicator of UTI, reported sensitivity of 75%–90%; results not valid in neutropenic patients; decreased sensitivity with increased urinary glucose concentration, high urinary SG, and presence of antimicrobial in urine
Nitrites	Surrogate marker for bacteriuria; presence indicates bacterial reduction of dietary nitrates to nitrites by select gram-negative uropathogens including *E. coli, Proteus* spp. Normally absent in sterile urine and infection caused by enterococci, staphylococci	Best done on well-concentrated urine such as first AM void; for nitrites to be present, urine should be held in bladder for ≤1 hr for nitrate-to-nitrite conversion to occur; dietary nitrate intake must be adequate; false-negative result possible with low colony–count UTI
Protein	Dipstick testing most sensitive for albumin	Common in febrile response or represents presence of protein-containing substance such as WBCs, bacteria, mucus; in UTI, usually trace to 30 mg/dL (1$^+$), seldom ≥100 mg/dL
pH	Average pH 5–6 Acid pH 4.5–5.5 Alkaline pH 6.5–8	If alkaline urine is found in presence of UTI symptoms and positive leukocyte esterase, likely that a urea splitting organism such as *Proteus* is allowing urea to be split into CO_2 and ammonia, causing increase in urine's normally acid pH
Red blood cells (RBCS)	Low number of RBCs noted Gross hematuria rare in uncomplicated UTI, but may be present in infection complicated by nephrolithiasis	Microscopic hematuria common with UTI, but not in urethritis or vaginitis

UTI, urinary tract infection; WBCs, white blood cells.

women with a shorter urethra-to-anus length seem to be at increased UTI risk. In contrast to the periurethral area in women, the male periurethral area does not support bacterial growth. Zinc-rich prostatic secretions are antibacterial, further discouraging pathogen growth.

In either sex, efficient emptying helps prevent urine stagnation and minimizes UTI risk. Factors that alter efficient bladder emptying, such as cystocele, rectocele, and benign prostatic hyperplasia, increase UTI risk. In addition, robust fucosyltransferase activity, an enzyme found in the periurethral and perivaginal area, discourages bacterial adherence; the presence of relatively few bacterial adhesion receptor sites in the bladder and urethra has a similar effect.

Women with these receptors who do not have mucosal secretion of the fucosyltransferase enzyme to help block bacterial adherence are more likely to have colonization with *E. coli* and other coliforms from the rectum and less likely to have lactobacilli in the periurethral area; this situation results in frequent episodes of cystitis. The uroepithelial receptors can also be found in the upper urinary tract, increasing the risk of pyelonephritis. Women who are nonsecretors of ABH blood group antigens show enhanced adherence of pathogenic *E. coli* to uroepithelial cells compared with women who are secretors of these antigens; this becomes a major UTI risk factor when coupled with spermicide use or frequent vaginal sexual intercourse.

A woman who is exposed to the spermicide nonoxynol 9, either through vaginal use or with a male partner who uses condoms with this spermicide, is at increased risk of UTI. The proposed mechanism of this risk is the antibacterial effect of the spermicide: reducing lactobacilli, a normal component of the periurethral flora. Lactobacilli produce hydrogen peroxide and lactic acid, providing the periurethral area and vagina with a pH that inhibits bacterial growth, blocks potential sites of attachment, and is toxic to uropathogens. Voiding at regular intervals with efficient bladder emptying, wiping patterns, and postcoital voiding have not been shown to provide UTI protection. In addition, use of hot tubs, wearing pantyhose, douching, and obesity have not been shown to increase UTI risk.

In postmenopausal women, estrogen deficiency leads to a marked reduction in lactobacilli colonization in the vaginal-perineal areas; topical estrogen use results in re-establishment of the normal protective flora and a reduction of UTI risk. Recent antimicrobial use potentially increases UTI risk by the same mechanism. In children and elderly adults, constipation has been noted to contribute to bladder instability and may encourage UTI.

Most episodes of community-acquired cystitis in women, the most commonly encountered UTI, are caused by enteric gram-negative rods from the Enterobacteriaceae group, such as *E. coli*, *P. mirabilis*, and less commonly encountered *K. pneumoniae*. *Staphylococcus saprophyticus*, a gram-positive organism, and *E. coli* accounted for more than 90% of the uropathogens in one study of more than 4000 urine isolates obtained from women with cystitis during a 5-year period. These organisms are usually sensitive to a fluoroquinolone such as ciprofloxacin and nitrofurantoin. Growing rates of resistance to trimethoprim-sulfamethoxazole (TMP-SMX, Bactrim) have been exhibited by the organisms that most often cause UTI, potentially reducing the usefulness of this inexpensive, standard medication. Long-standing resistance to the beta-lactams, including ampicillin, compounds the problem.

Factors influencing the development of multidrug-resistant *E. coli* strains include liberal use of TMP-SMX to treat UTI in adults and to provide prophylaxis against *Pneumocystis carinii* pneumonia in patients with HIV. In children, attendance at day care, age younger than 3 years, and repeated antimicrobial use, particularly TMP-SMX and beta-lactams for respiratory infections, are risk factors for infection with a resistant uropathogen; child-to-child and child-to-parent transmission of the organism often occurs. Also, the more liberal use of ciprofloxacin in recent years, triggered in part by the decrease in cost when this medication became available in a generic form, is a great cause for alarm.

Current treatment recommendations for UTI therapy in younger women without comorbid conditions include the use of a short course (3 to 7 days) of an antimicrobial with significant activity against gram-negative (*E. coli*) and select gram-positive (*S. saprophyticus*) organisms. Treatment for pyelonephritis is also focused on coverage of gram-negative pathogens, usually for 1 week with a fluoroquinolone or 2 weeks with certain other antimicrobials (Table 6–8).

Although *E. coli* is the most common uropathogen in the community and in long-term care–dwelling elderly persons, *P. mirabilis* and *K. pneumoniae* account for approximately one-third of all infections in this age group. Length of antimicrobial treatment in elderly persons with uncomplicated UTI should be 7 to 10 days for women and 10 to 14 days for men; short-course therapy is not recommended. First-line therapy includes TMP-SMX or fluoroquinolones; nitrofurantoin should not be used in elderly patients because safe use of the product requires a minimal creatinine clearance of 40 mL/min. In an elderly patient with impaired renal function, the fluoroquinolone dosage potentially needs adjustment, but is considered to be a safe, effective, first-line intervention.

UTI prophylaxis may be indicated for women who experience two or more symptomatic UTIs within 6 months or three or more UTIs over 12 months and for women with fewer infections but with severe discomfort. Continuous prophylaxis, in which an antimicrobial is taken daily for 6 months or more, and postcoital prophylaxis, in which an antimicrobial is taken with each act of coitus, have been shown to be effective in the management of recurrent uncomplicated cystitis. Before UTI prophylaxis is initiated, resolution of the previous UTI should be confirmed by a negative urine culture 1 to 2 weeks after treatment. The method prescribed depends on the frequency and pattern of recurrences and on patient preference.

Choice of an antimicrobial agent for recurrent UTI should be based on susceptibility patterns of the strains causing the patient's previous UTIs and on patient history of drug allergies or intolerance. Long-term TMP-SMX or nitrofurantoin therapy has been used successfully for many years. Compared with TMP-SMX, nitrofurantoin has the advantage of lower rates of resistance by the more common UTI pathogens. The use of a fluoroquinolone for UTI prophylaxis has gained some popularity; concern about emerging resistance is an issue. UTI prophylaxis in a postmenopausal woman should also include a topical estrogen to encourage lactobacilli recolonization.

Cranberry and blueberry juice intake has been touted as a helpful measure to reduce the rate of recurrent infections. These juices were initially believed to cause high levels of benzoic acid that resulted in urinary acidification and bacteriostatic action; however, further study failed to support this hypothesis, with mixed results on efficacy in UTI prevention.

Discussion Sources

Cunha B. Urinary tract infections in women. In: Rakel R, Bope E, eds. *Conn's Current Therapy*. Philadelphia, PA: Saunders Elsevier; 2009:682–685.

Ferri F. Dysuria. In: *Ferri's Best Test: A Practical Guide to Clinical Laboratory Medicine and Diagnostic Imaging*. 2nd ed. Philadelphia, PA: Elsevier Mosby; 2009:227.

TABLE 6–8
Urinary Tract Infection Therapies

Type of Infection	Usual Pathogens	Regimens
Acute, uncomplicated UTI (cystitis, urethritis) in nonpregnant women	*E. coli* (gram-negative, most common pathogen), *S. saprophyticus* (gram-positive), enterococci (gram-positive)	**PRIMARY** If local *E. coli* resistance to TMP-SMX <20% and no allergy, then TMP-SMX-DS bid × 3 days If local *E. coli* resistance to TMP-SMX >20% or sulfa allergy, nitrofurantoin × 5 days or fosfomycin × 1 dose. **ALTERNATIVE** If local *E. coli* resistance to TMP-SMX >20% or sulfa allergy, ciprofloxacin 250 mg bid, ciprofloxacin ER 500 mg qd, levofloxacin 250 mg qd, all for 3 days. Moxifloxacin and gemifloxacin not labeled for use in UTI
Recurrent UTI (≥3/yr)	*E. coli, S. saprophyticus,* enterococci, other pathogens possible	**PRIMARY** Eradicate organisms, then TMP-SMX SS qd long-term **ALTERNATIVE** TMP-SMX DS post coitus or 2 DS tablets at first sign of UTI For recurrent UTI in postmenopausal women, consider use of estrogen cream, also consider urological factor, such as cystocele, residual urine volume, incontinence
Acute uncomplicated pyelonephritis suitable for outpatient therapy (Note: Obtain urine and blood cultures before initiating antimicrobial therapy)	*E. coli,* enterococci	**PRIMARY** Ciprofloxacin 500 mg bid, ciprofloxacin ER 1000 mg qd, levofloxacin 250 mg qd, ofloxacin 400 mg bid, all for 7 days. Moxifloxacin and gemifloxacin not labeled for use in UTI **ALTERNATIVE** Amoxicillin with clavulanate, cephalosporin, TMP-SMX-DS, all for 14 days

TMP-SMX, trimethoprim-sulfamethoxazole; UTI, urinary tract infection.
Source: Gilbert D, Moerlling R, Eliopoulos G, Chambers H, Saag M. *The Sanford Guide to Antimicrobial Therapy.* 39th ed. Sperryville, VA: Antimicrobial Therapy, Inc; 2009:30.

Gilbert D, Moerlling R, Eliopoulos G, Chambers H, Saag M. *The Sanford Guide to Antimicrobial Therapy.* 39th ed. Sperryville, VA: Antimicrobial Therapy, Inc; 2009.

QUESTIONS

94. Diagnostic criteria for irritable bowel syndrome (IBS) include abdominal pain that is associated with all of the following except:

   A. improvement with defecation.
   B. a change in frequency of stool.
   C. a change of stool form.
   D. unexplained weight loss.

95. Altering the gut pain threshold in IBS is a possible therapeutic outcome with the use of:

   A. loperamide (Imodium).
   B. dicyclomine (Bentyl).
   C. bismuth subsalicylate (Pepto-Bismol).
   D. amitriptyline (Elavil).

96. Tenesmus is defined as which of the following?

   A. rectal burning with defecation
   B. a sensation of incomplete bowel emptying that is distressing and sometimes painful
   C. weight loss that accompanies many bowel diseases
   D. appearance of frank blood in the stool

97. Concerning IBS, which of the following statements is most accurate?

   A. Patients most often report chronic diarrhea as the most distressing part of the problems.
   B. Weight gain is often reported.
   C. Patients can present with bowel issues ranging from diarrhea to constipation.
   D. The condition is associated with a strongly increased risk of colorectal cancer.

98. An example of a medication with prokinetic activity is:

   A. dicyclomine (Bentyl).
   B. metoclopramide (Reglan).
   C. loperamide (Imodium).
   D. psyllium (Metamucil).

99. Diagnostic testing in IBS often reveals:

   A. evidence of underlying inflammation.
   B. anemia of chronic disease.
   C. normal results on most testing.
   D. mucosal thickening on abdominal radiologic imaging.

100. The clinical indication for the use of lubiprostone (Amitiza) is for:

   A. the treatment of constipation that is not amenable to standard therapies.
   B. intervention in intractable diarrhea.
   C. control of intestinal inflammation.
   D. the relief of intestinal spasms.

101. Diagnostic testing in inflammatory bowel disease (IBD) often reveals:

   A. evidence of underlying inflammation.
   B. notation of intestinal parasites.
   C. normal results on most testing.
   D. a characteristic intra-abdominal mass on radiologic imaging.

102. Which of the following best describes the hemogram results in a person with anemia of chronic disease that often accompanies IBD?

   A. microcytic, hypochromic
   B. macrocytic, normochromic
   C. normocytic, normochromic
   D. hyperproliferative

103. IBD is a term usually used to describe:

   A. ulcerative colitis and irritable bowel syndrome.
   B. C. difficile colitis and Crohn disease.
   C. Crohn disease and ulcerative colitis.
   D. inflammatory colitis and ileitis.

104. "Skip lesions" are usually reported in:

   A. irritable bowel syndrome.
   B. ulcerative colitis.
   C. Crohn disease.
   D. C. difficile colitis.

105. Immune modulators are often used for intervention in:

   A. ulcerative colitis.
   B. irritable bowel syndrome.
   C. Crohn disease.
   D. ulcerative colitis and Crohn disease.

106. After a decade of disease, a person with ulcerative colitis is at increased risk of malignancy involving the:

   A. small bowel.
   B. large intestine.
   C. duodenum.
   D. stomach.

107. to 117. Which of the following statements is most consistent with IBD, IBS, or both conditions?

____ 107. Onset of symptoms is before age 30 to 40 years in most cases.

____ 108. The patient population predominately female.

____ 109. The condition is often referred to as spastic colon by the general population.

____ 110. Extraintestinal manifestations occasionally include nondestructive arthritis and renal calculi.

____ 111. This is a potentially life-threatening condition.

____ 112. The etiology likely involves an autoimmune response to the GI tract.

____ 113. Patients should be advised to avoid trigger foods.

____ 114. Involvement can be limited to intestinal mucosa only, or the full thickness of the intestinal wall can be involved.

____ 115. The etiology is considered to be an alteration in small and large bowel motility.

____ 116. Potential complications include fistula formation and perineal disease.

____ 117. Potential complications include increased risk for colonic malignancy.

ANSWERS

94.	D	95.	D	96.	B
97.	C	98.	B	99.	C
100.	A	101.	A	102.	C
103.	C	104.	C	105.	D
106.	B	107.	Both	108.	IBS
109.	IBS	110.	IBD	111.	IBD
112.	IBD	113.	Both	114.	IBD
115.	IBS	116.	IBD	117.	IBD

DISCUSSION

Irritable bowel syndrome (IBS) is a functional GI disorder characterized by abdominal pain and altered bowel habits in the absence of specific and unique organic pathology. This condition is sometimes called spastic colon, irritable colon, or nervous colon. Diagnosis of the condition is usually made via careful history and clinical assessment, with a focus on excluding other conditions. The Rome III criteria for the diagnosis of IBS require that patients must have recurrent abdominal pain with two or more of the following: discomfort relieved by defecation, symptom onset associated with a change in stool frequency, or symptom onset associated with a change in stool form or appearance. Additional symptoms usually include altered stool frequency, form, or passage (or a combination of two or all three) usually accompanied by mucorrhea and abdominal bloating or the sensation of distention or both.

People with IBS often present with one of four typical bowel patterns: IBS, diarrhea prominent (IBS-D); IBS, constipation predominant (IBS-C); IBS, diarrhea and constipation alternating (IBS-A); and IBS, mixed diarrhea and constipation (IBS-M). Also, gut dysfunction occurs along a continuum, with most patients moving from type to type. Usually the patient reports that these symptoms have been present for many years before care was sought. Women are diagnosed with the condition more often. Most individuals with the condition have onset of symptoms before age 35 years, often reporting problems since childhood. Although IBS onset can occur after age 40 years, an alternative GI diagnosis, including malignancy, becomes more likely and should be carefully considered.

The etiology of IBS is unclear, but is likely multifactorial, featuring altered GI motility within the large and small intestine, visceral hypersensitivity, and psychological issues including mood disorders. Although the mood component of the disease has often been attributed to the resulting disease-induced suffering, in reality, anxiety or depression or both often predate IBS onset. More recent research suggests that inflammation and small bowel bacterial overgrowth, altered neurotransmitter and inflammatory mediator production and use are possible contributors to IBS development. Probiotic use is an emerging treatment option that likely helps to normalize the possibly altered gut flora.

On physical presentation, a person with IBS usually has tenderness in the sigmoid region; the remainder of the examination is usually normal. Laboratory analysis is usually directed at ruling out another cause for the condition and typically reveals a normal hemogram, a normal erythrocyte sedimentation rate, and a negative test for fecal occult blood. Stool analysis for ova, parasite, enteric pathogens, leukocytes, and *Clostridium difficile* toxin are negative. If imaging studies, such as GI barium study, ultrasound, or abdominal CT or endoscopy, are indicated by clinical presentation, the results are usually normal. Referral to a gastroenterology specialist should be considered, particularly if the diagnosis is in question; a gastroenterology specialist also can provide input to the treatment plan.

Intervention in IBS involves patient support and education about the nature of the condition, including information that life expectancy is not affected, the condition is usually chronic with periodic exacerbations, and stress is a common trigger. Nutritional intervention can be helpful, with adequate hydration, addition of dietary fiber, avoidance of trigger foods, and moderation of caffeine intake often reported as being helpful. Fiber supplementation is often helpful with diarrhea and constipation; polycarbophil-based products, such as Citracal or FiberCon, offer a potential advantage over psyllium by causing less flatulence. Although some patients report improvement with avoidance of lactose or fructose, others do not.

Intervention with medications is usually aimed at treating the predominant symptom. Loperamide (Imodium) and anticholinergics/antispasmodics such as dicyclomine (Bentyl) are prescribed to treat diarrhea; the use of these medications can result in constipation. Low-dose tricyclic antidepressant or selective serotonin reuptake inhibitor use can be helpful in altering the gut pain threshold, resulting in less abdominal pain; the anticholinergic effects of the tricyclic antidepressants can help with limiting stool frequency, but also worsen constipation. Prokinetic or promotility agents have been used for patients with constipation-dominant symptoms. Because of safety issues, many of these products have significant use limitations; some have been withdrawn from the market. Other prokinetics, such as metoclopramide (Reglan) and erythromycin, have not yielded consistent benefits in patients with IBS. Lubiprostone (Amitiza), approved for the treatment of constipation that is not amenable to standard therapies, promotes fluid secretion into the intestinal lumen and is a helpful option in constipation-dominant IBS.

Inflammatory bowel disease (IBD) is a disease of unclear etiology, but likely involves an autoimmune response to the GI tract. This condition has a genetic component; whether this is a predisposition or susceptibility is unclear. The two major types of IBD are ulcerative colitis (UC), in which the pathological changes are limited to the colon, and Crohn disease, in which the changes can involve any part of the GI tract. In contrast to IBS, the male-to-female ratio is approximately equal for UC and Crohn disease. Similar to IBS, IBD is most often diagnosed in late adolescence to early adulthood, with most individuals who develop the disease showing symptoms by their late 20s. Less commonly, new-onset IBD is diagnosed in a child or adult.

The diagnosis of IBD is usually made through a combination of careful health history; physical examination; and appropriate diagnostic investigations, including radiography, endoscopy, and biopsy. The manifestations of IBD generally depend on the area of the intestinal tract involved.

Patients with UC or Crohn colitis frequently have bloody diarrhea, occasionally with tenesmus. Patients with Crohn disease involving the small intestine frequently have abdominal pain and diarrhea, and occasionally they have symptoms of intestinal obstruction. In Crohn disease, a cobblestone mucosal pattern is often identified on endoscopy or contrast radiography. "Skip lesions," areas of affected mucosal tissue alternating with normal tissue, are common; the rectum is often spared with the terminal ileum and right colon involved in most cases. In UC, inflammation is limited to the mucosa, whereas in Crohn disease, the entire intestinal wall is involved.

During an IBD flare, serological markers of inflammation, including C-reactive protein (CRP) and erythrocyte sedimentation rate (ESR or sed rate) are usually elevated. Leukocytosis is often present. In Crohn disease, fistulas and perianal disease are often noted. Toxic colitis, characterized by nonobstructive colonic dilation with signs of systemic toxicity, can occur as a potentially life-threatening complication of either condition; this condition is usually infectious in origin, with *C. difficile* often implicated.

Anemia is a common problem in IBD; its etiology is often from multiple causes. Iron deficiency anemia, manifesting as a microcytic, hypochromic anemia, occurs as a result of chronic blood loss. Anemia of chronic disease, a normocytic, normochromic anemia, is a result of inflammation of IBD, whereas anemia associated with acute blood loss can occur as a result of GI hemorrhage during a flare. Vitamin B_{12} deficiency, manifesting as a macrocytic, normochromic anemia, can also result in Crohn disease, usually in the presence of significant terminal ileum disease. Because of the difficulty with micronutrient absorption, including iron and vitamin B_{12}, with Crohn disease, parenteral replacement therapy is often preferred over the oral route. Additional extraintestinal manifestations in IBD include a nondestructive axial or peripheral arthritis in 15% of cases. Renal calculi are often found with Crohn disease.

The care for a person with IBD is usually a combination of lifestyle support, medication, and occasionally surgery. A person with IBD should be counseled to keep track of dietary triggers. Lactose intolerance is common in Crohn disease, but no more common than in the general population in people with UC. Tobacco use is associated with greater Crohn disease, but not UC, activity. Smoking cessation should be encouraged for this and its numerous additional health benefits. Gut rest is often used during treatment of Crohn disease, but not UC flares. Although IBD is likely genetic, not psychological, in origin, mental health and social support are important treatment components as the patient and family cope with this chronic, life-altering, and potentially life-threatening disease.

Medication therapy in IBD is usually initiated at the time of a flare, often the most common point of disease diagnosis. In Crohn disease and UC, oral aminosalicylates, including sulfasalazine (Azulfidine) and mesalamine (Apriso) are usually the first-line therapy and are equally effective. Mesalamine is usually better tolerated and can be used in the presence of sulfa allergy. In UC, when disease is limited to the distal colon, mesalamine and corticosteroids can be administered rectally. Oral or parenteral corticosteroid use can provide rapid symptom relief because of potent anti-inflammatory effects. In Crohn disease, metronidazole and ciprofloxacin are used when perineal disease or an inflammatory mass is noted; antibiotic use in UC is discouraged because of the increased risk of *C. difficile* infection. Immune modulators including 6-mercaptopurine and azathioprine are often prescribed to provide long-term disease control. A monoclonal antibody against tumor necrosis factor alpha, infliximab (Remicade), is also a potentially helpful, although costly, treatment option, assisting in remission in about 80% of individuals with Crohn disease and about 50% of individuals with UC. Other immune modulators such as methotrexate and cyclosporine have been used with some success. Probiotic therapy is an emerging option, used to help normalize gut flora.

The course of IBD is quite variable. A person with UC has approximately a 50% chance of having a flare in 2 years after achieving disease remission; this number is lower, about 40%, for a person with Crohn disease. With UC, colorectal cancer risk is greatly increased after about a decade of disease; as a result, surveillance colonoscopy is recommended every 2 years after 8 to 10 years of disease. In contrast, with Crohn disease, there is an increased risk for small bowel malignancy. At present, no effective screening is available for IBD. Given the complexities in diagnosis and treatment for a person with IBD, expert consultation should be sought.

Table 6–9 compares IBS and IBD.

Discussion Sources

Crowell M, DiBaise J, Harris L. Irritable bowel syndrome. In: Rakel R, Bope E, eds. *Conn's Current Therapy*. Philadelphia, PA: Saunders Elsevier; 2009:521–525.

Lehrer J, Lichtenstein G. http://emedicine.medscape.com/article/180389, eMedicine: Irritable bowel syndrome, accessed 9/19/09.

Peppercorn M, Moss A. Inflammatory bowel disease. In: Rakel R, Bope E, eds. *Conn's Current Therapy*. Philadelphia, PA: Saunders Elsevier; 2009:515–521.

Rowe W. http://emedicine.medscape.com/article/179037, eMedicine: Inflammatory bowel disease, accessed 9/19/09.

TABLE 6–9

Irritable Bowel Syndrome (IBS) versus Inflammatory Bowel Disease (IBD)

What These Have in Common: History
Chronically recurring symptoms of abdominal pain, discomfort (urgency and bloating), and alterations in bowel habits

What Are Their Differences:

IBS	IBD (Ulcerative Colitis, Crohn Disease)
No detectable structural abnormalities Absence of rectal bleeding, fever, weight loss, elevated CRP, ESR Intervention • Lifestyle modification such as diet, fiber, fluids, exercise • Medications as indicated by symptoms (antidiarrheals or promotility agents)	Intestinal ulceration, inflammation • Crohn: Mouth to anus • UC: Colon only Rectal bleeding, diarrhea, fever, weight loss, elevated CRP, ESR, leukocytosis, especially during flares Intervention • Lifestyle modification such as diet, fluids, exercise • Immune modulators • Anti-inflammatory medications as indicated by clinical presentation and response • Surgical intervention often needed and careful ongoing monitoring for gastrointestinal malignancy

CRP, C-reactive protein; ESR, erythrocyte sedimentation rate.

7 Male Genitourinary System

QUESTIONS

1. Which of the following is inconsistent with the description of benign prostatic hyperplasia (BPH)?

   A. obliterated median sulcus
   B. size larger than 2.5 cm × 3 cm
   C. sensation of incomplete emptying
   D. boggy gland

2. When prescribing antihypertensive therapy for a man with BPH and hypertension, the NP considers that:

   A. loop diuretics are the treatment of choice.
   B. an alpha₁ antagonist should not be used as a solo or first-line therapeutic agent.
   C. angiotensin receptor antagonist use is contraindicated.
   D. beta-adrenergic antagonist use often enhances urinary flow.

3. When assessing a 78-year-old man with suspected BPH, the NP considers that:

   A. prostate size does not correlate well with severity of symptoms.
   B. BPH affects about 50% of men of this age.
   C. he is at increased risk for prostate cancer.
   D. limiting fluids is a helpful method of relieving severe symptoms.

4. Which of the following medications can contribute to acute urinary retention in an older man with BPH?

   A. amitriptyline
   B. loratadine
   C. enalapril
   D. lorazepam

5. A 78-year-old man presents with a 3-day history of new-onset fatigue and difficulty with bladder emptying. Examination reveals a distended bladder, but is otherwise unremarkable. Blood urea nitrogen level is 88 mg/dL (31.4 mmol/L); creatinine level is 2.8 mg/dL (247.5 μmol/L). The most likely diagnosis is:

   A. prerenal azotemia.
   B. acute glomerulonephritis.
   C. tubular necrosis.
   D. postrenal azotemia.

6. Surgical intervention in BPH should be considered with all of the following except:

   A. recurrent urinary tract infection.
   B. bladder stones.
   C. persistent obstruction despite medical therapy.
   D. acute tubular necrosis.

7. Finasteride (Proscar, Propecia) and dutasteride (Avodart) are helpful in the treatment of BPH because of their effect on:

   A. bladder contractility.
   B. prostate size.
   C. activity at select bladder receptor sites.
   D. bladder pressure.

8. Tamsulosin (Flomax) is helpful in the treatment of BPH because of its effect on:

   A. bladder contractility.
   B. prostate size.
   C. activity at select bladder receptor sites.
   D. bladder pressure.

See full color images of this topic on DavisPlus at http://davisplus.fadavis.com | Keyword: Fitzgerald

9. Concerning BPH, which of the following statements is true?

   A. Digital rectal examination is accurate in diagnosing the condition.

   B. The use of a validated patient symptom tool is an important part of diagnosing the condition.

   C. Prostate size directly correlates with symptoms and bladder emptying.

   D. Bladder distention is usually present in early disease.

10. Concerning herbal and nutritional therapies for BPH treatment, which of the following statements is false?

    A. The mechanism of action of the most effective and best studied products is similar to prescription medications for this condition.

    B. These therapies are currently considered emerging therapy by the American Urological Association.

    C. Major areas of concern with use of these therapies include issues of product purity and quality control.

    D. These therapies are safest and most effective when used with prescription medications.

ANSWERS

1.	D	2.	B	3.	A
4.	A	5.	D	6.	D
7.	B	8.	C	9.	B
10.	D				

DISCUSSION

Benign prostatic hyperplasia (BPH) is a common disorder in older men. Based on autopsy studies, the prevalence of BPH increases from approximately 8% in men 31 to 40 years old to approximately 50% in men 51 to 60 years old and to more than 80% in men 80 years old and older. Far fewer men have clinically symptomatic disease. This enlargement of the prostate not associated with malignancy can lead to bladder outlet obstruction, likely as a result of an enlargement in prostatic connective tissue and an increase in the number of epithelial and smooth muscle cells. To empty the bladder effectively in the face of increasing outflow tract obstruction, bladder detrusor hypertrophy occurs with occasional notation of subsequent diverticula. Chronic incomplete bladder emptying causes stasis and predisposes to calculus formation and infection with secondary inflammatory changes, including prostatitis and urinary tract infection. The cause of BPH is not fully understood, but it seems to be at least partly a response to androgenic hormones.

Diagnosis of BPH is based on numerous components of the evaluation. On rectal examination, the prostate usually is enlarged, has a rubbery consistency, and in many cases has lost the median sulcus or furrow. Digital rectal examination of prostate size is often misleading, however—a prostate that is apparently small on digital rectal examination causes significant symptoms. The use of a validated tool such as the American Urological Association Symptom Score for Benign Prostatic Hyperplasia (available at http://www.auanet. org/guidelines/main_reports/bph_management/chapt_1_ appendix.pdf, accessed 9.21.09) increases the likelihood of an accurate diagnosis. A systematic evaluation for prostate cancer must be done on any man who has an abnormal prostate examination with or without urinary symptoms.

BPH can lead to bladder outlet obstruction from urethral narrowing. As a result, men with BPH develop symptoms of increased frequency of urination, decreased force of urinary stream, nocturia, and the sensation of incomplete emptying. Prolonged obstruction can lead to hydronephrosis and compromised renal function; this is the etiology of postrenal azotemia, a potentially life-threatening condition. Postrenal azotemia accounts for about 5% of all renal failure. It is characterized by urea nitrogen and creatinine elevation, and evidence of urinary retention and outflow tract obstruction; other reasons for renal failure have been ruled out. Intervention in postrenal azotemia is focused on relieving the urinary outflow tract obstruction. When postrenal azotemia is promptly detected, renal function returns to baseline after treatment.

Patient education about BPH should include information on measures to avoid making symptoms worse. Drugs with anticholinergic effect, such as tricyclic antidepressants and first-generation antihistamines (e.g., diphenhydramine [Benadryl], chlorpheniramine [Chlor-Trimeton]), can cause acute urinary retention in men with BPH; opioid use and inactivity also increase the risk of urinary retention. In addition, urinary frequency occasionally becomes worse with ingestion of certain bladder irritants, such as caffeine, alcohol, and artificial sweeteners. Although men with BPH are often tempted to limit fluid intake to minimize urinary frequency, this can yield more concentrated and perhaps irritating urine, possibly leading to increased symptoms.

The prostate and bladder base contain numerous alpha$_1$ receptor sites. When these receptor sites are stimulated, the prostate contracts, increasing outflow tract obstruction. As a result, treatment with alpha$_1$ receptor antagonists (alpha blockers) including tamsulosin (Flomax) can be helpful in improving the symptoms of BPH. The use of alpha blockers as a solo or first-line antihypertensive agent has been associated with higher than expected rates of stroke and heart failure. Alpha blockers should be considered as a desirable agent in treating a man with hypertension and BPH, but only as medication added on to existing therapy; an alpha blocker that is specifically indicated for BPH therapy only, such as tamsulosin, has minimal effect on blood pressure. The use of finasteride (Proscar) and dutasteride (Avodart), 5-alpha-reductase inhibitors that block the conversion of testosterone to dihydrotestosterone, help to reduce the size of the prostate and ameliorate symptoms.

Surgical intervention in BPH should be considered when medication and lifestyle modification therapy is ineffective and any of the following are present and clearly secondary to the condition: recurrent urinary tract infection, recurrent or persistent gross hematuria, bladder stones, or renal insufficiency. A number of minimally invasive therapies, including thermal and laser interventions, are now available and offer an attractive alternative to surgery, although less is known about long-term outcomes.

Herbal and nutritional therapies, including saw palmetto, rye, and pumpkin, are considered emerging therapies by the American Urological Association, pending further study. The observed effect of these plant-based therapies is usually attributed to a mechanism of action similar to approved prescription BPH therapies. As with other herbal and nutritional therapies available over-the-counter (OTC), issues of product purity and strength and potential interaction with prescription and other OTC products remain a concern.

Discussion Sources

American Urology Association Practice Guidelines Committee. Diagnosis and treatment recommendations: AUA guideline on management of benign prostatic hyperplasia (2003). *J Urol.* 2003;170:530–547.

Leveillee R, Patel V. eMedicine. http://www.emedicine.com/MED/ topic1919.htm, Benign prostatic hyperplasia, accessed 9/21/09.

Merck Manual. http://www.merck.com/mmpe/sec17/ch240/ ch240b.html, Benign prostatic hyperplasia (BPH), accessed 9/21/09.

QUESTIONS

11. You examine a 32-year-old man with chancroid and anticipate finding:

   A. a verruciform lesion.
   B. a painful ulcer.
   C. a painless, crater-like lesion.
   D. a plaque-like lesion.

12. The causative organism of chancroid is:

   A. *Ureaplasma* species.
   B. *Chlamydia trachomatis.*
   C. *Mycoplasma hominis.*
   D. *Haemophilus ducreyi.*

13. Treatment options for chancroid include all of the following except:

   A. azithromycin.
   B. ciprofloxacin.
   C. ceftriaxone.
   D. amoxicillin.

14. When ordering laboratory tests to confirm chancroid, the NP considers that:

   A. concomitant infection with herpes simplex is often found.
   B. a disease-specific serum test is available.
   C. a white blood cell count with differential is indicated.
   D. dark-field examination is needed.

ANSWERS

11.	B	**12.**	D
13.	D	**14.**	A

DISCUSSION

The gram-negative bacillus *Haemophilus ducreyi* causes chancroid. ♂ The organism is most often contracted sexually (Table 7–1). Transmission to health-care providers and other caregivers through direct contact with chancroid lesions has also been documented. The chancroid lesion is typically found at the site of inoculation with a vesicular-form to pustular-form lesion that forms a painful, soft ulcer with a necrotic base. Multiple lesions, acquired through autoinoculation, are usually found. A dense, matted lymphadenopathy can be found on the ipsilateral side of the lesion. The affected nodes may spontaneously rupture. Diagnosis of the condition can be challenging because cultures often fail to reveal the offending organism. Polymerase chain reaction testing is 100% sensitive; drawbacks include the expense of the test. Treatment options include azithromycin, ciprofloxacin, and ceftriaxone.

As with all sexually transmitted infections (STIs), a critical part of care is discussion of prevention strategies, including condom use and limiting the number of sexual partners. The NP should offer and encourage testing for other STIs, including HIV. Concomitant infection with syphilis, herpes simplex, and HIV is often found.

Discussion Sources

Gilbert D, Moerlling R, Eliopoulos G, Chambers H, Saag M. *The Sanford Guide to Antimicrobial Therapy.* 39th ed. Sperryville, VA: Antimicrobial Therapy, Inc; 2009:21–25.

Workowski KA, Berman SM. Sexually transmitted disease treatment guidelines, 2006. *MMWR Morb Mortal Wkly Rep.* 2006;55(No. RR-11):1–94.

TABLE 7–1

Sexually Transmitted Male Genitourinary Infections

Conditions	Causative Organism	Clinical Presentation	Treatment Options
Chancroid	*H. ducreyi*	Painful genital ulcer, multiple lesions common, inguinal lymphadenitis	Primary: Azithromycin 1 g orally in a single dose, or ceftriaxone 250 mg intramuscularly (IM) in a single dose Alternative: Ciprofloxacin 500 mg orally twice a day for 3 days, or erythromycin base 500 mg orally three times a day × 7 days
Genital herpes	Human herpesvirus 2, also known as herpes simplex type 2 (rarely human herpesvirus 1)	Painful ulcerated lesions, lymphadenopathy, particularly with primary outbreak. Subsequent outbreaks often less severe	For primary infection (initial episode): Acyclovir 400 mg PO tid × 7–10 days or famciclovir 250 mg PO tid × 7–10 days or valacyclovir 1g PO bid × 7–10 days For episodic recurrent infection: Acyclovir 800 mg tid × 2 days or 400 mg PO tid × 5 days or famciclovir 1000 mg bid × 1 day or 125 mg PO bid × 5 days or valacyclovir 1 g PO qd × 5 days or valacyclovir 500 mg PO bid × 5 days For suppression of recurrent infection: Acyclovir 400 mg PO bid or famciclovir 250 mg PO bid or valacyclovir 1g PO qd For patient with <9 recurrences per year, another treatment option: Valacyclovir 500 mg qd with an increase to 1 g qd if breakthrough
Lymphogranuloma venereum	Invasive serovar L1, L2, L3 of *C. trachomatis*	Vesicular or ulcerative lesion on external genitalia with inguinal lymphadenitis or buboes	Primary therapy: Doxycycline 100 mg PO bid × 21 days Alternative therapy: Erythromycin 500 mg qid × 21 days
Nongonococcal urethritis	*C. trachomatis* (50%), *Mycoplasma hominis*, *Mycoplasma genitalium* Assume concomitant infection with *N. gonorrhoeae* unless ruled out by accurate diagnostic testing	Irritative voiding symptoms, rarely mucopurulent penile discharge, often asymptomatic	Primary therapy: Azithromycin 1 g PO as a single dose or doxycycline 100 mg PO bid × 7 days Alternative therapy: Erythromycin base 500 mg PO qid × 7 days or ofloxacin 300 mg bid × 7 days or levofloxacin 500 mg qd × 7 days
Gonococcal urethritis	*N. gonorrhoeae* Assume concomitant infection with *N. gonorrhoeae* unless ruled out by accurate diagnostic testing	Irritative voiding symptoms, occasional purulent discharge	Recommended therapy: Single-dose therapy for uncomplicated infection Cefixime 400 mg PO or ceftriaxone 125 mg IM Concurrently treat with azithromycin 1 g as a single dose or doxycycline 100 mg bid × 7 days if chlamydial infection has not been ruled out. Alternative therapy in the presence of severe beta-lactam allergy: Spectinomycin 2 g IM as a single dose

TABLE 7–1

Sexually Transmitted Male Genitourinary Infections—cont'd

Conditions	Causative Organism	Clinical Presentation	Treatment Options
Genital warts (condyloma acuminata)	Human papillomavirus	Verruca-form lesions or can be subclinical or unrecognized	Patient-applied therapy: Podofilox 0.5% solution or imiquimod 5% cream Provider-applied therapy: Liquid nitrogen or cryoprobe, trichloroacetic acid, podophyllin resin, or surgical removal
Balanitis (inflammation of glans of penis)	*Candida* (40%), Group B streptococcus, *Gardnerella*	Occurs in about ¼ of all male sex partners of women with *Candida vaginitis*. Can also occur in presence of immunosuppression or systemic antimicrobial use	Oral azole therapy, same as therapy for vulvovaginitis

Sources: Gilbert D, Moerlling R, Eliopoulos G, Chambers H, Saag M. *The Sanford Guide to Antimicrobial Therapy*. 39th ed. Sperryville, VA: Antimicrobial Therapy, Inc; 2009:21–25. Workowski KA, Berman SM. Sexually transmitted disease treatment guidelines, 2006. *MMWR Morb Mortal Wkly Rep*. 2006;55(No. RR-11):1–94.

QUESTIONS

15. The most common causative organism of lymphogranuloma venereum is:

  A. *Ureaplasma genitalium.*
  B. *C. trachomatis* types 1 to 3.
  C. *Neisseria gonorrhoeae.*
  D. *H. ducreyi.*

16. Physical examination findings in lymphogranuloma venereum include:

  A. verruciform lesions.
  B. lesions that fuse and create multiple draining sinuses.
  C. a painless crater.
  D. plaque-like lesions.

17. Treatment options for lymphogranuloma venereum include:

  A. tetracycline.
  B. penicillin.
  C. ceftriaxone.
  D. dapsone.

ANSWERS

15. B   16. B   17. A

DISCUSSION

Lymphogranuloma venereum is an STI caused by *Chlamydia trachomatis* types L1 to L3. The clinical presentation, usually occurring approximately 1 to 4 weeks after contact with an infected host, consists of a vesicular or ulcerative lesion on the external genitalia, often not noted by the patient, which progresses to cause inguinal lymphadenitis or buboes. These may fuse and then drain, forming multiple sinus tracts with resultant scarring. Polymerase chain reaction assays have been used to aid in the diagnosis, but have had availability limited to reference laboratories. Treatment options include tetracycline, doxycycline, and erythromycin (see Table 7–1). As with all STIs, a critical part of care is discussion of prevention strategies, including condom use and limiting the number of sexual partners. The NP should offer and encourage testing for other STIs, including HIV.

Discussion Sources

Gilbert D, Moerlling R, Eliopoulos G, Chambers H, Saag M. *The Sanford Guide to Antimicrobial Therapy*. 39th ed. Sperryville, VA: Antimicrobial Therapy, Inc; 2009:21–25.

Workowski KA, Berman SM. Sexually transmitted disease treatment guidelines, 2006. *MMWR Morb Mortal Wkly Rep*. 2006;55(No. RR-11):1–94.

QUESTIONS

18. The presentation of acute epididymitis includes:

    A. the presence of a positive Prehn sign.
    B. low back pain.
    C. absent cremasteric reflex.
    D. diffuse abdominal pain.

19. The most likely causative pathogens in a 26-year-old man with acute epididymitis include:

    A. *Escherichia coli.*
    B. *Enterobacteriaceae.*
    C. *C. trachomatis.*
    D. *Pseudomonas* species.

20. Which of the following is part of a reasonable treatment option for a 30-year-old man with acute epididymitis?

    A. doxycycline
    B. amoxicillin
    C. metronidazole
    D. clindamycin

ANSWERS

18. A   19. C   20. A

DISCUSSION

Acute epididymitis is a male upper reproductive tract infectious disease caused by various pathogens. In men younger than 35 years, it is usually caused by *C. trachomatis* or *N. gonorrhoeae*; the organism is acquired through sexual contact. In men older than 35 years, acute epididymitis is often seen secondary to prostatitis and is typically caused by a gram-negative organism. This condition manifests with irritative voiding symptoms; fever; and an acutely painful, enlarged epididymis. Pain often radiates up the spermatic cord to the ipsilateral lower abdomen. The Prehn sign, a reduction in pain when the scrotum is elevated above the symphysis pubis, is usually noted. Urethritis, scrotal swelling, and penile discharge are often found. As the disease progresses, the ipsilateral testis may become involved, swelling so that the two testes cannot be distinguished; this is known as epididymo orchitis.

Treatment options differ according to age and risk factors. In younger men with low risk for epididymo-orchitis as a complication of urinary tract infection, particularly with risk for STI, antimicrobials effective against gonorrhea and chlamydia such as ceftriaxone followed by doxycycline should be used (Table 7–2). In men at risk for epididymo-orchitis as a complication of urinary tract infection, the choice of antimicrobial agent should be directed by urine culture. A fluoroquinolone such as ciprofloxacin is likely to be effective. As with all STIs, a critical part of care is discussion of prevention strategies, including condom use and limiting the number of sexual partners. The NP should offer and encourage testing for other STIs, including HIV.

Discussion Sources

Gilbert D, Moerlling R, Eliopoulos G, Chambers H, Saag M. *The Sanford Guide to Antimicrobial Therapy*. 39th ed. Sperryville, VA: Antimicrobial Therapy, Inc; 2009:21–25.

Workowski KA, Berman SM. Sexually transmitted disease treatment guidelines, 2006. *MMWR Morb Mortal Wkly Rep*. 2006;55(No. RR-11):1–94.

QUESTIONS

21. Gram stain of the urethral discharge of a 37-year-old man with dysuria reveals gram-negative cocci. This most likely represents:

    A. *C. trachomatis.*
    B. *U. genitalium.*
    C. *N. gonorrhoeae.*
    D. *E. coli.*

22. Treatment options for uncomplicated gonococcal proctitis include:

    A. ceftriaxone, 125 mg intramuscularly as a single dose.
    B. erythromycin, 500 mg bid for 7 days.
    C. norfloxacin, 400 mg bid for 3 days.
    D. azithromycin, 1 g as a single dose.

23. Which of the following is recommended by the Centers for Disease Control and Prevention as single-dose therapy for uncomplicated urethritis caused by *N. gonorrhoeae*?

    A. cefixime
    B. metronidazole
    C. azithromycin
    D. amoxicillin

24. In gonococcal infection, which of the following statements is true?

    A. Risk of transmission from an infected woman to a male sexual partner is about 20% to 30% with a single coital act.
    B. Most men have symptomatic infection.
    C. The incubation period is about 2 to 3 weeks.
    D. The organism rarely produces beta-lactamase.

ANSWERS

21. C   22. A
23. A   24. A

TABLE 7–2

Assessment and Treatment of Male Genitourinary Infections

Conditions	Causative Organism	Clinical Presentation	Treatment Options
Epididymitis Epididymo orchitis Age ≤35 y.o.	*N. gonorrhoeae, C. trachomatis*	Irritative voiding symptoms, fever and painful swelling of epididymis and scrotum	Primary: Ceftriaxone 250 mg intramuscularly (IM) as a single dose plus doxycycline 100 mg bid × 10 days Advise scrotal elevation to help with symptom relief.
Epididymitis Epididymo orchitis Age >35 y.o. or insertive partner in anal intercourse	*Enterobacteriaceae* (coliforms)	Irritative voiding symptoms, fever and painful swelling of epididymis and scrotum	Primary: Ciprofloxacin 500 mg qd or levofloxacin 750 mg qd × 10–14 days Alternative: Intravenous ampicillin with sulbactam, third generation cephalosporin, other parenteral agents as indicated by severity of illness
Acute bacterial prostatitis (≤35 y.o.)	*N. gonorrhoeae, C. trachomatis*	Irritative voiding symptoms, suprapubic, perineal pain, fever, tender, boggy prostate, leukocytosis	Primary: Ceftriaxone 250 mg IM as one-time dose then doxycycline 100 mg PO bid × 10 days
Acute bacterial prostatitis (>35 y.o.)	Enterobacteriaceae (coliforms)	Irritative voiding symptoms, suprapubic, perineal pain, fever, tender, boggy prostate, leukocytosis	Ciprofloxacin 500 mg PO bid or ofloxacin 200 mg PO qd mg × 14 days
Chronic bacterial prostatitis	Enterobacteriaceae (coliforms) (80%), enterococci(15%), *P. aeruginosa*	Irritative voiding symptoms, dull, poorly localized, suprapubic, perineal pain	Ciprofloxacin 500 mg PO bid × 4 weeks or levofloxacin 500 mg PO qd × 6 weeks Alternative: TMP-SMX DS 1 tab bid × 1–3 mo With treatment failure, consider prostatic stones

Sources: Workowski KA, Berman SM. Sexually transmitted disease treatment guidelines, 2006. *MMWR Morb Mortal Wkly Rep.* 2006;55 (No. RR-11):1–94. Gilbert D, Moerlling R, Eliopoulos G, Chambers H, Saag M. *The Sanford Guide to Antimicrobial Therapy.* 39th ed. Sperryville, VA: Antimicrobial Therapy, Inc; 2009:30–32.

DISCUSSION

Gonorrhea, caused by the gram-negative diplococcus *N. gonorrhoeae,* is one of the most common STIs. This pathogen has a short incubation period, 1 to 5 days, and is likely to cause infection in approximately 20% to 30% of men who have sexual contact with an infected woman and approximately 60% to 80% of women who have sexual contact with an infected man. Male-to-male and female-to-female rates of transmission are not as well documented.

In men, presentation typically includes dysuria with a milky, occasionally blood-tinged penile discharge. Most men are asymptomatic, however. With anal-insertive sex, rectal infection leading to proctitis is often seen. Gonorrheal infection is usually confirmed by amplification testing of the DNA present in the organism.

Because the organism frequently produces beta-lactamase, therapeutic agents should include agents with beta-lactamase stability and a cephalosporin, such as injectable ceftriaxone or oral cefixime (see Table 7–1). Increasing prevalence of fluoroquinolone-resistant gonococcus limits the usefulness of these medications; fluoroquinolone is no longer recommended for gonorrheal infection. As with all STIs, a critical part of care is discussion of prevention strategies, including condom use and limiting the number of sexual partners. The NP should offer and encourage testing for other STIs, including HIV.

Discussion Sources

Gilbert D, Moerlling R, Eliopoulos G, Chambers H, Saag M. *The Sanford Guide to Antimicrobial Therapy.* 39th ed. Sperryville, VA: Antimicrobial Therapy, Inc; 2009:21–25.

Workowski KA, Berman SM. Sexually transmitted disease treatment guidelines, 2006. *MMWR Morb Mortal Wkly Rep.* 2006;55(No. RR-11):1–94.

QUESTIONS

25. When choosing an antimicrobial agent for the treatment of chronic bacterial prostatitis, the NP considers that:
    A. gram-positive organisms are the most likely cause of infection.
    B. cephalosporins are the first-line choice of therapy.
    C. choosing an antibiotic with gram-negative coverage is critical.
    D. length of antimicrobial therapy is typically 5 days.

26. All of the following are likely to be reported by patients with acute bacterial prostatitis except:
    A. perineal pain.
    B. irritative voiding symptoms.
    C. penile discharge.
    D. fever.

27. During acute bacterial prostatitis, the digital rectal examination usually reveals a gland described as:
    A. boggy.
    B. smooth.
    C. irregular.
    D. cystic.

28. Symptoms in chronic bacterial prostatitis often include:
    A. fever.
    B. gastrointestinal upset.
    C. low back pain.
    D. penile discharge.

29. The most common causative organisms in chronic bacterial prostatitis include:
    A. gram-negative rods.
    B. gram-positive cocci.
    C. gram-negative cocci.
    D. gram-positive coccobacilli.

30. Which of the following is the best choice of therapy in chronic bacterial prostatitis?
    A. trimethoprim-sulfamethoxazole for 2 weeks
    B. amoxicillin for 4 weeks
    C. ciprofloxacin for 4 weeks
    D. gentamicin for 8 weeks

31. The best diagnostic test to identify the offending organism in acute bacterial prostatitis is:
    A. a urine culture.
    B. a urethral culture.
    C. antibody testing.
    D. a urine Gram stain.

ANSWERS

25.	C	26.	C	27.	A
28.	C	29.	A	30.	C
31.	A				

DISCUSSION

Infection with a gram-negative rod such as *E. coli* and *Pseudomonas* species usually causes acute bacterial prostatitis in older men. In younger men or men at risk for STIs, gonorrhea or chlamydia or both are most often implicated. Less often, gram-positive organisms such as enterococci are implicated. Irritative voiding symptoms, suprapubic pain, and perineal pain are typically reported. Objective findings include fever; a tender, boggy prostate; leukocytosis; and a urine culture positive for the causative organism. Urine Gram stain usually fails to identify the offending organism.

Treatment for acute bacterial prostatitis is similar to treatment for acute pyelonephritis—an antimicrobial agent with activity against gram-negative organisms and excellent tissue penetration. In men younger than 35 years, ofloxacin or ceftriaxone followed by doxycycline is recommended; causative organisms are usually the sexually transmitted organisms *C. trachomatis* and *N. gonorrhoeae*. Length of therapy is usually 10 to 14 days. In men 35 years old and older, *Enterobacteriaceae* strains (coliforms) are usually implicated as the causative organsim in acute bacterial prostatitis. Antimicrobial therapy with a higher dose fluoroquinolone, such as ciprofloxacin, for 14 days is advised.

In patients with chronic bacterial prostatitis, irritative voiding symptoms, low back and perineal pain, and a history of urinary tract infection are typically reported. Objective findings include a tender, boggy prostate. Urinalysis results are usually normal from a freshly voided specimen. Urinalysis and culture after prostatic massage usually yields leukocytes and the causative organism; prostatic massage is not recommended if acute prostatitis is known to be present. Antimicrobial therapy for 4 to 12 weeks using a product with excellent tissue penetration and strong gram-negative coverage is usually required (see Table 7–2).

Discussion Sources

Gilbert D, Moerlling R, Eliopoulos G, Chambers H, Saag M. *The Sanford Guide to Antimicrobial Therapy.* 39th ed. Sperryville, VA: Antimicrobial Therapy, Inc; 2009:30–32.

Hedayati T, Kwon D. eMedicine. http://www.emedicine.com/emerg/topic488.htm, Prostatitis, 2007, accessed 8/8/08.

Workowski KA, Berman SM. Sexually transmitted disease treatment guidelines, 2006. *MMWR Morb Mortal Wkly Rep.* 2006;55(No. RR-11):1–94.

QUESTIONS

32. You perform a rectal examination on a 72-year-old man and find a lesion suspicious for prostate cancer. The findings are described as:
    A. a rubbery, enlarged prostatic lobe.
    B. an area of prostatic induration.
    C. a boggy gland.
    D. prostatic tenderness.

33. Which of the following prostate-specific antigen (PSA) results is most consistent with prostate cancer?
    A. a single elevated PSA result in a man recovering from prostatitis
    B. a doubling of PSA value in serial annual tests in the presence of a normal prostatic digital rectal examination
    C. an elevated, unchanged serial PSA level in a man with BPH
    D. a markedly abnormal PSA result immediately after cystoscopy

34. Risk factors for prostate cancer include all of the following except:
    A. African ancestry.
    B. history of genital trauma.
    C. family history of prostate cancer.
    D. high-fat diet.

35. The average American man has an approximately ____% lifetime risk of prostate cancer and an approximately ____% likelihood of clinical disease.
    A. 15, 5
    B. 25, 8
    C. 40, 10
    D. 60, 15

ANSWERS

| 32. | B | 33. | B |
| 34. | B | 35. | C |

DISCUSSION

Prostate cancer is the most common noncutaneous cancer in men in the United States. Although clinically detectable prostate cancer is a cause of considerable mortality and morbidity, most cancers are likely occult and limited to the prostate with little risk of metastasis. Prostate cancer has been found on autopsy in two-thirds of men 80 to 89 years old. The average American man has a 40% lifetime risk of latent prostate cancer, an approximate 10% risk of clinically significant disease, and an approximate 3% risk of dying of prostate cancer; prostate cancer is the third cause of male cancer death in the United States, after lung and colorectal cancer.

Most men with prostate cancer are asymptomatic unless the disease is advanced. Consequently, prostate cancer screening is important. The prostate-specific antigen (PSA) blood test and digital rectal examination (DRE) should be offered annually, beginning at age 50, to men who have at least a 10-year life expectancy; some experts advise discontinuing prostate cancer screening when men reach age 75 years, owing to the high prevalence of clinically nonsignificant disease in this age group. Men at high risk (African ancestry and men with a strong family history of one or more first-degree relatives [father, brothers] diagnosed before age 65) should begin testing at age 45 years. Men at even higher risk because of multiple first degree relatives affected at an early age could begin testing at age 40. Depending on the results of this initial test, no further testing might be needed until age 45. Not offering or discouraging testing is not considered to be appropriate practice, although emerging studies will likely influence practice.

Although periodic DRE and PSA testing is advised for some men, there are limitations to the effectiveness of this screening protocol. The prostatic DRE can reveal a discrete, painless lesion or area of induration, but is often normal until disease is advanced. PSA is a glycoprotein produced in benign and malignant prostate cells. Nearly two-thirds of men with PSA levels greater than 10 ng/mL (normal PSA <4 ng/mL in an older man, <2.5 ng/mL in a younger man) have prostate cancer, whereas about 25% of men with PSA values of 4 to 10 ng/mL have disease, and approximately the same percentage of men in the at-risk age group have evidence of prostate cancer with a normal PSA. Correlating an abnormal prostate examination finding with an abnormal PSA level increases the likelihood of a diagnosis of prostate cancer. PSA level can also be elevated transiently in conditions other than prostate cancer, including prostatitis or immediately after prostatic instrumentation such as cystoscopy. Levels often remain chronically elevated in patients with BPH. Serial increases even in the presence of a normal prostate examination should be evaluated further.

Because of its low sensitivity and specificity, transrectal ultrasound should not be used as a first-line screening test for prostate cancer. This test can be helpful, however, when coupled with PSA and DRE findings and for guiding prostatic biopsy, the usual next step when a diagnosis of prostate cancer is considered. Pathology and disease staging guide prostate cancer treatment options. Watchful waiting is often a reasonable option for older men with local disease.

Discussion Sources

American Cancer Society. http://www.cancer.org/docroot/ped/content/ped_2_3x_acs_cancer_detection_guidelines_36.asp, 2009 Guidelines for the early detection of cancer, accessed 9/21/09.

American Urological Association. http://www.auanet.org/
guidelines/patient_guides/pc08.pdf, The management of
localized prostate cancer, 2008, accessed 9/22/09.

Cookson M, Change S. Malignant tumors of the urogenital tract.
In: Rakel R, Bope E, eds. *Conn's Current Therapy*. Philadelphia,
PA: Elsevier Saunders; 2008:722–726.

QUESTIONS

36. A 19-year-old man presents with sudden onset of left-sided scrotal pain and unilateral loss of the cremasteric reflex. This most likely represents:

   A. acute epididymitis.

   B. testicular torsion.

   C. testicular neoplasia.

   D. incarcerated hernia.

37. In assessing a man with testicular torsion, the NP is most likely to note:

   A. relief of pain with scrotal elevation.

   B. white blood cells reported in urinalysis.

   C. a swollen, tender testicle.

   D. increased testicular blood flow by color-flow Doppler ultrasound.

38. Anticipated organ survival exceeds 85% with testicular decompression within how many hours of torsion?

   A. 1

   B. 6

   C. 16

   D. 24

39. To prevent a recurrence of testicular torsion, which of the following is recommended?

   A. use of a scrotal support

   B. avoidance of testicular trauma

   C. orchiopexy

   D. limiting the number of sexual partners

ANSWERS

| 36. | B | 37. | C |
| 38. | B | 39. | C |

DISCUSSION

Testicular torsion is a urological emergency caused by a twisting of the testis and spermatic cord around a vertical axis; experimental modeling of the event reveals that a 720-degree twist is needed to occlude arterial and venous blood flow and cause the resulting testicular swelling and testicular tissue death. Findings include severe unilateral scrotal pain and swelling, the affected testicle held high in the scrotum, absent cremasteric reflex, and lack of pain relief with scrotal elevation. Approximately 50% of men presenting with torsion report intermittent unilateral testicular pain in the past, perhaps caused by partial, reversible torsion. The left testicle is most often affected. Radionuclide testicular scan and color-flow Doppler ultrasound usually show reduction of blood flow.

Prompt referral to a urological surgeon for detorsion of the organ and restoration of testicular blood flow is indicated. Testicular survival surpasses 85% if detorsion is accomplished within 6 hours. Manual manipulation of the testicle to unwind the torsion is occasionally helpful, although surgical intervention is more common. A bilateral orchiopexy, a procedure in which both testes are brought down and tacked lower in the scrotum, is usually performed to avoid subsequent torsion.

Discussion Source

Rupp T. eMedicine. http://www.emedicine.com/emerg/
TOPIC573.HTM, Testicular torsion, accessed 9/21/09.

QUESTIONS

40. A 42-year-old man has a nontender "bag of worms" mass within the left scrotum that disappears when he is in the supine position. This is most consistent with:

   A. testicular neoplasm.

   B. varicocele.

   C. inguinal hernia.

   D. epididymitis.

41. Which of the following is a common finding in a man with varicocele?

   A. lower sperm count with increased number of abnormal forms

   B. increased rate of testicular cancer

   C. recurrent scrotal pain

   D. BPH

ANSWERS

| 40. | B | 41. | A |

DISCUSSION

A varicocele is an abnormally dilated spermatic vein within the scrotum. Typically described as a "bag of worms" lesion, and most often found in the left scrotum, a varicocele is present while the man is standing and disappears in the supine position. A decreased sperm count with an increase in abnormal forms is noted in about two-thirds of men with the condition. Although varicocele is considered one of the most common correctable forms of male infertility, some men with the condition have normal fertility. Surgery or varicocele embolization is curative. A scrotal support can be helpful for relief of discomfort associated with varicocele.

Discussion Source

Men's Health. http://www.mayoclinic.com/health/Varicocele/ DS00618, Varicocele, accessed 9/21/09.

QUESTIONS

42. How long after contact does the onset of clinical manifestations of syphilis typically occur?

    A. less than 1 week
    B. 1 to 3 weeks
    C. 2 to 4 weeks
    D. 4 to 6 weeks

43. Which of the following is not representative of the presentation of primary syphilis?

    A. a painless ulcer
    B. palpable inguinal nodes
    C. flu-like symptoms
    D. a spontaneously healing lesion

44. Which of the following is representative of the presentation of secondary syphilis?

    A. generalized rash
    B. chancre
    C. pupillary alterations
    D. aortic regurgitation

45. Which of the following is found in tertiary syphilis?

    A. arthralgia
    B. lymphadenopathy
    C. maculopapular lesions involving the palms and soles
    D. gumma

46. Syphilis is most contagious at which of the following times?

    A. before onset of signs and symptoms
    B. during the primary stage
    C. during the secondary stage
    D. during the tertiary stage

47. First-line treatment options for primary syphilis include:

    A. penicillin.
    B. ciprofloxacin.
    C. erythromycin.
    D. ceftriaxone.

ANSWERS

42.	C	43.	C	44.	A
45.	D	46.	C	47.	A

DISCUSSION

Caused by the spirochete *Treponema pallidum*, syphilis is a complex, multiorgan disease. Sexual contact is the usual route of transmission. The initial lesion forms ♂ about 2 to 4 weeks after contact; contagion is greatest during the secondary stage. Treatment is guided by the stage of disease and clinical manifestation (Table 7–3). As with all STIs, a critical part of care is discussion of prevention strategies, including condom use and limiting the number of sexual partners. The NP should offer and encourage testing for other STIs, including HIV.

Discussion Sources

Gilbert D, Moerlling R, Eliopoulos G, Chambers H, Saag M. *The Sanford Guide to Antimicrobial Therapy*. 39th ed. Sperryville, VA: Antimicrobial Therapy, Inc; 2009:21–25.

Workowski KA, Berman SM. Sexually transmitted disease treatment guidelines, 2006. *MMWR Morb Mortal Wkly Rep*. 2006;55(No. RR-11):1-94.

QUESTIONS

48. Sequelae of genital human papillomavirus (HPV) infection in a man can include:

    A. anorectal carcinoma.
    B. low sperm count.
    C. paraphimosis.
    D. Reiter syndrome.

49. Which of the following best describes the lesions associated with condyloma acuminatum?

    A. verruciform
    B. plaque-like
    C. vesicular
    D. bullous

50. Treatment options for patients with condyloma acuminatum include:

    A. imiquimod.
    B. penicillin.
    C. acyclovir.
    D. metronidazole.

TABLE 7–3

Stages of Syphilis, Clinical Manifestations, and Recommended Treatment

Stage of Syphilis	Clinical Manifestations	Treatment Options	Comment
Primary syphilis	Painless genital ulcer with clean base and indurated margins, localized lymphadenopathy	Recommended therapy: • Benzathine penicillin G 2.4 million U intramuscularly (IM) as a one-time dose Alternative therapy in penicillin allergy: • Doxycycline 100 mg PO bid × 2 weeks *or* • Tetracycline 500 mg PO qid × 2 weeks *or* Ceftriaxone 1 g IM or intravenously q24h × 8–10 days	Azithromycin 2 g as a one-time dose has been suggested, although issues of emerging resistance are concerning
Secondary syphilis	Diffuse maculopapular rash involving palms and soles, generalized lymphadenopathy, low-grade fever, malaise, arthralgias and myalgia, headache	Recommended therapy: • Benzathine penicillin G 2.4 million U IM as a one-time dose Alternative therapy in penicillin allergy: • Doxycycline 100 mg PO bid × 2 weeks *or* • Tetracycline 500 mg PO qid × 2 weeks	Also treatment for latent syphilis of <1 yr duration
Late or tertiary syphilis	Gumma (granulomatous lesions involving skin, mucous membranes, bone), aortic insufficiency, aortic aneurysm, Argyll Robertson pupil, seizures	Recommended therapy: • Benzathine penicillin G 2.4 million U IM × 3 weekly doses Alternative therapy in penicillin allergy: • Doxycycline 100 mg PO bid × 4 weeks *or* • Tetracycline 500 mg PO qid × 4 weeks Expert consultation advisable, especially in the face of neurosyphilis	Also treatment for latent syphilis of >1 yr or unknown duration

Source: Workowski KA, Berman SM. Sexually transmitted disease treatment guidelines, 2006. *MMWR Morb Mortal Wkly Rep.* 2006;55 (No. RR-11):1–94.

---

51. Which HPV types are most likely to cause colorectal carcinoma?

   A. 1 and 3
   B. 6 and 11
   C. 16 and 18
   D. 72 and 81

52. Which HPV types are most likely to cause condyloma acuminatum?

   A. 1, 2, and 3
   B. 6 and 11
   C. 16 and 19
   D. 22 and 24

ANSWERS

48.	A	49.	A	50.	A
51.	C	52.	B		

DISCUSSION

Condyloma acuminatum, the verruciform lesion seen in genital warts, is an STI. The causative agent is human papillomavirus (HPV), and multiple HPV types are usually seen with genital infection. Anal, penile, and cervical carcinoma can be consequences of HPV infection. Not all HPV types are correlated with malignancy, however. HPV types with a high malignancy risk include types 16, 18, 31, 33, 35, 39, and 45, whereas low malignancy risk is seen with infection from types 6, 11, 40, 42, 43, 44, 54, 61, 70, 72, and 81. HPV types 6 and 11 most often cause genital warts.

About 50% of patients have a spontaneous regression of warts without intervention. Treatment options include podofilox, imiquimod, trichloroacetic acid, and cryotherapy. Patient-administered therapies such as imiquimod (Aldara) or podofilox save on the cost and inconvenience of office visits. Surgical intervention is typically reserved for complicated, recalcitrant lesions.

Primary prevention of HPV disease is now available through immunization. As with all STIs, a critical part of care is discussion of prevention strategies, including condom use and limiting the number of sexual partners. The NP should offer and encourage testing for other STIs, including HIV.

Discussion Sources

Gilbert D, Moerlling R, Eliopoulos G, Chambers H, Saag M. *The Sanford Guide to Antimicrobial Therapy*. 39th ed. Sperryville, VA: Antimicrobial Therapy, Inc; 2009:21–25.

Workowski KA, Berman SM. Sexually transmitted disease treatment guidelines, 2006. *MMWR Morb Mortal Wkly Rep*. 2006;55(No. RR-11):1–94.

QUESTIONS

53. Which of the following is not a common risk factor for erectile dysfunction (ED)?
    A. diabetes mellitus
    B. hypertension
    C. cigarette smoking
    D. testosterone deficiency

54. Patient education about the use of sildenafil (Viagra) includes the following:
    A. A spontaneous erection occurs about 1 hour after taking the medication.
    B. This medication helps nearly all men who use it regain erectile function.
    C. With the use of the medication, sexual stimulation also is needed to achieve an erection.
    D. Nitrates can be safely used concurrently.

55. When discussing ED with a 70-year-old man, the NP considers that:
    A. it is a normal consequence of aging.
    B. most cases have an underlying cause.
    C. although depression is common in older men, it is usually not correlated with increased rates of ED.
    D. treatment options for younger men are seldom effective in older men.

56. Which of the following medications for ED treatment has the longest half-life?
    A. sildenafil (Viagra)
    B. tadalafil (Cialis)
    C. vardenafil (Levitra)

ANSWERS

53.	D	54.	C
55.	B	56.	B

DISCUSSION

Erectile dysfunction (ED), also known as impotency, is defined as the repeated inability to get or keep a penile erection firm enough for sexual intercourse. The spectrum of ED includes the total inability to achieve erection, an inconsistent ability to do so, and a tendency to sustain only brief erections. Achieving and sustaining a penile erection requires a precise sequence of events that depend on healthy nervous system function (brain, spinal column, and penile innervation), appropriate muscle response, and intact blood flow via patent veins and arteries in and near the corpora cavernosa. Any disorder that causes injury to the nerves or impairs blood flow in the penis has the potential to cause ED. Diabetes mellitus, kidney disease, chronic alcoholism, vascular disease, tobacco use, neuropathy, and urological surgery such as radical prostatectomy are implicated in at least 70% of cases of ED. Certain medications, such as antihypertensives, antidepressants, and cimetidine, can produce ED as an adverse effect. The presence of a mood disorder significantly contributes to the risk of ED. Hormonal disorders, particularly testosterone deficiency, pose a significant but uncommon ED risk.

The incidence of ED increases with age; it is found in about 5% of 40-year-old men and 15% to 25% of 65-year-old men. ED should not be thought to be an inevitable consequence of aging, however. Although most ED in older men has a physical cause, such as disease, injury, or adverse effects of drugs, treatment can often help the patient regain satisfactory sexual function.

Intervention in ED starts with treating or minimizing the underlying cause. With currently available therapies, effective treatment can be provided for most men with ED. Medications such as the phosphodiesterase-5 (PDE-5) inhibitors, sildenafil, vardenafil, and tadalafil, work by enhancing the effects of nitric oxide, a chemical that relaxes smooth muscles in the penis during sexual stimulation and allows increased blood flow. Use of these agents does not trigger an automatic erection, and they should be taken about 1 hour before the anticipated onset of sexual activity. The half-life of sildenafil and vardenafil is approximately 4 to 5 hours, whereas tadalafil has a longer half-life of approximately 17 hours. The concomitant use of a drug such as sildenafil with a nitrate is contraindicated because of the risk of profound hypotension; the duration of an adverse effect of a PDE-5 inhibitor is likely to persist for a period related to the drug's duration of action and half-life.

Drugs injected directly into the penis, such as alprostadil (Caverject), cause vasodilation and are highly effective. An alprostadil pellet inserted into the urethra (Muse) can achieve the same effect. Mechanical vacuum devices cause erection by creating a partial vacuum, which draws blood into the penis, engorging and expanding it. An elastic band is placed around the base of the penis to maintain the erection after the cylinder is removed and during intercourse by preventing blood from flowing back into the body. This mechanical method of ED treatment is particularly helpful when other methods fail to achieve desired results. Surgical options include vessel repair to treat the underlying ED; it should be kept in mind, however, that atherosclerosis is a widespread disease, and outcomes are unpredictable. Implantation of devices such as prostheses or pumps is another option, albeit with the associated risks and costs of any surgical procedure.

Discussion Source

Kolodny L. Erectile dysfunction. In: Rakel R, Bope E, eds. *Conn's Current Therapy*. Philadelphia, PA: Elsevier Saunders; 2008:704–709.

8
Musculoskeletal Disorders

QUESTIONS

1. The most common cause of acute bursitis is:
   A. inactivity.
   B. joint overuse.
   C. fibromyalgia.
   D. bacterial infection.

2. First-line treatment options for bursitis usually include:
   A. corticosteroid bursal injection.
   B. heat to area.
   C. weight-bearing exercises.
   D. nonsteroidal anti-inflammatory drugs (NSAIDs).

3. Patients with olecranon bursitis typically present with:
   A. swelling and redness over the affected area.
   B. limited elbow range of motion (ROM).
   C. nerve impingement.
   D. destruction of the joint space.

4. Patients with subscapular bursitis typically present with:
   A. limited shoulder ROM.
   B. heat over affected area.
   C. localized tenderness under the superomedial angle of the scapula.
   D. cervical nerve root irritation.

5. Patients with gluteus medius or deep trochanteric bursitis typically present with:
   A. increased pain from resisted hip abduction.
   B. limited hip ROM.
   C. sciatic nerve pain.
   D. heat over the affected area.

6. Likely sequelae of intrabursal corticosteroid injection include:
   A. irreversible skin atrophy.
   B. infection.
   C. inflammatory reaction.
   D. soreness at the site of injection.

7. First-line therapy for prepatellar bursitis should include:
   A. bursal aspiration.
   B. intrabursal corticosteroid injection.
   C. acetaminophen.
   D. knee splinting.

ANSWERS

1.	B	2.	D	3.	A
4.	C	5.	A	6.	D
7.	A					

DISCUSSION

Bursitis, inflammation of the fluid-filled sacs that act as a cushion between tendons and bones, most commonly affects the subdeltoid, olecranon, ischial, trochanter, and prepatellar bursae. In contrast to most forms of arthritis, bursitis typically has an abrupt onset with focal tenderness and swelling. The joint range of motion (ROM) is usually full, but is often limited by pain (Table 8–1).

Risk factors for acute bursitis include joint overuse, trauma, infection, or arthritis conditions such as rheumatoid arthritis or osteoarthritis. Because recurrence is common, prevention of further joint overuse and trauma should be emphasized.

With prepatellar bursitis, bursal aspiration should be considered as a first-line therapy because this procedure affords significant pain relief and allows the bursa to reapproximate. In other sites, first-line therapy includes minimizing or eliminating the offending activity, applying ice to the affected area for 15 minutes at least four times per day, and the use of nonsteroidal anti-inflammatory drugs (NSAIDs). If these conservative measures have not worked after approximately 4 to 8 weeks, intrabursal corticosteroid injection should be performed. Before injection, patients should be informed of the risks of this procedure, especially

See full color images of this topic on DavisPlus at http://davisplus.fadavis.com | Keyword: Fitzgerald

TABLE 8–1

Clinical Presentation of Bursitis

Location of Bursitis	Clinical Presentation	Comments
Prepatellar (knee)	Knee swelling and pain in the front of the knee, normal ROM	Risk factors include frequent kneeling (house-maid's knee)
Olecranon (elbow)	Pain, swelling behind the elbow, swelling in same area, often described as ball or sac hanging from the elbow	Risk factors include prolonged pressure or trauma to the elbow (draftsman's elbow)
Trochanter (hip)	Gait disturbance, local trochanter tenderness, pain on hip rotation and resisted hip abduction with normal hip ROM	Risk factors include back disease, leg-length discrepancy, and leg problems that lead to altered gait OA seldom implicated
Subscapular (shoulder)	Local tenderness under superomedial angle of the scapula over the adjacent rib, normal shoulder ROM, no nerve root impingement	Risk factors include repeated back-and-forth motion Common in assembly-line workers
Pre-Achilles (heel)	Pain and localized swelling behind the heel, minimal pain with dorsiflexion, normal ankle ROM	Usually not disabling and does not contribute to tendon rupture Often confused with Achilles tendonitis
Retrocalcaneal (heel)	Pain behind ankle worsened by walking Patient often runs fingers along both sides of Achilles tendon	Risk factors include wearing high-heeled shoes and repetitive ankle motion such as stair-climbing, running, jogging, and walking

OA, osteoarthritis; ROM, range of motion.
Sources: Anderson B. *Office Orthopedics for Primary Care: Diagnosis*. Philadelphia, PA: Saunders; 2006.
Anderson B. *Office Orthopedics for Primary Care: Treatment*. Philadelphia, PA: Saunders; 2006.

the most common problem, soreness at the injection site. After corticosteroid injection, infection, tissue atrophy, and inflammatory reaction are possible, but rarely encountered, complications.

Discussion Sources

Anderson B. *Office Orthopedics for Primary Care: Diagnosis*. Philadelphia, PA: Saunders Elsevier; 2006.

Anderson B. *Office Orthopedics for Primary Care: Treatment*. Philadelphia, PA: Saunders Elsevier; 2006.

QUESTIONS

8. Patients with lateral epicondylitis typically present with:

   A. electric-like pain elicited by tapping over the median nerve.
   B. reduced joint ROM.
   C. pain that is worst with elbow flexion.
   D. decreased hand grip strength.

9. Risk factors for lateral epicondylitis include all of the following except:

   A. repetitive lifting.
   B. playing tennis.
   C. hammering.
   D. gout.

10. Initial therapy for treatment of lateral epicondylitis includes:

    A. a long arm cast.
    B. a short arm cast with a thumb spica.
    C. a wrist splint with metal stays.
    D. a shoulder sling.

11. Patients with medial epicondylitis typically present with:

    A. forearm numbness.
    B. reduction in ROM.
    C. pain on elbow flexion.
    D. decreased grip strength.

12. Risk factors for medial epicondylitis include playing:

    A. tennis.

    B. golf.

    C. baseball.

    D. volleyball.

ANSWERS

8.	D	9.	D	10.	C
11.	D	12.	B		

DISCUSSION

The painful condition that arises as a result of injury to the extensor tendon at the lateral epicondyle is called tennis elbow or lateral epicondylitis. Patients usually give a history of an aggravating activity followed by forearm weakness and point to tenderness over the inner aspect of the humerus (Table 8–2). Medial epicondylitis is often called golfer's elbow.

Conservative therapy in the first 3 to 4 weeks should include avoidance of the precipitating activity, application of appropriate splints, and use of NSAIDs. If symptoms persist, a short arm cast can be used to limit arm movement further.

Local corticosteroid injection may be helpful if symptoms persist beyond 6 to 8 weeks or are particularly severe. The use of a tennis elbow band can help prevent recurrence.

Discussion Sources

Anderson B. *Office Orthopedics for Primary Care: Diagnosis.* Philadelphia, PA: Saunders Elsevier; 2006.

Anderson B. *Office Orthopedics for Primary Care: Treatment.* Philadelphia, PA: Saunders Elsevier; 2006.

QUESTIONS

13. Risk factors for acute gouty arthritis include:

    A. thiazide diuretic use.

    B. female gender.

    C. rheumatoid arthritis.

    D. joint trauma.

14. The clinical presentation of acute gouty arthritis affecting the base of the great toe includes:

    A. slow onset of discomfort over many days.

    B. greatest swelling and pain along the median border of the joint.

    C. improvement of symptoms with joint rest.

    D. fever.

TABLE 8–2

Clinical Presentation of Epicondylitis

Condition	Presentation	Comments
Medial epicondylitis	Patient complains of pain over medial epicondyle or inner aspect of lower humerus. Pain worsens with wrist flexion and pronation activities. Local epicondylar tenderness, elbow pain, forearm weakness, pain aggravated by wrist flexion, and pronation activities with decreased grip strength and full ROM	Often called golfers' elbow; results from repetitive activity such as lifting, tooling, sports involving a tight grip. Prevent recurrence by using palm-up lifting, using a tennis elbow band, avoiding precipitating causes, proper use of tools, use of proper body mechanics, and developing flexibility and strength of the involved musculature
Lateral epicondylitis	Patient complains of pain over lateral epicondyle or outer aspect of lower humerus, increases with resisted wrist extension, especially with elbow. Hand grip often weak on affected side. Elbow ROM usually normal	Often called tennis elbow; results from repetitive activity such as lifting, tooling, sports involving a tight grip. Prevent recurrence by avoiding precipitating causes, proper use of tools, proper body mechanics, and development of flexibility and strength of the involved musculature

ROM, range of motion.

Sources: Gibbs S. eMedicine. http://www.emedicine.com/pmr/topic74.htm, Medial epicondylitis, accessed 10/10/08.

Lorenzo C. http://www.emedicine.com/orthoped/topic510.htm, Lateral epicondylitis, accessed 10/10/08.

15. The most helpful diagnostic test to perform during acute gouty arthritis is:

    A. measurement of erythrocyte sedimentation rate (ESR).

    B. measurement of serum uric acid.

    C. analysis of aspirate from the affected joint.

    D. joint radiography.

16. First-line therapy for treating patients with acute gouty arthritis includes:

    A. aspirin.

    B. naproxen sodium.

    C. allopurinol.

    D. probenecid.

17. Which of the following patients with acute gouty arthritis is the best candidate for local corticosteroid injection?

    A. a 66-year-old patient with a gastric ulcer

    B. a 44-year-old patient taking a thiazide diuretic

    C. a 68-year-old patient with type 2 diabetes mellitus

    D. a 32-year-old patient who is a binge drinker

18. The most common locations for tophi include all of the following except:

    A. the auricles.

    B. the elbows.

    C. the extensor surfaces of the hands.

    D. the shoulders.

19. Dietary recommendations for a person with gouty arthritis include avoiding foods high in:

    A. artificial flavors and colors.

    B. purine.

    C. vitamin C.

    D. protein.

ANSWERS

13.	A	**14.**	B	**15.**	C
16.	B	**17.**	A	**18.**	D
19.	B				

DISCUSSION

Gouty arthritis, often simply called gout, manifests as acute monoarticular arthritis, usually triggered by a disorder in uric acid excretion that allows an accumulation of urates in joints, bones, and subcutaneous tissues. Urate precipitates out of biological fluids when levels are elevated, a condition that usually follows the inability of the kidney to eliminate uric acid. About 90% of patients presenting with primary gout ♂ are men; the condition is rarely seen in women before menopause. Gout risk factors include obesity, diabetes mellitus, and a family history of the condition. Less often, acute gout is caused by excessive uric acid production, usually coupled with decreased urate excretion. The use of select medications, including thiazide diuretics, niacin, aspirin, and cyclosporine, can precipitate gout by causing hyperuricemia; alcohol use is also a possible precipitant. Other causes of secondary gout include conditions characterized by increased catabolism and purine turnover, such as psoriasis, myeloproliferative and lymphoproliferative diseases, and chronic hemolytic anemia, and conditions with decreased renal uric acid clearance, such as intrinsic kidney disease and renal failure.

This acutely painful condition typically affects the metacarpophalangeal joint of the great toe. The onset is sudden and is accompanied by significant distress. Although the disease manifests acutely, the metabolic disorder behind the problem is typically present for months to years before the clinical presentation. Patients report the inability to walk, move the joint, or even tolerate the weight of a bed sheet on the affected joint because of severe pain. The entire great toe is usually reddened and enlarged with the greatest amount of swelling noted along the median border of the joint; this usually is also the point of greatest discomfort. Although the clinical presentation of gout can mimic that of an acutely infected joint, gout is 100 times more common than monoarticular septic arthritis. With repeated episodes, nontender firm nodules known as tophi can develop in soft tissue. Because the gouty crystals that fill tophi precipitate more easily in cooler areas of the body, these lesions often develop in the external ear; less common locations include nasal cartilage, extensor surfaces of the hands and feet, and over the elbows.

The diagnosis of acute gouty arthritis is usually straightforward, particularly with repeated episodes. With the first episode, an initial uric acid level is usually obtained, but is usually normal. Uric acid levels are often reduced during the acute phase, or the etiology of the attack is largely poor urate excretion. Analysis of joint aspirate for urate crystals is diagnostic; the ESR or C-reactive protein (CRP) is usually high, but these findings are neither sensitive nor specific for gout and simply reflect the inflammation associated with the condition. Radiographs are not needed, unless a concurrent history of trauma and risk of fracture are present.

The treatment of acute gouty arthritis should include minimizing or removing contributing factors, such as alcohol use or use of certain medications. Treatment should be aimed at reducing inflammation first and then treating hyperuricemia, trying to avoid a rapid reduction in serum uric acid, which can make the episode worse. A loading dose of an NSAID, such as naproxen, 750 mg, or indomethacin, 50 mg, followed by lower doses, can be helpful. Because aspirin can precipitate gout, its use in the presence of the condition is contraindicated. Colchicine, 0.6 mg every hour up to 2.4 mg total dose in 24 hours or when gastrointestinal symptoms occur, can be used, but is often poorly tolerated. A short course of a systemic corticosteroid, such as prednisone, 40 to 60 mg daily until pain relief is achieved (usually achieved in 3 to 4 days, slowly tapered over 6 to 7 days for a total of 10 days of use), is a helpful alternative to colchicine. Local injection with corticosteroids can provide significant relief and offers a treatment alternative to NSAIDs, particularly in the presence of warfarin use, renal failure, or peptic ulcer disease.

Dietary modification to avoid foods with high purine content is an important and often overlooked intervention to minimize the risk of future gout episodes. Examples of high-purine foods include certain seafood (scallops, mussels), organ and game meats, beans, spinach, asparagus, and baker's and brewer's yeasts when taken as dietary supplements.

After the acute flare has subsided, a 24-hour urine collection for uric acid helps assess whether the patient overproduces or undersecretes uric acid. Long-term care to avoid future attacks is directed by the result: Undersecretors benefit from probenecid, and overproducers benefit from allopurinol. Other medications not specifically designated for gout treatment, including fenofibrate and losartan, have been studied and found to be helpful in helping with urate excretion and can be used as therapeutic adjuncts.

Discussion Sources

http://www.drugs.com/cg/low-purine-diet.html, Low purine diet, accessed 9/29/09.

Kaplan J. eMedicine. http://www.emedicine.com/emerg/TOPIC221.HTM, Gout and pseudogout, accessed 9/29/09.

Mandell B. Hyperuricemia and gout. In: Rakel R, Bope E, eds. *Conn's Current Therapy 2008*. Philadelphia, PA: Saunders Elsevier; 2008:588–591.

QUESTIONS

20. Which of the following joints is most likely to be affected by osteoarthritis (OA)?
    A. wrists
    B. elbows
    C. metacarpophalangeal joint
    D. distal interphalangeal joint

21. Deformity of the proximal interphalangeal joints found in an elderly patient with OA is known as:
    A. Heberden nodes.
    B. Bouchard nodes.
    C. hallus valgus.
    D. Dupuytren contracture.

22. Which of the following best describes the presentation of a patient with OA?
    A. worst symptoms in weight-bearing joints later in the day
    B. symmetrical early morning stiffness
    C. sausage-shaped digits with associated skin lesions
    D. back pain with rest and anterior uveitis

23. As part of the evaluation of patients with OA, the NP anticipates finding:
    A. anemia of chronic disease.
    B. elevated CRP level.
    C. narrowing of the joint space on radiograph.
    D. elevated antinuclear antibody (ANA) titer.

24. First-line pharmacological intervention for milder OA should be a trial of:
    A. acetaminophen.
    B. naproxen.
    C. celecoxib.
    D. intra-articular corticosteroid injection.

25. In caring for a patient with OA of the knee, you advise that:
    A. straight-leg raising should be avoided.
    B. heat should be applied to painful joints after exercise.
    C. quadriceps-strengthening exercises should be performed.
    D. physical activity should be avoided.

26. Glucosamine and chondroitin are over-the-counter nutritional supplements that are usually taken to help with the management of:
    A. rheumatoid arthritis.
    B. OA.
    C. Reiter syndrome.
    D. gouty arthritis

ANSWERS

20.	D	21.	B	22.	A
23.	C	24.	A	25.	C
26.	B				

DISCUSSION

Osteoarthritis (OA) ♂ is the most common joint disease in North America; it is a degenerative condition that manifests without systemic manifestations or acute inflammation. The most problematic joint involvement is in the hip and knee. Worst symptoms are reported with use of the joints. As a result, discomfort typically increases as the day progresses, and there is minimal morning stiffness; in contrast, with rheumatoid arthritis (RA), morning stiffness is usually most problematic. Risk factors for OA include a positive family history of the condition and contact sport participation. Obesity is likely the most common personal risk factor, especially with hip and knee involvement. In OA, the articular cartilage becomes rough and wears away. Bone spurs may form, and the synovial membrane thickens. Consequently, the joint space narrows. The clinical presentation in patients with OA includes an insidious onset of symptoms, including use-related joint pain that is relieved by rest, and joint stiffness that occurs with rest, but resolves with less than 15 minutes of activity. Physical examination usually reveals smooth, cool joints and coarse crepitus. Particularly when the knee is affected, joint effusion is common and can be minimal to severe with up to 20 mL of fluid. Patients cannot achieve full knee flexion in the effused joint. The knee often locks, or a pop is heard, which suggests a degenerative meniscal tear.

Radiological findings in patients with OA include narrowing of the joint space and increased density of subchondral bone. Bone cysts and osteophytes are often present, developed as part of the body's repair process. Only about 50% of patients with radiological findings have symptoms, however. Because OA is typically a noninflammatory disease, ESR and CRP levels, both markers of inflammation, are typically normal. In contrast to RA and systemic lupus erythematosus (SLE), ANAs, rheumatoid factor, and other markers of systemic arthritis syndromes are absent from the serum unless there is concomitant disease.

Therapeutic goals for patients with OA include preventing further articular cartilage destruction, minimizing pain, and enhancing mobility. Therapies for symptom control include lifestyle modifications, such as weight loss and exercise with minimal weight-bearing, such as swimming or water-based activities, and exercise to maintain joint flexibility and enhance strength in the surrounding muscles (Table 8–3). Application of heat to minimize pain and stiffness in the morning before activity can be helpful, and applying ice to the joint after activity can minimize discomfort; the use of heat or ice should be directed by patient response. Acetaminophen and NSAIDs have long been used as arthritis drug treatments. These medications are helpful in controlling pain. Although NSAIDs also have potential anti-inflammatory activity, this mechanism of drug action is seldom needed in OA therapy because inflammation is a minor contributor to symptoms. Because of the gastropathy potential associated with long-term use of NSAIDs, a trial of acetaminophen is warranted for symptom control in less severe cases of OA, recognizing that NSAIDs are usually associated with superior analgesic effect. Long-acting opioids may be required if symptom control cannot be achieved.

Glucosamine, an amino acid, is usually used as first-line treatment for OA in many European nations and is available as an over-the-counter nutritional supplement in the United States. The results of research studies have differed on the effectiveness of its use, with many reporting no improvement in arthritis symptoms and others reporting a reduction in pain, increased joint flexion, and increased articular function. Glucosamine must be used consistently for a minimum of 2 weeks and likely 3 months before therapeutic effect is seen. Although no drug interactions or hepatotoxicity has been noted with its use, glucosamine should be used with caution because there is a risk of bronchospasm. Chondroitin is often used in conjunction with glucosamine because the two seem to have synergistic activity, although this has been disputed in limited studies. The mechanism of action of these products is not well understood. Although chondroitin is generally well tolerated, it should be used with caution because of a potential

TABLE 8–3

Exercise Regimens in Osteoarthritis

Joint Condition	Exercise Regimen	Comments
Osteoarthritis in the knee	• Straight-leg raises without weights, advance to using weights as tolerated • Quadriceps sets • Non–weight-bearing or limited weight-bearing aerobic activity	Avoid squatting and kneeling, high-impact exercise
Osteoarthritis of the hip	• Straight-leg raises without weights, advance to using weights as tolerated • Stretching exercises of adductors, rotator and gluteus muscles • Isometric exercises of iliopsoas and gluteus muscles • Non–weight-bearing or limited weight-bearing aerobic activity	Avoid high-impact exercise

anticoagulant effect. As with all nutritional supplements, using a preparation that is supplied by a manufacturer with *United States Pharmacopeia* or other similar verification is advised.

Intra-articular corticosteroid joint injection is often helpful when therapy that is more conservative has failed. In particular, with OA in the knee, corticosteroid injection can help when joint effusion is present. Hip injection is a technically challenging procedure that can be done with fluoroscopic guidance.

Joint replacement should be considered when pain cannot be adequately controlled, when function is severely compromised, or when more than 80% of the articular cartilage is worn away. The ideal candidate for joint replacement is able to tolerate a surgical procedure that lasts for several hours, followed by an aggressive postoperative course of rehabilitation. Many patients with OA who have been debilitated by poor mobility have improved health when ambulation becomes possible after hip or knee replacement. A patellar restraining brace, walker, or motorized assisted mobility aid may be needed for patients with advanced OA of the knee and hip that cannot be surgically repaired.

Discussion Sources

American College of Rheumatology. http://www.rheumatology.org/publications/guidelines/ oa-mgmt/oa-mgmt.asp?aud=mem, Recommendations for the medical management of osteoarthritis of the hip and knee, accessed 9/29/09.

Anderson B. *Office Orthopedics for Primary Care: Diagnosis.* Philadelphia, PA: Saunders Elsevier; 2006.

Anderson B. *Office Orthopedics for Primary Care: Treatment.* Philadelphia, PA: Saunders Elsevier; 2006.

Ehrlich G. Osteoarthritis. In: Rakel R, Bope E, eds. *Conn's Current Therapy 2008*. Philadelphia, PA: Saunders Elsevier; 2008:975–978.

QUESTIONS

27. Which of the following is not characteristic of rheumatoid arthritis (RA)?

    A. more common in women at a 3:1 ratio
    B. family history of rheumatoid disease often reported by patient
    C. peak age for disease onset in individuals age 50 to 70 years
    D. wrists, ankles, and toes often involved

28. Which of the following best describes the presentation of a person with RA?

    A. worst symptoms in weight-bearing joints later in the day
    B. symmetrical early-morning stiffness
    C. sausage-shaped digits with characteristic skin lesions
    D. back pain with rest and anterior uveitis

29. NSAIDs cause gastric injury primarily by:

    A. direct irritative effect.
    B. slowing gastrointestinal motility.
    C. thinning of the protective gastrointestinal mucosa.
    D. enhancing prostaglandin synthesis.

30. Of the following individuals, who is at highest risk for NSAID-induced gastropathy?

    A. a 28-year-old man with an ankle sprain who has taken ibuprofen for the past week and who drinks four to six beers every weekend
    B. a 40-year-old woman who smokes and takes about six doses of naproxen sodium per month to control dysmenorrhea
    C. a 43-year-old man with dilated cardiomyopathy who uses ketoprofen one to two times per week for low back pain
    D. a 72-year-old man who takes aspirin four times a day for pain control of osteoarthritis

31. Which of the following is the preferred method of preventing NSAID-induced gastric ulcer?

    A. a high-dose histamine 2 receptor antagonist
    B. timed antacid use
    C. sucralfate (Carafate)
    D. misoprostol (Cytotec)

32. Taking a high dose of aspirin or ibuprofen causes:

    A. an increase in the drug's half-life.
    B. enhanced renal excretion of the drug.
    C. a change in the drug's mechanism of action.
    D. a reduction of antiprostaglandin effect.

33. Which of the following statements is most accurate concerning RA?

    A. Joint erosions are often evident on radiographs or MRI.
    B. RA is seldom associated with other autoimmune diseases.
    C. A butterfly-shaped facial rash is common.
    D. Parvovirus B_{19} infection can contribute to its development.

34. Principles of treating patients with RA include:

    A. initial therapy with an NSAID, then adding other medications as directed by clinical response.
    B. early use of disease-modifying antirheumatic drugs (DMARDs) to slow or halt joint damage.
    C. pain relief as the chief therapeutic goal.
    D. recognizing that joint splinting is seldom advisable.

35. Which of the following tests is most specific to the diagnosis of RA?

   A. elevated levels of rheumatoid factor
   B. abnormally high ESR
   C. depressed total white blood cell count
   D. positive ANA titer

36. A 52-year-old woman has RA. She now presents with decreased tearing, "gritty"-feeling eyes, and a dry mouth. You consider a diagnosis of:

   A. systemic lupus erythematosus.
   B. vasculitis.
   C. Sjögren syndrome.
   D. scleroderma.

37. Cyclooxygenase-1 (COX-1) contributes to:

   A. inflammatory response.
   B. pain transmission.
   C. maintenance of gastric protective mucosal layer.
   D. renal arteriole function.

38. Cyclooxygenase-2 (COX-2) contributes to all of the following except:

   A. inflammatory response.
   B. pain transmission.
   C. maintenance of gastric protective mucosal layer.
   D. renal arteriole constriction.

39. Which of the following special examinations should be periodically obtained during hydroxychloroquine sulfate use?

   A. dilated eye retinal examination
   B. bone marrow biopsy
   C. pulmonary function tests
   D. exercise tolerance test

ANSWERS

27.	C	28.	B	29.	C
30.	D	31.	D	32.	A
33.	A	34.	B	35.	A
36.	C	37.	C	38.	C
39.	A				

DISCUSSION

Rheumatoid arthritis (RA) ♂ is a disease that causes chronic systemic inflammation, including the synovial membranes of multiple joints. As with most autoimmune diseases, RA is more common in women (ratio approximately 3:1); RA is often seen in people with other autoimmune diseases. Although new-onset RA can occur at any age, peak age at onset is 20 to 40 years. A family history of rheumatoid disease is often noted. Initial presentation may be with acute polyarticular inflammation. A clinical picture of slowly progressive malaise, weight loss, and stiffness is more common, however (Table 8–4). The stiffness is symmetrical, is typically worst on arising, lasts about 1 hour, involves at least three joint groups, and can recur after a period of inactivity or exercise. The hands (with sparing of the distal interphalangeal joints), wrists, ankles, and toes are most often involved. Soft tissue swelling or fluid is also present, as are subcutaneous nodules. The disease is characterized by periods of exacerbation and remission. Although in the past RA was believed to be a debilitating condition with little impact on longevity, more recent research shows that RA is now known potentially to shorten the life span while producing considerable disability, particularly without optimal treatment (Table 8–5).

The diagnosis of RA can be made only when clinical features are supported by laboratory testing. Usually initial diagnostic tests include ANA, ESR, and rheumatoid factor measurements and radiographs, with additional testing often ordered because of diagnostic uncertainty. When interpreting results, the NP should bear in mind the following:

• Radiographs typically reveal joint erosion and loss of normal joint space. Classic radiographic changes are not present in about 30% at disease onset. Musculoskeletal ultrasound and joint magnetic resonance imaging (MRI) are helpful in revealing RA-associated erosions.

• ESR and CRP are nonspecific tests of inflammation. In general, the higher the values, the greater the degree and intensity of the inflammatory process. Although ESR and CRP are frequently elevated in patients with RA, abnormal results are diagnostic of this or other conditions. In addition, a single elevated ESR or CRP is seldom helpful; however, following trends during flare and regression of disease often aids in charting the therapeutic course and response.

• Rheumatoid factor, an immunoglobulin M antibody, is present in approximately 50% to 90% of patients with RA. The level of the titer often corresponds to the severity of disease.

• An antibody to cyclic citrullinated peptide (anti-CCP), a ring-form amino acid that is usually not measurable in health, is a more specific, although less sensitive marker of RA.

• ANAs are antibodies against cellular nuclear components that act as antigens. ANA is occasionally present in healthy adults, but it is usually found in individuals with systemic rheumatic or collagen vascular disease. ANA is the most sensitive laboratory marker for SLE, detected in approximately 95% of patients, but it is found in only 30% to 50% of patients with RA. Patterns of immunofluorescence vary and have been given misplaced credence as to type of disease. Following are some examples of ANA patterns:

   • Homogeneous, diffuse, or solid pattern to DNA: High titers strongly associated with SLE

TABLE 8–4

American College of Rheumatology Criteria for Diagnosis of Rheumatoid Arthritis

Criterion*	Comment
Morning stiffness	Lasting ≥1 hour in and around joint
Symmetrical arthritis	Simultaneous involvement of joint areas on both sides
Hands involved	Wrist, PIP, and MCP involvement with evidence of fluid, joint swelling
Rheumatoid nodules	Subcutaneous nodules over bony prominences, extensor surfaces, or juxta-articular regions
Arthritis of three or more joints	Simultaneous soft tissue swelling or fluid in 14 possible areas (right or left PIP, MCP, wrist, elbow, knee, ankle, MTP)
Serum rheumatoid factor	Abnormal amounts present in serum
	Although noted in ~85% with RA, false-positive and false-negative test results are possible
Radiographic changes	Include juxta-articular osteopenia, joint erosions, narrowing of joint space, most marked in involved joints

*Four of the seven criteria must be present for ≥6 weeks.
MCP, metacarpophalangeal; MTP, metatarsophalangeal; PIP, proximal interphalangeal; RA, rheumatoid arthritis.
Source: Adapted from American College of Rheumatology.
http://www.rheumatology.org/public/factsheets/diseases_and_conditions/ra.asp?aud=pat, Fact sheet on rheumatoid arthritis, accessed 9/29/09.

- Peripheral or rim pattern: Associated with anti–double-stranded DNA and strongly correlated with SLE
- Nucleolar pattern: Associated with antiribonucleoprotein and strongly correlated with scleroderma
- Speckled pattern: Further antigen testing should be ordered with this result.

- Cytoplasmic pattern is often found in the presence of biliary cirrhosis.
- Hemogram usually reveals normocytic, normochromic, hypoproliferative anemia associated with chronic disease.

The goal of treatment of patients with RA is to reduce inflammation and pain, while preserving function and preventing deformity. Behavioral management is important because physiological and psychological stress precipitate RA flares. Allowing for proper rest periods is critical. Physical therapists can help develop a reasonable activity plan. Maintenance of physical activity through appropriate exercise is of greatest importance. Water exercise in particular is helpful because it includes mild resistance and buoyancy. Splints may provide joint rest while maintaining function and preventing contracture.

As helpful as NSAIDs are in symptom control, these products do not alter the underlying disease process; joint destruction continues despite control of symptoms and reduction in swelling. DMARDs help minimize the risk of joint damage and disease progression and should be started as soon as the diagnosis of RA is made (see Table 8–4). As the number and types of DMARDs available increase, knowledge of current RA therapy is critical for providing optimal patient care.

If a patient fails to achieve control of pain or symptoms with an adequate trial of a DMARD and an NSAID, additional therapy should be added. One option is intra-articular corticosteroid injection. This therapy can be quite helpful, but should be limited to not more than two to three injections per joint per year, to minimize risk of joint deterioration. Systemic corticosteroids can be most helpful in relieving inflammation, but use should not exceed 2 to 8 weeks, if possible, because of adverse reactions associated with these agents.

TABLE 8–5

Treatment of Rheumatoid Arthritis

Medication	Examples
Anti-inflammatory agents	NSAIDs, COX-2 inhibitors, corticosteroids
Analgesics	NSAIDs, COX-2 inhibitors, acetaminophen, opioids, topical agents
DMARDs	Traditional DMARDS—methotrexate, leflunomide, azathioprine, hydroxychloroquine, minocycline, others
	Biological response modifiers—infliximab, rituximab, adalimumab, abatacept, anakinra, etanercept, others

COX-2, cyclooxygenase 2; DMARDs, disease-modifying antirheumatic drugs; NSAIDs, nonsteroidal anti-inflammatory drugs.
Source: Matteson E. Rheumatoid arthritis. In: Rakel R, Bope E, eds. *Conn's Current Therapy 2008*. Philadelphia, PA: Saunders; 2008:955–961.

Aspirin and other NSAIDs have been the backbone of RA drug treatment for years. These medications are helpful in controlling inflammation and pain. Aspirin and ibuprofen are two more commonly used products. With many of the NSAIDs, the half-life of the drug is increased as the dose is increased.

A significant amount of peptic ulcer disease, particularly gastric ulcer and gastritis, is caused by NSAID use. NSAIDs inhibit synthesis of prostaglandins from arachidonic acid, yielding an anti-inflammatory effect. This effect is caused in part by the action of these products against cyclooxygenase (COX). COX-1 is an enzyme found in gastric mucosa, small and large intestine mucosa, kidneys, platelets, and vascular epithelium. This enzyme contributes to the health of these organs through numerous mechanisms, including the maintenance of the protective gastric mucosal layer and proper perfusion of the kidneys. COX-2 is an enzyme that produces prostaglandins important in the inflammatory cascade and pain transmission. The standard NSAIDs and corticosteroids inhibit the synthesis of COX-1 and COX-2, controlling pain and inflammation, but with gastric and renal complications. NSAIDs such as celecoxib (Celebrex) that spare COX-1 and are more COX-2-selective afford control of the potential for arthritis symptoms. The gastrointestinal benefit of the COX-2 inhibitors is likely attenuated with long-term use, whereas the cardiovascular risk associated with their use is increased.

Sjögren syndrome is an autoimmune disease that usually occurs in conjunction with another chronic inflammatory condition, such as RA or SLE. Complaints usually concern problems related to decreased oral and ocular secretions. In addition, mouth ulcers and dental caries are common, and ESR is elevated in more than 90% of patients. A salivary gland biopsy for the presence of mononuclear cell infiltration is useful. Intervention for patients with Sjögren syndrome includes management of presenting symptoms with appropriate lubricants. Treating the underlying disease is critical.

Discussion Sources

American College of Rheumatology. http://www.rheumatology.org/public/factsheets/diseases_and_conditions/ra.asp?aud=pat, Fact sheet on rheumatoid arthritis, accessed 9/29/09.

Ferri F. *Ferri's Best Test: A Practical Guide to Laboratory Testing and Diagnostic Imaging*. Philadelphia, PA: Mosby Elsevier; 2004.

Matteson E. Rheumatoid arthritis. In: Rakel R, Bope E, eds. *Conn's Current Therapy 2008*. Philadelphia, PA: Saunders Elsevier; 2008:955–961.

QUESTIONS

40. To confirm the results of a McMurray test, you ask the patient to:
    A. squat.
    B. walk.
    C. flex the knee.
    D. rotate the ankle.

41. Which of the following best describes the presentation of a patient with complete median meniscus tear?
    A. joint effusion
    B. heat over the knee
    C. inability to kneel
    D. loss of smooth joint movement

42. To help prevent meniscal tear, you advise:
    A. limiting participation in sports.
    B. quadriceps-strengthening exercises.
    C. using a knee brace.
    D. applying ice to the knee before exercise.

43. Initial treatment for meniscal tear includes all of the following except:
    A. NSAIDs.
    B. applying ice.
    C. elevation.
    D. joint aspiration.

ANSWERS

40.	A	**41.**	C
42.	B	**43.**	D

DISCUSSION

A meniscal tear results from a disruption of the meniscus, the C-shaped fibrocartilage pad located between the femoral condyles and the tibial plateaus. This injury is often seen in athletes because of a hyperextension or twist-type injury. This condition can also be found in older, sedentary adults; in this case, the injury is usually due to degenerative changes. Because the purpose of the fibrocartilage pad is shock absorption and smooth joint mobility, patients with larger tears often report that the knee locks, makes a popping sound or "gives out". Effusion is also common, with the patient reporting a sensation of knee tightness and stiffness. With certain positions, there is often sudden-onset, sharp, localized pain, usually on the median aspect of the knee. Over time, premature OA is often seen as the normal joint space is compromised.

Meniscal tears are typically classified as complex or partial; traumatic or degenerative; lateral, posterior, horizontal, or vertical; and radial, parrot-beak, or bucket-handle. Patients with partial, horizontal, and anterior tears often have relatively normal examination findings because the knee's mechanics are relatively unchanged even though these patients continue to have knee locking and pain with certain positions. The McMurray test, ♂ a palpable popping on the joint line, is highly specific but poorly sensitive for meniscal tear; the Apley grinding test ♂ gives similar results. Squatting or kneeling is nearly impossible for patients with a large, complete, or bucket-handle meniscal tear. Joint effusion is typical, with ROM being limited by discomfort.

Knee radiographs, which can reveal osteoarthritic changes, foreign bodies, or other injuries, are reasonable as initial evaluation. Because the meniscus does not contain calcium, the structure is not visible on a plain film. MRI can identify the type and extent of the tear and should be considered if milder symptoms do not resolve within 2 to 4 weeks, or if severe symptoms do not resolve earlier.

Initial treatment includes rest, elevation, ice application, and analgesia. Because joint effusion is nearly always present but is relatively mild, aspiration should be considered only if there is no improvement after 2 to 4 weeks of conservative therapy. Crutch walking should be encouraged, and a patellar stabilizer may be needed when significant knee instability is present. Straight-leg–raising exercises help strengthen the quadriceps and stabilize the joint. Arthroscopy, which provides the most accurate diagnosis with the possibility of concurrent treatment through débridement and repair, should be considered at 4 to 6 weeks if there is no improvement, and earlier if joint locking, giving out, and effusion are particularly problematic.

Discussion Sources

Achar S, Espinoza A. Common sports injuries. In: Rakel R, Bope E, eds. *Conn's Current Therapy 2008*. Philadelphia, PA: Saunders Elsevier; 2009:984–990.

Anderson B. *Office Orthopedics for Primary Care: Diagnosis*. Philadelphia, PA: Saunders Elsevier; 2006.

Anderson B. *Office Orthopedics for Primary Care: Treatment*. Philadelphia, PA: Saunders Elsevier; 2006.

QUESTIONS

44. The Phalen test is described as:
    A. reproduction of symptoms with forced flexion of the wrists.
    B. abnormal tingling when the median nerve is tapped.
    C. pain on internal rotation.
    D. palmar atrophy.

45. The Tinel test is best described as:
    A. reproduction of symptoms with forced flexion of the wrists.
    B. abnormal tingling when the median nerve is tapped.
    C. pain on internal rotation.
    D. palmar atrophy.

46. Risk factors for carpal tunnel syndrome (CTS) include all of the following except:
    A. pregnancy.
    B. untreated hypothyroidism.
    C. repetitive motion.
    D. multiple sclerosis.

47. Which of the following is least likely to be reported by patients with CTS?
    A. worst symptoms during the day
    B. burning sensation in the affected hand
    C. tingling pain that radiates to the forearm
    D. nocturnal numbness

48. Initial therapy for patients with CTS includes:
    A. intra-articular injection.
    B. joint splinting.
    C. systemic corticosteroids.
    D. referral for surgery.

49. Primary prevention of CTS includes:
    A. screening for thyroid dysfunction.
    B. treatment of osteoarthritis.
    C. stretching and toning exercises.
    D. wrist splinting.

ANSWERS

44.	A	45.	B	46.	D
47.	A	48.	B	49.	C

DISCUSSION

Carpal tunnel syndrome (CTS) is a painful syndrome caused by compression of the median nerve between the carpal ligament and other structures within the carpal tunnel. This compression leads to an entrapment neuropathy, causing symptoms in the distribution of the median nerve. The resulting symptoms are likely due to nerve ischemia rather than nerve damage.

The most common risk factor is repetitive motion; the condition is common with protracted computer keyboard use and in workers such as cake decorators and soldiers, who must consistently grasp a small object. CTS may also be part of the manifestation of a systemic disease, such as RA and sarcoidosis. Primary prevention of CTS includes limiting time spent in these activities, ensuring proper work breaks, and encouraging toning and stretching exercises.

Patients with CTS, the most commonly encountered peripheral compression neuropathy, usually report a burning, aching, or tingling pain radiating to the forearm in the distribution of the median nerve, occasionally to the shoulder, neck, and chest. Symptoms are often worst at night. A classic finding is the report of acroparesthesia, awakening at night with numbness and burning pain in the fingers. Physical examination findings occasionally include positive Tinel ♂ and Phalen ♂ tests, although the carpal compression test, in which symptoms are induced by direct application of pressure over the carpal tunnel, is likely a more sensitive and specific test. In later disease, muscle weakness and thenar atrophy are often noted. Diagnostic tests for patients suspected to have CTS include electromyography and nerve conduction studies that can confirm the median neuropathy. Although plain x-rays are of little diagnostic value, MRI and high-resolution ultrasound results often support the diagnosis.

Treatment of patients with CTS includes limiting the activity that caused the condition and elevating the affected extremity; application of a volar splint in a neutral position helps relieve the increase in intracanal pressure caused by wrist flexion and extension. NSAIDs and acetaminophen provide pain relief. Corticosteroid injection into the carpal tunnel at 6-week intervals can help reduce swelling and symptoms, but should be performed only by a skilled practitioner. Surgery to release the transverse carpal ligament provides symptom relief in most patients who do not respond to conservative therapy. About 10% of patients do not respond, however, because of nerve damage or new pressure within the carpal tunnel that results from recurrent compression caused by scar formation. Vitamin B_6 and other nutraceutical therapy have been reported to be helpful in minimizing CTS symptoms, although some studies have not supported their use.

CTS is often noted transiently at the end of pregnancy and in patients with untreated hypothyroidism. Pregnancy-induced CTS usually resolves quickly after the woman gives birth, and thyroxine supplements quickly ameliorate CTS caused by hypothyroidism. In the interim, splinting and analgesia can be helpful.

Discussion Sources

Anderson B. *Office Orthopedics for Primary Care: Diagnosis.* Philadelphia, PA: Saunders Elsevier; 2006.

Anderson B. *Office Orthopedics for Primary Care: Treatment.* Philadelphia, PA: Saunders Elsevier; 2006.

Turner S. Musculoskeletal system. In: Goolsby M, Grubbs L, eds. *Advanced Assessment: Interpreting Findings and Formulating Differential Diagnosis.* Philadelphia, PA: FA Davis; 2006:321–353.

QUESTIONS

50. Most episodes of low back pain are caused by:
    A. an acute precipitating event.
    B. disk herniation.
    C. muscle or ligamentous strain.
    D. nerve impingement.

51. With the straight-leg–raising test, the NP is evaluating tension on which of the following nerve roots?
    A. L1 and L2
    B. L3 and L4
    C. L5 and S1
    D. S2 and S3

52. During acute lumbosacral strain, which of the following is the best advice to give about exercising?
    A. You should not exercise until you are free of pain.
    B. Back-strengthening exercises may cause mild muscle soreness.
    C. Electric-like pain is to be expected.
    D. Conditioning exercises should be started immediately.

53. Early neurological changes in patients with lumbar radiculopathy include:
    A. loss of deep tendon reflexes.
    B. poor two-point discrimination.
    C. reduced muscle strength.
    D. footdrop.

54. In the evaluation of a patient with low back pain, the loss of bowel and bladder control most likely indicates:
    A. cauda equina syndrome.
    B. muscular spasm.
    C. vertebral fracture.
    D. sciatic nerve entrapment.

55. Loss of posterior tibial reflex may indicate a lesion at:
    A. L3.
    B. L4.
    C. L5.
    D. S1.

56. Loss of Achilles tendon reflex most likely indicates a lesion at:
    A. L1 to L2.
    B. L3 to L4.
    C. L5 to S1.
    D. S2 to S3.

57. Which test is demonstrated when the examiner applies pressure to the top of the head with the neck bending forward, producing pain or numbness in the upper extremities?
    A. Spurling
    B. McMurray
    C. Lachman
    D. Newman

58. Which of the following tests yields the greatest amount of information in a patient with acute lumbar radiculopathy?

   A. lumbosacral radiograph series
   B. ESR measurement
   C. MRI
   D. bone scan

59. The most common site for a cervical disk lesion is:

   A. C3 to C4.
   B. C4 to C5.
   C. C5 to C6.
   D. C6 to C7.

60. The most common sites for lumbar disk herniation are:

   A. L1 to L2 and L2 to L3.
   B. L2 to L3 and L4 to L5.
   C. L4 to L5 and L5 to S1.
   D. L5 to S1 and S1 to S2.

ANSWERS

50.	C	51.	C	52.	B
53.	A	54.	A	55.	C
56.	C	57.	A	58.	C
59.	C	60.	C		

DISCUSSION

Low back pain is at least an occasional problem for nearly all adults, with a lifetime prevalence of 60% to 90%. In about 90% of patients with low back pain, symptoms are short-lived and resolve within 1 month without specific therapy. A few individuals have recurrent or chronic low back pain, however, and significant disability.

Lumbosacral strain or disk herniation and resulting lumbar radiculopathy and sciatica can cause musculoskeletal low back pain. Most often, contributing factors include muscle or ligamentous strain, degenerative joint disease, or a combination of these factors. Lumbosacral strain is the most common reason for a patient to present to the primary care practitioner with acute low back pain. In the typical scenario, the patient complains of stiffness, spasm, and reduced ROM. The erector spinae muscle is most often implicated. Sitting usually aggravates the pain, but there may be some relief if the patient lies supine on a firm surface. A precipitating event is reported by only a few patients because lumbosacral strain is usually the culmination of many events, including repeated use of improperly stretched muscles in patients with overall poor conditioning. In addition, poor posture, scoliosis, and spinal stenosis can be predisposing factors. The physical examination usually reveals a straightening of the lumbosacral curve, paraspinal muscle tenderness, spasm worst at the level of L3 to L4, and decreased lumbosacral flexion and lateral bending. The neurological examination findings are typically normal, unless radiculopathy is present.

Diagnostic tests in lumbosacral strain vary according to the length and severity of symptoms. Radiographs can be helpful if spondylolisthesis, scoliosis, or degenerative joint disease is suspected. In the absence of these conditions, little is likely to be revealed. Lumbosacral radiographs should not be routinely obtained. Computed tomography (CT) scanning or MRI should be considered if radiculopathy is present and clinical presentation does not improve after a reasonable trial of conservative therapy because these studies might reveal contributing factors, such as spinal stenosis and disk herniation. MRI is a superior study for revealing soft tissue problems, whereas CT provides superior information on bony structures.

Lumbosacral disk herniation usually occurs after years of episodes of back pain caused by repeated damage to the annular fibers of the disk and is less common than lumbosacral strain as a cause of low back pain. Lumbar disk herniation often leads to sciatica, neurological changes, and significant distress. Because the intravertebral disks contain less water and are more fibrous, the risk of disk rupture decreases after age 50 years. The most common sites of lumbosacral disk herniation are L4 to L5 and L5 to S1, with the posterolateral aspect of the disk protruding.

Neuralgia along the course of the sciatic nerve is known as sciatica. The cause of sciatica is usually pressure on lumbosacral nerve roots from a herniated disk, spinal stenosis, or a compression fracture. Occasionally, sciatica can be caused by external pressure on the sciatic nerve, such as that often found in people who carry a wallet in a rear pants pocket and develop symptoms after prolonged sitting. Patients with sciatica complain of shooting pain that starts over the hip and radiates to the foot, often accompanied by leg numbness and weakness. The degree of pain can vary according to the degree of nerve involvement; it ranges from mildly bothersome and occasionally reported to be more itchy than painful to incapacitating pain.

Neck pain, a common clinical complaint, can result from abnormalities in the soft tissues such as muscles, ligaments, and nerves, and in bones and joints of the spine. The most common causes of neck pain are soft tissue abnormalities caused by injury or prolonged wear and tear; rare causes of neck pain include infection and tumors. The most common site for a cervical disk lesion is C5 to C6.

In patients who have herniated disks, whether in the neck or back, the degree of neurological involvement ranges from more minor symptoms of numbness to loss of extremity function. Deep tendon reflexes may be absent. With cauda equina involvement, there is compression of the lower portion of the nerve root inferior to the spinal cord, usually secondary to disk herniation. This compression leads to rectal or perineal pain and disturbance in bowel and bladder function. Signs of lumbosacral strain are present, and the straight-leg–raising maneuver reproduces pain.

Management of patients with low back pain differs according to presentation. In most patients with acute low back pain and intact neurological examination, a short course of 2 to 4 days of bed rest may be helpful; longer periods of immobilization may contribute to deconditioning and are potentially harmful. Intervention for acute neck pain is similar. Application of cold packs for 20 minutes three to four times a day can help with pain control, and heat applications may help before gentle stretching exercise. NSAIDs or acetaminophen should be prescribed for pain control. Muscle relaxants have been shown to be helpful in some patients. These medications are usually sedating, however, and need to be used with caution; occasionally, these are used as drugs of abuse. Treatment should also include initiation of aerobic and toning exercises and teaching the patient to minimize back stress through appropriate use of body mechanics.

Prompt referral to specialty care is needed when there is limb, bowel, or bladder dysfunction. Surgery is usually considered only if severe symptoms persist beyond 3 months. In addition, early referral is indicated in certain conditions that are particularly worrisome (Table 8–6).

Discussion Sources

Chou R, Qaseem A, Snow V, Casey V, Cross JT, Shekelle P, Owens D; Clinical Efficacy Assessment Subcommittee of the American College of Physicians and the American College of Physicians/American Pain Society Low Back Pain Guidelines Panel. http://www.annals.org/cgi/content/full/147/7/478, Diagnosis and treatment of low back pain: a joint clinical practice guideline from the American College of Physicians and the American Pain Society, 2007, accessed 9/29/09.

Turner S. Musculoskeletal system. In: Goolsby M, Grubbs L, eds. *Advanced Assessment: Interpreting Findings and Formulating Differential Diagnosis.* Philadelphia, PA: Davis; 2006:321–353.

QUESTIONS

61. A 22-year-old man presents with new onset of pain and swelling in his feet and ankles, conjunctivitis, oral lesions, and dysuria. The most important test to obtain is:
    A. ANA analysis.
    B. ESR measurement.
    C. rubella titer measurement.
    D. urethral cultures.

62. Treatment for reactive arthritis (also known as Reiter syndrome) in a sexually active man usually includes:
    A. antimicrobial therapy.
    B. corticosteroid therapy.
    C. antirheumatic medications.
    D. immunosuppressive drugs.

63. In reference to reactive arthritis (also known as Reiter syndrome), which of the following statements is false?
    A. When the disease is associated with urethritis, the male:female ratio is about 9:1.
    B. When the disease is associated with infectious diarrhea, the male and female incidences are approximately equal.
    C. ANA analysis reveals a speckled pattern.
    D. Results of joint aspirate culture are usually unremarkable.

ANSWERS

61.   D   **62.**   A   **63.**   C

TABLE 8–6

Low Back Pain: Potentially Serious Conditions

Possible Fracture	Possible Tumor or Infection	Cauda Equina Syndrome
History of recent trauma, particularly fall from significant height or motor vehicle accident	Age <20 y.o. or >50 y.o.	Bladder dysfunction, perineal sensory loss, or anal laxity
In person with or at risk for osteoporosis, minor trauma or strenuous lifting	Constitutional symptoms such as unexplained weight loss, fever	Neurological deficit in lower extremities
	Recent bacterial infection, injection drug use, immunosuppression	Lower extremity motor weakness
	Increased pain with rest	
	History of cancer	

Source: Chou R, Qaseem A, Snow V, Casey V, Cross JT, Shekelle P, Owens D; Clinical Efficacy Assessment Subcommittee of the American College of Physicians and the American College of Physicians/American Pain Society Low Back Pain Guidelines Panel. http://www.annals.org/cgi/content/full/147/7/478, Diagnosis and treatment of low back pain: a joint clinical practice guideline from the American College of Physicians and the American Pain Society, 2007, accessed 9/29/09.

DISCUSSION

Reactive arthritis refers to acute nonpurulent arthritis complicating an infection elsewhere in the body; Reiter syndrome also refers to this condition. Two or more of the following findings are required to make the diagnosis, with at least one musculoskeletal finding needed: asymmetrical oligoarthritis, predominantly of the lower extremity; sausage-shaped finger (dactylitis); toe or heel pain, or other enthesitis; cervicitis or acute diarrhea within 1 month of onset of the arthritis; conjunctivitis or iritis; and genital ulceration or urethritis. The knees and ankles are most often involved, and sacroiliitis is less common.

This condition is typically seen many days to weeks after an episode of acute bacterial diarrhea caused by *Shigella* species, *Salmonella* species, *Campylobacter* species, or a sexually transmitted infection such as *Chlamydia trachomatis* or *Ureaplasma urealyticum*. When seen with infectious diarrhea, the disease is found equally in both genders. When it is seen with urethritis, there is a male predominance of 9:1, with most being HLA-B27 positive. Cultures of joint aspirates in Reiter syndrome typically have negative results. Diagnostic testing is aimed at finding the underlying cause, such as urethral or stool cultures. Because this is an inflammatory condition, ESR is elevated, but this is not particularly sensitive or specific for the condition. Laboratory tests for rheumatic disease, such as ANA and rheumatoid factor analyses, are not affected by the disease.

Treatment includes the use of anti-inflammatory drugs such as NSAIDs. When reactive arthritis occurs with urethritis, the use of an antibiotic such as a tetracycline (e.g., doxycycline) shortens the duration of symptoms. Early antimicrobial treatment of infectious urethritis seems to limit a patient's risk of developing reactive arthritis. No change in symptoms is usually seen with antibiotic use if infectious diarrhea was the precipitating event.

Discussion Source

Scoggins T. eMedicine.
http://www.emedicine.com/emerg/topic498.htm, Reactive arthritis, accessed 9/29/09.

QUESTIONS

64. During a preparticipation sports examination, you hear a grade 2/6 early to mid systolic ejection murmur, heard best at the second intercostal space of the left sternal border, in an asymptomatic young adult. This most likely represents:

A. an innocent flow murmur.
B. mitral valve incompetency.
C. aortic regurgitation.
D. mitral valve prolapse (MVP).

65. You are examining an 18-year-old man who is seeking a sports clearance physical examination. You note a midsystolic murmur that gets louder when he stands. This may represent:

A. aortic stenosis.
B. hypertrophic cardiomyopathy.
C. a physiologic murmur.
D. a Still murmur.

66. A Still murmur:

A. is an indication to restrict sports participation selectively.
B. has a buzzing quality.
C. is usually heard in patients who experience dizziness when exercising.
D. is a sign of cardiac structural abnormality.

67. A 22-year-old woman wants to know whether she can start a walking program. She has a diagnosis of MVP, with echocardiogram revealing trace mitral regurgitation. You respond that:

A. she should have an exercise tolerance test.
B. an ECG should be obtained.
C. she may proceed in the absence of symptoms of activity intolerance.
D. running should be avoided.

68. You hear a fixed split second heart sound (S_2) in a 28-year-old woman who wants to start an exercise program and consider that it is:

A. a normal finding in a younger adult.
B. occasionally found in uncorrected atrial septal defect.
C. the result of valvular sclerosis.
D. often found in patients with right bundle branch block.

69. A 19-year-old man presents with stage 1 hypertension. Which of the following statements is correct concerning sports participation?

A. Full activity should be encouraged.
B. Weight lifting is contraindicated.
C. An exercise tolerance test is advisable.
D. A beta-adrenergic antagonist should be prescribed.

70. A 25-year-old woman presents with sinus arrhythmia. Which of the following statements is correct concerning sports participation?

A. Full activity should be encouraged.
B. Weight lifting is contraindicated.
C. An exercise tolerance test is advisable.
D. A calcium channel antagonist should be prescribed.

ANSWERS

64.	A	65.	B	66.	B
67.	C	68.	B	69.	A
70.	A				

DISCUSSION

Cardiovascular evaluation is an important component of the sports participation evaluation. Reducing the risk of exercised-induced sudden cardiac death and the progression or deterioration of cardiovascular function caused by exercise are the primary goals of preparticipation evaluation. The precise conditions responsible for athletic field deaths differ considerably according to age. In victims younger than 35 years, most sudden deaths are caused by several congenital cardiac malformations. Hypertrophic cardiomyopathy ♂ is the predominant abnormality in about one-third of cases, and congenital coronary anomalies rank as the second most common etiology. Most of these deaths occur while the victims are playing team sports. In athletes 35 years or older, most deaths are caused by atherosclerotic coronary artery disease, usually while the victims are participating in an individual endeavor such as long-distance running.

The preparticipation cardiovascular history should include questions about the following:
- Prior occurrence of exertional chest pain/discomfort or syncope/near-syncope
- Excessive, unexpected, and unexplained shortness of breath or fatigue associated with exercise
- Past detection of a heart murmur or high blood pressure
- Family history of the following: premature death (sudden or otherwise), significant disability from cardiovascular disease in one or more close relatives younger than 50 years, or specific knowledge of the occurrence of certain conditions (hypertrophic cardiomyopathy, dilated cardiomyopathy, long QT syndrome, Marfan syndrome, or clinically important arrhythmias)

The cardiovascular physical examination should include the following:
- Precordial auscultation in the supine and standing positions to identify heart murmurs consistent with dynamic left ventricular outflow obstruction
- Assessment of the femoral artery pulses to exclude coarctation of the aorta
- Recognition of the physical stigmata of Marfan syndrome
- Blood pressure measurement in the sitting and standing positions

If any abnormalities in the history or physical examination are revealed, further evaluation or appropriate referral should follow. The ability to participate in athletic activities is determined by the results of these studies.

Hypertension is a common clinical problem. Because of the cardiovascular benefit of exercise, activity restriction is usually not advisable, unless severely elevated hypertension or target organ damage is present. Certain antihypertensive agents may influence exercise tolerance. Generally, the use of angiotensin-converting enzyme inhibitors, angiotensin receptor blockers, calcium channel antagonists, and alpha-adrenergic blockers has little to no impact on exercise tolerance. Use of a beta-adrenergic antagonist can reduce the ability to exercise, however, because of its ability to blunt the normal increase in heart rate in response to exercise. Diuretic use should be avoided if possible because of increased risk of dehydration and hypokalemia.

Cardiac rhythm disturbances are common and are usually benign. In particular, the presence of sinus arrhythmia in a younger adult is a normal finding and is not an indication for curtailing activity. Dysrhythmias associated with ischemic heart disease and certain supraventricular and ventricular rhythms may preclude sports participation.

A systolic cardiac murmur is often benign. The examiner simply hears the blood flowing through the heart, but no cardiac structural abnormality exists. Certain cardiac structural problems, such as valvular and myocardial disorders, can contribute to the development of a murmur, however (Table 8–7).

Normal heart valves allow one-way, unimpeded forward blood flow through the heart. The entire stroke output is able to pass freely during one phase of the cardiac cycle (diastole with the atrioventricular valves, systole with the others), and there is no backward flow of blood. When a heart valve fails to open to its normal size, it is stenotic. When it fails to close appropriately, the valve is incompetent, causing regurgitation of blood to the previous chamber or vessel. Both of these events place patients at significant risk for embolic disease.

Physiologic murmurs, also known as functional or innocent flow murmurs, are present in the absence of cardiac pathology. There is no obstruction to flow, and there is a normal gradient across the valve. This type of murmur can be heard in 80% of thin adults or children if the cardiac examination is performed in a soundproof booth, and it is best heard at the left sternal border. It occurs in early to middle systole, leaving the two heart sounds intact. In addition, patients with a benign systolic ejection murmur deny having cardiac symptoms and have otherwise normal cardiac examination results, including an appropriately located point of maximal impulse and full pulses. Because no cardiac pathology is present in patients with a physiologic murmur, full activity should be encouraged.

Aortic stenosis is the inability of the aortic valves to open to optimal size. The aortic valve normally opens to 3 cm²; aortic stenosis usually does not cause significant symptoms until the valvular orifice is limited to 0.8 cm². In children and younger adults, aortic stenosis is occasionally found, usually caused by a congenital bicuspid (rather than tricuspid) valve or by a three-cusp valve with leaflet fusion. This defect is most often found in boys and men and is commonly accompanied

TABLE 8–7
Cardiac Conditions: Findings and Impact on Sports Participation

Cardiac Condition	Important Examination Findings	Additional Findings	Impact on Sports Participation
Hypertension	Elevated BP	With target organ damage: S_3, S_4 heart sounds; PMI displacement; hypertensive retinopathy	With all but markedly elevated BP or evidence of target organ damage, full participation should be encouraged because of cardiovascular benefit of exercise
Physiologic murmur (also called innocent or functional murmur)	Grade 1–3/6 early to mid systolic murmur, heard best at LSB, but usually audible over precordium	No radiation beyond precordium Softens or disappears with standing, increases in intensity with activity, fever, anemia S_1, S_2 intact, normal PMI	Full participation Patient should be asymptomatic, with no report of chest pain, heart failure (HF) symptoms, palpitations, syncope, and activity intolerance
Aortic stenosis (AS)	Grade 1–4/6 harsh systolic murmur, usually crescendo-decrescendo pattern, heard best at second RICS, apex	Radiates to carotids; may have diminished S_2, slow filling carotid pulse, narrow pulse pressure, loud S_4 Softens with standing The greater the degree of stenosis, the later the peak of murmur	Impact in participation varies with degree of stenosis Mild: Full participation Moderate: Selected participation Severe: No participation In younger adults, usually congenital bicuspid valve In older adults, usually calcific, rheumatic in nature Dizziness and syncope are ominous signs, pointing to severely decreased cardiac output
Mitral stenosis (MS)	Grade 1–3/4 low-pitched late diastolic murmur heard best at the apex, localized Short crescendo-decrescendo rumble, similar to a bowling ball rolling down an alley or distant thunder	Often with opening snap, accentuated S_1 in the mitral area Enhanced by left lateral decubitus position, squat, cough, immediately after Valsalva maneuver	Impact in participation varies with degree of stenosis Mild: Full participation Moderate: Selected participation Mild with atrial fibrillation: Selected participation Severe: No participation Nearly all cases rheumatic in origin Protracted latency period, then gradual decrease in exercise tolerance, leading to rapid downhill course as a result of low cardiac output Atrial fibrillation common
Mitral regurgitation (MR)	Grade 1–4/6 high-pitched blowing systolic murmur, often extending beyond S_2 Sounds like long "haaa," "hooo" Heard best at RLSB	Radiates to axilla, often with laterally displaced PMI Decreased with standing, Valsalva maneuver Increased by squat, hand grip	Impact in participation varies with ventricular size and function MR with normal LV size and function: Full participation MR with mild LV enlargement but normal function at rest: Selected participation MR with LV enlargement or any LV dysfunction at rest: No participation Origin: Rheumatic, ischemic heart disease, endocarditis Often with other valve abnormalities (AS, MS, AR)

Continued

TABLE 8–7

Cardiac Conditions: Findings and Impact on Sports Participation—cont'd

Cardiac Condition	Important Examination Findings	Additional Findings	Impact on Sports Participation
Aortic regurgitation (AR)	Grade 1–3/4 high-pitched blowing diastolic murmur heard best at third LICS	May be enhanced by forced expiration, leaning forward Usually with S₃, wide pulse pressure, sustained thrusting apical impulse	Impact in participation varies with ventricular size, function, and dysrhythmias AR with normal or mildly increased LV size and function: Full participation AR with moderate LV enlargement, premature ventricular contractions at rest and with exercise: Selected participation Mild to moderate AR with symptoms, severe AR, AR with progressive LVH: No participation More common in men, usually caused by rheumatic heart disease but occasionally by tertiary syphilis
Mitral valve prolapse (MVP)	Grade 1–3/6 late systolic crescendo murmur with honking quality, heard best at apex Murmur follows mid systolic click	With Valsalva maneuver or standing, click moves forward into earlier systole, resulting in a longer sounding murmur With hand grasp or squat, click moves back further into systole, resulting in a shorter murmur	Impact in participation varies with ventricular function and dysrhythmia. MVP alone: Full participation MVP with mild to moderate regurgitation, dysrhythmias such as repetitive supraventricular tachycardia, complex ventricular dysrhythmias: Selected participation
Hypertrophic cardiomyopathy	Harsh mid systolic crescendo-decrescendo murmur heard best at LLSB or at the apex	Murmur may increase with standing, squat, or Valsalva maneuver Triple apical impulse, loud S₄, bisferiens carotid pulse	Often seen with minor thoracic deformities such as pectus excavatum, straight back, and shallow anteroposterior diameter Dyspnea, chest pain, postexertional syncope often reported Sports participation should be determined on an individual basis according to degree of ventricular function and symptoms
Still murmur (also called vibratory innocent murmur)	Grade 1–3/6 early systolic ejection, musical or vibratory, short, often buzzing, heard best midway between apex and LLSB	Softens or disappears when sitting or standing or with Valsalva maneuver Usual onset, 2–6 y.o.; may persist through adolescence Benign condition	Benign finding No limitation on sports participation

Atrial septal defect (without surgical intervention)	Grade 1–3/6 systolic ejection murmur heard best at ULSB with widely split fixed S_2 May be accompanied by a mid diastolic murmur heard at the fourth ICS LSB common, caused by increased flow across tricuspid valve	Twice as common in girls Child may be entirely well or present with HF Often missed in the first few months of life or even entire childhood Watch for child with easy fatigability	With correction, full sports participation is typical Without correction, sports participation should be determined on an individual basis according to degree of pulmonary hypertension, right-to-left shunt, and symptoms
Ventricular septal defect (without surgical intervention)	Grade 2–5/6 regurgitant systolic murmur heard best at LLSB Occasionally holosystolic, usually localized	Usually without cyanosis With small to moderate-sized left-to-right shunt and without pulmonary hypertension, likely to have minimal symptoms Larger shunts may result in HF with onset in infancy	With correction, full sports participation is typical Without correction, sports participation should be determined on an individual basis according to degree of pulmonary hypertension, right-to-left shunt, and symptoms

BP, blood pressure; HF, heart failure; ICS, intercostal space; LICS, left intercostal space; LLSB, lower left sternal border; LSB, left sternal border; LV, left ventricular; LVH, left ventricular hypertrophy; PMI, point of maximal impulse; RICS, right intercostal space; RLSB, right lower sternal border; S_1, S_2, S_3, and S_4, first to fourth heart sounds; ULSB, upper left sternal border.

by a long-standing history of becoming excessively short of breath with increased activity such as running. The physical examination results are usually normal except for the murmur. The ability to participate in sports or other vigorous activity is dictated by the degree of aortic stenosis and patient symptoms (see Table 8–7).

In older adults, calcification aortic stenosis leading to the inability of the valve to open to its normal size is usually the problem. In middle-aged adults without congenital aortic stenosis, the disease is usually sequelae of rheumatic fever, representing about 30% of cases of valvular dysfunction seen in patients with rheumatic heart disease. As with patients who have congenital aortic stenosis, the ability to participate in sports or an exercise program is dictated by the degree of valvular dysfunction, ventricular enlargement, and patient symptoms.

The murmur of mitral regurgitation arises from mitral valve incompetency, or the inability of the mitral valve to close properly. This incompetency allows a retrograde flow from a high-pressure area (left ventricle) to an area of lower pressure (left atrium). Mitral regurgitation is most often caused by the degeneration of the mitral valve, most commonly by rheumatic fever, endocarditis, calcific annulus, rheumatic heart disease, ruptured chordae, or papillary muscle dysfunction. In mitral regurgitation from rheumatic heart disease, some mitral stenosis is usually present. After a patient becomes symptomatic and without intervention, the disease progresses in a downhill course of chronic heart failure over the next 10 years. Sports or other vigorous activity participation is dictated by the degree of mitral regurgitation and ventricular chamber enlargement.

Mitral valve prolapse (MVP) is likely the most common valvular heart problem; it is present in perhaps 10% of the general population. Most patients with MVP have a benign condition in which one of the valve leaflets is unusually long and buckles or prolapses into the left atrium, usually in mid systole. At that time, a click occurs, followed by a short murmur caused by regurgitation of blood into the atrium. Cardiac output is usually not compromised, and the event goes unnoticed by patients. Echocardiography fails to reveal any abnormality, simply noting the valve buckling, followed by a small-volume or trace mitral regurgitation. If there are no cardiac complaints, and the rest of the cardiac examination, including ECG, is normal, no further evaluation is needed. One way of describing this variation from the norm is to inform patients that one leaflet of the mitral valve is a bit longer than usual. The "holder" (valve orifice) is of average size, however. This variation causes the valve to buckle a bit, just as a person's foot would if forced into a shoe that is one or two sizes too small. The heart makes an extra set of sounds (click and murmur), but is not diseased or damaged.

MVP is often found in people with minor thoracic deformities, such as pectus excavatum, a dish-shaped concave area at T1, and scoliosis. The second and much smaller group with MVP has systolic displacement of one or more of the mitral leaflets into the left atrium along with valve thickening and redundancy, usually accompanied by mild to moderate mitral regurgitation. These people typically have additional health problems, such as Marfan syndrome or other connective tissue disease. Because structural cardiac abnormality is present in these people, there is increased risk of bacterial endocarditis.

Barring other health problems, patients with MVP usually have normal cardiac output and tolerate a program of aerobic exercise well. A program of regular aerobic activity should be encouraged to promote health and well-being. Maintaining a high level of fluid intake should be encouraged in patients with MVP because the mitral valve prolapses more, increasing the murmur, when circulating volume is low. Treatment with beta-adrenergic agonists (beta blockers) is indicated only when symptomatic recurrent tachycardia or palpitations are an issue. Although this degree of distress (i.e., chest pain, dyspnea) may depend in part on the degree of mitral regurgitation, some studies have failed to reveal any difference in the rates of chest pain in patients with or without MVP. The potentially biggest threat is the rupture of chordae, which is usually seen only in individuals with connective tissue diseases (especially Marfan syndrome).

Hypertrophic cardiomyopathy is a disease of the cardiac muscle. The ventricular septum is thick and asymmetrical, leading to potential outflow tract blockade. Patients with hypertrophic cardiomyopathy often exhibit symptoms of cardiac outflow tract blockage with activity because the hypertrophic ventricular walls better approximate with the increased force of myocardial contraction associated with exercise. The presentation of hypertrophic cardiomyopathy is occasionally sudden cardiac death. Idiopathic hypertrophic subaortic stenosis is a type of cardiomyopathy. A strong family history is often present in individuals who have this autosomal dominant disorder. The typical patient is a young adult with a history of dyspnea with activity, but persons with hypertrophic cardiomyopathy may also be asymptomatic.

In individuals with congenital heart disease such as atrial or ventricular septal defect, recommendations for sports participation vary according to patient presentation and surgical intervention. Most often, if the defect has been surgically repaired with little residual dysfunction, full sports participation is allowed. If the defect is uncorrected, or if there is significant alteration in cardiac function despite repair, the degree of participation should be assessed on an individual basis with expert consultation.

Discussion Sources

American Heart Association Council on Nutrition, Physical Activity, and Metabolism. http://circ.ahajournals.org/cgi/content/full/115/12/1643, Recommendations and considerations related to preparticipation screening for cardiovascular abnormalities in competitive athletes: 2007 update, accessed 9/29/09.

Kurowski K, Chandran S. http://www.aafp.org/afp/20000501/2683.html, The preparticipation athletic evaluation, 2000, accessed 9/29/09.

QUESTIONS

71. All of the following are common sites of fracture in patients with osteoporosis except:

    A. the proximal femur.
    B. the distal forearm.
    C. the vertebrae.
    D. the clavicle.

72. Osteoporosis is more common in individuals:

    A. with type 2 diabetes mellitus.
    B. on long-term systemic corticosteroid therapy.
    C. who are obese.
    D. of African ancestry.

73. Osteoporosis screening tests include all of the following except:

    A. quantitative ultrasound measurement.
    B. dual-energy x-ray absorptiometry.
    C. qualitative CT.
    D. wrist, spine, and hip radiographs.

74. Osteoporosis prevention measures include all of the following except:

    A. calcium supplementation.
    B. selective estrogen receptor modulator use.
    C. vitamin B$_6$ supplementation.
    D. weight-bearing exercise.

75. Early disease presentation in osteoporosis often includes:

    A. greater than 1-inch loss in terminal adult height.
    B. hip fracture.
    C. kyphosis.
    D. patient report of back pain.

76. In counseling a postmenopausal woman, you advise her that hormone therapy users may experience:

    A. an increase in breast cancer rates with long-term use.
    B. reduction in high-density lipoprotein cholesterol.
    C. a 10% increase in bone mass.
    D. no change in the occurrence of osteoporosis.

77. When counseling a patient taking a bisphosphonate such as alendronate (Fosamax), you advise that the medication should be taken with:

    A. a bedtime snack.
    B. a meal.
    C. other medications.
    D. a large glass of water.

ANSWERS

71. D   72. B   73. D
74. C   75. D   76. A
77. D

DISCUSSION

Osteoporosis ♂ is a disorder of bone thinning in which bone absorption exceeds bone formation to the degree that bone density is insufficient to meet skeletal needs. Osteoporosis is also defined as bone density more than 2.5 standard deviations below the average bone mass for women who are younger than 35 years. For every reduction of bone mass by 1 standard deviation, the relative risk of fracture rises by 1.5-fold to 3-fold.

Estrogen deficiency is a potent risk factor, and osteoporosis is most common in postmenopausal women; by age 80 years, the average woman has lost more than 30% of her premenopausal bone density. Men seem to be at significantly less risk; this is partly because of inherently greater bone density. Body habitus and ethnicity can influence the risk of osteoporosis; the condition is most common in small-framed women of Asian and European ancestry, who usually have lower bone density in adulthood. All ethnic groups are at risk. Obesity seems to minimize osteoporosis risk, in part because of high endogenous estrogen production by fatty tissue and increased bone weight-bearing. Additional risk factors for osteoporosis include disorders such as thyrotoxicosis, Cushing disease, and RA; inactivity; and prolonged therapy with certain medications, including some anticonvulsants, heparin, and systemic corticosteroids.

In patients with osteoporosis, hip, wrist, and spinal fractures most commonly occur, but all bones are at risk. Early disease usually does not have symptoms, but backache is commonly reported. Although hip fracture is often the first clinical manifestation of osteoporosis, it usually indicates advanced disease, as does loss of terminal adult height.

In patients with osteoporosis, the bone lost is from the baseline bone density. A small amount of loss may be of great significance against poor bone density, but of little consequence with greater density. Primary prevention of osteoporosis includes ensuring the development of maximal adult bone density. Because maximal bone density is achieved in the early adult years, encouraging adequate calcium intake and weight-bearing exercise throughout the teen and adult years is important. The calcium intake goal should be the equivalent of 1000 mg/d for men and premenopausal women, increased to 1200 to 1500 mg/d or more in postmenopausal women. Vitamin D (minimal dose 600 to 900 IU daily and likely safe up to daily dose of 2000 IU/d) is also recommended. Foods should be one source of this important micronutrient, although few foods are abundant vitamin D sources. Exposing the skin to sunlight is the most important vitamin D source because the body readily synthesizes this nutrient in response to sunlight. Given current lifestyles and dietary habits, supplements are often needed to meet recommended requirements.

Many tests are available to evaluate osteoporosis risk or detect progression of the disease (Table 8–8). Dual-energy x-ray absorptiometry is considered a reliable measure. Qualitative CT is precise, but uses more radiation than dual-energy x-ray absorptiometry. Quantitative ultrasound is relatively inexpensive and can be performed with portable equipment. Plain radiographic films should not be used for screening or evaluation of osteoporosis because disease cannot be detected until 40% to 50% of bone mass is lost.

When taken with calcium supplements, postmenopausal hormone therapy (estrogen supplementation with or without a progestin) can help reduce the risk of postmenopausal

fracture by 50% by minimizing further bone loss; the benefit must be balanced against the noted increased risk of breast cancer and other problems with short-term and long-term use. A selective estrogen receptor modulator such as raloxifene (Evista) helps preserve bone density. Because raloxifene does not attach to estrogen receptor sites in the breast or uterus, a selective estrogen receptor modulator is often considered an alternative to hormone therapy. Bisphosphonates such as alendronate (Fosamax) inhibit the resorptive activity of osteoclasts, can help modestly increase bone mass, and can significantly reduce fracture risk. To minimize the risk of drug-induced esophagitis, patients taking an oral bisphosphonate should be cautioned to take the medication in the morning with a full glass of water. At least 30 minutes must elapse before food, other liquids, or medications are ingested. In addition, patients should remain upright for at least 1 hour. Calcitonin (Miacalcin) is another

---

TABLE 8–8
Osteoporosis: Risks, Screening Guidelines, and Treatment

RISK FACTORS FOR OSTEOPOROSIS

- Female gender
- Advancing age
- Family history of osteoporosis or broken bones
- Small, thin body frame
- Certain race or ethnicity such as northern European, Asian, or Hispanic/Latino; African Americans are also at risk
- History of bone fracture
- Low estrogen levels in women, including menopause, and low levels of testosterone and estrogen in men
- Diet
  - Low calcium intake
  - Low vitamin D intake
  - Excessive intake of protein, sodium, and caffeine
- Inactive lifestyle
- Tobacco use
- Alcohol abuse
- Use of certain medications, such as long-term corticosteroids, some anticonvulsants
- Certain diseases and conditions, such as anorexia nervosa, rheumatoid arthritis, gastrointestinal diseases

RECOMMENDATIONS FOR OSTEOPOROSIS SCREENING

- Postmenopausal woman <65 y.o., with one or more risk factors for osteoporosis
- Man 50–70 y.o., with one or more risk factors for osteoporosis

- Woman ≥65 y.o., without any risk factors
- Man ≥70 y.o., without any risk factors
- Woman or man >50 y.o. who has broken a bone
- Woman going through menopause with certain risk factors
- Postmenopausal woman who has stopped taking estrogen therapy or hormone therapy
- Individuals with the above-mentioned risk factors

AVAILABLE SCREENING TESTS FOR OSTEOPOROSIS

- Dual-energy x-ray absorptiometry (DXA) of the hip and spine. Using DXA to measure bone density of the hand, wrist, forearm, and heel also seems to detect women who are at increased risk for fracture
- Other tests to measure bone mineral density: Ultrasound, radiographic absorptiometry, single-energy x-ray, absorptiometry, peripheral DXA, and peripheral quantitative computed tomography

OSTEOPOROSIS TREATMENT

- All to be used with appropriate calcium and vitamin D supplementation
- Bisphosphonates, such as alendronate, risedronate, and zoledronic acid
- Other antiresorptive medications including selective estrogen receptor modulators (SERMs), such as raloxifene, calcitonin, and estrogen
- Bone-forming (anabolic) medications such as teriparatide (parathyroid hormone)

Source: National Osteoporosis Foundation. http://www.nof.org/professionals/NOF_Clinicians_Guide.pdf, Clinician's Guide to Prevention and Treatment of Osteoporosis, accessed 11/20/09.

antiresorptive medication that is most helpful in building vertebral bone. Because it also has analgesic properties, calcitonin can help in the treatment of vertebral fracture pain and can help minimize the risk of future fracture. With all therapies, calcium supplementation should be continued, and vitamin D deficiency should be appropriately treated.

Discussion Sources

National Osteoporosis Foundation. http://www.nof.org/professionals/NOF_Clinicians_Guide.pdf, Clinician's guide to prevention and treatment of osteoporosis, accessed 9/29/09.

Turner S. Musculoskeletal system. In: Goolsby M, Grubbs L, eds. Advanced Assessment: Interpreting Findings and Formulating Differential Diagnosis. Philadelphia, PA: FA Davis; 2006:321–353.

QUESTIONS

78. The most common site of sprain is the:

   A. wrist.
   B. shoulder.
   C. ankle.
   D. knee.

79. A grade II ankle sprain is best described as:

   A. minor swelling and minimal joint instability.
   B. moderate joint instability without swelling or ecchymosis.
   C. moderate swelling, mild to moderate ecchymosis, and moderate joint instability.
   D. complete ankle instability, significant swelling, and moderate to severe ecchymosis.

80. A person with a grade III ankle sprain presents with:

   A. minor swelling and minimal joint instability.
   B. moderate joint instability without swelling or ecchymosis.
   C. moderate swelling, mild to moderate ecchymosis, and moderate joint instability.
   D. complete ankle instability, significant swelling, and moderate to severe ecchymosis.

81. Patients with a grade III ankle sprain should be advised that full recovery is likely to take:

   A. a few days.
   B. 2 to 3 weeks.
   C. 4 to 6 weeks.
   D. many months.

82. Which of the following is usually not part of treatment of a sprain?

   A. immobilization
   B. applying ice to the area
   C. joint rest
   D. local corticosteroid injection

ANSWERS

78.	C	**79.**	C	**80.**	D
81.	D	**82.**	D		

DISCUSSION

A sprain is a partial or complete injury of a ligament either within the ligament body or at its site of attachment to the bone. Inversion injuries of the ankle cause about 85% of all sprains and are the most common injury sustained while jumping or running. Sprains can also involve the wrist, elbow, and knee. Wearing appropriate footwear, improved conditioning, pre-exercise warm-up exercises, and taping can be helpful in avoiding sprains.

Sprains are often graded according to presentation and proposed underlying degree of ligamentous injury (Table 8–9). The ankle anterior drawer test is used to assess for excessive laxity of the tibiotarsal joint. Excessive anterior motion is usually seen with a grade III sprain. Immobilization is important in helping appropriate healing and minimizing sequelae. Grade II and III injuries are occasionally associated with persistent joint laxity and a risk of future sprain.

Discussion Sources

Anderson B. *Office Orthopedics for Primary Care: Diagnosis.* Philadelphia, PA: Saunders Elsevier; 2006.

Anderson B. *Office Orthopedics for Primary Care: Treatment.* Philadelphia, PA: Saunders Elsevier; 2006.

Turner S. Musculoskeletal system. In: Goolsby M, Grubbs L, eds. *Advanced Assessment: Interpreting Findings and Formulating Differential Diagnosis.* Philadelphia, PA: FA Davis; 2006:321–353.

QUESTIONS

83. The diagnosis of tendonitis is usually made from:

   A. clinical presentation.
   B. plain radiographic films.
   C. MRI.
   D. laboratory diagnosis.

84. Complications of Achilles tendonitis include:

   A. tendon rupture.
   B. neurological sequelae.
   C. stress fracture.
   D. bursitis.

TABLE 8–9

Ligamentous Sprains: Grading, Presentation, and Intervention

Grade of Injury	Pathology and Presentation	Intervention
Grade I	Partial tear No instability	RICE (rest, ice, compression, elevation) Immobilizer Limit weight-bearing Analgesia Length of disability usually limited to a few days
Grade II	Partial ligamentous tear Moderate joint instability Moderate swelling Mild to moderate ecchymosis	RICE Immobilizer Limit weight-bearing Analgesia Length of disability usually several weeks to a few months
Grade III	Complete ligamentous tear Complete ankle instability Significant swelling Moderate to severe ecchymosis	Orthopedic referral RICE Immobilizer Limit weight-bearing Analgesia Length of disability may be many months

RICE, rest, ice, compression, and elevation.
Sources: Anderson B. *Office Orthopedics for Primary Care: Diagnosis*. Philadelphia, PA: Saunders; 2006.
Anderson B. *Office Orthopedics for Primary Care: Treatment*. Philadelphia, PA: Saunders; 2006.
Turner S. Musculoskeletal system. In: Goolsby M, Grubbs L. *Advanced Assessment: Interpreting Findings and Formulating Differential Diagnosis*.
Philadelphia, PA: FA Davis; 2006:321–353.

85. Which of the following is often found with rotator cuff tendonitis?

A. osteoarthritis
B. tendon rupture
C. bursitis
D. joint effusion

86. First-line therapy for biceps tendonitis usually includes:

A. applying ice to the area.
B. local corticosteroid injection.
C. orthopedic referral.
D. nerve block.

ANSWERS

83.	A	**84.**	A
85.	C	**86.**	A

DISCUSSION

The most common sites for tendonitis are the rotator cuff, elbow, biceps (shoulder), wrist, and heel. In most cases, a microscopic tear causes tendon inflammation; the resulting swelling and inflammation in the tendon are a result of overuse. The clinical presentation usually includes a report of reduced ROM caused by joint stiffness and discomfort and a dull, aching pain over the affected tendon, especially with joint use. This pain can become sharp and acute when the tendon is squeezed. With rotator cuff involvement, abduction and elevation of the shoulder joint worsen symptoms.

The diagnosis of tendonitis is usually straightforward, with no special studies required. If it occurs with a history of recent trauma, plain radiographic films of the affected area may reveal calcium deposits on the tendon. Because bursitis and tendonitis often occur concurrently, assessment often reveals both conditions. If there is a question about accompanying soft tissue injury, MRI is the most helpful diagnostic test.

Treatment of tendonitis includes limiting or discontinuing the contributing activity. Applying ice to the region is helpful. When the hand or wrist is affected, splinting and NSAIDs are reasonable first-line therapies. Achilles tendonitis may necessitate treatment with a posterior splint to immobilize the heel and heel cord stretching and orthotics after the acute phase to prevent recurrence. There is a 10% risk of tendon rupture with recurrent Achilles tendonitis; the risk can exceed 12% with biceps tendonitis. With rotator cuff involvement, the likelihood of concurrent bursitis is high; treatment includes limiting overhead movement and intrabursal corticosteroid injection.

Discussion Sources

Anderson B. *Office Orthopedics for Primary Care: Diagnosis.* Philadelphia, PA: Saunders Elsevier; 2006.

Anderson B. *Office Orthopedics for Primary Care: Treatment.* Philadelphia, PA: Saunders Elsevier; 2006.

Turner S. Musculoskeletal system. In: Goolsby M, Grubbs L, eds. *Advanced Assessment: Interpreting Findings and Formulating Differential Diagnosis.* Philadelphia, PA: FA Davis; 2006:321–353.

QUESTIONS

87. Which of the following statements is most consistent with fibromyalgia?

   A. It is diagnosed with equal frequency in men and women.
   B. It affects less than 1% of the general population.
   C. It is four to seven times more common in women than in men.
   D. It is most often initially diagnosed in adults younger than 20 years old and older than 55 years.

88. Which of the following is inconsistent with the clinical presentation of fibromyalgia?

   A. widespread body aches
   B. joint swelling
   C. fatigue
   D. cognitive changes

89. When discussing physical activity with a 40-year-old woman with fibromyalgia, you advise that:

   A. limiting exercise is an important component of symptom management.
   B. weight-bearing exercise would be most helpful.
   C. physical activity aimed at increasing flexibility is an important part of treatment.
   D. although possibly helpful in minimizing pain, physical activity usually significantly worsens fatigue.

90. Which of the following medications is approved by the U.S. Food and Drug Administration (FDA) for pain management in a person with fibromyalgia?

   A. trazodone
   B. nortriptyline
   C. pregabalin
   D. gabapentin

ANSWERS

87.	C	88.	B
89.	C	90.	C

DISCUSSION

Fibromyalgia is a common, complex disorder composed of a specific set of signs and symptoms that likely affects at least 2% of the general population; the condition is one of the most common central pain-related syndromes. Although its etiology is not fully understood, central nervous system dysfunction and central sensitization are likely the source of the multiple clinical findings associated with this condition. Biochemical changes noted in the central nervous system in a person with fibromyalgia include low serotonin levels, elevated levels of substance P, and other biological markers; these changes likely contribute to the diffuse hypersensitivity to pain. Genetic factors and a history of physical or emotional trauma (or both) predispose to fibromyalgia.

Fibromyalgia is four to seven times more common in women than in men; the reason for this finding is not understood. Symptom onset is usually between ages 20 and 55 years. Fibromyalgia is found in all ethnic groups.

No particular test is diagnostic for fibromyalgia. The diagnosis is made after careful consideration of the patient's health history and physical examination. The patient usually presents with a complaint of persistent fatigue combined with nonrefreshing sleep. Chronic, often migratory, pain, usually described as burning, aching, soreness, or feeling bruised (without objective evidence of bruising), is usually reported. Occasionally, a patient has a single painful area, such as the back or neck.

According to the American College of Rheumatology criteria, the diagnosis of fibromyalgia is supported by the presence of tender points in specific locations; the tenderness is triggered at the area where pressure, enough to cause the examiner's nail bed to blanch, or about 4 kg, is applied, and there is no referred pain. The locations of the tender points are as follows on the anterior body, usually bilaterally: at the fifth through seventh intertransverse spaces of the cervical spine, in the pectoral muscle at the second costochondral junctions, approximately 3 finger breadths (2 cm) below the lateral epicondyle, and at the medial fat pad proximal to the joint line. Posteriorly, bilateral findings are as follows: tenderness at the upper border of the shoulder in the trapezius muscle midway from the neck to the shoulder joint, the craniomedial border of the scapula at the origin of the supraspinatus, in the upper outer quadrant of the gluteus medius, and just posterior to the prominence of the greater trochanter at the piriformis insertion. The diagnostic is supported by the presence of pain in all four quadrants of the body and in the axial skeleton for 3 or more months and is noted in 11 or more of 18 anatomically specific tender points. Additional patient complaints often include chronic gastrointestinal problems, including intermittent diarrhea and constipation, cognitive changes, and altered mood.

Intervention in fibromyalgia is complex and requires a comprehensive, interdisciplinary approach; simply attempting to treat the pain associated with the condition is inadequate. Patient education should include information about the need for physical activity, which has been shown to reduce pain and increase function, such as flexibility exercises, progressive stretching, and low-impact activities such aquatic exercise. Trigger point injection has been noted to be helpful in certain patients. Medications such as trazodone can be helpful in improving sleep latency and duration. Tricyclic antidepressants such as nortriptyline and antiepileptics including gabapentin have been shown to minimize symptoms in fibromyalgia and numerous other chronic pain conditions; these medications can be helpful in treating the concomitant altered mood that often accompanies, but is not the cause of, fibromyalgia. Pregabalin (Lyrica) and duloxetine (Cymbalta) are approved by the FDA for pain reduction in fibromyalgia. Topical treatments such as capsaicin are often helpful treatment adjuncts.

Discussion Sources

American College of Rheumatology. http://www.rheumatology.org/public/factsheets/diseases_and_conditions/fibromyalgia.asp?aud=pat, Fibromyalgia, 2008, accessed 9/29/09.
Gilliland R. eMedicine. http://www.emedicine.com/pmr/topic47.htm, Fibromyalgia, accessed 9/29/09.

QUESTIONS

91. Which of the following provides the most abundant source of vitamin D?

    A. fortified dairy products
    B. fatty fish
    C. exposure of the skin to the sun
    D. leafy green vegetables

92. The vitamin D needs for a 36-year-old person who is taking phenytoin are best described as:

    A. easily met by a well-balanced diet.
    B. equivalent to what is required by other adults in this age group.
    C. markedly increased by twofold to fivefold from the age norm.
    D. reduced from baseline because of the drug's vitamin D–preserving qualities.

93. Clinical manifestations of vitamin D deficiency include all of the following except:

    A. rickets.
    B. osteomalacia.
    C. antigravity muscle weakness.
    D. azotemia.

94. Treatment for documented vitamin D deficiency should be initiated with which of the following vitamin D dosing regimens?

    A. 400 IU twice a day
    B. 1000 IU daily
    C. 10,000 IU twice a week
    D. 50,000 IU weekly

ANSWERS

91.	C	**92.**	C
93.	D	**94.**	D

DISCUSSION

Vitamin D has long been recognized as essential for the efficient use of dietary calcium and for bone and muscle health. More recent studies have highlighted the importance of the multiple roles of this micronutrient. As an inhibitor of abnormal cellular growth, vitamin D is needed to help with cell differentiation, minimizing abnormal cell proliferation, a key step in cancer development. A stimulator of insulin secretion in response to increased insulin demands, vitamin D plays a role in the maintenance of normoglycemia. Because vitamin D receptors are expressed by most cells of the immune system, the micronutrient plays an important role as an immune modulator. When vitamin D is available in physiological amounts, this micronutrient produces renin, contributing to blood pressure control.

Dietary intake of vitamin D–rich foods and regular periods of skin exposure to the sun should provide the body with an adequate supply of this important micronutrient; however, vitamin D deficiency is a common problem. Studies find this problem in different populations. In Boston, 36% of healthy adults 18 to 29 years old have vitamin D deficiency by winter's end, and in the United Kingdom, 27% of otherwise healthy, Asian children have vitamin D deficiency. Studies also found vitamin D deficiency in 57% of patients on a hospital medical ward and in 93% of patients with nonspecific musculoskeletal pain at a Minneapolis pain clinic. Vitamin D deficiency is a common problem in the well and the sick.

Fatty fish and vitamin D–enriched dairy products can supply a small amount of the estimated 3000 to 5000 IU/d of vitamin D the body needs per day; the average U.S. dietary intake is typically less than 5% of the body's requirement. Skin exposure to the sun's rays should supply 95% or greater of the daily requirements by triggering the body's natural ability to synthesize vitamin D. The ability of the body to synthesize vitamin D is determined by numerous factors, including the skin's melanin pigmentation. A person with a darker skin tone synthesizes less vitamin D with sun exposure compared with a person with lighter skin tone. The use of sunscreen, although helpful in limiting the risk of certain skin cancers, likely increases the risk of vitamin D deficiency because the application of a sunscreen with sun protection factor 8 reduces the capacity of the skin to produce vitamin D by 95%. Individuals who spend little time outdoors have significant risk of vitamin D deficiency. Time of year and place of residence also influence sun-induced vitamin D synthesis, with winter sun and northern latitudes providing the weakest effect. Even people who are regularly involved in outdoor activities that facilitate exposure to sunshine can have vitamin D deficiency if little skin is exposed to the sun. Exposing the hands, face, and arms or legs to about 5 to 15 minutes of sun at a strength found in northern latitude between the hours of 11 a.m. and 2 p.m. would help provide an adequate amount of vitamin D synthesis. This level of sun exposure is unlikely to induce sunburn or increase skin cancer risk. Recommended dietary allowances for vitamin D differ by age and gender and are currently being re-evaluated; the current guidelines of 400 to 800 IU/d for adults is likely inadequate.

Risk factors for vitamin D deficiency include poor diet and limited sun exposure, a common problem given indoor-oriented lifestyles and the use of sunscreen when outdoors. The use of certain medications, including phenytoin (Dilantin) and phenobarbital, is potentially vitamin D–depleting; as a result, patients taking these medications require two to five times the recommended daily amount of vitamin D. Vitamin D deficiency is also common in the presence of hepatic or renal disease and after gastric bypass.

In infants and children, severe vitamin D deficiency results in the failure of growing bone to mineralize, resulting in the condition known as rickets. Even though adult bones are no longer growing, they are in a state of constant cell renewal and are susceptible to problems related to vitamin D deficiency, including persistent, nonspecific musculoskeletal pain.

The clinical effects of vitamin D deficiency are many. Without sufficient amounts of vitamin D, intestinal calcium absorption is inadequate. The resulting calcium deficiency prompts an increase in production and secretion of parathyroid hormone (PTH). PTH acts at the level of the kidney by facilitating an increase in tubular calcium reabsorption and stimulating renal production of 1,25-dihydroxyvitamin D, the hormonally active form of vitamin D. With continued deficiency, unusually high levels of PTH allow osteoclast activation so that bone can serve as a calcium source. In addition, the continued presence of high levels of circulating PTH causes phosphate to be wasted via the kidney. The calcium phosphate product in the circulation decreases and becomes inadequate to mineralize the bone properly, potentially leading to osteopenia and osteoporosis. At the same time, osteoblasts deposit a rubbery collagen matrix layer on the skeleton. This surface cannot provide

sufficient structural support; the clinical effect is osteomalacia. This abnormal collagen matrix can absorb fluids and expand. With expansion, pressure builds under the richly innervated periosteal covering. This process likely explains in part the origin of the constant dull bone ache often reported in patients with osteomalacia. In these patients, minimal pressure applied with a fingertip on the sternum, anterior tibia, radius, or ulna elicits a painful response. Because vitamin D deficiency symptoms overlap considerably with symptoms of fibromyalgia, one condition is often mistaken for the other.

Vitamin D deficiency has also been long recognized as a cause of muscle weakness and muscle aches and pain in all ages. Aside from osteomalacia and localized bone pain, antigravity muscle weakness, difficulty rising from a chair or walking, and pseudofractures are also noted in a person with vitamin D deficiency. These findings resolve with appropriate treatment. Vitamin D deficiency also contributes to the development of hypocalcemia and hypophosphatemia. In this situation, unless the vitamin D deficiency is addressed, replacing calcium or phosphate alone does not restore the body to homeostasis.

Serum 25-hydroxyvitamin D is the most commonly accepted measure of vitamin D status. Opinions differ on what constitutes deficiency. A physiological deficiency is defined at a level of serum 25-hydroxyvitamin D sufficiently low to cause an increase in the PTH levels to correct calcium levels via increased bone turnover and accelerated bone loss—clearly a point later in the disease process. According to expert opinion, the clinician should consider a biologically based reference, with a level of serum 25-hydroxyvitamin D concentration below which PTH serum levels increase and calcium homeostasis is preserved. A measure of 25-hydroxyvitamin D less than 8 ng/mL is sometimes reported as deficient per laboratory norms. In reality, clinical studies have revealed increased PTH levels with 25-hydroxyvitamin D levels of 20 ng/mL (50 nmol/L). According to data published in the *Mayo Clinic Proceedings,* a serum 25-hydroxyvitamin D level of at least 20 ng/mL is necessary minimally to satisfy the body's vitamin D requirement, and maintenance of a serum level of 30 to 50 ng/mL is preferred.

Because of its ability to be stored in fat and long half-life, low-dose (400 to 800 IU) vitamin D supplementation is insufficient to correct a deficiency. According to Holick's recommendations, a dose of 50,000 IU of vitamin D once a week for 8 weeks is likely to be needed, with long-term prevention accomplished by giving 50,000 IU of vitamin D once or twice a month. Daily lower-dose supplementation is also needed. Increasing sun exposure is also helpful. Eating a diet rich in vitamin D–containing foods and exposing the skin to a sensible and safe level of sunlight can aid in preventing vitamin D deficiency. Excessive supplementation, although not excessive sun exposure, can result in vitamin D toxicity, leading to various problems, including calcium deposition into solid organs.

Discussion Sources

Holick M. Vitamin D deficiency: what a pain it is. *Mayo Clin Proc.* 2003;78:1457–1459. http://www.mayoclinicproceedings.com, accessed 9/29/09 .

Linus Pauling Institute. Micronutrient Information Center. http://lpi.oregonstate.edu/infocenter/vitamins/vitaminD/, Vitamin D, accessed 9/29/09.

Lyman D. Undiagnosed vitamin D deficiency in the hospitalized patient. *Am Fam Physician.* January 15, 2005. http://www.aafp.org/afp/20050115/299.html, accessed 9/29/09.

Plotnikoff G, Quigley J. Prevalence of severe hypovitaminosis D in patients with persistent, nonspecific musculoskeletal pain. *Mayo Clin Proc.* 2003;78:1463–1470. http://www.mayoclinicproceedings.com, accessed 9/29/09.

Tangpricha V. eMedicine. http://www.emedicine.com/med/topic3729.htm, Vitamin D deficiency and related disorders, accessed 9/29/09.

9

Peripheral Vascular Disease

QUESTIONS

1. Who is most likely to have new-onset primary Raynaud phenomenon?

   A. a 68-year-old man
   B. a 65-year-old woman
   C. a 25-year-old man
   D. an 18-year-old woman

2. All of the following are associated with secondary Raynaud phenomenon except:

   A. hypertension.
   B. scleroderma.
   C. repeated use of vibrating tools.
   D. use of beta-adrenergic antagonists.

3. Lifestyle modification for patients with Raynaud phenomenon includes:

   A. discontinuing cigarette smoking.
   B. increasing fluid intake.
   C. avoiding placing hands in warm water.
   D. discontinuing aspirin use.

4. Medications that are often helpful in relieving symptoms associated with Raynaud phenomenon include:

   A. nonsteroidal anti-inflammatory drugs (NSAIDs).
   B. angiotensin-converting enzyme inhibitors.
   C. beta-adrenergic antagonists.
   D. diuretics.

5. Which of the following is the most common presentation in a patient with Raynaud phenomenon?

   A. digital ulceration
   B. worsening of symptoms in warm weather
   C. a period of intense itchiness after blanching
   D. unilateral symptoms

ANSWERS

1. D   2. A   3. A   4. B   5. C

DISCUSSION

Raynaud phenomenon, also known as Raynaud disease, is characterized by paroxysmal digital vasoconstriction that results in bilateral symmetrical pallor or cyanosis. The hands are nearly always involved; foot involvement is rare. A period of rubor follows this initial response. Primary Raynaud phenomenon, also known as Raynaud disease, is idiopathic in origin in most patients and is most often found in women. The condition usually appears between the ages of 15 and 45 years. Vasoconstriction triggers include exposure to cold relieved by warmth and, less commonly, emotional upset. Symptoms tend to be progressive, with vasospasm becoming more frequent and prolonged. There are no specific studies to help diagnose primary Raynaud disease. The diagnosis is made if recurrent episodes occur for more than 3 years without notation of associated disease or secondary cause.

Secondary Raynaud phenomenon is seen in the presence of an underlying condition, such as atherosclerosis, collagen vascular disease, and select autoimmune disease such as scleroderma; in scleroderma, this concomitant condition is a nearly universal finding. In addition, the use of vibrating tools, repeated sharp digit movement such as piano playing or typing, frostbite, tobacco, ergotamine, and beta blocker use can be contributing factors. The presentation of secondary Raynaud phenomenon is the same as that of the idiopathic condition; the degree and length of vasospasm are often more severe. Rarely, distal digital ulceration is seen.

Whatever the cause, intervention in Raynaud phenomenon is aimed primarily at preventing vasospasm by avoiding cold and other known triggers. At the onset of an

See full color images of this topic on DavisPlus at http://davisplus.fadavis.com | Keyword: Fitzgerald

episode, submerging the hands in warm water may be helpful in limiting the length and severity of vasospasm; hot water should not be used because of risk of burn. Because wound healing may be delayed, and infection is common, the hands should be protected from even minor injury. Keeping the skin well lubricated can help avoid small fissures. Tobacco use exacerbates vasospasm. As a result, all forms of tobacco use should be discouraged; smoking cessation is usually associated with a stabilization of or improvement in symptoms. Biofeedback can be helpful because the patient can be taught to envision warming the digits, reducing symptoms. The dihydropyridine calcium channel blockers ("-ipine" suffix, such as amlodipine or nifedipine) and angiotensin-converting enzyme inhibitors ("-pril" suffix, such as lisinopril or fosinopril) can be used for their vasodilator effect when lifestyle modification is inadequate. In patients with secondary Raynaud phenomenon, treatment of the associated condition is important and often helps minimize episodes. Surgical intervention with distal digital sympathectomy and arterial reconstruction should be considered when more conservative therapy is unsuccessful in managing the condition.

Discussion Sources

Lisse J. eMedicine. http://www.emedicine.com/med/TOPIC1993. HTM, Raynaud phenomenon, accessed 9/30/09.

QUESTIONS

6. Which of the following does not directly contribute to the development of varicose veins?
   A. leg crossing
   B. pregnancy
   C. heredity
   D. Raynaud disease

7. When advising a woman with varicose veins about the use of support stockings, you consider that the preferred type:
   A. can be purchased in the hosiery section of a department store.
   B. is a lightweight pair and available over-the-counter.
   C. is a medium-weight to heavy-weight prescription product.
   D. is used with a panty girdle.

8. In patients with varicose veins, which vessel is most often affected?
   A. femoral vein
   B. posterior tibial vein
   C. peroneal vein
   D. saphenous vein

9. Which of the following statements is most accurate in the assessment of a patient with varicose veins?
   A. The degree of venous tortuosity is well correlated with the amount of leg pain reported.
   B. As the number of affected veins increases, so does the degree of patient discomfort.
   C. Symptoms are sometimes reported with minimally affected vessels.
   D. Lower extremity edema is usually seen only with severe disease.

10. Spider varicosities are:
    A. usually symptomatic.
    B. a potential site for thrombophlebitis.
    C. responsive to laser obliteration.
    D. caused by sun exposure.

ANSWERS

6.	D	7.	C	8.	D
9.	C	10.	C		

DISCUSSION

Varicose veins are seen in 15% of the adult population and are most often found in the lower extremities. Tortuous, dilated, superficial veins are characteristic. An inherited venous defect of either a valvular incompetence or a weakness in the walls of the vessel likely plays a significant role. In addition, situations that cause high venous pressure, such as leg crossing, wearing of constricting garments, prolonged standing, heavy lifting, and pregnancy, contribute to their development. Women are affected twice as often as men.

The vessel most often affected is the great saphenous vein and its tributaries. Often asymptomatic, varicose veins may also be associated with leg aching, but usually not severe pain. The degree of discomfort is poorly correlated with the number and appearance of the affected veins. Mild edema in the ankle area, particularly at the end of the day and in warm weather, is common. When palpated, the vein compresses easily and without pain. No specific diagnostic tests are needed with typical presentation. Various diagnostic tests are available, however, including duplex ultrasound and magnetic resonance venography; these tests are usually used to rule out deep vein obstruction as a contributor of the severity of varicose veins.

With uncomplicated varicose veins, lifestyle modification usually helps minimize the symptoms and disease progress. Attaining and maintaining normal weight helps to reduce intravenous pressure and discourage the development and progression of varicose veins. Periodic leg elevation is helpful in minimizing edema and encouraging venous return. The use of medium-weight to heavy-weight elastic support hose such as Jobst stockings should be encouraged. Support hose purchased in a department store or drugstore does not supply enough compression. Wearing possibly constricting garments such as panty girdles and garters should be avoided.

Various minimally invasive interventions, including endovenous laser venous ablation, are now also available for varicose vein treatment. Sclerotherapy is a common procedure done for vein obliteration and involves injecting a sclerosing agent into the affected vein, followed by a period of compression, which results in vessel obliteration. Surgery is often needed for symptomatic varicose veins that do not respond to conservative therapy. Patients often prefer more aggressive treatment in this condition to yield the best noncosmetic, such as relief of discomfort, and cosmetic outcome.

Possible complications of varicose veins include superficial thrombophlebitis. Over time, varicose veins tend to dilate progressively, which can lead to secondary changes in the lower extremities, including chronic edema, skin hyperpigmentation, and development of chronic venous insufficiency. Spider varicosities ♂ are visible surface vessels usually seen with varicose veins. These vessels do not usually cause symptoms and pose no thromboembolic risk. Vessel obliteration with laser or other modalities is helpful in reducing the appearance of spider varicosities and is considered a cosmetic procedure.

Discussion Source

Lew W, Weaver F, Feied C. eMedicine. http://www.emedicine.com/med/topic2788.htm, Varicose veins, accessed 9/30/09.

QUESTIONS

11. Which of the following is not a contributing factor to development of venous thrombophlebitis?

    A. venous status
    B. injury to vascular intima
    C. malignancy-associated hypercoagulation states
    D. isometric exercise

12. Presentation of superficial venous thrombophlebitis usually includes:

    A. positive Homans' sign.
    B. diminished dorsalis pedis pulse.
    C. a dilated vessel.
    D. dependent pallor.

13. Treatment of superficial venous thrombophlebitis in a low-risk, stable patient includes use of:

    A. compression stockings.
    B. acetaminophen.
    C. warfarin.
    D. heparin.

14. In providing care for a patient with superficial thrombophlebitis, the NP considers that:

    A. it is a benign, self-limiting disease.
    B. the linear pattern of induration can help differentiate the process from cellulitis or other inflammatory processes.
    C. a chest radiograph should be obtained.
    D. limited activity enhances recovery.

15. Which of the following is the most likely to be found in deep vein thrombophlebitis (DVT)?

    A. unilateral leg edema
    B. leg pain
    C. warmth over the affected area
    D. positive Homan sign

16. A positive Homans' sign is present in approximately what percentage of patients with DVT?

    A. 25%
    B. 33%
    C. 50%
    D. 75%

17. The initial diagnostic evaluation of a clinically stable patient with suspected DVT most often includes obtaining a/an:

    A. impedance plethysmography.
    B. iodine 125 fibrinogen scan.
    C. contrast venography.
    D. duplex ultrasonography.

18. Which of the following is the preferred medication to reverse the anticoagulant effects of unfractionated heparin?

    A. vitamin K
    B. protamine sulfate
    C. platelet transfusion
    D. plasma components

19. Which of the following is the preferred medication to reverse the anticoagulant effects of warfarin?

    A. vitamin K
    B. protamine sulfate
    C. platelet transfusion
    D. plasma components

20. The onset of anticoagulation effect of warfarin usually occurs how soon after the initiation of therapy?

    A. immediately
    B. 1 to 2 days
    C. 3 to 5 days
    D. 5 to 7 days

21. Compared with unfractionated heparin, characteristics of low-molecular-weight heparin (LMWH) include all of the following except:
    A. more antiplatelet effect.
    B. decreased need for monitoring of anticoagulant effect.
    C. longer half-life.
    D. superior bioavailability.

22. Which of the following is least likely to be found in patients with pulmonary embolus (PE)?
    A. pleuritic chest pain
    B. tachypnea
    C. DVT signs and symptoms
    D. hemoptysis

23. The most commonly used method of preventing venous thromboembolism in higher risk surgical patients is:
    A. antiplatelet therapy.
    B. LMWH.
    C. vena cava filter.
    D. warfarin.

24. When taken with warfarin, which of the following causes a possible increased anticoagulant effect?
    A. clarithromycin
    B. carbamazepine
    C. oral contraceptives
    D. sucralfate

25. When taken with warfarin, which of the following causes a possibly decreased anticoagulant effect?
    A. cholestyramine
    B. allopurinol
    C. cefpodoxime
    D. chloral hydrate

26. What is the international normalized ratio (INR) range recommended during warfarin therapy as part of the management of a patient with DVT?
    A. 1.5 to 2.0
    B. 2.0 to 3.0
    C. 2.5 to 3.5
    D. 3.0 to 4.0

ANSWERS

11.	D	12.	C	13.	A
14.	B	15.	A	16.	B
17.	D	18.	B	19.	A
20.	C	21.	A	22.	D
23.	B	24.	A	25.	A
26.	B				

DISCUSSION

Blood coagulation can be activated by various pathways via the tissue factor (TF) pathway (formerly known as the extrinsic pathway) and the contact activation pathway (formerly known as the intrinsic pathway). Expressed by injured endothelial cells, TF is the clinically most significant initiator of coagulation. TF binds to and activates coagulation factor VII; the TF/factor VIIa complex then activates factor X and factor IX to factors Xa and IXa. In the presence of factor XIIa, factor IXa can also convert factor X to factor Xa. The contact activation pathway is activated when factor XII comes in contact with a foreign surface. The resulting factor XIIa activates factor XI, which activates factor IX. Factor IXa activates factor X. These pathways work together to provide maximal stimulation of factor X, which, in the presence of factor V, activates prothrombin to thrombin; this is also known as the common pathway.

Equally as important as blood coagulation is the ability of blood to avoid clot formation. In the larger arteries, clot risk is usually limited because aggregating platelets are dislodged by high-velocity blood flow, and thrombus formation is avoided. In smaller arteries and veins, blood flow is slower, with platelet aggregation more likely to occur and clot risk higher. Working against thrombus formation, TF pathway inhibitor binds to and inactivates the TF/factor VIIa/factor Xa complex. Antithrombin III inactivates circulating thrombin, whereas proteins C and S are contributors to a complex process that downregulates thrombin activity by preventing the activation of factor V. If a clot does form, circulating plasminogen is incorporated into the thrombus; healthy endothelial cells adjacent to the vessel injury site release tissue plasminogen activator and activate plasminogen to plasmin, causing thrombolysis on the clot surface and minimizing thrombus size. Meanwhile, numerous factors, including plasminogen activator inhibitor, produced by the liver and endothelial cells, inhibit fibrin degradation by plasmin to limit thrombolysis.

The Virchow triad of stasis, injury to the vascular intima, and abnormal coagulation leading to clot usually contributes to the development of vessel inflammation and the resulting thrombophlebitis. The lower extremities are most often affected.

Thrombophlebitis, presence of coagulated blood or thrombus in a vein with resulting inflammation, can occur in superficial or deep veins. Risk factors for superficial thrombophlebitis include local trauma, prolonged travel or rest, presence of varicose veins, history of prior episodes, and use of estrogen-containing hormonal contraceptives or postmenopausal hormone therapy. Owing to the increased platelet stickiness noted in late pregnancy through the first 6 weeks postpartum, this time also marks a period for increased thrombotic risk.

Characteristics of superficial thrombophlebitis usually include a localized, tender, dilated, thrombosed vessel, causing a linear area of redness, often in the popliteal fossa. Homans' sign ♂ is absent. Having the patient stand for 2 minutes before examination enhances the findings because less severe cases might be missed on supine examination. Superficial thrombophlebitis is often considered a benign condition. Extension into a deep vein, the vessels that act as conduits to return blood to the heart, is typically present, however, in 45% of patients with the condition. In particular, superficial, noninfectious thrombophlebitis in hospitalized patients is more likely to be associated with DVT and PE. Until proven otherwise, a patient with superficial thrombophlebitis should be assumed to have deep vein involvement. Compression duplex venous ultrasonography should be performed to help rule out concurrent DVT.

Because disordered coagulation tends to occur in multiple locations simultaneously, superficial thrombophlebitis is often accompanied by DVT in a different location or extremity; the study should not be limited to the affected area. Serial studies are often needed if initial examination findings are negative, but symptoms persist. Although direct venography is the most sensitive and specific test, its use has been limited because these less invasive tests have become available. Magnetic resonance direct thrombus imaging provides an accurate noninvasive modality in DVT diagnosis.

Further PE evaluation should be undertaken based on clinical findings, such as shortness of breath or friction rub. Coagulation studies should be obtained, particularly if there is a history of previous episodes without such evaluation. D-dimer, a degradation product produced by plasmin-mediated proteolysis of cross-linked fibrin, is often elevated in DVT and PE. The test has significant limitations, however, because d-dimer levels can be elevated whenever the coagulation and fibrinolytic systems are activated and are falsely elevated in the presence of high rheumatoid factor levels.

After the diagnosis of superficial thrombophlebitis is confirmed, intervention is dictated by DVT risk factors and patient history. In the absence of risk factors and history of similar episodes, warm packs, compression hose, and NSAIDs can be used to treat superficial thrombophlebitis. Ambulation should be encouraged because rest promotes stasis and enhances coagulation. In the presence of prior episodes, a history of DVT, decreased mobility, hypercoagulability, or extensive saphenous vein involvement, subcutaneous LMWH therapy should be initiated, with consideration for long-term warfarin use. The inflammation associated with superficial thrombophlebitis usually subsides over 2 weeks, with a firm cord remaining for a much longer period. As with DVT, collateral venous flow develops over the next few months.

Acute DVT usually involves the veins of the lower extremities and pelvis. PE, a potentially fatal condition, is largely a sequela of DVT. Long-term sequelae of DVT include chronic venous insufficiency and venous ulceration.

Because the triad of venous stasis, vessel wall injury, and altered coagulation state is the primary mechanism underlying DVT (as noted with superficial thrombophlebitis), risk factors include prolonged rest, recent trauma, recent surgery

(especially hip replacement), pregnancy, and the peripartum period. The hypercoagulation state associated with many malignancies also presents considerable risk. The use of hormone-containing contraceptives (combined oral contraceptive, topical patch, or vaginal ring) and postmenopausal hormone therapy can increase DVT risk, particularly in cigarette smokers. Disorders of coagulation, such as factor V Leiden mutation and protein C and S and antithrombin III deficiencies, are recognized as a cause of DVT in otherwise healthy adults.

Because the presentation of DVT varies, making the diagnosis from clinical presentation alone is problematic (Table 9–1). Only a few patients with suspected DVT have the diagnosis supported, unless the Virchow triad of venous stasis, vessel wall injury, and coagulation abnormalities is present. With regard to risk and clinical presentation, Table 9–2 provides a guide for estimating clinical suspicion.

To establish the diagnosis and develop an appropriate plan of intervention, a thorough diagnostic evaluation is needed in patients suspected to have DVT. Contrast venography has the greatest sensitivity and specificity for the condition. Because of cost and the invasive nature of the test and the risk of allergy to the contrast medium, noninvasive tests are used more commonly. Compression duplex ultrasound is the most common first-line diagnostic technique in DVT. Magnetic resonance direct thrombus imaging is the diagnostic test of choice for suspected iliac vein or inferior vena caval thrombosis. In the second or third trimester of pregnancy, magnetic resonance imaging (MRI) is also more accurate than duplex ultrasound because the gravid uterus alters Doppler venous flow characteristics.

Levels of d-dimer are elevated in DVT with high sensitivity but low specificity; similar results are found with recent surgery, trauma, myocardial infarction, pregnancy, and metastatic cancer. When findings are positive in DVT, the degree of d-dimer elevation depends on the size of the clot. A lower risk patient with a normal d-dimer level is unlikely to have DVT. A growing body of knowledge compels the NP to consider an underlying clotting disorder in a person with DVT, and testing for protein S, protein C, antithrombin III, fibrinogen, lupus anticoagulant, factor V Leiden, prothrombin 20210A mutation, antiphospholipid antibodies, and other thrombophilia forms is appropriate. These tests should be obtained before initiating anticoagulation therapy.

Therapy for patients with DVT should be aimed at minimizing the risk of PE and extension of peripheral thrombus. Anticoagulation therapy with medications, usually heparin first followed by warfarin (Coumadin), should be prescribed. These products are aimed at allowing natural fibrinolysis action and clot resolution to occur and minimizing risk for clot extension; heparin and warfarin do not have intrinsic thrombolytic activity.

Because rapid anticoagulation is needed in DVT therapy, heparin is usually the initial treatment (Table 9–3). A naturally occurring acidic carbohydrate, heparin potentiates antithromboplastin III (a naturally occurring antithrombotic

TABLE 9–1

Clinical Presentation of Deep Vein Thrombophlebitis (DVT)

Finding	Comment
Edema	Usually unilateral
	Most specific finding
	Bilateral calf measurement with comparative readings helpful in clinical assessment
Leg pain	Usually described as a tugging pain, heaviness, ache
	Present in ~50% of patients with DVT
	Degree of pain does not correlate well with extent of thrombus
Homans' sign	Pain on dorsiflexion of the foot
	Present in about one-third of patients with DVT and up to half without DVT
Pulmonary embolus (PE) signs and symptoms	Present in ~10% of patients with DVT, but likely PE concurrently present in a higher percentage
Warmth over area of thrombosis	Relatively rare
Venous distention and prominence of subcutaneous veins	Relatively uncommon
Fever	If present, typically mild
Tenderness	Found in ~75% of patients with DVT
	May also be found in many conditions other than DVT
	Degree of tenderness does not correlate well with extent of thrombus

Source: Hoffer E, Bloch R, Messiner M, Fontaine A, Borsa J. eMedicine. http://emedicine.medscape.com/article/420457, Deep vein thrombosis, lower extremity, accessed 9/30/09.

TABLE 9–2

Wells Clinical Prediction Guide in Deep Vein Thrombophlebitis (DVT)

Clinical Parameter	Score
Active cancer (treatment ongoing, within 6 mo, or palliative therapy)	1
Paralysis or recent plaster immobilization	1
Recently bedridden for >3 days or major surgery <4 weeks earlier	1
Localized tenderness along distribution of the deep venous system	1
Entire leg swelling	1
Calf swelling >3 cm compared with asymptomatic leg	1
Pitting edema (greater in the symptomatic leg)	1
Collateral superficial veins (nonvaricose)	1
Alternative diagnosis (as likely or greater than that of DVT)	−2

TOTAL OF SCORES

High probability: Score ≥3
Moderate probability: Score 1–2
Low probability: Score 0

Wells Clinical Prediction Guide in Pulmonary Embolus (PE)

Clinical Parameter	Score
Clinical signs/symptoms of DVT	3
No alternative diagnosis likely or more likely than PE	3
Heart rate >100 bpm	1.5
Immobilization or surgery in the last 4 weeks	1.5
Previous history of DVT or PE	1.5
Hemoptysis	1
Cancer actively treated within past 6 months	1

SCORING

Probability of PE is high if total score >6; moderate, if 2–6; and low, if <2.

Source: Adapted from Anand SS, Wells PS, Hunt D, et al. Does this patient have deep vein thrombosis? *JAMA*. 1998;279:1094–1099.

agent) and inhibits the activity of numerous coagulating factors. Its effect on thrombus formation is immediate, in contrast to warfarin, which usually requires 3 to 5 days of use before therapeutic effect is seen.

Heparin is available in the standard unfractionated form, with an average molecular weight of 15,000 daltons, and a low molecular weight heparin (LMWH), with a molecular weight of 4000 to 6500 daltons. Enoxaparin (Lovenox), dalteparin (Fragmin), and ardeparin (Normiflo) are examples of LMWH. LMWH selectively enhances factor Xa and accelerates antithrombin III activity; because of limited bleeding risk, monitoring of partial thromboplastin time is not required during its use. LMWH has additional advantages,

including superior bioavailability, a longer half-life that allows for twice-a-day dosing, ease of calculating dosage, and limited antiplatelet effect. LMWH is more expensive, however, than unfractionated heparin. Patients with an isolated calf vein DVT who are clinically stable with few risks for a further embolic process and with access to careful provider follow-up should be considered for initial outpatient treatment with self-administered injections of LMWH twice a

TABLE 9–3

Indications and Length of Warfarin Treatment

Condition	INR	Duration of Therapy
Acute venous thrombosis		
• First episode	• 2.0–3.0	• 3–6 mo
• High risk of recurrence	• 2.0–3.0	• Indefinitely
• With antiphospholipid syndrome or other thrombophilia or coagulopathy	• 3.0–4.0	• Lifelong
Prevention of systemic embolus		
• Tissue heart valves	• 2.0–3.0	• 3 mo
• Valvular heart disease with history of thrombotic event	• 2.0–3.0	• Indefinitely
• Mechanical heart valve (if initially indicated by valve type)	• 2.5–3.5	• Indefinitely
• Acute myocardial infarction	• 2.0–3.0	• As deemed by concomitant clinical problems
Atrial fibrillation		
• Chronic or intermittent	• 2.0–3.0	• Lifelong for chronic or intermittent atrial fibrillation
• Cardioversion	• 2.0–3.0	• With cardioversion, for 3 weeks before and 4 weeks after conversion to sinus rhythm

INR, international normalized ratio.

Sources: Family Practice Notebook. http://www.fpnotebook.com/HEM183.htm, Warfarin protocol, accessed 10/1/09. http://www.globalrph.com/warfarin.htm, Warfarin dosing, accessed 10/1/09.

day. In the absence of this scenario, inpatient admission and heparin anticoagulation are indicated. Length of therapy is usually about 5 days, and therapy is discontinued when heparin has been given for 5 days or until international normalized ratio (INR) is greater than 2.0 as a result of the concomitant warfarin therapy. LMWH is often used for DVT prophylaxis for high risk surgical and medical patients.

Long-term warfarin therapy usually follows an initial heparin course. Warfarin acts against coagulation factors II, VII, IX, and X as a result of vitamin K antagonism. Warfarin is highly (99%) protein bound, primarily to albumin, and has a narrow therapeutic range. To avoid problems with warfarin therapy, patients must be well informed of the drug-to-drug and drug-to-food interactions (Table 9–4). Because cigarette smoking likely increases thrombotic risk while reducing efficacy of warfarin, developing a smoking cessation plan is important.

Prothrombin time is used as the measure of the efficacy of warfarin and is reported as an INR. INR prolongation is seen in about 48 to 72 hours after the first warfarin dose (Table 9–5). Warfarin anticoagulant therapy is usually prescribed for at least 3 to 6 months after the first DVT episode. Studies have supported long-term low-intensity (INR 1.5 to 2.0) warfarin anticoagulation to minimize thrombus risk even after a first DVT episode. With a second episode, abnormal clotting should be suspected, and anticoagulant therapy should be lifelong. In the presence of a clotting disorder, such as factor V Leiden mutations or antiphospholipid antibodies, anticoagulation should also be lifelong.

Approximately 2% to 10% of patients taking warfarin develop hemorrhage. This complication is rarely seen, however, in patients with INR of 2.0 to 3.0. In the presence of significant bleeding in patients taking warfarin, the drug should be discontinued, and vitamin K should be given promptly. Vitamin K has little effect on hemostasis, however, until 24 hours after its administration. If immediate action is needed, such as in the case of hemorrhage or bleeding into an enclosed space, fresh frozen plasma must be given. If anticoagulation therapy is continued after the bleeding crisis, response to warfarin may fluctuate, which necessitates close monitoring.

Thrombolytic therapy with streptokinase or a similar product is also a therapeutic option for DVT. This treatment is usually reserved for patients with extensive iliofemoral venous thrombus and low risk for bleeding.

With a mortality rate of 20% to 40%, PE is a feared complication of DVT. The diagnosis is often missed, however, because the presentation is nonspecific. PE presentation usually includes dyspnea, pleuritic chest pain, pleural friction rub, and accentuation of the pulmonic component of S_2 heart sound; tachypnea (respiratory rate >16/min) and tachycardia are nearly universal findings. DVT signs and symptoms are often noted, but their absence should not

TABLE 9–4
Warfarin: Drug and Food Interactions

Note: The concomitant use of warfarin with one of the following medications is not contraindicated. The prescriber and patient need to be aware, however, of the impact of concurrent use on anticoagulation state

Increased Anticoagulant Effect	Decreased Anticoagulant Effect	Variable Effects
Alcohol (particularly with liver disease)	Barbiturates	Phenytoin—increased and decreased effects noted, and increase in phenytoin level
Amiodarone	Carbamazepine	
Cimetidine	Chlordiazepoxide	
Clofibrate	Cholestyramine	
Cotrimoxazole	Griseofulvin	
Erythromycin	Rifampin	
Clarithromycin	Sucralfate	
Fluconazole	Azathioprine	
Isoniazid	Cyclosporine	
Metronidazole	Trazodone	
Miconazole		
Omeprazole		
Piroxicam		
Propafenone		
Propranolol		
Acetaminophen (inconsistent)		
Ciprofloxacin		
Dextropropoxyphene		
Disulfiram		
Itraconazole		
Quinidine		
Tamoxifen		
Tetracyclines including doxycycline, minocycline		

Source: Indiana University School of Medicine Division of Clinical Pharmacology. http://medicine.iupui.edu/clinpharm/ddis/table.asp, P450 drug interaction table, accessed 9/30/09.

eliminate the consideration of PE. Hemoptysis, cyanosis, and change in level of consciousness are rarely encountered, but are often considered to be an expected part of the presentation. The use of the Wells predictive scale can helpful in forming the diagnosis (see Table 9–2). The use of d-dimer testing in PE diagnosis has the same limitations as noted in DVT diagnosis. Imaging with spiral CT pulmonary angiography is a helpful confirmatory test.

In treating patients with PE, thrombolytic therapy is often used, followed by heparin and then warfarin therapy for a minimum of 3 to 6 months. If the patient is not a candidate for long-term anticoagulation therapy, or if clotting occurs despite adequate anticoagulation therapy, a vena cava filter is usually used to minimize the risk of future PE. Follow-up is recommended as needed to monitor INR and the underlying clinical condition.

Discussion Sources

Ferri F. *Ferri's Best Test: A Practical Guide to Clinical Laboratory Medicine and Diagnostic Imaging.* 2nd ed. Philadelphia, PA: Elsevier Mosby; 2009.

Ferri F. Pulmonary thromboembolism. In: Ferri F. *Practical Guide to the Care of the Medical Patient.* 7th ed. Philadelphia, PA: Elsevier Mosby; 2007:796–804.

Ferri F. Deep vein thrombosis. In: Ferri F. *Practical Guide to the Care of the Medical Patient.* 7th ed. Philadelphia, PA: Elsevier Mosby; 2007:851–858.

Hillman R, Ault K. Normal hemostasis. In: *Hematology in Clinical Practice.* 3rd ed. New York, NY: McGraw-Hill; 2002: 301–307.

Hoffbrand A, Pettit J, Moss P. Thrombosis and antithrombotic therapy. In: *Essential Hematology.* 4th ed. London, UK: Blackwell Scientific; 2001:273–288.

QUESTIONS

27. Which of the following is the most potent risk factor for lower extremity vascular occlusive disease?

    A. hypertension
    B. older age
    C. cigarette smoking
    D. leg injury

28. Clinical presentation of advanced lower extremity vascular disease includes all of the following except:

    A. resting pain.
    B. absent posterior tibialis pulse.
    C. blanching of the foot with elevation.
    D. spider varicosities.

29. Drug therapy that can potentially worsen symptoms in lower extremity arterial vascular disease includes:

    A. aspirin.
    B. cilostazol.
    C. pentoxifylline.
    D. propranolol.

30. Typically, the earliest sign of lower extremity venous insufficiency is:

    A. edema.
    B. altered pigmentation.
    C. skin atrophy.
    D. shiny skin.

TABLE 9–5

Warfarin: Initiation of Therapy and Long-Term Management

- Warfarin's anticoagulation effect takes at least 3–4 days of use to achieve. If immediate anticoagulation effect is needed, initiate heparin therapy while also starting warfarin 5–10 mg qd for 2 days, then reduce to 5 mg qd. Check INR daily; when at goal, discontinue heparin
- If there is no need for immediate anticoagulation, warfarin should be initiated at 5 mg/d, anticipating therapeutic effect in ~4 days. In older adults, initiate warfarin at 4 mg/d, anticipating therapeutic effect in 6–7 days
- If INR is not within goal during warfarin therapy, check for adherence to recommended therapy before adjusting dose and use of medications or foods that may interfere with warfarin effect

INR Goal 2.0–3.0	Action
At desired range	Repeat INR at interval determined by duration of therapeutic INR and underlying condition • 4–6 weeks if stable condition and typically therapeutic INR • At least weekly when underlying condition can affect coagulation state (e.g., malignancy, clotting disorder, use of medications that can influence warfarin effect)
INR <2.0	• Increase total weekly dose by 5%–20% • Repeat INR two to three times/week until within desired range
INR 3.0–3.5	• Decrease total weekly dose by 5%–15% • Repeat INR two to three times/week until within desired range
INR 3.6–4.0	• Consider withholding 1 daily dose, decrease total weekly dose by 10%–15% • Repeat INR two to three times/week until within desired range
INR >4.0 without complications and no indication for rapid reversal of anticoagulation effect	• Consider withholding 1 daily dose, decrease total weekly dose by 10%–20% • Repeat INR two to three times/week until within desired range
INR >4.0 and need for rapid reversal of anticoagulant effect	• Vitamin K 2.5–5 mg PO × 1–2 doses or 3 mg subcutaneous (SC) or slow intravenous (IV) route

INR Goal 2.5–3.5	Action
At desired range	• Repeat INR at interval determined by duration of therapeutic INR and underlying condition 4–6 weeks if stable. Repeat INR at interval determined by duration of therapeutic INR and underlying condition • 4–6 weeks if stable condition and typically therapeutic INR. • At least weekly when underlying condition can affect coagulation state (e.g., malignancy, clotting disorder, use of medications that can influence warfarin effect)
INR <2.0	• Increase weekly dose by 10%–20% • Repeat INR two to three times/week until within desired range
INR 2.0–2.4	• Increase weekly dose by 5%–15% • Repeat INR two to three times/week until within desired range
INR 3.5–4.6	• Decrease weekly dose by 5%–15% • Repeat INR two to three times/week until within desired range
INR 4.7–5.2	• Consider withholding 1 dose, decrease weekly dose by 10%–20% • Repeat INR two to three times/week until within desired range
INR >5.2 without complications and no indication for rapid reversal of anticoagulation effect	• Withhold 1–2 doses, decrease weekly dose by 10%–20% • Repeat INR two to three times/week until within desired range
INR >5.2 or need for rapid reversal of anticoagulant effect	• Vitamin K 2.5 mg PO × 1–2 doses or 3 mg SC or slow IV route

INR, international normalized ratio.
Source: Family Practice Notebook. http://www.fpnotebook.com/HEM183.htm, Warfarin protocol, accessed 9/30/09.

31. Comprehensive treatment for a person with peripheral occlusive arterial disease and diabetes mellitus includes all of the following except:

    A. daily aspirin use.

    B. lipid lowering with an HMG-CoA reductase inhibitor (statin).

    C. application of a topical antimicrobial to the affected area.

    D. maintenance of glycemic control.

32. Treatment options for venous stasis ulcers in the lower extremities include:

    A. cleansing with hydrogen peroxide.

    B. applying Burow solution.

    C. prescribing oral corticosteroids.

    D. applying a moisture-retaining dressing.

33. Cilostazol (Pletal) should be used with great caution in the presence of which of the following diagnoses?

    A. diabetes mellitus

    B. heart failure

    C. hypertension

    D. dyslipidemia

34. Clinical presentation of acute lower extremity atherosclerotic arterial disease most likely includes:

    A. pain and paresthesia.

    B. pallor and pulselessness.

    C. poikilothermy.

    D. paralysis or loss of limb strength.

35. More common etiologies of acute lower extremity atherosclerotic arterial disease include:

    A. arterial embolism with underlying atrial fibrillation.

    B. chronic venous insufficiency.

    C. extension of venous thrombosis.

    D. vessel trauma.

36. Compared with standard arteriography, potential benefits of magnetic resonance angiography include:

    A. superior visualization of small vessel disease.

    B. the use of a relatively non-nephrotoxic contrast material.

    C. more accurate estimation of degree of stenosis.

    D. significantly less expense.

ANSWERS

27.	C	**28.**	D	**29.**	D
30.	A	**31.**	C	**32.**	D
33.	B	**34.**	A	**35.**	A
36.	B				

DISCUSSION

Peripheral vascular disease refers to a group of conditions in which there is a reduction of blood flow to the extremities. In people with peripheral vascular disease, the venous, arterial, or lymphatic system is often affected. Risk factors for arterial occlusive disease, caused by extensive atherosclerosis, include diabetes mellitus, hypertension, and hyperlipidemia; tobacco use is the most potent risk factor, in particular in progressive disease. In the absence of these risk factors, peripheral arterial occlusive disease is rare except in advanced age; the condition is found in 10% of older adults. Clinical presentation usually includes a patient complaint of claudication, a reproducible ischemic muscle pain. Claudication is caused by the inability of the diseased vessel to vasodilate and allow for increased blood flow to handle the metabolic demands associated with physical activity.

Disease caused by atherosclerosis in the distal aorta or iliac, femoral, or popliteal arteries results in the most common clinical form and is typically called lower extremity occlusive disease. Presentation varies according to the area of vessel disease and dysfunction (Table 9–6). Atherosclerotic and calcific lesions usually cause occlusive disease of the aorta and its branches. Disease is often asymmetrical because the distribution of obstructive lesions usually occurs in segments, rather than continuously.

The diagnosis of lower extremity occlusive disease is made from clinical presentation and select diagnostic studies. Magnetic resonance angiography and duplex ultrasonography help confirm the diagnosis and monitor disease progress. Angiography, although an invasive procedure, gives the best measure of the extent of the disease; the information gained from angiography is sometimes needed before the clinicians proceed with percutaneous treatment or surgery.

Because patients with lower extremity arterial occlusive disease usually have other health problems, prevention and intervention measures, such as aggressive risk factor reduction—including cessation of tobacco use and blood pressure, glucose, and lipid control—help improve overall well-being. In addition, the presence of concomitant disease, such as cardiovascular or cerebrovascular disease, often limits the patient's ability to be physically active. Exercise such as walking helps to minimize symptoms and should be encouraged; although exercise was previously thought to enhance collateral blood flow, the benefit is now recognized as being a result of improving oxygen extraction for the skeletal muscles. Meticulous skin care is needed, and periodic podiatric care is recommended.

Pharmacotherapy for individuals with lower extremity arterial occlusive disease often yields variable results. The use of pentoxifylline (Trental), a medication thought to reduce blood viscosity and improve blood flow by altering the ability of red blood cells to pass through diseased vessels, can be helpful in increasing exercise tolerance. Outcomes with pentoxifylline use are variable; patients without diabetes mellitus

TABLE 9–6

Clinical Presentation of Lower Extremity Vascular Occlusive Disease

Patient Presentation	Clinical Significance
Burning sensation or ache with walking	Usually indicates femoropopliteal arterial disease
Pain in calf, hip, or buttock with activity, relieved by rest	Classic report in intermittent claudication
Foot pain at rest	Blood flow to extremity ≤10% of normal; indicates profound disease and gangrene risk
Numbness, coldness, pain in extremity	More common than claudication report in the older adult
Absent posterior tibialis pulse	This pulse is always present in a healthy adult
	Dorsalis pedis pulse absent in ~5% of healthy adults
Nail thickening	Because numbness is often also a problem, meticulous nail hygiene while minimizing injury is needed
	Onychomycosis is often seen in PVD
Absent dorsalis pedis and tibial pulses	Proximal pulses may remain palpable even in presence of significant occlusive disease
Blanching of foot with elevation, poor capillary return, dependent rubor	≤10% of normal blood flow to extremity
Ache in anterior tibial muscles, foot, and metatarsal arch with activity	Most common with long-standing poorly controlled diabetes mellitus
	Can be confused with peripheral neuropathy
Sexual dysfunction	Most common in presence of smoking, hyperlipidemia, diabetes mellitus
	PVD contributes to its development, but is likely one of many influencing factors

PVD, peripheral vascular disease.

Source: Lopez Rowe V. eMedicine. http://emedicine.medscape.com/article/460178,.08, Peripheral arterial occlusive disease, accessed 10/1/09.

and milder symptoms seem to gain the most benefit. Cilostazol (Pletal), a medication that impairs platelet aggregation and increases vasodilation, is often helpful, but has limitations. Its use is contraindicated in heart failure and carries an approximately 20% rate of adverse effects, with headache, dizziness, and diarrhea. The use of these medications does not alter the course of the disease, but rather reduces symptoms. Daily aspirin and statin therapy is usually indicated as part of a comprehensive plan to reduce cardiovascular risk; concomitant control of diabetes mellitus, which is often present, is critical. The use of beta blockers has been occasionally noted to worsen claudication symptoms. Beta blockers are often recommended, however, to treat the concomitant conditions found in the person with PVD.

Clopidogrel (Plavix) has been used in therapy for lower extremity arterial occlusive disease, particularly in patients who are allergic to aspirin or do not tolerate aspirin, or have an underlying hypercoagulable state; it prevents fibrinogen binding and may reduce the risk of thrombus formation. Warfarin therapy with a goal INR of 2.0 to 3.0 is occasionally used for certain patients with high thrombus risk, particularly patients who have undergone a vascular procedure. The use of vasodilators and anticoagulants does not seem to alter the natural history of the disease.

Surgical evaluation for percutaneous or open procedures should be part of the care of patients with lower extremity occlusive disease; medical management of concomitant problems, such as cardiovascular disease and diabetes mellitus, needs to be optimized preoperatively, and surgical intervention for other forms of vascular disease also needs to be considered. Angioplasty and grafting procedures can help improve blood flow and minimize symptoms and complications. Owing to the complexity of care, intervention in peripheral arterial ulcers usually requires specialty consultation.

Although lower extremity arterial occlusive disease is characterized by a predictable, slower, progressive process, acute occlusion can occur. Caused by embolic, thrombotic, or traumatic events, acute limb ischemia usually manifests with the so-called six Ps: pain, paresthesia (the two most common manifestations), pallor, pulselessness, poikilothermy (variation in limb temperature), and paralysis. When acute limb ischemia is caused by arterial embolism, the origin of the clot is usually the heart with underlying atrial fibrillation. When caused by arterial thrombosis, chronic arteriosclerotic occlusive disease is usually at the core of the problem. Prompt assessment is needed to support the diagnosis. Arteriography is usually considered the diagnostic "gold standard," but carries the risk of exposure to potentially nephrotoxic contrast material and ionizing radiation. Magnetic resonance angiography is likely replacing diagnostic angiography, owing to its less invasive nature without ionizing radiation exposure; the contrast agent used is relatively non-nephrotoxic. Drawbacks include the limited depiction of small vessels, and the possible overestimation of the degree of stenosis.

Chronic venous insufficiency is a common sequela of DVT and leg trauma, although the absence of this history is noted in about 25% of patients. There is decreased venous return because of vessel damage, and lower extremity edema is usually the earliest sign. Symptoms usually include leg aching and itchiness. Over time, the edema progressively worsens; this results in the development of thin, shiny, atrophic skin, often with brown pigmentation. Subcutaneous tissue thickens and becomes fibrous.

The stage is set for stasis ulceration. Inflamed pruritic patches usually precede the formation of an irregular ulceration with a clean base. Yellow eschar is occasionally found. Compression therapy has long been considered an important part of venous ulcer therapy; high compression bandages, exerting 30 to 30 mm Hg at the ankle, are most effective. The use of a flexible compression bandage is preferred over a rigid compression dressing such as an Unna boot. Although no particular wound care regimen has been associated with more rapid ulcer healing, various products are available with some notable advantages. Slow-release antiseptic bandages are helpful in reducing bacterial burden. Moisture-retaining dressings improve pain and have utility in autolytic débridement. Surgical débridement is occasionally needed, especially if an advanced therapy such as a bioengineered skin graft is being considered. High-dose pentoxifylline therapy is associated with decreased time for wound healing when compression therapy has been inadequate. If wound healing is not noted with a usually helpful therapy, a biopsy specimen of the lesion should be obtained to rule out malignancy. Given the complexity of care in patients with venous ulcer, referral to specialty wound care is usually indicated.

Discussion Sources

Lew W, Weaver F, Feied C. eMedicine. http://www.emedicine.com/med/topic2788.htm, Varicose veins, accessed 9/30/09.

Lopez Rowe V. eMedicine. http://emedicine.medscape.com/article/460178,.08, Peripheral arterial occlusive disease, accessed 9/30/09.

Panuncialman J, Flanaga V. Venous leg ulcers. In: Rakel R, Bope E, eds. *Conn's Current Therapy 2009*. Philadelphia, PA: Saunders Elsevier; 2009:855–857.

10
Endocrine Disorders

QUESTIONS

1. Which of the following characteristics applies to type 1 diabetes mellitus (DM)?

   A. Significant hyperglycemia and ketoacidosis result from lack of insulin.
   B. This condition is commonly diagnosed on routine examination or work-up for other health problems.
   C. Initial response to oral sulfonylureas is usually favorable.
   D. Insulin resistance (IR) is a significant part of the disease.

2. Which of the following characteristics applies to type 2 DM?

   A. Major risk factors are heredity and obesity.
   B. Pear-shaped body type is commonly found.
   C. Exogenous insulin is needed for control of disease.
   D. Exercise increases IR.

3. You consider prescribing insulin glargine (Lantus) because of its:

   A. extended duration of action.
   B. rapid onset of action.
   C. ability to prevent diabetic end-organ damage.
   D. ability to preserve pancreatic function.

4. After use, the onset of action of lispro (Humalog) occurs in:

   A. less than 15 minutes.
   B. approximately 1 hour.
   C. 1 to 2 hours.
   D. 3 to 4 hours.

5. Which of the following medications should be used with caution in a person with suspected or known sulfa allergy?

   A. metformin
   B. glyburide
   C. rosiglitazone
   D. NPH insulin

6. The mechanism of action of metformin (Glucophage) is as:

   A. an insulin-production enhancer.
   B. a product virtually identical in action to sulfonylureas.
   C. a drug that increases insulin action in the peripheral tissues and reduces hepatic glucose production.
   D. a facilitator of renal glucose excretion.

7. Generally, testing for type 2 DM in asymptomatic, undiagnosed individuals older than 45 years should be conducted every _____.

   A. year.
   B. 3 years
   C. 5 years
   D. 10 years

8. You are seeing 17-year-old Cynthia. As part of the visit, you consider her risk factors for type 2 DM would likely include all of the following except:

   A. obesity.
   B. member of certain ethnic groups (Native American, African American, Latino, Asian American, Pacific Islander).
   C. family history of type 1 DM.
   D. personal history of polycystic ovary syndrome.

9. Criteria for the diagnosis of type 2 DM include:

   A. classic symptoms regardless of fasting plasma glucose measurement.
   B. plasma glucose level of 126 mg/dL (7 mmol/L) as a random measurement.
   C. a 2-hour glucose measurement of 156 mg/dL (8.6 mmol/L) after a 75-g anhydrous glucose load dissolved in water.
   D. a plasma glucose level of 126 mg/dL (7 mmol/L) or greater after an 8-hour or greater fast on more than one occasion.

See full color images of this topic on DavisPlus at http://davisplus.fadavis.com | Keyword: Fitzgerald

10. The mechanism of action of rosiglitazone is as:

   A. an insulin-production enhancer.
   B. a reducer of pancreatic glucose output.
   C. an insulin sensitizer.
   D. a facilitator of renal glucose excretion.

11. Which of the following should be the goal measurement in treating a person with DM and hypertension?

   A. blood pressure less than or equal to 130 mm Hg systolic and less than or equal to 80 mm Hg diastolic
   B. hemoglobin A1c equal to or greater than 7%
   C. triglyceride 200 to 300 mg/dL (11.1 to 16.6 mmol//L)
   D. high-density lipoprotein (HDL) 35 to 40 mg/dL (0.9 to 1.03 mmol/L)

12. In caring for a patient with DM, microalbuminuria measurement should be obtained:

   A. annually if urine protein is present.
   B. periodically in relationship to glycemia control.
   C. yearly if urinalysis is negative for protein.
   D. with each office visit related to DM.

13. The mechanism of action of sulfonylureas is as:

   A. an antagonist of insulin receptor site activity.
   B. a product that enhances insulin release.
   C. a facilitator of renal glucose excretion.
   D. an agent that can reduce hepatic glucose production.

14. When caring for a patient with DM and hypertension, the NP considers prescribing:

   A. furosemide.
   B. methyldopa.
   C. fosinopril.
   D. nifedipine.

15. Clinical presentation of type 1 DM usually includes all of the following except:

   A. report of recent weight gain.
   B. ketosis.
   C. thirst.
   D. polyphagia.

16. Which of the following should be periodically monitored with the use of a biguanide?

   A. creatine kinase (CK)
   B. alkaline phosphatase (ALP)
   C. alanine aminotransferase (ALT)
   D. creatinine (Cr)

17. Which of the following should be periodically monitored with the use of a thiazolidinedione?

   A. CK
   B. ALP
   C. ALT
   D. Cr

18. All of the following are risks for lactic acidosis in individuals taking metformin except:

   A. renal insufficiency.
   B. dehydration.
   C. radiographic contrast dye use.
   D. chronic obstructive pulmonary disease.

19. Secondary causes of hyperglycemia include the use of all of the following medications except:

   A. niacin.
   B. corticosteroids.
   C. thiazide diuretics.
   D. angiotensin receptor blockers.

20. Hemoglobin A1c provides information on glucose control over the past:

   A. 21 to 47 days.
   B. 48 to 63 days.
   C. 64 to 90 days.
   D. 90 to 120 days.

21. Which of the following statements is not true concerning the effects of exercise and IR?

   A. Approximately 80% of the body's insulin-mediated glucose uptake occurs in skeletal muscle.
   B. With regular aerobic exercise, IR is reduced by approximately 40%.
   C. The IR-reducing effects of exercise persist for 48 hours after the activity.
   D. Hyperglycemia can occur as a result of aerobic exercise.

22 to 25. With an 8:00 a.m. dose of the following drugs and inadequate dietary intake or excessive energy use, at approximately what time would hypoglycemia be most likely to occur?

22. Lispro _____

23. Regular insulin _____

24. NPH insulin _____

25. Insulin glargine (Lantus) _____

26. The meglitinide analogues are particularly helpful adjuncts in type 2 DM care to minimize risk of:

   A. fasting hypoglycemia.
   B. nocturnal hyperglycemia.
   C. postprandial hyperglycemia.
   D. postprandial hypoglycemia.

27. What is the most common adverse effect noted with alpha-glucosidase inhibitor use?

   A. gastrointestinal upset
   B. hepatotoxicity
   C. renal impairment
   D. symptomatic hypoglycemia

28. Which of the following statements best describes the Somogyi effect?

A. Insulin-induced hypoglycemia triggers excess secretion of glucagon and cortisol, leading to hyperglycemia.
B. Early morning elevated blood glucose levels result in part from growth hormone and cortisol-triggering hepatic glucose release.
C. Late evening hyperglycemia is induced by inadequate insulin dose.
D. Episodes of postprandial hypoglycemia occur as a result of inadequate food intake.

29. Intervention in microalbuminuria for a person with DM includes:

A. improved glycemic control.
B. strict dyslipidemia control.
C. use of an angiotensin-converting enzyme inhibitor or angiotensin receptor blocker.
D. all of the above.

30. Hemoglobin A1c should be tested:

A. at least annually for all patients.
B. at least two times a year in patients who are meeting treatment goals and who have stable glycemic control.
C. monthly in patients whose therapy has changed or who are not meeting glycemic goals.
D. only via standardized laboratory testing because of inaccuracies associated with point-of-service testing.

31. The mechanism of action of sitagliptin (Januvia) is as:

A. a drug that increases levels of incretin, increasing synthesis and release of insulin from pancreatic beta cells.
B. a product virtually identical in action to sulfonylureas.
C. a drug that increases insulin action in the peripheral tissues and reduces hepatic glucose production.
D. a facilitator of renal glucose excretion.

32. The mechanism of action of exenatide (Byetta) is as:

A. a drug that stimulates insulin production in response to increase in plasma glucose.
B. a product virtually identical in action to sulfonylureas.
C. a drug that increases insulin action in the peripheral tissues and reduces hepatic glucose production.
D. a facilitator of renal glucose excretion.

33. You see an obese 25-year-old man with acanthosis nigricans and consider ordering:

A. FBS.
B. LFT.
C. RPR.
D. ESR.

34. The use of a thiazolidinedione is not recommended in all of the following clinical scenarios except:

A. a 57-year-old man who is taking a nitrate.
B. a 62-year-old woman with heart failure.
C. a 45-year-old man who is using insulin.
D. a 35-year-old patient with newly diagnosed type 2 DM.

35. In an older adult with type 2 DM with gastroparesis, the use of which of the following medications should be avoided?

A. insulin glargine (Lantus)
B. insulin aspart (NovoLog)
C. glimepiride (Amaryl)
D. exenatide (Byetta)

36. Metformin should be discontinued for the day of and at least 48 hours after surgery because of risk of:

A. hypoglycemia.
B. hepatic impairment.
C. lactic acidosis.
D. interaction with most inhaled anesthetic agents.

37. All the following medications are recommended by JNC-7 for treatment of concomitant hypertension when seen with type 2 DM except:

A. beta blockers.
B. angiotensin-converting enzyme inhibitors.
C. alpha blockers.
D. angiotensin receptor blockers.

ANSWERS

1. A	2. A	3. A
4. A	5. B	6. C
7. B	8. C	9. D
10. C	11. A	12. C
13. B	14. C	15. A
16. D	17. C	18. D
19. D	20. D	21. D

22. Approximately 8:30 to 9:30 a.m. (with peak of insulin dose)
23. Approximately 10 to 11 a.m. (with peak of insulin dose)
24. Approximately 12 to 6 p.m. (with peak of insulin dose)
25. Because insulin glargine (Lantus) has no peak, an episode of hypoglycemia is unlikely. If hypoglycemia were to occur, the episode could be protracted if left untreated because of the protracted duration of activity of the medication.

26.	C	27.	A	28.	A
29.	D	30.	B	31.	A
32.	A	33.	A	34.	D
35.	D	36.	C	37.	C

DISCUSSION

Type 1 diabetes mellitus (DM) is a disease of insulin deficiency. This disease usually occurs in persons younger than 30 years, with symptomatic presentation often comprising the classic "polys": polydipsia, polyphagia, and polyuria. If type 1 DM is associated with ketoacidosis, DM presentation can be dramatic, with severe dehydration, abdominal pain, vomiting, and decreased level of consciousness. In any event, prompt intervention with appropriate insulin therapy is indicated.

Insulin resistance (IR) is a genetically predetermined condition that is central to the pathogenesis of type 2 DM. In IR, there is a reduced sensitivity in the tissues to insulin's action at a given concentration, which causes a subnormal effect on glucose metabolism. Hyperglycemia results, which stimulates pancreatic insulin production to reduce the blood glucose level. Euglycemia occurs, albeit in the presence of hyperinsulinemia. Elevated fasting insulin levels are noted to be an independent predictor for ischemic heart disease. When coupled with acquired or lifestyle characteristics that contribute to IR, such as obesity, physical inactivity, and high-carbohydrate (>60% total calories) diet, the body has greater difficulty maintaining a normal blood glucose level. Over time, generally after many years of IR, pancreatic beta cell deficiency usually occurs, resulting in impaired glucose tolerance, hyperglycemia, and the diagnosis of type 2 DM.

Numerous conditions are seen in conjunction with IR. Increased IR is inversely related to decreased urinary uric acid clearance; this leads to a dramatic increase in the rate of gout. Most women with polycystic ovary syndrome have IR. Acanthosis nigricans, hyperpigmentation of the skin often in the neck and axilla, is also correlated with IR. This finding is most common in children and young adults with IR and DM risk. Birth weight that is low for gestational age is also correlated with increased risk of IR.

Although the correlation of obesity with IR and DM type 2 is well established, not all body fat types and distribution are equally problematic. Some persons with IR and DM type 2 are of normal weight, whereas others with IR never develop hyperglycemia. Obesity dramatically increases the risk of diabetes in a person with IR, however. "Apple-shaped" or central abdominal obesity comprises metabolically active fat and is associated with high insulin levels, IR, and high mobilization rate of free fatty acids; high insulin levels are often associated with increased appetite. This genetic makeup helped increase the likelihood of survival in times of famine. In these times of plentiful food, however, IR helps promote fat storage (Tables 10–1 and 10–2).

Patients with type 2 DM are most often asymptomatic at onset. As a result, the American Diabetes Association (ADA) recommends periodic fasting plasma glucose screening every 3 years in all adults, regardless of appearance of risk;

TABLE 10–1
Diabetes Mellitus Testing Recommendations

Type 2 diabetes mellitus testing should be considered in all adults who are overweight (BMI ≥25 kg/m²*) and have additional risk factors:
- Physical inactivity
- First-degree relative with diabetes
- Members of a high-risk ethnic population (e.g., African American, Latino, Native American, Asian American, Pacific Islander)
- Women who delivered an infant weighing >9 lb or were diagnosed with gestational diabetes mellitus
- Hypertension (≥140/90 mm Hg or on therapy for hypertension)
- HDL cholesterol level <35 mg/dL (<0.90 mmol/L) or triglyceride level >250 mg/dL (>2.82 mmol/L)
- Women with polycystic ovarian syndrome
- Impaired glucose tolerance or impaired fasting glucose on previous testing
- Other clinical conditions associated with insulin resistance (e.g., severe obesity, acanthosis nigricans)
- History of cardiovascular disease

In the absence of the above criteria, testing for prediabetes and diabetes should begin at age 45 yr. If results are normal, testing should be repeated at least at 3-yr intervals, with consideration of more frequent testing depending on initial results and risk status

Source: American Diabetes Association. http://care.diabetesjournals.org/cgi/content/full/32/Supplement_1/S13/T3, Criteria for testing for pre-diabetes and diabetes in asymptomatic adult individuals, accessed 9/26/09.

TABLE 10–2

Testing for Type 2 Diabetes Mellitus in Asymptomatic Children

Age of initiation: 10 y.o. or at onset of puberty, if puberty occurs at a younger age
Recommended testing frequency: Every 3 yr

CRITERIA

- Overweight (BMI >85th percentile for age and sex, weight for height >85th percentile, or weight >120% of ideal for height)

Plus any two of the following risk factors:

- Family history of type 2 diabetes in first-degree or second-degree relative
- Race/ethnicity (Native American, African American, Latino, Asian American, Pacific Islander)
- Signs of insulin resistance or conditions associated with insulin resistance (acanthosis nigricans, hypertension, dyslipidemia, polycystic ovarian syndrome, or small-for-gestational-age birth weight)
- Maternal history of diabetes or gestational diabetes mellitus during child's gestation

Source: http://care.diabetesjournals.org/cgi/content/full/32/Supplement_1/S13/T4, accessed 9/27/09.

the rationale for this testing interval is that type 2 DM is unlikely to develop in a 3-year interval if initial glucose was normal. Testing should be considered at a younger age or be done more frequently in individuals with or with acquisition of type 2 DM risk factors (see Table 10–2).

When a fasting plasma glucose threshold level of equal to or greater than 126 mg/dL (≥7.0 mmol/L) after an 8-hour fast is used, this testing is 98% specific and 40% to 88% sensitive for type 2 DM. Typically, wide-scale screening done according to these guidelines yields a 6% true-positive rate. Additional ADA diagnostic criteria for type 2 DM include a casual (random) plasma glucose level greater than 200 mg/dL (>11.1 mmol/L) with classic diabetic symptoms and an oral glucose tolerance result of greater than 200 mg/dL (>11.1 mmol/L) at 2 hours.

Glycosylated (or glycated) hemoglobin, also known as hemoglobin A1c (or simply A1c), increases in proportion to the amount of circulating glucose. The most abundant glycohemoglobin subtype of hemoglobin A_1 is A1c, which constitutes about 4% to 6% of the body's total hemoglobin. Glycohemoglobin circulates as part of the red blood cell for about 90–120 days, the length of the red blood cell's life span. As a result, measurement of hemoglobin A_{1c} provides a method for evaluating glucose control over time; the measurement best reflects blood glucose trends over the preceding 4 to 6 weeks. Correlation with average plasma glucose and hemoglobin A1c is an important clinical tool and can be

used for reinforcement in patient counseling. The ADA now advises that hemoglobin A1c can be used as a tool for diagnosing DM, with a measure equal to or greater than 6.5% consistent with the diagnosis. The test should be repeated in an asymptomatic adult with glucose less than or equal to 200 mg/dL (≤11.1 mmol/L). A repeat test is not needed in the presence of DM symptoms or glucose levels greater than 200 mg/dL (>11.1 mmol/L). (This change in recommendations resulted from numerous factors, most importantly improved standardization in hemoglobin A1c measurement. In addition, hemoglobin A1c measurement takes no special patient preparation because it can be done in a nonfasting state and avoids the protracted time needed for an evaluation such as the glucose tolerance test (Table 10–3).

Therapeutic lifestyle changes are critically important for a person with DM. Tobacco use in any form should be discouraged. Because approximately 80% of the body's insulin-mediated glucose uptake occurs in muscle and is enhanced by physical activity, a regular program of aerobic exercise should be prescribed. Exercise reduces IR by approximately 40%, with the effects persisting for up to 48 hours after the activity, and aids in weight maintenance. For a person with type 1 or type 2 DM, current ADA recommendations advise a diet of 300 mg or less of cholesterol per day, 8% to 9% or less of total dietary calories per day from saturated fat with similar proportions of polyunsaturated and monounsaturated fats, and 25 to 30 g of dietary fiber per day. Calories from protein should be no more than 10% to 20% of the daily total. Reinforcement of proper foot care and a clinical foot examination should be a part of every DM-related visit (Table 10–4).

Insulin therapy is indicated for all patients with type 1 DM and patients with type 2 DM with insulinopenia; short-term insulin therapy is indicated when type 2 DM is initially diagnosed, particularly with glucose values greater than 250 to 300 mg/dL (>13.9 to 16.7 mmol/L). Insulins come in many forms, from shorter acting to long-acting forms with different onsets, peaks, and durations of action (Tables 10–5 and 10–6). The clinician needs to be aware of the characteristics of each insulin form and how these different products contribute to glycemic control.

With insulin use, two conditions that can result in early morning hyperglycemia can occur. The Somogyi effect occurs when an insulin-induced hypoglycemia triggers excess secretion of glucagon and cortisol; this leads to hyperglycemia. Intervention is aimed at lowering the inappropriately high insulin dose, usually the dinnertime dose of intermediate-acting insulin. The dawn phenomenon is a result of reduced insulin sensitivity developing between 5:00 and 8:00 a.m., caused by earlier spikes in growth hormone. The net result is cortisol release, which triggers hepatic glucose secretion and early morning hyperglycemia. Intervention for the dawn phenomenon includes splitting the evening intermediate insulin dose between dinner and bedtime. Alternative interventions include switching to a bedtime dose of insulin glargine or an insulin pump.

TABLE 10–3

Diagnosing Prediabetes and Diabetes Mellitus in Adults and Adolescents

	Plasma Glucose	Oral Glucose Tolerance Test (OGTT)	A1c
Diabetes mellitus	Fasting (no caloric intake for ≥8 hr) ≥126 mg/dL (≥7.0 mmol/L) Random ≥200 mg/dL (≥11.1 mmol/L) with symptoms including polyphagia, polyuria, polydipsia, and unexplained weight loss	2-hr plasma glucose ≥200 mg/dL (≥11.1 mmol/L) after a 75 g glucose load	A1c ≥6.5% Recommendation as of mid-2009 for the following reasons: No special patient preparation, can be done nonfasting, no protracted time needed to test like OGTT, improved standardization of A1c measurement. A1c repeat recommended in asymptomatic adult with glucose ≤200 mg/dL (≤11.1 mmol/L). Repeat not needed in presence of DM symptoms and/ or glucose levels greater than 200 mg/dL (11.1 mmol/L).
Impaired fasting glucose (IFG), impaired glucose tolerance (IGT), prediabetes	IFG = 100 mg/dL (5.6 mmol/L) to 125 mg/dL (6.9 mmol/L)	IGT = 140 to 199 mg/dL (7.8–11.0 mmol/L) on the 75 g OGTT	DM prevention efforts should be intensified with A1c ≥6% but less than 6.5%.

Source: American Diabetes Association. Standards of medical care in diabetes, 2009. Available at professional.diabetes.org/CPR_Search.aspx. Accessed 10/20/09.

Source: International expert report on the role of the A1c assay in the diagnosis of diabetes. Available at care.diabetesjournals.org/site/misc/DC09-9033.pdf. Accessed 10/20/09.

Various oral and noninsulin injectable therapies are available for the treatment of type 2 DM. To prescribe these medications appropriately and effectively, the prescriber must know the mechanism of action, indications, anticipated adverse effects, contraindications, and anticipated benefit with the available medications (Table 10–7).

DM is the leading cause of chronic renal failure. After the diagnosis of DM is made, periodic screening of renal function should be done (see Table 10–4). Often serum creatinine measurement is used for this purpose. An increase in creatinine is not seen, however, until at least 50% of the nephrons are not functioning. An elevated creatinine level is a late rather than early indicator of renal damage. A far more sensitive indicator of diabetic nephropathy is the presence of proteinuria, a harbinger of progressive renal failure. Urine protein consists of many forms, including the most abundant, albumin, and immunoglobulin, haptoglobin, and light chains. The standard dipstick test is sensitive to 100 to 150 mg/L of urine albumin, an earlier marker of progressive renal failure than serum creatinine, but still a later disease marker. The presence of a small amount of albumin (microalbumin, or >20 mg/L albumin, or >30 to 40 mg/d) is considered a predictor of glomerular dysfunction associated with diabetic nephropathy.

Microalbuminuria can precede development of DM by 10 years. With type 2 DM, the patient should be screened for microalbuminuria at onset of disease, with an annual recheck if results are normal. Collection of a first morning specimen is important because normal daily activity may cause a low level of protein spillage into the urine, creating a false-positive result. The diagnosis of microalbuminuria should be confirmed by obtaining at least two positive results from three collections in a 3- to 6-month period; results should be correlated with serum creatinine level. Intervention includes tightening of glycemic control, to A1c of less than 7%; controlling elevated blood pressure (<130 mm Hg systolic and <80 mm Hg diastolic, per the Seventh Report of the Joint National Committee on the Prevention, Detection, Evaluation, and Treatment of Hypertension [JNC-7] guidelines); aggressive treatment of dyslipidemia; and addition of

TABLE 10–4

Guidelines for Adult Diabetes Mellitus Care

		Frequency	Description/Comments
HEALTH HISTORY AND PHYSICAL EXAMINATION	Blood pressure (BP), height and weight	Every 3–6 mo	If BP >130/80 mm Hg, initiate measures to lower
	Dilated eye examination	Annual, more often with progressive retinopathy	Refer to eye care specialist
	Foot examination	Every 3–6 mo	Visual examination without shoes and socks every routine diabetes visit
	Comprehensive lower extremity sensory examination	Initial/annual	Teach protective foot behavior if sensation diminished. Refer to podiatrist if indicated
	Dental examination	Every 6 mo	Refer to a dentist, reinforce ongoing dental care
	Smoking status	Ongoing	Check every visit. Encourage smoking cessation
LABORATORY TESTS	A1c	Every 3–6 mo	Goal ≤6.9% (ADA) or ≤6.5% (AACE)
	Fasting/casual blood glucose	As indicated	Compare laboratory results with glucose self-monitoring
	Fasting lipid profile	Annual, consider less often with stable levels	As part of comprehensive plan to reduce cardiovascular disease risk
	Urine microalbumin/ creatinine	Initial/annual	If abnormal, recheck × 2 in a 3-mo period, then treat if 2 out of 3 collections show elevated levels
	Serum creatinine	Annual	Measure annually for estimation of glomerular filtration rate
	EKG	Initial	If patient ≥40 years of age or DM ≥10 yr
	Thyroid assessment	Initial/as indicated	Thyroid palpitation, thyroid function test(s) if indicated
RECOMMENDED IMMUNIZATIONS	Influenza	Every fall in anticipation of seasonal influenza	
	Antipneumococcal vaccine	Recommended	Also revaccination × 1 if ≥65 y.o. and the first vaccine >5 yr ago *and* patient <65 y.o. at time of first vaccine
SELF-MANAGEMENT SKILLS AND PATIENT COUNSELING	Review self-management skills	Initial/ongoing	Reinforce healthy habits, monitoring, sick day care
	Review treatment plan	Initial/ongoing	Check self-monitoring log book, diet, physical activity, and medications
	Review education plan	Initial/ongoing	Refer for diabetes self-management education if indicated
	Review nutrition plan	Initial/ongoing	Refer for medical nutrition therapy if indicated
	Review physical activity plan	Initial/ongoing	Assess/prescribe based on patient's health status
	Tobacco use	Annual/ongoing	Assess readiness, counsel about cessation. Refer to smoking cessation program
	Psychosocial adjustment	Initial/ongoing	Suggest diabetes support group. Counsel and refer as indicated
	Sexuality/erectile dysfunction	Annual/ongoing	Discuss diagnostic evaluation and therapeutic options
	Preconception/pregnancy	Initial/ongoing	Need for tight glucose control 3–6 mo preconception. Consider early referral to high risk prenatal care

Source: Adapted from Massachusetts guidelines for adult diabetic care. http://www.maclearinghouse.com/PDFs/Diabetes/GuidelinesFY07/ DB723_2007.pdf, accessed 11/20/09.

TABLE 10–5

Insulins: Onset, Peak, and Duration of Action

Type	Onset of Action	Peak	Duration of Action
Short-acting, rapid onset of action (insulin lispro solution, Humalog)	15–30 min, give within 15 min or right after meals	30 min–2.5 hr	3–6.5 hr
Short-acting, rapid onset of action (insulin aspart solution, NovoLog)	10–20 min, give 5–10 min before meals	1–3 hr	3–5 hr
Short-acting, rapid onset of action (insulin glulisine, Apidra)	10–15 min, give within 15 min or right after meals	1–1.5 hr	3–5 hr
Short-acting, rapid onset of action (human insulin for inhalation use, Exubera)*	10–20 min, use within 10 min of meal ingestion	30–90 mins	6 hr
Short-acting (regular, Humulin R, Novolin R)	½–1 hr	2–3 hr	4–6 hr
Intermediate-acting (Lente, Humulin L; NPH, Novolin N, Humulin N)	1–2 hr	6–14 hr	16–24 hr
Long-acting (insulin glargine solution, Lantus)	Clinical effect ~1 hr after injection	None	≥24 hr
Long-acting (insulin detemir solution, Levemir)	Unknown, not stated in product information, but seems to be ~1–2 h from PK graphics	6–8 hr (minimal peak)	Dose-dependent; 12 hr for 0.2 U/kg, 20 hr for 0.4 U/kg. Albumin bound

*Exubera is not currently available in United States.

Source: Prescribers Letter Detail—Document #220309. Prescribersletter.com, Comparisons of insulins based on U.S. product information, accessed 9/27/09.

TABLE 10–6

When to Use Insulin in Diabetes Mellitus Treatment

Type 1 DM	Type 2 DM
• All patients • Basal insulin with adjustments for meals via multiple injections or pump	• At time of diagnosis to help achieve initial glycemic control, particularly when glucose values >250–300 mg/dL (13.9–16.7 mmol/L) • When acutely ill: Per ADA recommendations, in critically or acutely ill patients with type 1 or type 2 DM, blood glucose levels should be kept as close to 110 mg/dL (6.1 mmol/L) as possible and generally <180 mg/dL (<10 mmol/L) • When ≥2 oral agents at optimized dose are inadequate to maintain glycemic control

a medication recommended for use in individuals with concomitant type 2 DM and hypertension, including angiotensin-converting enzyme inhibitors (drugs whose names have the "-pril" suffix—lisinopril, enalapril, others), angiotensin receptor blockers (drugs whose names have the "-sartan" suffix), beta blockers (drugs whose names have the "-lol" suffix—metoprolol, atenolol), alpha-beta blockers (also "-lol" suffix—carvedilol, others), and nondihydropyridine calcium channel blockers (diltiazem [Cardizem, others], verapamil [Calan, Verelan, others]). Although use of beta blockers in patients with DM was discouraged or contraindicated in the past, current practice supports the use of this drug class because of its ability to reduce the target population's considerable cardiovascular risk.

Discussion Sources

American Diabetes Association Clinical Practice Recommendations. http://care.diabetesjournals.org/content/vol32/Supplement_1/, 2009, accessed 9/28/09.

Implementation Conference for AACE Outpatient Diabetes Mellitus Consensus Conference Recommendations. www.aace.com/pub/pdf/guidelines/OutpatientImplementationPositionStatement.pdf, Position statement, accessed 9/27/09.

Massachusetts Guidelines for Adult Diabetic Care. http://www.maclearinghouse.com/PDFs/Diabetes/GuidelinesFY07/DB723_2007.pdf, accessed 9/27/09.

TABLE 10–7

Medications Used in the Treatment of Type 2 Diabetes Mellitus

Medication	Mechanism of Action A₁c Reduction	Comment
Sulfonylurea (SU) Examples: Glipizide (Glucotrol), glyburide (Diaβeta), glimepiride (Amaryl)	Insulin secretagogue Anticipated A_{1c} reduction with intensified use 1%–2%	Adjust dose in renal impairment Use with caution with sulfonamide allergy Potentially photosensitizing. Typically less effective after ≥5 yr T2DM diagnosis, older adults, in the presence of severe hyperglycemia Hypoglycemia possible when used alone or in combination with metformin or TZD or both One of the least expensive T2DM treatment options
Biguanide Example: Metformin (Glucophage)	Reduces hepatic glucose production and intestinal glucose absorption, insulin sensitizer via increased peripheral glucose uptake and use Anticipated A_{1c} reduction with intensified use 1%–2%	Monitor creatinine, do not initiate or continue with impaired renal function. Avoid use in presence of heart failure Rare risk of lactic acidosis, most often with impaired renal function, hypovolemia, low perfusion state, or advanced age (>80 y.o.) With radiocontrast use, surgery, omit day of and ≥48 hr post study, reinitiate when baseline renal function has been re-established Hypoglycemia possible when used with SU or insulin, but uncommon when used alone or with TZD Often used as a first-line medication in treatment of T2DM
Thiazolidinedione (TZD) Examples: Rosiglitazone (Avandia), pioglitazone (Actos)	Insulin sensitizer via action at PPAR-γ receptors found in muscle, adipose, and other tissue Anticipated A_{1c} reduction with intensified use 1%–2%	Rare risk (<0.5%) of hepatotoxicity with use. Monitor ALT periodically Edema risk, particularly when used with insulin or SU. TZD use can cause or exacerbate heart failure. Do not initiate use in presence of heart failure, monitor at-risk patients carefully In consideration of cardiovascular risk, use with insulin or nitrates not recommended Onset of action delayed, requires up to 12 weeks of use before maximal therapeutic effect Hypoglycemia possible when used with SU or insulin, but uncommon when used alone or with metformin

Continued

TABLE 10–7

Medications Used in the Treatment of Type 2 Diabetes Mellitus—cont'd

Medication	Mechanism of Action A_{1c} Reduction	Comment
Meglitinides Examples: Repaglinide (Prandin), nateglinide (Starlix)	Short-acting insulin secretagogue (non-SU) Anticipated A1c reduction with intensified use 1%–1.5%	Take medication 1–30 min before meal. Provides quick insulin burst with onset of action ~20 min after dose taken. Helpful in management of postprandial hyperglycemia No additional benefit if used with SU Use with caution in hepatic or renal impairment
Alpha-glucosidase inhibitors Examples: Acarbose (Precose), miglitol (Glyset)	Delays intestinal carbohydrate absorption by reducing postprandial digestion of starches and disaccharides via enzyme action inhibition Anticipated A1c reduction with intensified use 0.3%–0.9%	Taken with first bite of a meal Helpful in management of postprandial hyperglycemia Does not enhance insulin secretion or sensitivity Gastrointestinal side effects are an issue. Avoid use in inflammatory bowel disease and impaired renal function
Amylin analogue Example: Pramlintide (Symlin) Injection only	Modulates gastric emptying and glucagon release postprandially. Increased feeling of satiety often results in decreased caloric intake and weight loss Anticipated A1c reduction with intensified use 1%–2%	Contraindicated in gastroparesis, inability to recognize hypoglycemia symptoms Boxed warning about hypoglycemia risk. Only use with meal ≥250 kcal, 30 g carbohydrate. Adjunct for patients who use mealtime insulin and have inadequate glucose control despite optimal insulin therapy
Incretin mimetics Example: Exenatide (Byetta) Injection only	Stimulates insulin production in response to increase in plasma glucose, inhibits glucagon release postprandially. Slows gastric emptying, often leading to appetite suppression and weight loss Anticipated A1c reduction with intensified use 1%–2%	Major adverse effect: Nausea/vomiting usually better with dose adjustment, continued use Contraindicated in gastroparesis Adjunct to improve glycemic control in T2DM when not adequately controlled with biguanide or SU or both
Dipeptidyl peptidase-4 (DPP-4) inhibitor Examples: Sitagliptin (Januvia), saxagliptin (Onglyza)	Increases levels of incretin, increasing synthesis and release of insulin from pancreatic beta cells and decreasing release of glucagon from pancreatic alpha cells Anticipated A1c reduction with intensified use 0.6%–1.4%	Dose adjustment required in renal impairment Well tolerated, little hypoglycemia risk, weight neutral Indicated to improve glycemic control, in combination with metformin or TZD

QUESTIONS

38. Risk factors for heatstroke include all of the following except:

- **A.** obesity.
- **B.** use of beta-adrenergic antagonists.
- **C.** excessive activity.
- **D.** use of a vasodilator.

39. Possible adverse outcomes from heatstroke include:

- **A.** rhabdomyolysis.
- **B.** anemia.
- **C.** hypernatremia.
- **D.** leukopenia.

40. Laboratory findings in heatstroke usually include:

- **A.** elevated total creatine kinase level.
- **B.** anemia.
- **C.** metabolic alkalosis.
- **D.** hypokalemia.

41. Intervention for patients with heatstroke includes:

- **A.** total body ice packing.
- **B.** rehydration.
- **C.** fluid restriction.
- **D.** potassium supplementation.

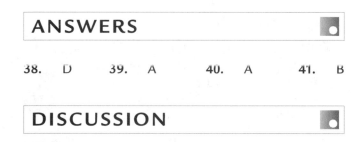

ANSWERS

| 38. | D | 39. | A | 40. | A | 41. | B |

DISCUSSION

Heatstroke is a life-threatening emergency caused by a failure of the body's thermoregulatory system, usually in response to extreme environmental and personal factors. In exertional heatstroke, the illness has been triggered by exercise in a warm environment that adds to the thermal load produced by the muscular contraction. In addition, a protracted period of exercise, such as running a marathon or participating in a long football practice, usually poses greatest risk. Nonexertional heatstroke is noted in the presence of extreme environmental heat, usually defined as more than 10°F (-12.2° C) greater than is typical for the given geographic area for more than 3 days, and poses a particular risk to segments of the population who have the most difficulty with body temperature self-regulation including the very young (infants) and the elderly.

Risk factors for heatstroke include the use of medications that alter adrenergic activity and possibly decrease cardiac output (negative inotrope), such as tricyclic antidepressants (drugs whose names have the "-triptyline" suffix); beta-adrenergic antagonists, or beta blockers (drugs whose names have the "-lol" suffix); and vasoconstrictors, such as oral decongestants. The use of these products negates the body's normal attempts to decrease core temperature, such as increasing cardiac output and cutaneous vasodilation. Obesity limits the ability of the body to dissipate heat and is considered a heatstroke risk factor. In addition, as mentioned previously, extremes of age, very young or very old, with the associated difficulties in maintaining body temperature, increases heatstroke risk. Alcohol use also increases risk. Adequate hydration with nonalcoholic fluids, particularly water, coupled with dressing lightly helps to minimize heatstroke risk.

Individuals who participate in strenuous activity during hot weather should be warned about early heatstroke symptoms, such as extreme increase in heart rate, usually described as pounding; headache; and difficulty breathing. If any of these symptoms occur, the physical activity should be discontinued immediately, and the person should move to a shady location and drink cool water. If symptoms do not dissipate rapidly, help should be sought.

Assessment of a patient with heatstroke includes a complete evaluation of electrolytes, hematologic parameters, and liver enzymes. Total creatine kinase (CK) level is typically elevated, owing to skeletal muscle injured by muscle cramping and convulsion releasing this enzyme. Because of the release of this intracellular electrolyte with tissue damage, hyperkalemia is common; potentially life-threatening levels can be reached. Heatstroke can lead to a transient polycythemia caused by volume constriction, hyponatremia with Na^+ level of less than 120 mEq/L (<120 mmol/L), and stress-induced leukocytosis.

Intervention for a patient with heatstroke includes controlled cooling by the use of tepid sprays and fanning or by the application of cold packs to selected areas such as the axillae, neck, and groin. Rapid cooling by ice packing is discouraged because this can stimulate cutaneous vasoconstriction, inhibiting heat loss. Rehydration should be aggressive, but with careful monitoring because of the risk of pulmonary edema from reduced cardiac output.

Optimally, a patient with heatstroke should be admitted to the hospital for at least 24 hours after stabilization because of the risk of late complications, including one of the most feared complications: rhabdomyolysis, a condition of rapid muscle tissue destruction. As the muscle breaks down, large amounts of myoglobin and other cellular products are released into circulation to be excreted by the kidney. Renal hypoperfusion from low blood pressure is common. As a result, about 50% of patients with rhabdomyolysis develop acute renal failure. In heatstroke, the presence of myoglobinuria is an early indicator of rhabdomyolysis. Typically, the patient also complains of muscle pain and weakness. Treatment of rhabdomyolysis is aimed at treating the potentially life-threatening consequences, such as renal failure and profound hyperkalemia.

Discussion Sources

Centers for Disease Control and Prevention. http://www.bt.cdc.gov/disasters/extremeheat/heat_guide.asp, Extreme heat: a prevention guide to promote your personal health and safety, accessed 9/29/09.

Hellman R, Habal R. eMedicine. http://emedicine.medscape.com/article/166320-overview, Heatstroke, accessed 9/27/09.

QUESTIONS

42. A 62-year-old woman has hypertension, a 100–pack-year history of cigarette smoking, and peripheral vascular disease. Triglyceride level is 280 mg/dL (3.164 mmol/L), high-density lipoprotein (HDL) level is 38 mg/dL (1 mmol/L), and low-density lipoprotein (LDL) level is 135 mg/dL (3.5 mmol/L). Which of the following represents the most appropriate pharmacological intervention for this patient's lipid disorders?

   A. No further intervention is required.
   B. Multidrug therapy will likely be needed.
   C. A resin should be prescribed.
   D. The use of ezetimibe (Zetia) will likely be sufficient to achieve dyslipidemia control.

43. You examine a 46-year-old male smoker with hypertension. His lipid profile is as follows: HDL level is 48 mg/dL (1.24 mmol/L), LDL level is 192 mg/dL (4.9 mmol/L), and triglyceride level is 110 mg/dL (1.3 mmol/L). He had been on a low-cholesterol diet for 6 months when these tests were taken. Which of the following represents the best next step?

   A. No further intervention is required.
   B. A fibrate should be prescribed.
   C. A 3-hydroxy-3-methylglutaryl–coenzyme A (HMG-CoA) reductase inhibitor should be prescribed.
   D. A resin is the best choice of lipid-lowering agent for this patient.

44. You examine a 64-year-old man with hypertension and type 2 DM. Lipid profile results are as follows: HDL level is 38 mg/dL (1 mmol/), LDL level is 135 mg/dL (3.5 mmol/L), and triglyceride level is 180 mg/dL (1.9 mmol/L). His current medications include a sulfonylurea, a biguanide, an angiotensin-converting enzyme inhibitor, and a thiazide diuretic, and he has acceptable glycemic and blood pressure control. He states, "I really watch the fats and sugars in my diet." Which of the following is the most appropriate advice?

   A. No further intervention is needed.
   B. His lipid profile should be repeated in 6 months.
   C. Lipid-lowering drug therapy with a statin should be initiated.
   D. The patient's dietary intervention seems adequate.

45. When providing care for a patient taking an HMG-CoA reductase inhibitor, periodic monitoring of which of the following is recommended?

   A. potassium
   B. aspartate aminotransferase
   C. creatine kinase
   D. blood urea nitrogen

46. When prescribing a fibrate, the NP expects to see which of the following changes in lipid profile?

   A. marked decrease in LDL level
   B. increase in HDL level
   C. no effect on triglyceride level
   D. increase in very-low-density lipoprotein (VLDL) level

47. When prescribing niacin, the NP expects to see which of the following changes in lipid profile?

   A. marked decrease in LDL level
   B. increase in HDL level
   C. no effect on triglyceride level
   D. increase in VLDL level

48. In prescribing niacin therapy for a patient with hyperlipidemia, the NP considers that:

   A. postdose flushing is often reported.
   B. hepatic monitoring is not warranted.
   C. low-dose therapy is usually effective in increasing LDL level.
   D. drug-induced thrombocytopenia is a common problem.

49. With the use of ezetimibe (Zetia), the NP expects to see:

   A. a marked increase in HDL cholesterol.
   B. a reduction in LDL cholesterol.
   C. a significant reduction in triglyceride levels.
   D. increased rhabdomyolysis when the drug is used in conjunction with HMG-CoA reductase inhibitor.

50. With ezetimibe (Zetia), which of the following should be periodically monitored?

   A. ALP
   B. LDH
   C. CPK
   D. No special laboratory monitoring is recommended.

51. With the use of a lipid-lowering resin, which of the following enzymes should be periodically monitored?

   A. ALP
   B. LDH
   C. AST
   D. No particular monitoring is recommended.

52. All of the following are risks for statin-induced myositis except:

   A. advanced age.
   B. use of a statin with a resin.
   C. low body weight.
   D. high statin dose.

53. What is the average LDL reduction achieved with a change in diet as a single lifestyle modification?

   A. less than 5%
   B. 5% to 10%
   C. 11% to 15%
   D. 16% to 20% or more

54. You are seeing a patient who is taking atorvastatin and cholestyramine and provide the following advice:

   A. "Take both medications together."

   B. "You need to have extra blood tests while on this combination."

   C. "Separate the cholestyramine from other medications by at least 2 hours."

   D. "Make sure you take these medications on an empty stomach."

55. Which of the following medications is most effective against lipoprotein (a)?

   A. HMG-CoA reductase inhibitors

   B. niacin

   C. bile acid sequestrants

   D. fibrates

56. All of the following are common causes of secondary hypertriglyceridemia except:

   A. hypothyroidism.

   B. ACE inhibitor use.

   C. poorly controlled DM.

   D. excessive alcohol use.

57. Untreated hypothyroidism can result in which of the following changes in the lipid profile?

   A. increased HDL and decreased triglycerides

   B. increased LDL and total cholesterol

   C. increased LDL, total cholesterol, and triglycerides

   D. decreased LDL and HDL

58. Regular vigorous physical activity can yield which of the following changes in the lipid profile?

   A. increases HDL, lowers VLDL and triglycerides

   B. lowers VLDL and LDL

   C. increases HDL, lowers LDL

   D. lowers HDL, VLDL, and triglycerides

59. The most potent anticipated effect on the lipid profile with high-dose omega-3 fatty acid use includes:

   A. increase in HDL.

   B. decrease in LDL.

   C. decrease in total cholesterol.

   D. decrease in triglycerides.

60. The most potent anticipated effect on the lipid profile with plant stanol and sterol use includes:

   A. increase in HDL.

   B. decrease in LDL.

   C. decrease in total cholesterol.

   D. decrease in triglycerides.

61. For patients with documented coronary heart disease, the American Heart Association advises intake of approximately _____ of eicosapentaenoic acid (EPA) and docosahexaenoic acid (DHA) per day, preferably from oily fish.

   A. 500 mg

   B. 1 g

   C. 2 g

   D. 4 g

62. Which of the following statins has the greatest per milligram potency?

   A. fluvastatin

   B. atorvastatin

   C. simvastatin

   D. pravastatin

ANSWERS

42.	B	**43.**	C	**44.**	C
45.	B	**46.**	B	**47.**	B
48.	A	**49.**	B	**50.**	D
51.	D	**52.**	B	**53.**	B
54.	C	**55.**	B	**56.**	B
57.	C	**58.**	A	**59.**	D
60.	B	**61.**	B	**62.**	B

DISCUSSION

Treatment of hyperlipidemia is an important part of cardiovascular and cerebrovascular risk reduction. Intensive therapeutic lifestyle changes should be the first line of therapy. Dietary advice includes reducing saturated fat and cholesterol intake and adding dietary options to enhance LDL lowering, such as adding plant stanols and sterols and increasing intake of viscous or soluble fiber. Most adults achieve only a 5% to 10% reduction in LDL cholesterol with dietary advice as a single intervention. Weight management and a program of regular aerobic exercise should be prescribed for overall health. Dietary lipid improvement is often enhanced if coupled with exercise; because physical activity reduces insulin resistance, the anticipated improvement in the lipid profile includes an increase in HDL and reduction of triglycerides.

Pharmacological intervention in hyperlipidemia is likely to be needed in patients with considerable cardiovascular and cerebrovascular risk, including patients with DM, hypertension, and existing vascular disease. The choice of a lipid-lowering agent should be guided by the effect of the agent on the lipid profile and the desired lipid levels (Tables 10–8 and 10–9). Causes of secondary dyslipidemia should be considered and eliminated or minimized, usually through lifestyle intervention or treatment of the underlying cause, or both (Table 10–10).

TABLE 10–8

Effect of Medications on Lipid Levels

Medication	Effect	Comment
HMG-CoA reductase inhibitor (statin) Examples: Atorvastatin (Lipitor), simvastatin (Zocor), lovastatin (Mevacor), rosuvastatin (Crestor)	↓LDL: 18%–55% ↑HDL: 5%–15% ↓TG: 7%–30%	Small risk (≤0.5%) of hepatic enzyme increase with use. Check hepatic enzymes before initiation, periodically after initiation or dose adjustment as recommended in product information Consider checking creatine kinase (CK) at initiation to establish baseline. Ongoing CK evaluation in the absence of symptoms not warranted Adverse effects: Rhabdomyolysis, myositis, rare but most often noted with higher statin dose, in combination with fibrate, in renal impairment, multiple comorbidities, low body weight, advanced age
Resins (also known as bile acid sequestrants) Examples: Cholestyramine (Questran), colestipol (Colestid), colesevelam (WelChol)	↓LDL: 15%–30% ↑HDL: 3%–5%	Nonsystemic with no hepatic monitoring required Minimal effect on triglyceride (TG) with the exception of potential to increase TG if >400 mg/dL (>4.5 mmol/L) Adverse effects: Gastrointestinal distress, constipation, decreased absorption of other drugs if taken within 2 hr of many medications
Niacin (Niaspan, others)	↑HDL: 15%–35% ↓TG: 20%–50% ↓LDL: 5%–25%	Particularly effective against highly atherogenic lipoprotein (a) Adverse effect: Flushing (potentially minimized by taking aspirin 1 hr before niacin dose), hyperglycemia, hyperuricemia, upper gastrointestinal distress, hepatotoxicity
Fibric acid derivatives Examples: Gemfibrozil (Lopid), fenofibrate (TriCor, others)	↑HDL: 10%–20% ↓TG: 20%–50% ↓LDL: 5%–20% (with normal TG) May increase LDL-cholesterol (with high TG)	Contraindications: Active liver disease, severe gout, peptic ulcer Adverse effects: Dyspepsia, gallstones, myopathy including rhabdomyolysis if taken with a statin, in particular with gemfibrozil use, less risk with statin and fenofibrate use Contraindications: Severe renal or hepatic disease
Ezetimibe (Zetia)	↓LDL-C: 15%–20% ↑HDL-C: 3%–5%	Minimal effect on TG. Most often prescribed with another lipid-lowering agent such as a statin to enhance LDL reduction Adverse effects: Few because of limited systemic absorption

Source: Adult Treatment Panel III (ATP III) Guidelines. www.nhlbi.nih.gov/guidelines/cholesterol/index.htm, National Cholesterol Education Program Adult Treatment Panel III guidelines for lipid goals, accessed 9/26/09.

TABLE 10–9

Risk Categories That Modify Low-Density Lipoprotein (LDL)-Cholesterol Goals

Risk Categories	LDL Goal
CHD and CHD risk equivalents	<70–100 mg/dL (<1.18–2.6 mmol/L)
Multiple (>2) risk factors	<130 mg/dL (<3.36 mmol/L)
0–1 risk factor	<160 mg/dL (<4.4 mmol/L)

CHD, coronary heart disease.
From National Cholesterol Education Program Adult Treatment Panel III (ATP III) guidelines. www.nhlbi.nih.gov/ncep, accessed 9/29/09.

TABLE 10–10

Causes of Secondary Hyperlipidemia

Cause	Lipid Abnormality
Chronic inactivity	↓ HDL
Alcohol abuse	↑ TG, ↑ HDL, ↑ LDL
Type 2 diabetes mellitus associated with insulin resistance	↑ TG, ↓ HDL, ↑ TC
Undertreated or untreated hypothyroidism	↑ TG, ↑ TC, ↑ LDL
Higher dose thiazide diuretics	↑ TC, ↑ LDL, ↑ TG
Chronic renal insufficiency	↑ TC, ↑ TG

HDL, high-density lipoprotein; LDL, low-density lipoprotein; TC, total cholesterol; TG, triglyceride.

Discussion Sources

American Heart Association. http://www.americanheart.org/presenter.jhtml?identifier=4632, Fish oil and omega-3 fatty acids, accessed 9/25/09.

American Heart Association. http://circ.ahajournals.org/cgi/content/full/112/20/3184, Managing abnormal lipids: a collaborative approach, accessed 9/29/09.

Crouch M. Management of patient with dyslipoproteinemias (cholesterol and triglycerides disorders). In: Rakel R, Bope E, eds. *Conn's Current Therapy 2009.* Philadelphia, PA: Saunders Elsevier; 2009:601–606.

National Heart, Lung, and Blood Institute. www.nhlbi.nih.gov/guidelines/cholesterol/index.htm, Adult Treatment Panel III (ATP III) Guidelines: National Cholesterol Education Program Adult Treatment Panel III guidelines for lipid goals, accessed 9/18/09.

QUESTIONS

63. According to the ATP III guidelines, diagnosis of metabolic syndrome includes notation of:

    A. abdominal obesity.
    B. triglyceride level equal to or greater than 150 mg/dL ($\geq$1.7 mmol/L)
    C. HDL cholesterol level less than 40 mg/dL ($<$1.036 mmol/L) for men and less than 50 mg/dL ($<$1.295 mmol/L) for women.
    D. all of the above.

64. Which of the following characteristics applies to metabolic syndrome?

    A. IR is a common denominator in all individuals with the condition.
    B. Hypertension is an uncommon finding.
    C. Progression to type 2 DM occurs rapidly.
    D. Increased peripheral vascular resistance is uncommon.

65. Which of the following characteristics is not descriptive of plasminogen activator inhibitor?

    A. increased levels noted in atherosclerotic lesion
    B. produced by the pancreas
    C. inhibits fibrin degradation by plasmin
    D. enhances clot formation

66. When counseling obese patients, the clinician realizes that:

    A. a daily energy deficit of 500 to 1000 kcal/d leads to about a 1- to 2-lb (0.45- to 0.9-kg) weight loss per week.
    B. each 1 lb (0.45 kg) of body fat represents approximately 6000 stored calories.
    C. exercise enhances IR.
    D. thyroid dysfunction is found in most cases.

67. The International Diabetes Federation's diagnostic criteria for metabolic syndrome include:

    A. an obligatory finding of persistent hyperglycemia.
    B. notation of ethnic-specific waist circumference measurements.
    C. documentation of microalbuminuria.
    D. a family history of type 2 DM.

68. A 30-minute session of brisk walking can have an IR-modifying effect for up to:

    A. 12 hours.
    B. 24 hours.
    C. 36 hours.
    D. 48 hours.

69. Acanthosis nigricans is commonly noted in all of the following areas except:

    A. groin folds.
    B. axilla.
    C. nape of the neck.
    D. face.

70. Metformin has all of the following effects except:

    A. improved insulin-mediated glucose uptake.
    B. modest weight loss with initial use.
    C. enhanced fibrinolysis.
    D. increased LDL cholesterol production.

71. Cardiovascular effects of hyperinsulinemia include:

    A. decreased renal sodium reabsorption.
    B. constricted circulating volume.
    C. greater responsiveness to angiotensin II.
    D. diminished sympathetic activation.

72. Which of the following is an unlikely consequence of untreated metabolic syndrome and IR in a woman of reproductive age?

    A. hyperovulation
    B. irregular menses
    C. acne
    D. hirsutism

ANSWERS

63.	D	**64.**	A	**65.**	B
66.	A	**67.**	B	**68.**	D
69.	D	**70.**	D	**71.**	C
72.	A				

DISCUSSION

Synonymous with numerous other names, such as syndrome X, Reaven syndrome, the "deadly quartet," metabolic cardiovascular syndrome, atherothrombogenic syndrome, and cardiovascular dysmetabolic syndrome, the term metabolic syndrome is now most commonly used to describe a complex health problem that usually includes three or more of the following: obesity, blood pressure problems, dyslipidemia, and glucose intolerance (Table 10–11). Various definitions for metabolic syndrome have been offered by well-regarded groups, including the World Health Organization (WHO), the European Group for the Study of Insulin Resistance (EGIR), and U.S.-based Adult Treatment Panel III (ATP III). Although the definitions offered by these groups are similar, the nuanced differences in them have led to confusion, particularly when attempting to compare data from studies using different definitions. Also uncertain was which, if any, of the definitions best detected persons at risk of cardiovascular disease (CVD) and DM.

To facilitate the use of a single definition, the International Diabetes Federation (IDF) has issued a global consensus statement, proposing a consensus definition of metabolic syndrome that reflects input from experts on six continents in the fields of diabetes, cardiology, endocrinology, genetics, and nutrition. This definition blends criteria from WHO, EGIR, and ATP III. The IDF diagnostic criteria for metabolic syndrome closely resemble the current ATP III definition, but with stricter criteria for glucose intolerance and ethnic differences when defining central obesity; this definition does not include any measure of IR, and hyperglycemia is not an obligatory component, which sets it apart from the definitions offered by WHO and EGIR.

As mentioned, metabolic syndrome arises from numerous causes, including predetermined genetic factors, such as IR, and acquired or lifestyle characteristics, such as obesity, physical inactivity, and high-carbohydrate (>60% of total calories) diets. In IR, there is a reduced sensitivity in the tissues to insulin's action at a given concentration, which causes a subnormal effect on glucose metabolism. This effect results in

TABLE 10–11
Diagnostic Criteria for Metabolic Syndrome

World Health Organization	Adult Treatment Panel (ATP) III	International Diabetes Federation
Insulin resistance (type 2 diabetes mellitus or impaired fasting glucose) plus ≥2 of the following • Abdominal/central obesity defined as a waist-to-hip ratio >0.90 (men), >0.85 (women), or BMI >30 kg/m² • Hypertriglyceridemia ≥150 mg/dL (≥1.7 mmol/L) • Low HDL cholesterol <35 mg/dL (<0.9 mmol/L) for men, <39 mg/dL (<1 mmol/L) or women <40 mg/dL (<1.036 mmol/L) • High BP ≥140/90 mm Hg or documented use of antihypertensive therapy • Microalbuminuria with urinary albumin-to-creatinine ratio 30 mg/g, or albumin excretion rate 20 mcg/min	≥3 of the following • Waist circumference: >102 cm (>40 inches) in men, >88 cm (35 inches) in women • Hypertriglyceridemia ≥150 mg/dL (≥1.7 mmol/L) • Low HDL cholesterol <40 mg/dL (<1.036 mmol/L) for men, <50 mg/dL (<1.295 mmol/L) for women • BP ≥130/85 mm Hg or documented use of antihypertensive therapy • Fasting glucose ≥100 mg/dL (≥5.6 mmol/L)	Central obesity, defined as ethnic-specific waist circumference European, sub-Saharan African, Eastern Mediterranean, Middle Eastern (Arabic) ancestry • Men ≥94 cm (≥37 inches) • Women ≥80 cm (≥31.5 inches) South Asian, Chinese, ethnic South and Central American ancestry • Men ≥90 cm (≥35.5 inches) • Women ≥80 cm (≥31.5 inches) Japanese ancestry • Men ≥85 cm (≥33.5 inches) • Women ≥90 cm (≥35.5 inches) with ≥2 of the following • Abnormal triglycerides ≥150 mg/dL (≥1.7 mmol/L) • HDL-cholesterol <40 mg/dL (<1.04 mmol/L) in men, <50 mg/dL (<1.29 mmol/L) in women • BP ≥130 mm Hg systolic or ≥85 mm Hg diastolic or treatment of previously diagnosed hypertension • Fasting glucose ≥100 mg/dL (≥5.6 mmol/L) or previous diagnosis of type 2 diabetes or impaired glucose tolerance

BMI, body mass index; BP, blood pressure; HDL, high-density lipoprotein.

hyperglycemia, which stimulates pancreatic insulin production to reduce the blood glucose levels. Euglycemia occurs, albeit in the presence of hyperinsulinemia. High fasting insulin levels are noted to be an independent predictor for ischemic heart disease in men. Over time, usually many years, pancreatic beta cell deficiency generally occurs, resulting in impaired glucose tolerance, hyperglycemia, and subsequent type 2 DM with dyslipidemia and hypertension.

Although present in nearly all persons with type 2 DM, IR is also found in many people who never develop clinically evident glucose intolerance. Also, although this condition is more common and severe as weight increases, some persons with IR are of normal weight. Obesity dramatically increases the risk of diabetes, however, in a person with IR.

Numerous conditions are seen in conjunction with IR. Increased IR is inversely related to decreased urinary uric acid clearance; this leads to a dramatic increase in the rate of gout. Acanthosis nigricans, hyperpigmentation of the skin often in the neck and axilla, is also correlated with IR. This finding is most common in children and young adults with IR and DM risk and should alert the NP to work aggressively with such patients on developing or maintaining a healthy lifestyle. In addition, many women with polycystic ovary syndrome have IR. Intervention to minimize IR through lifestyle modification and the use of medications that enhance insulin sensitivity can modify this condition. The resumption of ovulation and enhanced fertility is often the end result. In addition, when IR is reduced, acne and hirsutism, usually a consequence of hyperandrogenism, are usually improved.

Although the correlation of obesity with IR and type 2 DM is well established, not all body fat types and distribution are equally problematic. "Apple-shaped" or central abdominal obesity comprises metabolically active fat and is associated with high insulin levels, IR, and high mobilization rate of free fatty acids; high insulin levels are often associated with increased appetite. This genetic makeup helped increase the likelihood of survival in times of famine. In these times of plentiful food, IR helps increase insulin levels, however, and promotes fat storage.

IR and resulting metabolic syndrome are now recognized as contributing to a prothrombotic and proatherogenic state. Plasminogen activator inhibitor, produced by the liver and endothelial cells, inhibits fibrin degradation by plasmin and enhances clot formation; increased levels are found in atherosclerotic lesions. High levels of triglyceride, VLDL, and oxidized LDL stimulate the production of plasminogen activator inhibitor. Plasminogen activator inhibitor levels are significantly correlated with increased body mass and high plasma insulin levels, whereas levels are reduced when endogenous insulin levels are reduced by exercise, weight loss, or insulin-sensitizing medications, such as metformin and thiazolidinediones.

The ADA guidelines for the diagnosis of DM include a plasma glucose level greater than 126 mg/dL (>7 mmol/L) after an 8-hour fast. Most people without IR or glucose intolerance have a fasting blood glucose level in the range of 70 to 100 mg/dL (3.9 to 5.6 mmol/L); however, seeing a gradual increase in a patient's glucose level over the years should be considered an early warning sign of metabolic syndrome and future DM type 2.

Hypertension is usually seen in a person with IR. In contributing to the development of increased blood pressure, hyperinsulinemia leads to increased renal sodium reabsorption, which potentially expands circulating volume and increases vascular resistance. Additional cardiovascular effects include increased vascular smooth muscle proliferation, greater responsiveness to angiotensin II, and greater sympathetic activation. Endothelial dysfunction is correlated with decreased nitric oxide production and peripheral vasoconstriction in the muscle tissue, which can potentially increase blood pressure. IR also contributes significantly to dyslipidemia; a person with persistent hypertriglyceridemia is likely to have significant IR.

A major goal of treating a person with metabolic syndrome is to work with the patient to minimize the core defect, IR. Cigarette smoking increases IR, as does inactivity and obesity. Conversely, most patients note an improvement in HDL cholesterol with smoking cessation and exercise. Also, the benefits of smoking cessation on lung and vascular health cannot be overstated. Because approximately 80% of the body's insulin-mediated glucose uptake occurs in muscle and is enhanced by physical activity, the positive effects of a program of regular aerobic exercise are significant. Exercise—20 to 30 minutes of brisk walking—reduces IR by approximately 40%, with the effects persisting for up to 48 hours after the activity. In addition, exercise aids in weight loss, reduces blood pressure, and improves lipid levels, modifying many metabolic component parameters. Regular aerobic physical activity is one of most effective therapies to help decrease IR and prevent the development of DM.

Weight loss improves insulin sensitivity and reduces blood pressure; improvement is not related to the degree of weight loss. Eating frequent, small, high-fiber meals and foods with a low glycemic index and smaller serving sizes should be encouraged. Dietary fat should be limited, but not eliminated, with emphasis on decreasing saturated fats, while using monounsaturated fat. A pound of fat contains approximately 3500 stored calories. A deficit of 500 to 1000 calories per day would lead to a 1- to 2-lb (0.45- to 0.9-kg) weight loss per week.

Many medications are now available for the treatment of IR and metabolic syndrome (see Table 10–7). Thiazolidinediones (pioglitazone, rosiglitazone) help improve insulin sensitivity and metabolic parameters such as lipids and blood pressure, and decrease intra-abdominal fat mass. These products should be prescribed only when cardiovascular risk is carefully considered; these medications should not be used in conjunction with insulin or nitrates. Metformin, a biguanide, improves insulin-mediated glucose uptake and metabolic parameters such as fibrinolysis. An increased body of knowledge demonstrates that metformin use in early metabolic syndrome can help in delaying the onset of type 2 DM. Insulin secretagogues such as a sulfonylurea or injectable insulin are likely to be needed as pancreatic insulin production wanes. Dyslipidemia and hypertension must be aggressively treated to minimize risk of cardiovascular disease. Daily aspirin use is recommended to counteract the proinflammatory and prothrombotic effects of IR.

Discussion Sources

American Diabetes Association Clinical Practice Recommendations. http://care.diabetesjournals.org/content/vol32/Supplement_1/, 2009, accessed 9/28/09.

Implementation Conference for AACE Outpatient Diabetes Mellitus Consensus Conference Recommendations. www.aace.com/pub/pdf/guidelines/OutpatientImplementation PositionStatement.pdf, Position statement, accessed 9/28/09.

International Diabetes Federation. http://www.idf.org/home/index.cfm?unode=32EF2063-B966-468F-928C-A5682A4E3910, A new worldwide definition of the metabolic syndrome, accessed 9/28/09.

National Heart, Lung, and Blood Institute. www.nhlbi.nih.gov/guidelines/cholesterol/index.htm, Adult Treatment Panel III (ATP III) Guidelines National Cholesterol Education Program Adult Treatment Panel III guidelines for lipid goals, accessed 9/28/09.

QUESTIONS

73. Obesity is usually defined as having a body mass index (BMI) equal to or greater than _____ kg/m².

   A. 25
   B. 30
   C. 35
   D. 40

74. An example of an appropriate question to pose to a person with obesity who is in the precontemplation stage is:

   A. "How do you feel about your weight?"
   B. "What are barriers you see to losing weight?"
   C. "What is your personal goal for weight loss?"
   D. "How do you envision my helping you meet your weight loss goal?"

75. An example of an appropriate question to pose to a person with obesity who is in the contemplation stage is:

   A. "How do you feel about your weight?"
   B. "What are barriers you see to losing weight?"
   C. "What is your personal goal for weight loss?"
   D. "How do you envision my helping you meet your weight loss goal?"

76. When advising a person who will be using orlistat (Xenical, Alli) as part of a weight loss program, the NP provides the following information about when to take the medication:

   A. within an hour of each meal that contains fat
   B. before any food with high carbohydrate content
   C. only in the morning, to avoid sleep disturbance
   D. up to 3 hours after any meal, regardless of types of food eaten

77. The action of which of the following is believed to be responsible for satiety?

   A. norepinephrine
   B. epinephrine
   C. dopamine
   D. serotonin

78. Potential adverse effects of sibutramine (Meridia) use include:

   A. bradycardia.
   B. somnolence.
   C. blood pressure increase.
   D. diarrhea.

79. In a person with obesity, weight loss of _____% or more yields an immediate reduction in death rates from cardiovascular and cerebrovascular disease.

   A. 5
   B. 10
   C. 15
   D. 20

80. When counseling about bariatric surgery, the NP provides the following information:

   A. Most people achieve ideal BMI postoperatively.
   B. The most dramatic weight losses are seen in the first few postoperative months.
   C. The death rate directly attributable to surgery is about 20%.
   D. Weight loss will continue for years postoperatively in most patients, unless a carefully planned refeeding diet is prescribed.

81. The use of which of the following medications is often associated with weight gain?

   A. risperidone (Risperdal)
   B. topiramate (Topamax)
   C. metformin (Glucophage)
   D. phentermine (Fastin)

82. The commonly recommended physical activity level of 8000 to 10,000 steps per day is roughly the equivalent of walking _____ miles.

   A. 1 to 2
   B. 2 to 3
   C. 3 to 4
   D. 4 to 5

ANSWERS

73.	B	74.	A	75.	B
76.	A	77.	D	78.	C
79.	B	80.	B	81.	A
82.	D				

DISCUSSION

Rates of obesity, usually defined as a body mass index (BMI) of 30 kg/m² or greater (Table 10–12), in North America are currently at record levels and are projected to double over the next 30 years; this mirrors the overall increase in overweight and obesity rates worldwide. Although no specific endocrine disorder, including thyroid dysfunction, is usually found in obese individuals, the cause of the overweight and obese condition is likely a combination of environmental, genetic, and behavioral influences. Consequences of overweight and obesity include increased risk of all-cause morbidity and mortality, greater health care cost, lower workforce productivity, and increased workplace absentee rates and employer costs. Direct health care cost increases related to obesity are attributable largely to well-known obesity-related disease, including gallbladder disease, coronary heart disease, DM, osteoarthritis, and dyslipidemia. Less commonly known consequences of obesity include an increase in certain cancers and sleep apnea risk, a reduction in fertility, and fatty liver. Less tangible are issues of social and workplace discrimination.

Often, persons who are overweight or obese assume that only dramatic weight loss can produce healthy results. In reality, a 10% body weight loss yields a nearly immediate improvement of death rates from heart disease and stroke. Clinical improvement in osteoarthritis and asthma symptoms and a reduction in sleep apnea symptoms are usually noted.

The NP is well situated to help a person with obesity. For a person who desires weight loss, a first step is the discussion of achievable, reasonable goals. A first step can be simply to help the person halt weight gain or to lose 5% to 10% of total body weight. Slow, steady weight loss usually leads to long-term health benefit and risk reduction. A pound of fat contains approximately 3500 stored calories. A deficit of 500 to 1000 calories per day would lead to a 1- to 2-lb (0.45- to 0.9-kg) weight loss per week. Physical activity is often the most difficult part of a comprehensive weight reduction program. The idea of a protracted walking or other exercise regimen is quite daunting for a person who is obese. Although 30 minutes or more of aerobic activity on 5 days or more per week is typically recommended, an exercise prescription of 3 to 5 minutes of increased physical activity five to six times per day would likely yield the same results and be much better tolerated. A pedometer can also be used to measure objectively the number of steps taken; the goal should be 8000 to 10,000 per day, or the equivalent of walking 4 to 5 miles. A pedometer is one method of quantifying how physically active in day-to-day behavior and deliberate exercise the person is.

A comprehensive approach to obesity treatment that includes behavior modification and pharmacotherapy that result in decreased food intake and increased energy expenditure can lead to long-term success. Asking about readiness for change at every clinical visit can help facilitate success (Table 10–13).

Pharmacotherapy is an important tool in weight management. Many antiobesity drugs are available. Orlistat (Xenical, Alli) is taken with meals and contributes to weight loss by reducing dietary fat absorption by approximately 30%. The fat passes undigested, and weight loss is facilitated. The medication is taken three times daily with or within 1 hour of a meal that contains fat. The most common adverse effect is gastrointestinal disturbance, including loose stools and oily anal seepage. Sibutramine (Meridia) acts in areas of the brain that control not only mood and sense of well-being, but also appetite by influencing levels of norepinephrine, serotonin, and, to a lesser extent, dopamine that are available to neurons by interfering with the reabsorption of these substances. 5-Hydroxytryptamine (serotonin) facilitates satiety; norepinephrine and dopamine inhibit feeding. The result is diminished appetite and reduced food intake. Adverse effects include dry mouth, constipation, disturbed sleep, and mildly increased blood pressure. Valvuloplasty, which was noted with dexfenfluramine (Redux; no longer

TABLE 10–12

Classification of Overweight and Obesity

Body Mass Index (kg/m²)	WHO Classification	CDC Description
<18.5	Underweight	Underweight
18.5–24.9		Healthy weight
25–29.9	Grade 1 overweight	Overweight
30–39.9	Grade 2 overweight	Obesity
≥40	Grade 3 overweight	Extremely obese

TABLE 10–13

Facilitating Change in the Care of a Person Who Is Overweight or Obese

Stage	Questions to Ask	As the Provider, You Can:
Precontemplation (not interested in change)	• How do you feel about your weight? • How does your weight affect you? • Are you considering/planning weight loss now? • On a scale of 0–10, how ready are you to start a weight loss program?	Validate and acknowledge • This will take working together but can be done. Restate position, leave the door open • It's up to you to make the decision to lose weight. I cannot do this for you, but I am here to help you.
Contemplation (thinking about change)	• What are the pros and cons of weight loss? • Where are you on the scale of 0–10 as far as ready? • What are barriers/supports you envision? • How do you view me as helping?	Praise and validate • I am happy that you want to deal with this issue and feel ready to do so. Try to shift decisional balance • I am here to help you and point you in the direction of other sources of support. Arrange follow-up
Preparation for change	• What is your usual food and activity pattern? • What is your personal goal for weight loss? • Health goal? • Cosmetic goal?	Help set small behavioral goal related to diet, physical activity Assist in compiling food and activity diaries Begin to negotiate goal weight Identify support system Help set a date to start
Making change Maintaining change Dealing with relapse	• How can I help? • What is getting in your way? • What is making this work?	Teach nutritional tactics to help control obesity • Learn energy values of different foods Monitor food consumption by keeping a food diary; reduce portion size Read and understand nutrition labels on foods • Learn new habits of food purchasing • Eliminate high-calorie foods from grocery list Limit fats and oils in cooking, recipes; high-calorie or "calorie-dense" foods Increase physical activity

Source: Center for Chronic Disease Prevention and Health Promotion. http://www.cdc.gov/nccdphp/dnpa/obesity/, Overweight and obesity, accessed 9/24/09.

available in North America) use, has not been noted with sibutramine. As with many other weight-loss medications, weight loss plateaus and then may slowly increase, particularly if lifestyle modification does not include increased activity and decreased caloric intake. Sympathomimetics such as dexamphetamine and phentermine (Fastin, others) work with norepinephrine and dopamine, reducing the appetite, with resulting reduction in food intake. Sleep disturbances and nervousness rank among the most adverse effects associated with the use of these medications.

The use of certain medications can promote weight gain. These medications include atypical or second generation antipsychotics (risperidone [Risperdal], olanzapine [Zyprexa], others), select antiepileptics (valproate [Depakote], carbamazepine [Tegretol], others), and corticosteroids (prednisone, methylprednisolone, others). The use of these medications is occasionally necessary in a person with obesity. The patient should be advised about the risk, and weight-controlling efforts would need to be increased.

Numerous surgical options are available for obesity intervention. The most common options include gastric bypass and adjustable laparoscopic band. The ideal candidate for a bariatric surgical procedure is a person with BMI equal to or greater than 40 or BMI equal to or greater than 35 who also has DM, hypertension, obstructive sleep apnea, cardiovascular disease, gastroesophageal reflux, degenerative joint disease, or fatty liver (steatohepatitis), in whom behavioral and pharmacological therapy has failed. Contraindications to bariatric surgery include untreated or unstable mental health conditions, active drug or alcohol abuse, poor adherence to advised health regimens, and concomitant health conditions that would pose significant operative risk. Roux-en-Y gastroplasty, or gastric bypass, is a common surgical procedure that results in weight loss through stomach restriction. An additional mechanism of weight loss with gastroplasty is that, as a result of surgical manipulation, food no longer passes over the duodenum, the part of the gastrointestinal tract where calories are normally absorbed. The adjustable laparoscopic band procedure is an intervention that does not lead to malabsorption because food still passes through the duodenum, but rather restricts the amount of calories that can be ingested. High-calorie soft or liquid foods, such as milkshakes and ice cream, can pass through the band, however, and the calories in these foods are absorbed.

A person considering bariatric surgery must have a realistic idea regarding the anticipated outcome. In a well-selected patient population, the average weight loss with the gastric band procedure is approximately 40% to 60% of excess body weight. With gastric bypass, the expected weight loss is approximately 70% to 80% of excess body weight. With either procedure, most of that weight is lost within the first 3 years after surgery, and the most dramatic weight losses are seen in the first months postoperatively. With either procedure, future weight regain can occur if recommended dietary and physical activity guidelines are not followed. About 80% of patients lose a great deal of weight without major complications and maintain this loss long-term. About 15% have a significant short-term problem after the surgery (e.g., reoperation, long hospital stay, insufficient weight loss, persistent gastrointestinal upset), but most do well in the long-term. About 5% have major unresolved problems over time, including, for some and rarely, death as a direct result of the surgery. With gastric bypass, expert consultation on micronutrient supplementation should be sought to avoid anemia and other health problems.

Discussion Sources

Center for Chronic Disease Prevention and Health Promotion. http://www.cdc.gov/nccdphp/dnpa/obesity/, Overweight and obesity, accessed 9/28/09.

Still C, Jensen G. Obesity. In: Rakel R, Bope E, eds. *Conn's Current Therapy 2009*. Philadelphia, PA: Saunders Elsevier; 2009:606–612.

QUESTIONS

83. Risk factors for acute pancreatitis include all of the following except:

    A. hypothyroidism.
    B. dyslipidemia.
    C. abdominal trauma.
    D. thiazide diuretic use.

84. A 38-year-old woman with a long-standing history of alcohol abuse presents with a 4-day history of a mid-abdominal ache that radiates through to the back, remains relatively constant, and has been accompanied by nausea and three episodes of vomiting. She has tried taking antacids without relief. Abdominal examination reveals slightly hyperactive bowel sounds with upper abdominal tenderness without localization or rebound. Her skin is cool and moist with a blood pressure of 90/72 mm Hg, pulse rate of 120 bpm, and respiratory rate of 24/min. The most likely diagnosis is:

    A. gastric ulcer.
    B. acute pancreatitis.
    C. acute alcohol poisoning.
    D. viral hepatitis.

85. Your next best action in caring for the patient in the previous question is to:

    A. refer to the acute care hospital for admission.
    B. attempt office hydration after administration of an analgesic agent.
    C. initiate therapy with ranitidine (Zantac) and an antacid.
    D. obtain serum electrolyte levels.

86. Which of the following statements is true when evaluating a patient with acute pancreatitis?

    A. Diagnosis can be made by clinical assessment alone.
    B. The pancreas can be clearly visualized by abdominal ultrasound.
    C. Measuring serum lipase level along with amylase level increases diagnostic specificity in acute pancreatitis.
    D. Hypocalcemia is a nearly universal finding.

87. In assessing a person with suspected pancreatic cancer, the clinician anticipates which of the following findings?

    A. palpable midline abdominal mass
    B. mid-epigastric pain that radiates to the mid-back or lower back region
    C. Cullen sign
    D. positive obturator and psoas signs

88. The clinical presentation of pancreatic cancer involving the head of the pancreas usually includes:

    A. jaundice.
    B. polycythemia.
    C. hematuria.
    D. hyperkalemia.

89. Which of the following is unlikely to be found in a person with pancreatic cancer?

    A. history of chronic pancreatitis
    B. lesion identified on abdominal CT
    C. normocytic, normochromic anemia
    D. elevation of amylase level

ANSWERS

83.	A	**84.**	B	**85.**	A
86.	C	**87.**	B	**88.**	A
89.	D				

DISCUSSION

TABLE 10–14

Lipase and Amylase Evaluation in Acute Pancreatitis

Amylase	Lipase

• In pancreatitis
  • Appears 2–12 hr after symptom onset
  • Back to normal within 7 days of pancreatitis resolution
• Amylase level >1000 U/L
  • 80% cholelithiasis diagnosis
  • 6% alcoholic pancreatitis diagnosis
	• In pancreatitis
	  • Appears 4–8 hr after symptom onset
	  • Peaks at 24 hr, decreases 8–14 days after pancreatitis resolution

• Nonpancreatic amylase sources
  • Salivary glands
  • Ovarian cysts
  • Ovarian tumors
  • Tubo-ovarian abscess
  • Ruptured ectopic pregnancy
  • Lung cancer
	• Nonpancreatic reasons for elevated lipase
	  • Renal failure
	  • Perforated duodenal ulcer
	  • Bowel obstruction
	  • Bowel infarction

Pancreatitis, characterized by an acute or chronic inflammation of the organ, is a potentially life-threatening condition. The most common risks for pancreatitis include gallstones (45%), excessive alcohol use (35%), and elevated triglyceride levels and idiopathic causes (20% combined). Although alcohol abuse is commonly thought of as being one of the most common contributing factors for the disease, a small percentage of people who are problem drinkers develop the condition; likely the etiology of pancreatitis is multifactorial. Binge drinkers are at risk; most alcohol-related acute pancreatitis occurs in people with a minimum of 5 to 7 years of heavy ethanol ingestion, with binge drinkers having much lower risk. Less common risk factors are use of opioids, corticosteroid use, and thiazide diuretics; viral infection; and blunt abdominal trauma.

In a patient with acute pancreatitis, serum amylase level is typically elevated. Because elevated amylase level is often found in many other conditions, including perforated duodenal ulcer and other surgical abdominal emergencies, concurrently measuring serum lipase level increases diagnostic specificity (Table 10–14). Abdominal ultrasound can assist in diagnosing contributing gallbladder disease; this study does not typically help with diagnosing acute or chronic pancreatitis because of limited views of the organ. Abdominal computed tomography (CT) scan usually provides a diagnostic view of the inflamed pancreas. With expert consultation, additional studies are occasionally obtained if the diagnosis is unclear.

Significant pain and volume constriction are common in patients with acute pancreatitis. Intervention includes parenteral hydration and analgesia and gut rest. Treatment of the underlying cause, such as gallbladder disease or hypertriglyceridemia, or discontinuation of the causative agent, such as alcohol, corticosteroids, or thiazide diuretics, is also indicated. The clinical course of pancreatitis can range from a self-limiting condition to life-threatening illness. The Ranson criteria (Table 10–15) are usually used in assessing severity of pancreatitis. When three or more criteria are found on clinical presentation, a severe clinical course can be predicted with significant risk for pancreatic necrosis.

Persons with pancreatic cancer most commonly present with abdominal pain, weight loss, anorexia, nausea, and vomiting. In addition, when the disease involves the head of the pancreas, jaundice is often present, but usually without localized right upper quadrant abdominal tenderness seen in hepatic and biliary disorders such as cholecystitis and acute hepatitis. Pancreatic cancer has high mortality rates because clinical presentation usually occurs with late disease and the spread of the cancer. Risk factors for pancreatic cancer include a history of chronic pancreatitis, tobacco use, and DM. About 5% of the time, a genetic factor contributes to the disease. About 40% of cases occur sporadically with no identifiable risk factors.

Abdominal CT scan is helpful in identifying pancreatic cancer. The usefulness of abdominal ultrasound is limited by the presence of intestinal gas. Normochromic, normocytic

TABLE 10–15

Ranson Criteria of Severity of Acute Pancreatitis

At Time of Patient Presentation	Development of the Following Within First 48 Hours Indicative of Worsening Prognosis
Age >55 yr	Hematocrit decrease >10%
WBC >16,000 mm³	Arterial PO_2 <60 mm Hg
Blood glucose >200 mg/ dL (>11.1 mmol/L)	Serum Ca^{++} <8 mg/dL
AST >250 U/L	Base deficit >4 mEq/L
LDH >350 IU/L	Estimate fluid sequestration of >6 L
	BUN increase >5 mg/ dL over admission value

No. Criteria	Mortality Rate per Ranson Criteria
0-2	1%
3-4	16%
5-6	40%
>6	100%

AST, aspartate aminotransferase; BUN, blood urea nitrogen; LDH, lactate dehydrogenase; WBC, white blood cell count.
Source: http://ncemi.org/shared/etools_c/etools_c.pl, Ranson's criteria for pancreatitis mortality prediction, accessed 9/29/09.

anemia is a common finding, as is elevated total and direct bilirubin and alkaline phosphatase. An elevation in amylase is an uncommon finding, unless concomitant pancreatitis is present.

Discussion Sources

Erickson R, Larson C, Shabahang C. eMedicine. http:// emedicine.medscape.com/article/280605, Pancreatic cancer, accessed 9/29/09.

Solorzano C, Prinz R. Acute and chronic pancreatitis. In: Rakel R, Bope E, eds. *Conn's Current Therapy 2009*. Philadelphia, PA: Saunders Elsevier; 2009:545–552.

QUESTIONS

90. Increased risk of thyroid disorder is found in individuals who are:
    A. obese.
    B. hypertensive.
    C. treated with corticosteroids.
    D. elderly.

91. Which of the following is most consistent with subclinical hypothyroidism?
    A. elevated free thyroxine (T_4) and thyroid-stimulating hormone (TSH) levels
    B. normal free T_4 and elevated TSH levels
    C. elevated TSH and low free T_4 levels
    D. low TSH and free T_4 levels

92. The most common cause of hypothyroidism is:
    A. primary pituitary failure.
    B. thyroid neoplasia.
    C. autoimmune thyroiditis.
    D. radioactive iodine exposure.

93. Which is most likely to be found in Graves disease?
    A. decreased free T_4 level
    B. decreased TSH level
    C. "cold spot" on thyroid scan
    D. solid lesion on thyroid ultrasound

94. Physical examination findings in patients with Graves disease include:
    A. muscle tenderness.
    B. coarse, dry skin.
    C. eyelid retraction.
    D. delayed relaxation phase of the patellar reflex.

95. The mechanism of action of radioactive iodine in the treatment of Graves disease is to:
    A. destroy the overactive thyroid tissue.
    B. reduce production of TSH.
    C. alter thyroid metabolic rate.
    D. relieve distress caused by increased thyroid size.

96. Which of the following medications is a helpful treatment option for relief of tremor and tachycardia seen with untreated hyperthyroidism?
    A. propranolol
    B. diazepam
    C. carbamazepine
    D. verapamil

97. In prescribing levothyroxine therapy for an elderly patient, which of the following statements is true?
    A. Elderly persons require a rapid initiation of T_4 therapy.
    B. TSH should be checked about 2 days after dosage adjustment.
    C. T_4 dose needed by elderly persons is 75% or less of that needed by younger adults.
    D. TSH should be suppressed to a nondetectable level.

98. Physical examination findings in hypothyroidism likely include:

   A. muscle tenderness.
   B. exophthalmos.
   C. smooth, silky skin.
   D. delayed relaxation phase of the deep tendon reflex.

99. In the report of a thyroid scan done on a 48-year-old woman with a thyroid mass, a "cold spot" is reported. This finding is most consistent with:

   A. autonomously functioning adenoma.
   B. Graves disease.
   C. Hashimoto disease.
   D. thyroid cyst.

100. Which of the following is likely to be found in a person with untreated hypothyroidism?

   A. hypokalemia
   B. hypernatremia
   C. hypertriglyceridemia
   D. microcytic anemia

101. The findings of a painless thyroid mass and TSH level of less than 0.1 IU/mL in a 35-year-old woman is most consistent with:

   A. autonomously functioning adenoma.
   B. Graves disease.
   C. Hashimoto disease.
   D. thyroid malignancy.

102. A fixed, painless thyroid mass accompanied by hoarseness and dysphagia should raise the suspicion of:

   A. autonomously functioning adenoma.
   B. Graves disease.
   C. Hashimoto disease.
   D. thyroid malignancy.

103. Which of the following is the most cost-effective method of distinguishing malignant from benign thyroid nodules preoperatively?

   A. ultrasound
   B. magnetic resonance imaging
   C. fine-needle aspiration biopsy
   D. radioactive iodine scan

104. Possible consequences of excessive levothyroxine use include:

   A. bone thinning.
   B. fatigue.
   C. renal impairment.
   D. constipation.

105. Optimally, at what interval should TSH be reassessed after a levothyroxine dosage is altered?

   A. 1 to 2 weeks
   B. 2 to 4 weeks
   C. 4 to 6 weeks
   D. 6 to 8 weeks

106. As part of an evaluation of a 3-cm, round, mobile thyroid mass, you obtain a thyroid ultrasound scan revealing a fluid-filled structure. The most likely diagnosis is:

   A. adenoma.
   B. thyroid cyst.
   C. multinodular goiter.
   D. vascular lesion.

107. Periodic monitoring for hypothyroidism is indicated in the presence of which of the following clinical conditions?

   A. digoxin use
   B. male gender
   C. Down syndrome
   D. alcoholism

108. to 124. Identify each of the following findings as associated with hyperthyroidism, hypothyroidism, or both.

____ 108. heat intolerance

____ 109. smooth, silky skin

____ 110. thin nails that break with ease

____ 111. frequent, low-volume, loose stools

____ 112. chilling easily, cold intolerance

____ 113. amenorrhea or low-volume menstrual flow

____ 114. coarse, dry skin

____ 115. menorrhagia

____ 116. hyperreflexia with a characteristic "quick out–quick back" action at the patellar reflex

____ 117. proximal muscle weakness

____ 118. tachycardia with hypertension

____ 119. hyporeflexia with a characteristic slow relaxation phase, the "hung-up" reflex

____ 120. coarse hair with tendency to break

____ 121. thick, dry nails

____ 122. constipation

____ 123. atypical presentation in an elderly person

____ 124. change in mental status

ANSWERS

90.	D	**91.**	B	**92.**	C	**93.**	B
94.	C	**95.**	A	**96.**	A	**97.**	C
98.	D	**99.**	D	**100.**	C	**101.**	A
102.	D	**103.**	C	**104.**	A	**105.**	D
106.	B	**107.**	C				

108.	Hyperthyroidism	**109.**	Hyperthyroidism
110.	Hyperthyroidism	**111.**	Hyperthyroidism
112.	Hypothyroidism	**113.**	Hyperthyroidism
114.	Hypothyroidism	**115.**	Hypothyroidism
116.	Hyperthyroidism	**117.**	Hyperthyroidism
118.	Hyperthyroidism	**119.**	Hypothyroidism
120.	Hypothyroidism	**121.**	Hypothyroidism
122.	Hypothyroidism	**123.**	Both
124.	Both		

DISCUSSION

Thyroid hormone is essential to normal body function because it assists cells in energy-releasing activities. When assessing a patient with thyroid dysfunction, the NP should look for signs of excessive energy release in hyperthyroidism or decreased energy release in hypothyroidism. Hyperthyroidism or hypothyroidism signs and symptoms often are present in the history and physical examination (Table 10–16).

Although thyroid disease likely exists in less than 7% of the population, a high index of suspicion should be maintained for individuals at particular risk. Risk factors and associated conditions include the following:
- Down syndrome: Hypothyroidism
- Elderly age: Hypothyroidism or hyperthyroidism with a high propensity for atypical presentation in either situation
- Use of certain medications causing an alteration in thyroid hormone synthesis (including lithium, amiodarone): Hypothyroidism
- Female gender: Hyperthyroidism or hypothyroidism; because most thyroid dysfunction is autoimmune in

TABLE 10–16

Comparison of Hyperthyroidism With Hypothyroidism

	Hyperthyroidism	Hypothyroidism
Characteristics	Excessive energy release, rapid cell turnover	Reduced energy release, slow cell turnover
Causes	Graves disease, thyroiditis, metabolically active thyroid nodule	Post-thyroiditis (>90%), primary pituitary failure (rare)
Neurological	Nervousness, irritability, memory problems	Lethargy, disinterest, memory problems
Weight	Weight loss (usually modest, present in ~50%)	Weight gain (usually 5–10 lb)
Environmental response	Heat intolerance	Chilling easily, cold intolerance
Skin	Smooth, silky skin	Coarse, dry skin
Hair	Fine hair with frequent loss	Thick, coarse hair with tendency to break
Nails	Thin nails that break with ease	Thick, dry nails
Gastrointestinal	Frequent, low-volume, loose stools, hyper-defecation	Constipation
Menstrual	Amenorrhea or low-volume menstrual flow	Menorrhagia
Reflexes	Hyperreflexia with a characteristic "quick out–quick back" action	Overall hyporeflexia with characteristic slow relaxation phase, the "hung-up" patellar deep tendon reflex
Muscle strength	Proximal muscle weakness	Usually no change
Cardiac	Tachycardia	Bradycardia in severe cases

nature, these diseases are more common in women than in men, as are most autoimmune diseases

- Postpartum period: A transient hypothyroidism is common, as is a transient thyroiditis
- Personal and family history of autoimmune disease, such as pernicious anemia, vitiligo, and type 1 DM: Hyperthyroidism and hypothyroidism
- History of head and neck irradiation or surgery: Hypothyroidism

Highly sensitive (89% to 95%) and specific (90% to 96%), the measurement of TSH is the most helpful thyroid test, particularly when diagnosing the condition in the outpatient setting. TSH is produced by the anterior pituitary gland, with secretion stimulated by thyrotropin-releasing hormone through a negative feedback loop in response to amount of circulating thyroid hormone (T_4). Because only a small fraction of T_4 circulates free, with 99.7% bound to T_4-binding globulin or other plasma proteins, the unbound portion of T_4, or free T_4, is metabolically active. The measurement of free T_4 is the most helpful test to confirm an abnormal TSH level. Approximately 40% of T_4 is converted in periphery to triiodothyronine (T_3). Compared with T_4, T_3 is likely four times more metabolically active; T_4 is often referred to as a prodrug for T_3.

Serum total T_4 is a commonly performed test to assess thyroid function. Numerous factors can cause an increase or decrease in total T_4, however, that is not indicative of a change in metabolic status. These factors include a change in thyroxine-binding globulin (TBG) levels, the principal carrier protein of T_3 and T_4. The use of certain medications, including exogenous estrogen (oral contraceptives, postmenopausal hormone therapy), opioids, and selective estrogen receptor modifiers (tamoxifen, raloxifene) can cause an alteration in TBG levels, resulting in an increase or decrease in total T_4 (the total of protein-bound and free T_4), but no change in the metabolically active free T_4; these results are metabolically insignificant. As a result, the clinical usefulness of total T_4 measurement is limited.

The likelihood of normal free T_4 if TSH level is normal is greater than 98%. In the small remainder, pituitary disorder is the likely cause. If the clinician suspects thyroid disorder, and TSH level is normal, it should be assumed that the hypothalamic-pituitary-thyroid axis is intact, with no further testing required. TSH level is increased in hypothyroidism; a 50% decrease in T_4 concentration can yield a 90-fold increase in TSH. Conversely, TSH level is decreased in hyperthyroidism. If TSH level is elevated, hypothyroidism should be confirmed by obtaining free T_4 level. If TSH is low or undetectable, hyperthyroidism should be confirmed with a measurement of free T_4.

Because thyroid disease can produce low-level symptoms attributed to other conditions, especially stress, fatigue, and a variety of self-limiting illnesses, the issue of routine testing for thyroid disorder with TSH has been long debated. Clinical Preventive Services Guidelines advise that there is insufficient evidence to recommend for or against routine screening for thyroid disease.

Chronic lymphocytic thyroiditis, also known as Hashimoto thyroiditis, is the most common inflammatory disease of the thyroid and the leading cause of hypothyroidism. This condition likely has a genetic predisposition as an inherited dominant trait and is often linked with other autoimmune disorders, such as systemic lupus erythematosus, pernicious anemia, rheumatoid arthritis, DM, and Sjögren syndrome. The condition is most often seen in women 30 to 50 years old; clinical presentation often includes a diffusely enlarged, firm thyroid with fine nodules, neck pain, and tightness. This Hashimoto goiter may regress over time; many individuals first present with the condition in the hypothyroid state, which necessitates the use of T_4 replacement in the form of levothyroxine (Levothroid, Levoxyl, Synthroid, Unithroid). Antimicrosomal thyroid antibodies, likely reflecting cell-mediated immunity, are found in nearly all patients with Hashimoto thyroiditis.

With an 8:1 female-to-male ratio, Graves disease is the most common form of thyrotoxicosis, or hyperthyroidism. The age at onset is usually 20 to 40 years, and there is a significant correlation with autoimmune diseases such as pernicious anemia, myasthenia gravis, and DM. Clinical presentation of Graves disease includes diffuse thyroid enlargement, exophthalmos, nervousness, tachycardia, and heat intolerance. Thyroid scan reveals a large "hot" (metabolically active) gland with heterogeneous uptake. Treatment of Graves disease includes the use of antithyroid preparations such as methimazole or propylthiouracil, with eventual use of radioactive iodine for thyroid abblation. Subsequent hypothyroidism is the norm, necessitating the use of levothyroxine.

Subclinical hypothyroidism is diagnosed based on the presence of an elevated TSH level and a normal free T_4 level in the absence of or with minimal symptoms. Given that fatigue, often reported by a person with untreated or undertreated hypothyroidism, is so common in this condition, mild hypothyroidism is likely a more appropriate term for this condition. Goiter, or chronic thyroid enlargement usually caused by hypertrophic or degenerative changes, is a common finding, but is also found in many individuals with normal thyroid function.

The prevalence of subclinical hypothyroidism varies by age and gender, and ranges from estimations of 1% to 10% of the overall population to 20% in women 60 years and older. In men 74 years and older, the prevalence has been reported as more than 15%. Most of these patients have TSH values of 5 to 10 mIU/L; 50% to 80% have evidence of antithyroid or antithyroperoxidase antibodies. The estimated prevalence of this disorder is about 7% in women and 3% in men among community-dwelling individuals 60 to 89 years old. There is a 2% to 5% likelihood of development of overt hypothyroidism per year if clinical findings are consistent with subclinical hypothyroidism.

The treatment of subclinical hypothyroidism is a matter of differing approaches; some authorities recommend levothyroxine therapy in the presence of antithyroid antibodies versus a watch-and-wait approach, with periodic TSH and free T_4 testing every 6 months. When TSH level increases to more than 10 mIU/L, even in the presence of a normal free T_4 level, a significant increase in LDL, increasing cardiovascular disease risk, is often noted, and levothyroxine therapy should be initiated. The American Association of Clinical Endocrinologists guidelines recommend treatment of patients with TSH greater than 5 mIU/L if the patient has a goiter, or if thyroid antibodies are present. The presence of symptoms compatible with hypothyroidism, infertility, pregnancy, or plans to become pregnant in the near future also favors treatment.

In the treatment of subclinical hypothyroidism, T_4 replacement is prescribed in the form of levothyroxine (Levothroid, Levoxyl, Synthroid, Unithroid). The anticipated dosage of thyroid replacement with levothyroxine for an adult with clinically detected hypothyroidism is 1.6 mcg/kg/d, based on ideal body weight; a lower dose is recommended for older adults. In the presence of subclinical hypothyroidism, a lower dose is often sufficient because some thyroid function remains. Over time, thyroid failure progresses, and the patient's levothyroxine requirement typically increases.

In the treatment of hypothyroidism, T_4 replacement is needed in the form of levothyroxine (Levothroid, Levoxyl, Synthroid, Unithroid). The anticipated dosage of thyroid replacement for an adult is 75 to 125 mcg of levothyroxine, or about 1.6 mcg/kg/d. For an elderly person, the anticipated dosage is 75% or less of the adult dosage. Because this drug has a long half-life, the effects of a dosage adjustment would not cause a change in TSH for approximately five to six drug half-lives, or about 6 to 8 weeks.

Thyroid hormone requirements tend to remain stable over time. Certain factors can influence thyroid hormone requirements, however. When levothyroxine is taken at the same time as iron, calcium, aluminum-containing antacids, or sucralfate, its absorption can be impaired; ingestion of these medications should be separated by several hours.

When levothyroxine is taken with rifampin, phenytoin, carbamazepine, and phenobarbital, its metabolism can be increased with resulting reduction of free T_4.

The evaluation of a palpable thyroid nodule presents a challenge. In the absence of hyperthyroidism symptoms, the presentations of benign and malignant thyroid lesions are typically the same; the risk that any thyroid nodule is malignant is about 5%. A history of head or neck irradiation, localized pain, dysphonia, hemoptysis, regional lymphadenopathy, or a hard fixed mass should raise suspicion. Initial testing for a person with a thyroid nodule should include obtaining a TSH measurement. A metabolically active or "hot" nodule has a low risk of malignancy and can cause a reduction in TSH production from the pituitary. A thyroid scan can identify areas of increased uptake. Fine needle aspiration biopsy is advised, regardless of TSH results, and is more helpful and cost-effective in arriving at a definitive diagnosis than ultrasound or thyroid scan. A properly performed fine needle aspiration biopsy has a false-negative rate of less than 5% and a false-positive rate of about 1%.

Discussion Sources

American Association of Clinical Endocrinologists. http://www.aace.com/pub/pdf/guidelines/hypo_hyper.pdf, Medical guidelines for clinical practice for the evaluation and treatment of hyperthyroidism and hypothyroidism, accessed 9/28/09.

American Association of Clinical Endocrinologists. http://www.aace.com/pub/pdf/guidelines/thyroid_carcinoma.pdf, Medical/surgical guidelines for clinical practice: management of thyroid carcinoma, accessed 9/29/09.

Cooper D. Subclinical hypothyroidism. *N Engl J Med.* 2001;345:260–265.

Prinz R, Chen E. Thyroid cancer. In: Rakel R, Bope E, eds. *Conn's Current Therapy 2009*. Philadelphia, PA: Saunders Elsevier; 2009:670–673.

Shimshi M, Davies T. Hypothyroidism. In: Rakel R, Bope E, eds. *Conn's Current Therapy 2009*. Philadelphia, PA: Saunders Elsevier; 2009:661–665.

Singer P. Hyperthyroidism. In: Rakel R, Bope E, eds. *Conn's Current Therapy 2009*. Philadelphia, PA: Saunders Elsevier; 2009:665–670.

11

Hematological and Immunological Disorders

QUESTIONS

1. Tom is a 19-year-old man who presents with sudden onset of edema of the lips and face and a sensation of "throat tightness and shortness of breath," after a bee sting. Physical examination reveals inspiratory and expiratory wheezing. Blood pressure is 78/44 mm Hg; heart rate is 102 bpm; respiratory rate is 24/min. His clinical presentation is most consistent with the diagnosis of:

   A. urticaria.
   B. angioedema.
   C. anaphylaxis.
   D. reactive airway disease.

2. Your priority in caring for Tom (question 1) is to:

   A. administer a rapidly acting antihistamine.
   B. ensure airway patency.
   C. initiate vasopressor therapy.
   D. increase circulating volume.

3. Which of the following food-based allergies is likely to be found in adults and children?

   A. milk
   B. egg
   C. soy
   D. peanut

4. A person with latex allergy also often has a cross-allergy to all of the following except:

   A. banana.
   B. avocado.
   C. kiwi.
   D. romaine lettuce.

5. The most common clinical manifestation of systemic anaphylaxis is usually:

   A. dizziness.
   B. airway obstruction.
   C. urticaria.
   D. gastrointestinal upset.

6. First-line drug intervention in the presence of anaphylaxis should be:

   A. oral diphenhydramine.
   B. nebulized albuterol.
   C. parenteral epinephrine
   D. oral prednisone.

ANSWERS

1.	C	2.	B	3.	D
4.	D	5.	C	6.	C

DISCUSSION

Anaphylaxis is an acute, life-threatening, systemic antibody-antigen reaction that is an example of a type I immune response or a hypersensitivity or allergic reaction. This type of reaction occurs after a person has been exposed to an allergen and has subsequently developed antibodies. Common allergens include insect venoms, latex, and certain medications. Food allergens that occur more commonly in children but are often absent in adulthood include egg, soy, milk, and wheat. Shellfish, fish, tree nuts, and peanut allergies tend to manifest in childhood and persist throughout the life span.

See full color images of this topic on DavisPlus at http://davisplus.fadavis.com | Keyword: Fitzgerald

The immunoglobulin E (IgE) antibodies that develop in response to allergen exposure occupy receptor sites on mast cells, causing a degradation of the mast cell and subsequent release of histamine, vasodilation, mucous gland stimulation, and tissue swelling. Type I hypersensitivity reactions are composed of two subgroups: atopy and anaphylaxis.

Atopy is a group of localized allergic reactions, including allergic rhinitis and eczema, that are bothersome but not life-threatening. Anaphylaxis is typically manifested as a systemic IgE-mediated reaction in response to exposure to an allergen. Anaphylaxis is characterized by widespread vasodilation, urticaria, and angioedema, often accompanied by bronchospasm, creating a life-threatening condition of airway obstruction coupled with circulatory collapse (Table 11–1). The first symptom is usually apprehension, followed by tingling sensation, palpitations, urticaria, and angioedema.

First-line intervention in anaphylaxis includes avoiding or discontinuing use of the offending agent, if possible (Table 11–2). Simultaneously, maintaining airway patency is the greatest priority. Maintaining adequate circulation is also critical. Angioedema and urticaria are subcutaneous anaphylactic reactions that are not life-threatening unless tissue swelling impinges on the airway. Epinephrine must be administered promptly, usually along with a systemic antihistamine such as diphenhydramine (Benadryl). A person who is having an anaphylactic reaction should be observed for many hours after the event, even if signs and symptoms resolved with initial treatment; a late phase reaction is a common occurrence, necessitating repeat treatment. A person with a history of anaphylaxis should

be instructed on the use of an epinephrine self-injector such as EpiPen or Twinject; this should be kept with the person at all times. Education about avoiding the provoking agent is key.

Discussion Source

American Academy of Immunology Joint Task Force on Practice Parameters. www.aaaai.org/professionals/resources/pdf/anaphylaxis_2005.pdf, The diagnosis and management of anaphylaxis: an updated practice parameter, accessed 9/30/09.

TABLE 11–1

Clinical Manifestations of Anaphylaxis

Although urticaria and angioedema are most consistently reported, the clinical presentation of anaphylaxis can be quite variable

Urticaria	Angioedema
Upper airway edema	Flush
Dyspnea and wheezing	Dizziness and syncope
Hypotension	Gastrointestinal symptoms
Headache	Substernal pain
Itch without rash	Seizure

Source: www.anaphylaxis.com, www.aaaai.org/professionals/resources/pdf/anaphylaxis_2005.pdf, accessed 9/30/09.

TABLE 11–2

Treatment of Anaphylaxis in Patient with Currently Patent Airway

Intervention	Comment
Immediate administration of epinephrine SC or IM	No contraindications to epinephrine use in anaphylaxis
	Failure to or delay in use associated with fatalities
Administer antihistamine such as diphenhydramine (Benadryl)	Important part of anaphylaxis treatment, but should be used with, not instead of, epinephrine
Additional measures as dictated by patient response	Airway maintenance including supplemental oxygen
	IV fluids, vasopressor therapy
	Systemic corticosteroids
	Repeat epinephrine every 5 min if symptoms persist or increase
	Repeat antihistamine with or without H_2 blocker if symptoms persist
	Observe as dictated by patient response, recalling that anaphylaxis reactions often have a protracted or biphasic response
Arrange follow-up care	Provide instruction on avoidance of provoking agent
	Give EpiPen or Twinject with appropriate education about indications and safety of use

SC, subcutaneous; IM, intramuscular
Source: www.anaphylaxis.com, www.aaaai.org/professionals/resources/pdf/anaphylaxis_2005.pdf, accessed 9/30/09.

QUESTIONS

7. Worldwide, which of the following is the most common type of anemia?

    A. pernicious anemia
    B. folate-deficiency anemia
    C. anemia of chronic disease
    D. iron-deficiency anemia

8. Most of the body's iron is obtained from:

    A. animal-based food sources.
    B. recycled iron content from aged red blood cells (RBCs).
    C. endoplasmic reticulum production.
    D. vegetable-based food sources.

9. Which of the following is most consistent with iron-deficiency anemia?

    A. low mean corpuscular volume (MCV), normal mean corpuscular hemoglobin (MCH)
    B. low MCV, low MCH
    C. low MCV, elevated MCH
    D. normal MCV, normal MCH

10. One of the earliest laboratory markers in iron-deficiency anemia is:

    A. an increase in RBC distribution width (RDW).
    B. a reduced hemoglobin level.
    C. a low MCH level.
    D. an increased platelet count.

11. A 48-year-old woman developed iron-deficiency anemia after excessive perimenopausal bleeding, successfully treated by endometrial ablation. Her hematocrit (Hct) level is 25%, and she is taking iron therapy. At 5 days into therapy, you expect to find:

    A. a correction of mean cell volume.
    B. a 10% increase in Hct level.
    C. brisk reticulocytosis.
    D. a normal ferritin level.

12. A healthy 34-year-old man asks whether he should take an iron supplement. You respond that:

    A. this is a prudent measure to ensure health.
    B. iron-deficiency anemia is a common problem in men of his age.
    C. use of an iron supplement in the absence of a documented deficiency can lead to iatrogenic iron overload.
    D. excess iron is easily excreted.

13. Which of the following is the best advice on taking ferrous sulfate to enhance iron absorption?

    A. "Take with other medications."
    B. "Take on a full stomach."
    C. "Take on an empty stomach."
    D. "Do not take with vitamin C."

14. A 40-year-old woman with pyelonephritis who is taking ciprofloxacin and is being treated for iron-deficiency anemia with ferrous sulfate asks about taking both medications. You advise that:

    A. she should take the medications with a large glass of water.
    B. an inactive drug compound is potentially formed if the two medications are taken together.
    C. she can take the medications together to enhance adherence to therapy.
    D. the ferrous sulfate potentially slows gastrointestinal motility and results in enhanced ciprofloxacin absorption.

15. One month into therapy for pernicious anemia, you wish to check the efficacy of the intervention. The best laboratory test to order at this point is a:

    A. Schilling test.
    B. hemoglobin measurement.
    C. reticulocyte count.
    D. serum ferritin.

16. A woman who is planning a pregnancy should increase her intake of which of the following to minimize the risk of neural tube defect in the fetus?

    A. iron
    B. niacin
    C. folic acid
    D. vitamin C

17. Risk factors for folate-deficiency anemia include:

    A. menorrhagia.
    B. chronic ingestion of overcooked foods.
    C. use of nonsteroidal anti-inflammatory drugs.
    D. gastric atrophy.

18. Folate-deficiency anemia causes which of the following changes in the RBC indices?

    A. microcytic, normochromic
    B. normocytic, normochromic
    C. microcytic, hypochromic
    D. macrocytic, normochromic

19. Pernicious anemia is usually caused by:

    A. dietary deficiency of vitamin B_{12}.
    B. lack of production of intrinsic factor by the gastric mucosa.
    C. RBC enzyme deficiency.
    D. a combination of micronutrient deficiencies caused by malabsorption.

20. Pernicious anemia causes which of the following changes in the RBC indices?

    A. microcytic, normochromic
    B. normocytic, normochromic
    C. microcytic, hypochromic
    D. macrocytic, normochromic

21. Common physical examination findings in patients with pernicious anemia include:

    A. hypoactive bowel sounds.
    B. stocking-glove neuropathy.
    C. thin, spoon-shaped nails.
    D. retinal hemorrhages.

22. You examine a 47-year-old man with the following results on hemogram:
    Hemoglobin (Hgb) = 15 g
    Hct = 45%
    MCV = 108 fL
    These values are most consistent with:

    A. pernicious anemia.
    B. alcohol abuse.
    C. thalassemia minor.
    D. Fanconi disease.

23. You examine a 22-year-old woman of Asian ancestry. She has no presenting complaint. Hemogram results are as follows: Hgb 9.1 g (normal 12 to 14 g); Hct 28% (normal 36% to 42%); RBC 5 million (normal 3.2 to 4.3 million); MCV 68 fL (normal 80 to 96 fL); RBC distribution width (RDW) 13% (normal <15%). The most likely diagnosis is:

    A. iron-deficiency anemia.
    B. Cooley anemia.
    C. alpha-thalassemia minor.
    D. hemoglobin Bart.

24. A 68-year-old man is usually healthy, but presents with new onset of "huffing and puffing" with exercise. Physical examination reveals conjunctiva pallor and a hemic murmur. Hgb is 7.6 g; MCV is 71 fL. The most likely clinical problem is:

    A. poor nutrition.
    B. occult blood loss.
    C. malabsorption.
    D. microcytosis.

25. You examine a 57-year-old woman with rheumatoid arthritis and find the following results on hemogram:
    Hgb = 10.5 g
    Hct = 33%
    MCV = 88 fL
    The laboratory findings are most consistent with:

    A. pernicious anemia.
    B. anemia of chronic disease.
    C. beta-thalassemia minor.
    D. folate-deficiency anemia.

26. You examine a 27-year-old woman with menorrhagia and note the following results on hemogram:
    Hgb = 10.1 g
    Hct = 33%
    MCV = 72 fL
    Physical examination is likely to include:

    A. conjunctiva pallor.
    B. hemic murmur.
    C. tachycardia.
    D. no specific anemia-related findings.

27. Results of hemogram in anemia of chronic disease include:

    A. microcytosis.
    B. anisocytosis.
    C. reticulocytopenia.
    D. macrocytosis.

28. When prescribing erythropoietin supplementation, the NP considers that:

    A. the adrenal glands are its endogenous source.
    B. the addition of iron and other micronutrient supplementation is advisable.
    C. its use is as an adjunct in treating thrombocytopenia.
    D. with its use, the RBC life span is prolonged.

29. In the first weeks of pernicious anemia therapy with parenteral vitamin B_{12} in a 68-year-old woman, the patient should be carefully monitored for:

    A. hypernatremia.
    B. dehydration.
    C. hypokalemia.
    D. acidemia.

30. Which of the following conditions is unlikely to result in anemia of chronic disease?

    A. rheumatoid arthritis
    B. peripheral vascular disease
    C. chronic renal insufficiency
    D. chronic osteomyelitis

31. In health, the ratio of hemoglobin to hematocrit is usually:

A. 1:1.
B. 1:2.
C. 1:3.
D. 1:4.

ANSWERS

7.	D	8.	B	9.	B	10.	A
11.	C	12.	C	13.	C	14.	B
15.	B	16.	C	17.	B	18.	D
19.	B	20.	D	21.	B	22.	B
23.	C	24.	B	25.	B	26.	D
27.	C	28.	B	29.	C	30.	B
31.	C						

DISCUSSION

Anemia is defined as a decrease in the oxygen-carrying capability of the blood. This condition is not a disease, but rather a sign of an underlying process. Anemia occurs only in the presence of a clinical insult severe enough to disturb the normal hematological homeostatic mechanisms and exceed the body's ample hematological reserves.

The clinical presentation of anemia is highly variable, and compensation is common because most anemias are usually gradual in onset. In addition, the oxyhemoglobin-dissociation curve is moved to the right as the hemoglobin level decreases, with the oxygen molecule given up more freely by the RBC. As a result, symptoms of anemia seldom occur, unless the hemoglobin level decreases to less than 10 g/dL.

The health history usually reveals clues about the cause of the anemia (i.e., excessive menstrual flow, acute blood loss). Patients frequently report deep, sighing respiration with activity, often associated with a sensation of rapid, forceful heart rate; this is likely a reflection of the decreased oxygen-carrying capability of the blood and a corresponding compensatory mechanism. Fatigue and headache also may be present. In patients at risk for or who have coronary artery disease, anginal symptoms are commonly reported.

The physical examination usually contributes little to the diagnosis, unless the anemia is severe. Pallor of the skin and mucous membranes is an unreliable indicator and is usually seen only when the hemoglobin is less than 8 g/dL. In elderly persons and in individuals with coronary artery disease, signs of heart failure (i.e., distended neck veins, rales, tachycardia, right upper quadrant abdominal tenderness, hepatomegaly) may be seen with severe anemia. An early systolic murmur, also known as a hemic murmur, is often heard, owing in part to the increase in blood flow over the heart valves. Neurological findings, such as paresthesia, stocking-glove neuropathy, difficulty with balance, and, in extreme cases, confusion, can be found in patients with vitamin B_{12} deficiency or folate-deficiency anemia.

In evaluating the hemograms of patients with anemia, the following questions should be answered to ascertain the origin of the anemia (Table 11–3).

- What are hemoglobin (hgb), hematocrit (hct), and red blood cell (RBC) values? These values should be proportionately decreased. Normally, the hemoglobin-to-hematocrit ratio is 1:3, so that in health, 1 g of hemoglobin is equivalent to 3% points of hematocrit. The hematocrit value reflects the percentage of RBCs in a given volume of blood; the value is influenced by the body's hydration status. This ratio is usually violated only in severe dehydration, where the hematocrit is artificially elevated (e.g., hgb 12 g, hct 39%), or overhydration, where the hematocrit is artificially decreased (e.g., hgb 12 g, hct 32%).
- What is the cell size? Is the RBC abnormally small (microcytic or low MCV)? Because hemoglobin is a major contributor to cell size, microcytosis is usually seen in patients with anemia in whom hemoglobin synthesis is impaired, such as in patients with iron-deficiency anemia and thalassemias. In addition, because hemoglobin gives RBCs their characteristic red color, small (microcytic) and pale (hypochromic) go together. A microcytic cell is also hypochromic (low mean hemoglobin concentration).
- Is the RBC abnormally large (macrocytic)? Impaired RNA and DNA synthesis in young erythrocytes most commonly cause macrocytosis. Folic acid and vitamin B_{12} contribute significantly to RNA and DNA synthesis in the developing RBC. A lack of either or both of these micronutrients can result in macrocytic anemia. Because hemoglobin synthesis is not the issue, macrocytic cells are usually of normal color (normochromic).
- Is the RBC of normal size (normocytic)? In these anemias, the cells are made under ordinary conditions with sufficient hemoglobin; there is no problem with RNA, DNA, or hemoglobin synthesis. Acute blood loss and anemia of chronic disease result in a normocytic, normochromic anemia.
- What is the RDW? RDW reflects the degree of variation in RBC size; this is often reported as anisocytosis on RBC morphologic study. RDW measurement is elevated when RBCs are of varying sizes, which implies that cells were synthesized under varying conditions. In iron-deficiency anemia, normal-sized cells produced before iron depletion continue to circulate until their 90- to 120-day life span ends. Meanwhile, new, microcytic, iron-deficient cells containing less hemoglobin are produced. There is wide variation in cell size (newer cells are smaller, and older cells are larger) and an increase in RDW. Because minor variation in cell size is normal, RDW is considered increased only when it is greater than 15%. An elevated RDW is often the first abnormal finding in the hemogram of a person with an evolving microcytic or macrocytic anemia.

TABLE 11–3

Identifying Common Anemias

Anemia Type	Description	Example
Normocytic (MCV 80–96 fL), normochromic anemia with normal RDW Most common etiology: Acute blood loss or anemia of chronic disease	Cells made under ordinary conditions with sufficient hemoglobin. This yields cells that are normal size (normocytic), normal color (normochromic), and about the same size (normal RDW)	72 y.o. man with an acute gastro-intestinal bleed 32 y.o. woman with newly diag-nosed lupus erythematosus Hgb 10.1 g (12–14 g) Hct 32% (36%–43%) RBC 3.2 million (4.2–5.4 million) MCV 82 fL (81–96 fL) MCHC 34.8 g/dL (31–37 g/dL) RDW 12.1% (11.5%–15%)
Microcytic (MCV <80 fL) hypochromic anemia with elevated RDW Most common etiology: Iron-deficiency anemia	Small cell (microcytic) owing to insuf-ficient hemoglobin (hypochromic) with new cells smaller than old cells (elevated RDW)	68 y.o. man with erosive gastritis Hgb 10.1 g (12–14 g) Hct 32% (36%–43%) RBC 3.2 million (4.2–5.4 million) MCV 72 fL (81–96 fL) MCHC 26.8 g/dL (31–37 g/dL) RDW 18.1% (11.5%–15%)
Microcytic (MCV <80 fL) hypochromic anemia with normal RDW Most common etiology: Alpha or beta thalassemia minor At-risk ethnic groups for alpha tha-lassemia minor: Asian, African ancestry At-risk ethnic groups for beta thalassemia minor: African, Middle Eastern, Mediterranean ancestry	Through genetic variation, small (microcytic), pale (hypochromic) cells that are all around the same size (normal RDW)	27 y.o. man of African ancestry Hgb 11.6 g (14–16 g) Hct 36.7% (42%–48%) RBC 6.38 million (4.7–6.10 million) MCV 69.5 fL (81–99 fL) MCH 22 pg (27–33 pg) RDW 13.8% (11.5%–15%)
Macrocytic (MCV >96 fL) normochromic anemia with elevated RDW Most common etiology: Vitamin B₁₂ deficiency, pernicious anemia, folate-deficiency anemia	Abnormally large (macrocytic) cell owing to altered RNA:DNA ratio, hemoglobin content normal (normochromic), new cells larger than old cells (elevated RDW)	52 y.o. woman with untreated pernicious anemia Hgb 10.2 g (12–14 g) Hct 32% (36%–43%) RBC 3.2 million (4.2–5.4 million) MCV 125.5 fL (81–99 fL) MCH 31 pg (27–33 pg) RDW 18.8% (11.5%–15%)
Drug-induced macrocytosis usually without anemia Etiology: Use of medications such as carbamazepine (Tegretol), zidovudine (AZT), valproic acid (Depakote), phenytoin (Dilantin), alcohol, others. Reversible when use of offending medication is discontinued	Abnormally large (macrocytic) cell owing to altered RNA:DNA ratio, hemoglobin content normal (normochromic), new cells usually same size as old cells (normal RDW)	32 y.o. woman who is taking phenytoin Hgb 12 g (12–14 g) Hct 37% (36%–43%) RBC 4.2 million (4.2–5.4 million) MCV 105.5 fL (81–99 fL) MCH 31 pg (27–33 pg) RDW 12.8% (11.5%–15%)

- What is the hemoglobin content (color) of the cell? The hemoglobin content of the cell is reflected in the MCH, reported as a percentage of the cell's volume. Because hemo-globin gives RBCs their characteristic red color, the suffix "-chromic" is used to describe the MCH. When a cell has a normal MCH, it is of normal color, or normochromic. When there is an impairment of hemoglobin synthesis, such as in iron-deficiency anemia or thalassemia, the cells are pale or hypochromic, and the MCH is low. RBCs seldom are hyper-chromic, or containing excessive amounts of hemoglobin.

- What is the reticulocyte production index (RPI)? The body's normal response to anemia is to increase reticulocyte production to increase the hemoglobin level. An increase in the reticulocyte count, known as reticulocytosis, is an expected normal response to a decrease in hemoglobin; if it is absent, impaired marrow function or lack of erythropoietin stimulus should be suspected. RPI is an indicator of how rapidly new RBCs are produced and mature; RPI is calculated as the reticulocyte percentage (corrected) divided by correction factor (Fig. 11–1). RPI greater than 3 indicates adequate hematological and bone marrow responses to the anemia, whereas RPI less than 2 indicates inadequate response.

Worldwide, iron deficiency is the most common reason for anemia. Because an estimated 8 years of poor iron intake is needed in adults before iron-deficiency anemia occurs, diet is rarely the etiology. Chronic blood loss causing a wasting of the RBCs' recyclable iron, the body's most important iron source, is the most common cause. Occult gastrointestinal blood loss, such as from an oozing gastritis or gastrointestinal malignancy, is a common cause, as is excessive menstrual flow.

Men and postmenopausal women require 1 mg of iron each day. During reproductive years, women require 1.5 to 3 mg/d of iron, in part because of the monthly loss of RBCs with the menses. In all these circumstances, these iron requirements are achievable with a well-balanced diet. Because 1 mL of packed RBCs contains 1 mg of iron, losses of 2 to 3 mL of blood per day through chronic, low gastrointestinal bleeding or repeated phlebotomy can lead to iron deficiency.

The laboratory diagnosis of iron-deficiency anemia is supported by the following findings (Table 11–4):
- Early disease: Low to normal hgb, low hct, and low total RBC count; normocytic, possible hypochromic; RDW greater than 15%.
- Later disease: Microcytic, hypochromic anemia with low RBC count and elevated RDW greater than 15%.
- Low serum iron level: Reflecting iron concentration in circulation. Serum iron is reflective of iron intake during the past 24 to 48 hours and can be falsely elevated because of recent high levels of dietary iron ingestion or self-prescribed oral iron supplementation.
- Elevated total iron-binding capacity (TIBC): A measure of transferrin, a plasma protein that easily combines with

iron. When more of transferrin is available for binding, the TIBC level increases, reflecting iron deficiency.
- Iron saturation less than 15%: Calculated by dividing the serum iron level by the TIBC.
- Low serum ferritin level: The body's major iron storage protein.
- Absence of iron from bone marrow, if aspiration is done.

In iron-deficiency anemia, the order of the laboratory markers is as follows:
- Ferritin (decrease)
- Iron in marrow (absent)
- Serum iron (decrease)
- RDW (increase)
- TIBC (increase)
- Hemoglobin (decrease)
- RBC indices (decrease)

A decrease in hemoglobin or RBC indices is a late rather than an early marker of disease. Therapy for patients with iron-deficiency anemia involves not only iron replacement, but also treatment of the underlying cause. Drug interactions are common (Table 11–5).

Iron use without a distinct clinical indication, including the use of iron-fortified multiple vitamins, is not recommended because this can lead to an iatrogenic iron overload. Iron overload has been hypothesized to be a cardiovascular risk factor. A lower rate of cardiovascular disease has been noted in frequent blood donors with relatively low levels of stored iron compared with age-matched controls. In addition, cardiovascular disease rates in women equal rates in men 5 to 10 years after menopause, a time when ferritin levels in women and men are equal.

Reticulocytosis begins quickly after initiation of iron therapy, with the reticulocyte count peaking 7 to 10 days into therapy. Hemoglobin increases at a rate of 2 g/dL every 3 weeks in response to iron therapy and is likely to take 2 months to correct if the underlying cause of the anemia has been successfully treated. As a result, the following laboratory tests may be used to evaluate the resolution of iron-deficiency anemia: reticulocytes at 1 to 2 weeks to ensure marrow response to iron therapy, hemoglobin at 6 weeks to 2 months to ensure anemia recovery, and ferritin at 2 months after measure of normal hemoglobin (or 4 months after initiation of iron therapy) to ensure documentation of replenished iron stores.

Folic acid (pteroylglutamic acid) is a water-soluble B complex vitamin found in abundance in peanuts, fruits, and vegetables. Through a complex reaction, folic acid is reduced to folate. Folate donates 1 carbon unit to oxidation at various levels, reactions vital to proper DNA synthesis. During times of accelerated tissue growth and repair, such as in childhood, pregnancy, recovery from serious illness, and recovery from hemolytic anemia, folic acid requirements increase from the baseline of twofold to fourfold. Folate deficiency causes a macrocytic, normochromic anemia.

The most common causes of folic acid–deficiency anemia are inadequate dietary intake, seen in elderly, alcoholic, and

Correction factor table for calculating reticulocyte production index

Patient's hct (%)	Correction factor
40–45	1.0
35–39	1.5
25–34	2.0
15–24	2.5
<15	3.0

Figure 11–1 Correction table for calculating reticulocyte production index (RPI).

TABLE 11–4
Hemogram Evaluation in Anemia

Laboratory Parameter	Comment
What are hgb and hct, RBC values?	Values should be proportionately decreased. Normally, hgb:hct ratio 1:3 • 10 g 30% • 12 g 36% • 15 g 45%
What is the RBC size?	Wintrobe's classification of anemia by evaluation of mean corpuscle volume (MCV) • Microcytic: Small cell with MCV <80 fL • Normocytic: Normal size cell with MCV 80–96 fL • Macrocytic: Abnormally large cell with MCV >96 fL
What is the RBC's hemoglobin content?	Reflected by mean cell hemoglobin (MCH), mean cell hemoglobin concentration (MCHC) • Hemoglobin is the source of the cell's color ("-chromic") • Normochromic: Normal color—MCHC 31–37 g/dL • Hypochromic: Pale—MCHC <31 g/dL
What is the RDW?	Index of variation in RBC size (normal 11.5%–15%) Abnormal value: >15%, indicating that new cells differ in size (smaller or larger) compared with older cells. This is one of the earliest laboratory indicators of an evolving microcytic or macrocytic anemia
What is the reticulocyte count?	The body's normal response to anemia is to attempt correction via increasing the number of new cells (reticulocytes) Normal response to anemia is reticulocytosis Because the reticulocyte MCV >96 fL, marked reticulocytosis can cause RDW to increase transiently

TABLE 11–5
Drug Interactions With Oral Iron Therapy

Drug	Effect	Comment
Antacids	Decreased iron absorption	Separate use by ≥2 hr
Caffeine	Decreased iron absorption	Separate use by ≥2 hr
Fluoroquinolones (ciprofloxacin, ofloxacin, levofloxacin, others)	Decreased fluoroquinolone effect	Avoid concurrent use or separate doses by ≥6 hr
Levodopa	Decreased levodopa and iron effect	Separate medications by as much time as possible; increase levodopa dose as needed
Some antihypertensives (ACE inhibitor, methyldopa)	Decreased antihypertensive effect	Separate medications by ≥2 hr, monitor BP Additional effect with IV iron: when ACE inhibitors are given concurrently, increased risk of systemic reaction to iron (fever, arthralgia, hypotension); concurrent use should be avoided
Tetracyclines including doxycycline	Decreased tetracycline and iron effect	Do not use concurrently, or separate by ≥3–4 hr
Thyroid hormones	Decreased thyroxine effect	Take thyroid hormones ≥2 hr before or 4 hr after iron dose
Histamine-2 receptor antagonists	Decreased iron absorption	Minor interaction

ACE, angiotensin-converting enzyme; BP, blood pressure.
Source: Drug Digest. http://www.drugdigest.org/wps/portal/ddigest, Drug interactions, accessed 9/30/09.

impoverished persons and in persons with decreased ability to absorb folic acid, which occurs with malabsorption syndromes such as sprue and celiac disease. Folic acid deficiency can be avoided with a healthy diet featuring folate-rich fruits and vegetables.

Folic acid transfers readily through the placenta to the fetus, with fetal levels usually higher than maternal levels; there is evidence that pregnancy is a maternal folate–depleting event. Repeated or multiple pregnancies, in particular, cause depletion of maternal folate stores. Folate deficiency during pregnancy can be largely avoided through the consistent use of prescriptive prenatal vitamins, each tablet usually containing 0.8 to 1 mg of folic acid. Over-the-counter prenatal vitamins contain significantly less of this micronutrient, usually about 0.4 mg per tablet. Supplementation should continue through lactation because approximately 0.5 mg/d of folic acid is transferred to breast milk. Accumulation of the vitamin in human milk takes precedence over maintaining maternal folate levels.

Maternal folic acid deficiency is a teratogenic state, particularly during neural tube formation. To reduce the rate of neural tube defects in the fetus, a woman planning a pregnancy should be advised to take additional amounts of folic acid, 0.4 mg/d, for 3 months before conception. This recommendation should be extended to all women capable of conception. Over-the-counter multivitamin or diet supplementation with vitamin-fortified foods can easily supply the recommended folate dose. If a woman has a history of giving birth to an infant with a neural tube defect, the folic acid dose should be increased to 4 mg/d for 3 months before conception and continued at least through the first 12 weeks of pregnancy. If the pregnancy is unplanned or preconception counseling was not sought, initiating folic acid supplementation during the first 7 weeks of pregnancy seems to offer some neural tube protection. Folic acid supplementation can be supplied by a prescription prenatal vitamin supplement. If a pregnant woman cannot tolerate the prenatal vitamin supplement because of nausea, a common condition, she likely would be able to take folic acid alone without difficulty. A growing body of knowledge points to genetic factors in metabolizing and using folic acid as a possible contributor to the risk of neural tube defect.

Recommended doses for folic acid replacement for adults range from 0.5 to 1 to 5 mg/d, the usual dose being 1 mg/d. The underlying cause of the folate deficiency must also be treated.

Reticulocytosis occurs rapidly, with a peak at 7 to 10 days into folic acid therapy. The hematocrit level increases by 4% to 5% per week and generally returns to normal within 1 month. Leukopenia and thrombocytopenia resolve within 2 to 3 days of therapy. A repeat hemogram in 1 to 2 months assists in monitoring of therapeutic effect. Resolution of the related signs and symptoms generally follows the time frame needed for the resolution of the anemia.

Vitamin B_{12}, a member of the cobalamin family, is found in abundance in foods of animal origin and is essential to the development of the RBC. When vitamin B_{12} is ingested orally, it binds with intrinsic factor, a glycoprotein produced by the gastric parietal cells, and is transported systematically. Within the portal blood flow, the vitamin is attached to transcobalamin II, a polypeptide synthesized in the liver and ileum. Intrinsic factor is not absorbed, and the new compound is transported to the bone marrow and other sites, where it is available for use in RBC formation. Two additional glycoproteins, transcobalamin I and III, combine with vitamin B_{12} and are used in the formation of granulocytes. In synergy with folic acid, vitamin B_{12} plays an essential role to RBC DNA synthesis. When deficiencies of either of these micronutrients exist, DNA synthesis in the RBC is impaired, which leads to the distinct changes in the RBC, macrocytosis, and bone marrow.

Vitamin B_{12} therapy should be initiated when the diagnosis is made. Usually there is a brisk hematological response, and the anemia is resolved within 2 months. Reversal of neurological abnormalities is generally slower, but improvement is seen quickly.

Vitamin B_{12} is available generically and in oral and injectable forms. The parenteral form is preferred because of its excellent absorption. In oral form, vitamin B_{12} is erratically absorbed in the distal portion of the small intestine, which can potentially lead to treatment failure. The usual initial vitamin B_{12} dosage is 100 mcg/d intramuscularly for the first week, then weekly for the first month, and then 100 mcg monthly for the rest of the patient's life. Traditionally, doses of 1000 mcg per injection have been used. A cyanocobalamin dose of more than 100 mcg in a single injection exceeds the binding capacity of transcobalamin II, however; the excess is excreted via the kidney and wasted. Concomitant administration of folic acid, iron, vitamin C, and other micronutrients is often needed to help with hematological recovery. When vitamin B_{12} deficiency is to be treated orally, a higher dose, 1000 mcg/d, is needed. Vitamin B_{12} is also available in a nasal gel, usually used weekly at a dose of 500 mcg. When the cause of macrocytic anemia has not yet been established, a prudent course of action is to give parenteral vitamin B_{12} initially while giving folic acid, 1 to 2 mg/d. With this plan, no intervention time is lost. After the appropriate diagnosis is established, the correct vitamin supplement is continued; drug interactions should be noted (Table 11–6).

The hematological response is generally rapid after therapy is begun. Reticulocytosis is brisk and peaks at 5 to 7 days. Hypokalemia, caused by serum-to-intracellular potassium shifts, is common if the anemia was particularly severe and is most likely seen with the peak of reticulocytosis. Monitoring serum potassium daily during the first week of therapy is important, especially in patients receiving diuretic therapy, at other risk of hypokalemia, or taking digoxin. If hypokalemia occurs, oral potassium replacement at 40 mEq/d is usually sufficient. Concomitant oral iron therapy is indicated if there is an iron deficiency or low iron stores. Full hematological recovery usually takes about 2 months.

TABLE 11–6
Oral Vitamin B$_{12}$ Drug Interactions

Drug	Effect
Aminoglycosides	With concomitant use, decreased vitamin B$_{12}$ absorption
Colchicine	With concomitant use, decreased vitamin B$_{12}$ absorption
Potassium supplements	With concomitant use, decreased vitamin B$_{12}$ absorption
Ascorbic acid	May destroy vitamin B$_{12}$ if taken within 1 hr of vitamin B$_{12}$ ingestion

Source: Drug Digest. http://www.drugdigest.org/wps/portal/
ddigest, Drug interactions, accessed 9/30/09.

Reversal of the signs and symptoms of vitamin B$_{12}$ deficiency is generally rapid. A sense of improved well-being is usually reported within 24 hours of the onset of treatment. Neurological changes, if present for less than 6 months, reverse quickly. Neurological reversal is likely impossible, however, if these changes have been present for a protracted period.

Anemia is often noted in persons with select chronic health problems, such as acute and chronic inflammatory conditions (infection, arthritis), renal insufficiency, and hypothyroidism. In part, this condition, known as anemia of chronic disease, is caused by reduced erythropoietin response in the marrow, resulting in RBC hypoproliferation. Worldwide, anemia of chronic disease is second only to iron deficiency in occurrence. Bone marrow can be suppressed as a result of the use of certain drugs, including cancer chemotherapy agents. Because normal RBC death occurs without the production of new RBC forms, anemia can occur. When glomerular filtration rate declines to less than 30 to 40 mL/min, renal erythropoietin synthesis is reduced; a hypoproliferative normochromic, normocytic anemia develops, usually with hemoglobin level of 7 to 8 g/dL or greater. That is, as the kidney fails, erythropoietin production declines, and anemia of chronic disease develops.

Recombinant human erythropoietin (epoetin alfa) is used in the treatment of anemias associated with end-stage renal disease, HIV, and cancer chemotherapy and other forms of anemia of chronic disease. The drug can be administered parenterally (subcutaneously or intravenously) three times per week with an expected increase in hematocrit of approximately 4% over 2 weeks. Iron therapy is also needed, unless iron overload is present. Patient symptoms, such as altered exercise capacity and sexual function, which are often attributed to renal disease, are often attenuated if hemoglobin level is appropriately corrected to 11 to 12 g/dL with the use of recombinant human erythropoietin (epoetin alfa); correction beyond this hemoglobin level has been associated with increased thrombotic risk without additional health benefit.

Discussion Sources

Conrad M. eMedicine. http://www.emedicine.com/Med/topic1799.htm, Pernicious anemia, accessed 9/30/09.

Conrad M. eMedicine. http://www.emedicine.com/med/TOPIC1188.HTM, Iron deficiency anemia, accessed 9/30/09.

Desai, S. *Clinician's Guide to Laboratory Medicine.* 3rd ed. Hudson, OH: Lexi-Comp, Inc; 2004.

Fitzgerald M. Hematologic disorders. In: Youngkin E, Sawin K, Kissinger J, Israel D, eds. *Pharmacotherapeutics: A Primary Care Clinical Guideline.* 2nd ed. Saddle River, NJ: Prentice-Hall; 2005.

QUESTIONS

32. An 18-year-old woman presents with a chief complaint of a 3-day history of "sore throat and swollen glands." Her physical examination includes exudative pharyngitis, minimally tender anterior and posterior cervical lymphadenopathy, and maculopapular rash. Abdominal examination reveals right and left upper quadrant abdominal tenderness. This clinical presentation is most consistent with:

    A. group A beta-hemolytic streptococcal pharyngitis.
    B. infectious mononucleosis.
    C. rubella.
    D. scarlet fever.

33. Which of the following is most likely to be found in the laboratory data of a person with infectious mononucleosis?

    A. neutrophilia
    B. lymphocytosis with atypical lymphocytes
    C. presence of antinuclear antibody
    D. macrocytic anemia

34. You examine a 25-year-old man who has infectious mononucleosis with tonsillar hypertrophy, exudative pharyngitis, difficulty swallowing, and a patent airway. You prescribe:

    A. amoxicillin.
    B. prednisone.
    C. ibuprofen.
    D. acyclovir.

35. The rash associated with scarlet fever is usually described as:

    A. sandpaper-like.
    B. having lacelike borders.
    C. being limited to the trunk.
    D. starting with vesicular lesions.

36. What percentage of patients with Epstein-Barr virus mononucleosis has splenomegaly during the acute phase of the illness?

A. at least 10%
B. about 25%
C. at least 50%
D. nearly 100%

ANSWERS

32.	B	33.	B	34.	B
35.	A	36.	C		

DISCUSSION

Developing an accurate diagnosis of an acute febrile illness with associated rash and pharyngitis can be a daunting task. A few key points can help:

• Lymphadenopathy: Diffuse lymphadenopathy is most often seen in patients with widespread infection, such as a systemic viral illness. When associated with a localized bacterial infection such as streptococcal pharyngitis ("strep throat"), the affected lymph nodes are also localized (anterior cervical chain).

• Pharyngitis and associated symptoms: Systemic viral infection can cause pharyngitis, but also involves other mucous membranes such as the conjunctiva and the oral and respiratory mucosa. These signs and symptoms are usually absent with a more localized infection such as streptococcus pharyngitis.

Infectious mononucleosis is an acute systemic viral illness usually caused by Epstein-Barr virus, a DNA herpesvirus that typically enters the body via oropharyngeal secretions and infects B lymphocytes. After an incubation period of 30 to 50 days, an intense T cell–mediated response develops and coincides with the onset of clinical illness. A 3- to 5-day prodrome of headache, malaise, myalgias, and anorexia is followed by acute symptoms that last about 5 to 15 days. The clinical presentation of acute infectious mononucleosis includes fatigue, exudative pharyngitis and tonsillar enlargement, fever, headache, and posterior cervical lymphadenopathy. Splenomegaly develops in more than 50% of patients, and hepatomegaly develops in about 10%; these organs are also tender to palpation. Additional findings include jaundice, periorbital edema, soft palatal petechiae, generalized adenopathy, rubella-like rash, and a 30% incidence of concurrent streptococcal pharyngitis. Full recovery time varies, but is usually about 4 to 6 weeks.

Diagnostic testing for patients with infectious mononucleosis usually includes obtaining a heterophil antibody test (Monospot). This test is positive in only 60% of patients by the second week of illness, however, and can have a false-negative rate of 15%. To complicate this issue further, acute infection with cytomegalovirus, adenovirus, *Toxoplasma gondii*, HIV, and other agents can cause an infectious mononucleosis–like illness with a risk of heterophil antibody cross-reactivity rate and a resulting infectious mononucleosis false-positive rate of 5% to 15%. Leukopenia with lymphocytosis is present. The presence of atypical lymphocytes is not unique to infectious mononucleosis and is commonly found in systemic viral infection (see Table 15–7). Mild thrombocytopenia is seen in 50% of patients; 85% of infected individuals develop a twofold to threefold elevation in hepatic enzymes (aspartate and alanine aminotransferases) by the second and third weeks of the illness.

Treatment of infectious mononucleosis is usually supportive, with recovery slow but complete. There is a potential, however, for obstruction and respiratory distress when enlarged tonsils and lymphoid tissue impinge on the upper airway. A corticosteroid such as prednisone, 40 to 60 mg/day for 3 days, is the treatment of choice, although little evidence exists to support this practice. In uncomplicated infectious mononucleosis, neither the use of antiviral agents such as acyclovir nor routine prescribing of corticosteroid agents is indicated.

In a person who participates in contact or collision sports or other activities, the risk of splenic rupture, the most common cause of mortality and morbidity in patients with infectious mononucleosis, needs to be considered during acute and convalescent stages. The risk for splenic rupture is greatest in the second and third weeks of illness—hence the mandate of abstaining from collision or contact sports for at least 21 days. The risk of rupture is greatest in the enlarged spleen; the size of the normal spleen can be recalled by the "rules of odds": $1 \times 3 \times 5$ inches in size, weighing 7 oz (about 200 g), and lying between ribs 9 and 11. When the spleen is easily palpated, its size is usually increased by two or more times normal. The physical examination is a relatively insensitive measure of splenic size, however. Obtaining an ultrasound examination may be a prudent measure to ensure splenic regression before approving return to sports play. All persons with infectious mononucleosis are at risk of splenic rupture, however, regardless of spleen size.

Discussion Source

Omori M. eMedicine. http://www.emedicine.com/EMERG/topic319.htm, Mononucleosis, accessed 9/30/09.

QUESTIONS

37. A 29-year-old woman has a sudden onset of right-sided facial asymmetry. She is unable to close her right eyelid tightly or frown or smile on the affected side. Her examination is otherwise unremarkable. This likely represents paralysis of cranial nerve:

A. III.
B. IV.
C. VII.
D. VIII.

38. Which of the following represents the most important diagnostic test for the patient in the previous question?

    A. complete blood cell count with white blood cell differential
    B. serum testing for *Borrelia burgdorferi* infection
    C. computed tomography (CT) scan of the head with contrast enhancement
    D. serum protein electrophoresis

39. Which of the following findings is often found in a person with stage 1 Lyme disease?

    A. peripheral neuropathic symptoms
    B. high-grade atrioventricular heart block
    C. Bell palsy
    D. single painless annular lesion

40. Which of the following findings is often found in a person with stage 2 Lyme disease?

    A. peripheral neuropathic symptoms
    B. atrioventricular heart block
    C. conductive hearing loss
    D. macrocytic anemia

41. Preferred antimicrobials for the treatment of adults with Lyme disease include all of the following except:

    A. a tetracycline.
    B. an aminoglycoside.
    C. a cephalosporin.
    D. a penicillin.

ANSWERS

37.	C	38.	B	39.	D
40.	B	41.	B		

DISCUSSION

Lyme disease is a multisystem infection caused by *B. burgdorferi*, a tick-transmitted spirochete. Although original reports of this disease, also known as Lyme borreliosis, were clustered through select areas of the United States, primarily in the Northeast and Mid-Atlantic states, it has now been diagnosed in every state. The disease's name comes from the town of Old Lyme, Connecticut, where it was first diagnosed after a community epidemic of rash and arthritis. Lyme disease is the most common vector-borne disease in the United States. Overdiagnosis of Lyme disease is a problem, as is the issue of significant but understandable anxiety about any tick exposure. Infected ticks must feed on the human host for more than 24 hours to transmit the spirochete. In addition, not all ticks are infected, with rates varying from 15% to 65% in areas where Lyme disease is endemic.

Lyme disease is typically divided into three stages:
- Stage 1 (early localized disease): This is a mild flu-like illness, often with a single annular lesion with central clearing (erythema migrans). The lesion is rarely pruritic or painful. Signs and symptoms can resolve in 3 to 4 weeks without treatment.
- Stage 2 (early disseminated infection): Typically months later, the classic rash may reappear with multiple lesions, usually accompanied by arthralgias, myalgia, headache, and fatigue. Less commonly, cardiac manifestations such as heart block and neurological findings such as acute facial nerve paralysis (Bell palsy) and aseptic meningitis may also be present. Individuals with Bell palsy should undergo careful examination and serological testing for Lyme disease. Regression of symptoms can occur without treatment.
- Stage 3 (late persistent infection): Starting approximately 1 year after the initial infection, musculoskeletal signs and symptoms usually persist, ranging from joint pain with no objective findings to frank arthritis with evidence of joint damage. Neuropsychiatric symptoms can appear, including memory problems, depression, and neuropathy.

Serum testing for *B. burgdorferi* by enzyme-linked immunosorbent assay and a confirmatory Western blot assay for IgM antibodies help to support the clinical diagnosis of Lyme disease; IgM antibodies decline to low levels after 4 to 6 months of illness, whereas IgG is noted about 6 to 8 weeks after onset of symptoms and often persists at low levels despite successful treatment. Careful correlation of patient history and physical examination and astute interpretation of laboratory diagnostics are critical to prevent overdiagnosing and underdiagnosing this condition.

Effective antimicrobials for treatment of Lyme disease include doxycycline, cefuroxime axetil (Ceftin), amoxicillin, and select macrolides. The clinician needs to be aware of the latest recommendation for dosage and duration of treatment with these products; recommendations range from 14 days for earlier disease to 28 days or more with more advanced disease. Most adults with Lyme disease recover in weeks with appropriate treatment, although some have a late relapse.

Prevention of Lyme disease includes avoiding areas with known or potential tick infestation, wearing long-sleeved shirts and pants, and using insect repellents. Inspecting the skin and clothing for ticks with appropriate tick removal is also helpful. If a tick bite occurs, a single 200-mg dose of doxycycline taken orally seems to be effective in reducing Lyme disease risk; observation is also a reasonable option given the low rate of infection after tick bite.

Discussion Sources

American Lyme Disease Foundation. http://www.aldf.com/dosage.shtml, Treatment of Lyme disease, accessed 9/30/09.

Centers for Disease Control and Prevention. http://www.cdc.gov/ncidod/dvbid/Lyme/ld_prevent.htm, Lyme disease prevention and control, 2008, accessed 9/30/09.

12

Psychosocial Disorders

QUESTIONS

1. A 44-year-old man who admits to drinking "a few beers now and then" presents for examination. After obtaining a health history and performing a physical examination, you suspect he is a heavy alcohol user. Your next best action is to:

   A. obtain liver enzymes.
   B. administer the CAGE questionnaire.
   C. confront the patient with your observations.
   D. advise him about the hazards of excessive alcohol use.

2. During an office visit, a 38-year-old woman states, "I drink way too much but do not know what to do to stop." According to Prochaska's change framework, her statement is most consistent with a person at the stage of:

   A. precontemplation
   B. contemplation
   C. preparation
   D. action

3. Lorazepam is the preferred benzodiazepine for treating alcohol withdrawal symptoms when there is a concomitant history of:

   A. seizure disorder.
   B. folate-deficiency anemia.
   C. multiple substance abuse.
   D. hepatic disease.

4. Which of the following is the most helpful approach in the care of a patient with alcoholism?

   A. Tell the patient to stop drinking.
   B. Counsel the patient that alcohol abuse is a treatable disease.
   C. Inform the patient of the long-term health consequences of alcohol abuse.
   D. Refer the patient to Alcoholics Anonymous.

5. A 42-year-old man who has a long-standing history of alcohol abuse presents for primary care. He admits to drinking 12 to 16 beers daily for 10 years. He states, "I really do not feel like the booze is a problem. I get to work every day." Your most appropriate response is:

   A. "Work is usually the last thing to go in alcohol abuse."
   B. "Your family has suffered by your drinking."
   C. "I am concerned about your health and safety."
   D. "Alcoholics Anonymous can help you."

6. Which of the following agents offers an intervention for the control of tremor and tachycardia associated with alcohol withdrawal?

   A. phenobarbital
   B. clonidine
   C. verapamil
   D. naltrexone

7. Which of the following is most likely to be noted in a 45-year-old woman with laboratory evidence of chronic excessive alcohol ingestion?

   A. alanine aminotransferase (ALT, also known as SGPT) 202 U/L (0–31 U/L), mean corpuscular volume (MCV) 60 fL (80–96 fL)
   B. aspartate transaminase (AST, also known as SGOT) 149 U/L (0–31 U/L), MCV 81 fL (80–96 fL)
   C. ALT 88 U/L (0–31 U/L), MCV 140 fL (80–96 fL)
   D. AST 80 U/L (0–31 U/L), MCV 103 fL (80–96 fL)

8. Which of the following is the anticipated clinical effect of acamprosate (Campral) in the treatment of alcohol dependence?

   A. modifies intoxicating effects of alcohol
   B. causes unpleasant adverse effects of alcohol
   C. helps to reduce the urge to drink
   D. minimizes alcohol withdrawal symptoms

See full color images of this topic on DavisPlus at http://davisplus.fadavis.com | Keyword: Fitzgerald

ANSWERS

1.	B	2.	B	3.	D
4.	B	5.	C	6.	B
7.	D	8.	C		

DISCUSSION

Providing primary care for patients abusing alcohol presents many challenges; this is a complex disorder affecting an individual's family and social function, health, and employment. Often a person who is abusing alcohol minimizes its effect by pointing out that employment has not been affected. In reality, alcoholism is a progressive disease that usually affects family and personal relationships first, then health and, much later, employment. The use of an effective screening tool for alcohol abuse such as the CAGE questionnaire (Box 12–1) is critical for disease detection.

Counseling the patient and family about alcoholism as a lifelong but treatable disease is a helpful clinical approach. In addition, asking about current drinking habits and associated consequences to health with each visit is important. Consistently offering assistance in accessing treatment conveys the seriousness of this life-threatening condition. As with other health problems with a behavioral component, using statements beginning with "I" is important—"I continue to be very concerned about your health and safety when I hear that you are drinking every day."

In providing primary care, the NP must maintain an attitude that, as with any substance abuse, the patient is capable of changing and achieving sobriety. Change occurs dynamically and often unpredictably. A commonly used change framework is based on the work of Prochaska, who notes five stages of preparation for change:

- Precontemplation: The patient is not interested in change and might be unaware that the problem exists or minimizes the problem's impact.
- Contemplation: The patient is considering change and looking at its positive and negative aspects. The person often reports feeling "stuck" with the problem.
- Preparation: The patient exhibits some change behaviors or thoughts and often reports feeling that he or she does not have the tools to proceed.
- Action: The patient is ready to go forth with change, often takes concrete steps to change, but is inconsistent with carrying through.
- Maintenance/relapse: The patient learns to continue the change and has adopted and embraced the healthy habit. Relapse can occur, however, and the person learns to deal with backsliding.

As health counselor, the NP provides a valuable role in continually "tapping" the patient with a message of concern about health and safety, possibly moving the person in the precontemplation stage to the contemplation stage. After the patient is at this stage, presenting treatment options and support for change is a critical part of the NP's role.

In a person who drinks more than 1 pint of hard liquor or 6 beers per day, alcohol withdrawal symptoms typically begin about 12 hours after the last drink. Peak symptoms are seen at 24 to 48 hours with abatement over the next few days. Abrupt withdrawal of alcohol use in an addicted person can lead to potentially life-threatening problems with autonomic hyperactivity (i.e., agitation, hallucinations, disorientation) and seizures. The most serious presentation of alcohol withdrawal is known as delirium tremens, which has significant mortality in untreated patients. Use of a benzodiazepine is helpful in managing distressing symptoms and preventing seizures. Treatment of concurrent problems, such as dehydration, malnutrition, and infection, is also warranted.

A highly motivated person with adequate social support systems and a relatively low level of alcohol addiction is likely a good candidate for outpatient detoxification. In this type of detoxification, the patient and support person contract with the health care provider about a safe plan of detoxification. This plan includes daily office visits or contact; ongoing involvement in Alcoholics Anonymous (AA), Employee Assistance Program (EPA) or similar program; counseling services; and use of a limited supply of medications for managing withdrawal symptoms.

Benzodiazepines have long been used to treat alcohol withdrawal symptoms. Chlordiazepoxide (Librium) or diazepam (Valium), therapeutic agents with a long half-life, are reasonable treatment options for a patient with adequate hepatic function, but lorazepam or a similarly shorter acting benzodiazepine should be used in patients with hepatic dysfunction. Providing a higher dose long-acting benzodiazepine, such as diazepam 20 mg on day one, followed by a dosing schedule reduced by 5 mg daily

---

BOX 12–1

CAGE Questionnaire

Have you ever felt you ought to *Cut* down on drinking?

Have people *Annoyed* you by criticizing your drinking?

Have you ever felt bad or *Guilty* about your drinking?

Have you ever had a drink first thing in the morning to steady your nerves or get rid of a hangover? (*Eye-opener*)

■ This questionnaire can be modified for use with other forms of substance abuse by substituting N (Normal) for E (Eye-opener), i.e., Do you ever use heroin to keep from getting sick or withdrawing?

Source: Ewing JA. Detecting alcoholism: the CAGE questionnaire, *JAMA*. 1984;252:1905–1907.

(increased if symptoms are particularly severe), is often effective and is currently favored over a fixed-dosed dose schedule. If benzodiazepine allergy or intolerance is an issue, carbamazepine offers a therapeutic alternative; atypical or standard antipsychotics play no role in managing alcohol withdrawal symptoms. Alpha-adrenergic agonists (e.g., clonidine) or beta-adrenergic antagonists (i.e., propranolol) are helpful in managing the distressing physical manifestations of alcohol withdrawal such as tachycardia and tremor. The use of these medications does not prevent the progression of alcohol withdrawal, and these should not be used as monotherapy but only with appropriate use of a benzodiazepine. Attention must be focused on treating alcohol-induced nutritional deficiencies, in particular with high-dose B-vitamin supplementation, including thiamine, pyridoxine, and folic acid, and vitamin C. Magnesium deficiency is a common correctable problem in alcohol abuse.

Although it is tempting to rely on laboratory markers in assessing a person with alcohol abuse, typically few laboratory markers are abnormal (Table 12–1). Evaluation of hepatic function is often ordered by providers, who then have the dilemma of presenting an alcohol-abusing patient with a set of relatively normal test results. This situation can help reinforce further the patient's denial or minimization of the effect excessive alcohol use has on health. As previously mentioned, physical health is negatively affected by alcohol abuse later in the course of the abuse. All currently available hepatic tests indirectly measure liver function or capacity. The most commonly performed tests are measurement of

TABLE 12–1

Hepatic Enzyme Elevations and Their Significance

Enzyme Elevation	Comment, Associated Conditions	Example
Alanine aminotransferase (ALT, formerly known as SGPT)	Measure of hepatic cellular enzymes found in circulation, elevated when hepatocellular damage is present. Highly liver specific In hepatitis A, B, C, D, or E, and drug- or industrial chemical–associated hepatitis, ALT usually increases more than AST	A 22 y.o. woman with acute hepatitis A AST 678 U/L (normal 0–31 U/L) ALT 828 U/L (normal 0–31 U/L) AST:ALT ratio <1
Aspartate aminotransferase (AST, formerly known as SGOT)	Measure of hepatic cellular enzymes found in circulation, elevated when hepatocellular damage is present. Enzyme also present in lesser amounts in skeletal muscle and myocardium In alcohol-related hepatic injury, with HMG-CoA reductase inhibitor ("statin") use (rare finding in <1% statin users), acetaminophen overdose, or excessive use. AST increases more than ALT	A 38 y.o. man with a 10-yr history of increasingly heavy alcohol use AST 83 U/L (normal 0–31 U/L) ALT 50 U/L (normal 0–31 U/L) AST:ALT ratio >1
Alkaline phosphatase (ALP)	Enzyme found in rapidly dividing or metabolically active tissue such as liver, bone, intestine, placenta. Elevated levels can reflect damage or accelerated cellular division in any of these areas. Most in circulation is of hepatic origin. Levels increase in response to biliary obstruction and is a sensitive indicator of intrahepatic or extrahepatic cholestasis	A 40 y.o. woman with acute cholecystitis AST 45 U/L (normal 0–31 U/L) ALT 55 U/L (normal 0–31 U/L) ALP 225 U/L (normal 0–125 U/L)
Gamma glutamyl transferase (GGT)	Enzyme involved in transfer of amino acids across cell membranes, found primarily in the liver and kidney. In liver disease, usually parallels changes in alkaline phosphatase. Marked elevation often noted in obstructive jaundice, hepatic metastasis, intrahepatic cholestasis	A 40 y.o. woman with acute cholecystitis AST 45 U/L (normal 0–31 U/L) ALT 55 U/L (normal 0–31 U/L) ALP 225 U/L (normal 0–125 U/L) GGT 245 U/L (normal 0–45)

Source: Ferri F. *Ferri's Best Test: A Practical Guide to Clinical Laboratory Medicine and Diagnostic Imaging.* 2nd ed. Philadelphia, PA: Mosby; 2009.

hepatic enzymes, protein molecules acting as catalysts and regulating metabolism within liver cells.

Aspartate aminotransferase (AST, formerly known as SGOT) is found in large quantities in hepatocytes. Small amounts are typically found in circulation as a result of hepatic growth and repair. AST level increases in response to hepatocyte injury, as can occur in heavy alcohol use and acetaminophen misuse or overdose; a less common reason for AST elevation is the use of HMG-CoA reductase inhibitors, more commonly called the "statins," such as simvastatin (Zocor). This enzyme is also found in myocardium, brain, kidney, and skeletal tissue in smaller amounts; damage to these areas can result in a modest increase in AST. With a circulatory half-life (T½) of approximately 12 to 24 hours, AST levels increase rapidly in response to hepatic damage and clear quickly after damage ceases. AST elevation is generally found in only about 10% of problem drinkers. If AST is elevated, however, particularly coupled with normal alanine aminotransferase (ALT) and mild macrocytosis (MCV >100 fL), long-standing alcohol abuse is the likely cause. This finding is noted in about 30% to 60% of men who drink 5 or more drinks per day and in women at a threshold of 3 or more drinks per day.

Alanine aminotransferase (ALT, formerly known as SGPT) is more specific to the liver, having limited concentration in other organs. This enzyme has a longer T½ than AST at 37 to 57 hours. As a result, ALT levels increase slowly after the onset of hepatic injury, and elevation persists longer after hepatic damage has ceased. The greatest elevation of this enzyme is likely seen in liver injury caused by hepatitis induced by infection or drug reaction. This enzyme is unlikely to increase significantly if the only hepatic problem is related to alcohol abuse.

When evaluating a patient with suspected substance abuse causing hepatic dysfunction, the NP should note the degree of AST and ALT elevation. The AST-to-ALT ratio can also offer insight into the cause of hepatic enzyme elevations (see Table 12–1). The hepatic enzymes generally return to baseline after 2 to 3 months of sobriety. This is an important patient teaching point because a patient who has abused alcohol for many years often believes that little health benefit is gained from sobriety. The mild macrocytosis seen in alcohol abuse also resolves after about 2 to 3 months of alcohol abstinence.

In addition to psychosocial support and counseling, many medications are available to assist in preventing relapse in an alcohol-dependent person. These products can be divided into categories by anticipated clinical effect and include medications that modify the intoxicating effects of alcohol, such as naltrexone (ReVia); medications that help to reduce alcohol craving, such as acamprosate (Campral); and medications that induce unpleasant adverse effects if alcohol is ingested, such as disulfiram (Antabuse). Although these medications can be helpful, the therapeutic effect is generally seen only when they are used in a motivated patient who has adequate psychosocial support and is involved in counseling. Because of its significant adverse-effect profile, disulfiram use

has largely fallen out of favor. Treatment of underlying mental health problems such as depression with a selective serotonin reuptake inhibitor can also be helpful in maintaining sobriety.

Discussion Sources

Ferri F. Ferri's Best Test: *A Practical Guide to Clinical Laboratory Medicine and Diagnostic Imaging.* 2nd ed. Philadelphia, PA: Elsevier Mosby; 2008.

Ferri F. Management of alcohol withdrawal. In: Ferri F. *Practical Guide to the Care of the Medical Patient.* Philadelphia, PA: Elsevier Mosby; 2006:871–874.

Prochaska JO, Redding CA, Evers KE. The transtheoretical model and stages of change. In: Glanz K, Lewis FM, Rimer BK, eds. *Health Behavior and Health Education: Theory, Research, and Practice.* 2nd ed. San Francisco, CA: Jossey-Bass; 1997.

Mayo-Smith MF, Beecher LH, Fischer TL, Gorelick DA, Guillaume JL, Hill A, Jara G, Kasser C, Melbourne J. Management of alcohol withdrawal delirium: an evidence-based practice guideline. *Arch Intern Med.* 2004;164:1405–1412.

Pratt DS, Kaplan MM. Evaluation of abnormal liver-enzyme results in asymptomatic patients. *N Engl J Med.* 2000;342:1267.

Stein M. Alcohol and substance abuse. In: Goldberg R, ed. *Practical Guide to the Care of the Psychiatric Patient.* 3rd ed. Philadelphia, PA: Elsevier Mosby; 2006:287–316.

QUESTIONS

9. When providing primary care for a middle-aged woman with a history of prescription benzodiazepine dependence, you consider that:
   A. she is unlikely to have a problem with misuse of other drugs or alcohol.
   B. rapid detoxification is the preferred method of treatment for this problem.
   C. she likely has an underlying untreated or undertreated mood disorder.
   D. she is at significant risk for drug-induced hepatitis.

10. Risk of benzodiazepine misuse can be minimized by use of:
    A. agents with a shorter half-life.
    B. the drug as an "as-needed" rescue medication for acute anxiety.
    C. more lipophilic products.
    D. products with longer duration of action.

11. While counseling an adolescent about the risks of marijuana use, the NP considers that:
    A. symptoms of physical and psychological dependency are rarely reported by regular users.
    B. the development of chronic obstructive airway disease is often associated with regular use.
    C. use on a daily basis among teens is significantly less common than that of alcohol.
    D. driving ability is minimally impaired with its use.

12. When assessing a person with acute opioid withdrawal, you expect to find:

    A. constipation.
    B. hypertension.
    C. hypothermia.
    D. somnolence.

13. When providing care for a middle-aged man with acute cocaine intoxication, you inquire about:

    A. feelings of anxiety.
    B. difficulty maintaining sleep.
    C. chest pain.
    D. abdominal pain.

14. Use of flunitrazepam (Rohypnol) has been associated with:

    A. agitation.
    B. amnesia.
    C. increased appetite.
    D. hallucination.

ANSWERS

9.	C	10.	D	11.	B
12.	B	13.	C	14.	B

DISCUSSION

The misuse and overuse of various mood-altering products such as alcohol, opioids, cocaine, and amphetamines is often referred to as substance abuse. Substance abuse is a common problem, affecting 10% to 14% of primary care patients, with less than 10% being detected and appropriately treated.

The *Diagnostic and Statistical Manual of Mental Disorders*, 4th edition ((DSM-IV) defines substance abuse as a maladaptive pattern of substance use leading to significant impairment or distress as manifested by one or more of the following, occurring within a 12-month period: Recurrent substance use resulting in a failure to fulfill major role obligations at work, school, or home; recurrent substance use in situations in which it is physically hazardous such as driving an automobile or operating a machine when impaired; recurrent substance-related legal problems including arrests, and continued substance use despite having persistent or recurrent social or interpersonal problems caused or exacerbated by the effects of the substance.

DSM-IV describes substance dependence as a maladaptive pattern of use leading to clinically significant impairment or distress, directly attributed to substance misuse, within a 12-month period with three or more of the following noted:

- The person exhibits tolerance, shown by markedly increased intake of the substance being needed to achieve the same effect, or with continued use, the same amount of the substance has markedly less effect.
- The person exhibits withdrawal, shown by the substance's characteristic withdrawal syndrome, or the substance (or one closely related) is used to avoid or relieve withdrawal symptoms.
- The amount or duration of use is often greater than intended.
- The person repeatedly attempts to control or reduce substance use without success.
- The person spends much time using, recovering from its effects, or trying to obtain the substance.
- The person reduces or abandons important social, occupational, or recreational activities because of substance use.
- The person continues to use the substance, despite knowing that this has likely led to physical or psychological problems.

When providing primary care, the NP should remember that substance abuse and dependence commonly means misuse of multiple agents, including alcohol, prescription drugs, and illegal agents. Many substance abusers have an underlying psychiatric problem, such as a mood disorder. Substance abuse, including alcoholism, is often a method of self-treatment in patients with an undetected or untreated psychiatric illness.

Compared with men, women have higher rates of misuse of prescription medications, which is most likely related partly to their more frequent use of the health-care system. In addition, women are more likely to have mood disorders, including anxiety and depression, and consequently are more likely to have potential drugs of abuse such as benzodiazepines prescribed by a health-care provider. Benzodiazepine abuse is likely less common than perceived by prescribers, however, who often fear that many patients receiving these anxiolytic agents would abuse or misuse the medications (Table 12–2). Prescribers often hesitate to use these highly effective agents because of fear of providing the patient with a potentially habituating drug with the possibility of needing increasing doses. In reality, psychological dependence does occur occasionally, but careful prescribing practices can help avoid this.

Psychological dependence on benzodiazepines is usually associated with a rapid-onset agent, one that possibly gives a sensation of intoxication. In addition, prescribing at dosing intervals beyond duration of action of the drug gives alternating periods of drug effect and withdrawal. The perception of difference is significant and possibly perceived as a buildup of unpleasant anxiety followed by a period of relief or rescue provided by the patient, with the cycle repeated with each drug dose. Using a benzodiazepine as an "as-needed" product increases the likelihood of abuse because this heightens the patient's awareness of drug versus no-drug state. Psychological dependence on benzodiazepines can be avoided by using a slow-onset product with a long half-life, such as

TABLE 12–2

Psychotropic Medications Typically Prescribed to Treat Anxiety

Medications	Pharmacokinetics	Indications	Onset of Action	Comments
Buspirone (BuSpar)	Slow onset of action (>7 days), lipophilic, T½ of metabolite 16 hr	Generalized anxiety syndrome, social phobia May be used as adjunct in obsessive-compulsive disorder, post-traumatic stress disorder Less effective in panic disorder, acute anxiety Not helpful in alcohol withdrawal	2–4 weeks for some relief of anxiety 4–5 weeks for full therapeutic effect	5-HT$_{1A}$ receptor site agonist, not a benzodiazepine (BZD), not effective as a prn or sleep aid drug Minimal to no effect on performance, nonsedating. No tolerance, withdrawal syndrome No potentiation with alcohol Little abuse potential If anxiety is disabling, consider adding short-term BZD while awaiting other agent's action
Lorazepam (Ativan)	Plasma peak in 1–6 hr, about half as lipophilic as diazepam (Valium) No active metabolites T½ 10–20 hr	Generalized anxiety syndrome, social phobia, adjunct in obsessive-compulsive disorder, post-traumatic stress disorder, panic disorder. Helpful in acute anxiety, alcohol withdrawal	Slow onset of action, sustained effect	As with all BZDs, abuse and habituation potential
Oxazepam (Serax)	About half as lipophilic as diazepam, slower onset of action Plasma peak in 1–4 hr No active metabolites T½ 3–21 hr	Generalized anxiety syndrome, social phobia, adjunct in obsessive-compulsive disorder, post-traumatic stress disorder, panic disorder. Helpful in acute anxiety, alcohol withdrawal	Slow onset of action, relatively sustained effect	As with all BZDs, abuse and habituation potential Good choice for elderly patients with anxiety because of short elimination T½ and lack of active metabolites. BZDs should be used with caution in older adults because of increased risk of fall and potential for altering mental status
Alprazolam (Xanax)	Plasma peak in 1–2 hr About half as lipophilic as diazepam Parent compound T½ 12–15 hr	Generalized anxiety syndrome, social phobia, adjunct in obsessive-compulsive disorder, post-traumatic stress disorder, panic disorder. Helpful in acute anxiety, alcohol withdrawal	Slow onset of action, relatively sustained effect	As with all BZDs, abuse and habituation potential. When prescribed, sufficient daily doses should be allotted

Drug	Pharmacokinetics	Indications	Onset	Comments
Clonazepam (Klonopin)	Plasma peak in 1–2 hr; About one quarter as lipophilic as diazepam; No active metabolites; T½ 18–50 hr	Generalized anxiety syndrome, social phobia, adjunct in obsessive-compulsive disorder, post-traumatic stress disorder, panic disorder. Helpful in acute anxiety, alcohol withdrawal; Absence and petit mal seizures; Anxiety and panic	Slow onset of action, highly sustained effect	As with all BZDs, abuse and habituation potential; Protracted T½ may pose a problem when used in elderly adults, but helpful in younger adults to provide consistent anxiety relief
Diazepam (Valium)	Plasma peak in 0.5–2 hr; Highly lipophilic; Three active metabolites with various T½; Desmethyldiazepam T½ 30–200 hr; Oxazepam T½ 3–21 hr; 3-hydroxydiazepam T½ 5–20 hr	Generalized anxiety syndrome, social phobia, adjunct in obsessive-compulsive disorder, post-traumatic stress disorder, panic disorder. Helpful in acute anxiety, alcohol withdrawal Anxiety; Seizures; Musculoskeletal pain	Rapid onset of action, relatively sustained effect	As with all BZDs, abuse and habituation potential; Protracted T½ may pose a problem when used in elderly patients

Source: Goldberg R, Posner D. Anxiety disorders: Diagnosis and management. In: Goldberg R, ed. *Practical Guide to the Care of the Psychiatric Patient.* 3rd ed. Philadelphia, PA: Mosby; 2007:158–177.

clonazepam. If using short-acting products, an adequate number of doses per day should be given. If a benzodiazepine is being used on an as-needed basis, the practitioner should advise a maximum number of available or prescribed doses per week, such as three to four times per week, rather than once or twice a day. This approach may help avoid benzodiazepine tolerance, a situation where the patient requires increasingly higher doses to reach therapeutic effect. Tolerance may lead to physical dependence.

Physical dependence on benzodiazepines is a significant problem. When working with a patient to discontinue benzodiazepine use, the practitioner should consider reducing the dose by 25% per week. Rapid withdrawal can lead to tremors, hallucinations, seizures, and a delirium tremens–like state. The onset of withdrawal symptoms occurs a few days after the last dose in a benzodiazepine with a shorter half-life (e.g., lorazepam) and up to 3 weeks in one with a longer half-life (e.g., clonazepam).

Benzodiazepines rarely cause hepatic or renal impairment. When taken alone in overdose, benzodiazepines have a favorable toxicity profile. Sedation risk is enhanced, however, when benzodiazepines are combined with alcohol and barbiturates, leading to a potentially life-threatening condition. Accidental and intentional fatalities with benzodiazepine ingestion with alcohol often occur.

Opioid withdrawal shares many common characteristics with alcohol withdrawal. Hypertension, tachycardia, diarrhea, nausea, hyperthermia, restlessness, myalgia, lacrimation, and rhinorrhea are often reported. Although very distressing, the condition is not life-threatening and usually resolves within a few days. Clonidine, an alpha-adrenergic agonist, helps minimize opioid withdrawal symptoms. As with any chemical dependence, long-term rehabilitation therapy is usually needed, necessitating a high level of patient desire for sobriety. Methadone, a long-acting opioid, can help curb the use of illegal drugs when used in conjunction with a comprehensive counseling and monitoring program. Buprenorphine with naloxone (Suboxone) is a fixed-dose combination of an opioid agonist (buprenorphine) and antagonist (naloxone) that offers an alternative to methadone. Compared with methadone, this drug combination has clinically desirable qualities, such as lower abuse potential, less withdrawal discomfort, and greater safety in overdose. When used to treat addiction, methadone can be dispensed only through a qualified opioid treatment program, whereas buprenorphine with naloxone can be prescribed in private practices and outpatient clinics by qualified clinicians. Although this is a helpful option that potentially increases access to patients with opioid addiction, this medication is most helpful when used by a motivated patient who is actively involved in a comprehensive treatment program.

Marijuana has historically been considered a drug that has potential for psychological dependence, but with little potential for physical addiction. For teens in many communities, daily use of marijuana is more common than daily alcohol use. Marijuana currently being used is extremely potent, however, because of its high tetrahydrocannabinol (THC) content. After a period of abstinence, physical withdrawal symptoms are often reported among daily marijuana users. Chronic marijuana use can lead to airway obstruction similar to that found in heavy tobacco users. Individuals with marijuana intoxication while performing activities requiring concentration or physical skills such as operating a motor vehicle show significant impairment.

Cocaine is a potent sympathomimetic. After cocaine ingestion, the user has an increase in heart rate and myocardial contractility and generalized vasoconstriction, causing an increase in blood pressure. In addition, cocaine preferentially constricts the coronary and cerebral vessels, creating significant risk for cerebral ischemia and stroke and myocardial ischemia and infarction. Inquiring about chest pain is prudent in caring for a patient with cocaine abuse.

Flunitrazepam (Rohypnol) is a benzodiazepine, also known as Ruffies or the date rape drug. Flunitrazepam is particularly potent with a rapid onset of action and is not available for prescription use in North America. This product is a commonly prescribed sleep aid in other countries, however. Flunitrazepam has been misused as a drug to reduce sexual inhibition, often given without the knowledge of the recipient. Because its use can result in amnesia, sexual assault can occur, possibly without the victim's recalling the event.

Discussion Sources

Book S, Myrick H. http://www.psychiatrictimes.com/display/article/10168/47706, The diagnosis and treatment of substance abuse/dependence and co-occurring social anxiety disorder, accessed 9/30/09.

Stein M. Alcohol and substance abuse. In: Goldberg R, ed. *Practical Guide to the Care of the Psychiatric Patient.* 3rd ed. Philadelphia, PA: Elsevier Mosby; 2006:287–316.

QUESTIONS

15. Which of the following statements is true concerning anorexia nervosa?

    A. The disease affects men and women equally.

    B. Onset is usually in the mid-20s for men and women.

    C. Depression is often found concomitantly.

    D. Individuals with anorexia nervosa are aware of the extreme thinness associated with the disease.

16. Treatment for anorexia nervosa usually includes:

    A. referral for parenteral nutrition evaluation.

    B. antidepressant therapy.

    C. use of psychostimulants.

    D. psychoanalysis.

17. Physical examination findings in patients with bulimia nervosa often include:

    A. body mass index (BMI) less than 75% of anticipated.
    B. dental surface erosion.
    C. tachycardia.
    D. easily pluckable hair.

18. Which of the following is most consistent with the diagnosis of bulimia nervosa?

    A. Patients with bulimia nervosa usually present asking for treatment.
    B. Periods of anorexia often occur.
    C. Hyperkalemia often results from laxative abuse.
    D. Most patients with bulimia nervosa are significantly obese.

19. All of the following pharmacological interventions are used in the treatment of patients with bulimia nervosa except:

    A. fluoxetine (Prozac).
    B. desipramine (Norpramin).
    C. bupropion (Wellbutrin).
    D. paroxetine (Paxil).

20. Characteristics of binge eating disorder include all of the following except:

    A. lack of control over the amount and type of food eaten.
    B. behavior present for at least 6 months.
    C. marked distress, self-anger, shame, and frustration as a result of binging.
    D. purging activity after an eating binge.

21 to 25. Identify if the following characteristics are noted in anorexia nervosa, bulimia nervosa, or both disorders.

____ 21. Parotid gland enlargement

____ 22. Hypokalemia

____ 23. Lanugo

____ 24. Esophageal tears

____ 25. Dysrhythmias

ANSWERS

15.	C	16.	B	17.	B
18.	B	19.	C	20.	D

21. Bulimia nervosa, possible with anorexia nervosa if binge-purging type present

22. Both anorexia nervosa and bulimia nervosa

23. Anorexia nervosa

24. Bulimia nervosa, possible with anorexia nervosa if binge-purging type present

25. Both anorexia nervosa and bulimia nervosa

DISCUSSION

Anorexia nervosa (AN) is a potentially life-threatening disease. DSM-IV criteria for AN include the following:

- Inability or refusal to maintain body weight
- Body weight 85% or less of normal weight for age and height
- Intense fear of gaining weight and becoming fat despite low body weight
- Disturbance in perception of body weight and shape

A denial of the seriousness of the low body weight is often found in patients with AN. Often despite extreme thinness, a patient with AN looks in the mirror and comments on the need to lose "just a few more pounds." Amenorrhea, which is common in women with AN, contributes to establishing the diagnosis. The usual onset of AN in women is during the teens to early 20s, with ages 14 and 18 years being the most common; men with the condition typically present a few years later. AN is an overwhelmingly female disease (90%), with either gender often involved in an activity that has an emphasis on weight and shape, including wrestling, modeling, dancing, gymnastics, and swimming. Some of the activities are occasionally called appearance as well as performance sports.

Patients with AN usually exhibit one of two types of behavior. With the restricting type, a patient with AN severely limits food intake, but does not use binge eating or purging. In the binge-purging type, a patient with AN has cycles of these behaviors.

In contrast to bulimia nervosa (BN), which is a secretive disease with relatively few easily noted clinical findings, AN is usually easy to identify clinically. Besides the marked reduction in weight, muscle wasting, abdominal distention with hepatomegaly, cheilosis, oral and gum disease, coarse dry skin, and hypotension with bradycardia and hypothermia are commonly noted.

AN is a potentially life-threatening disease with a mortality rate of 5% to 20%. Hospitalization to correct fluid and electrolyte disorders and to initiate refeeding is often needed. When physiological stability is reached, AN treatment usually includes cognitive-behavioral and pharmacological and ongoing nutritional therapy. In cognitive-behavioral therapy, the focus is the disturbed eating and the patterns of thinking that help perpetuated the binge-purge cycle. To be effective, accessing care with a clinician or treatment team expert in eating disorders is critical.

Pharmacological therapy usually involves the use of antidepressants, which may have an effect because of the high rate of comorbid depression. The choice of a specific agent should be guided by the principles used in choosing therapy for depression. Benzodiazepines are also sometimes used to reduce anxiety associated with eating. Cyproheptadine (Periactin) can be used before meals to enhance appetite and reduce anxiety.

BN is more common in women and typically is present for many years before the patient presents for treatment or before the disorder is noted by a health-care provider seeing the patient for another issue. Because BN tends to be a secretive disease, few with the disease present directly requesting intervention.

According to DSM-IV criteria, a person with BN has episodes of binge eating characterized by eating excessive quantities of food in a discrete period, such as 2 hours. During this period, the person feels a lack of control over the eating for the amount and the type of food ingested. In addition, there is a recurrent compensatory behavior used to prevent excessive weight gain from a binge, such as self-induced vomiting, excessive exercise, laxative or diuretic abuse, or fasting. Body weight and shape excessively influence self-worth.

A patient with BN is often identified in the clinical setting by problems with erosion of the lingual surface of the upper teeth because of excessive exposure to gastric contents during induced vomiting. Hypokalemia, caused by laxative and diuretic use, is also common. Body weight provides few clues because a patient is typically of average to slightly above-average weight.

Treatment of a patient with BN usually includes cognitive-behavioral and pharmacological therapy. In cognitive-behavioral therapy, the focus is the disturbed eating and the thinking patterns that help perpetuate the binge-purge cycle. To be effective, accessing care with a clinician or treatment team expert in eating disorders is critical.

Pharmacological therapy usually involves the use of antidepressants such as selective serotonin reuptake inhibitors (SSRIs). SSRIs are usually highly successful in reducing the frequency and amount of binges, partly because of their activity at the $5\text{-}HT_{1A}$-receptor site. All antidepressants can be used except for bupropion (Wellbutrin), which can induce further bingeing or seizures in patients with BN. The choice of a specific agent should be guided by the principles used in choosing therapy for depression.

Binge eating disorder is characterized as a lack of control over the amount and type of food eaten, occurring two or more times per week for at least 6 months. The bingeing is accompanied by marked distress, self-anger, shame, and frustration as a result of the bingeing. Purging activity is not present; as a result, a person with binge eating disorder is usually obese. As with all eating disorders, treatment requires an interdisciplinary approach with contributions from health-care providers with expertise in this area.

Discussion Sources

Academy of Eating Disorders. http://www.aedweb.org/eating_disorders/treatment.cfm#IA, Treatment, accessed 9/30/09.

Elliot M. Eating disorders, obesity and nicotine dependence. In: Goldberg R, ed. *Practical Guide to the Care of the Psychiatric Patient,* 3rd ed. Philadelphia, PA: Elsevier Mosby; 2006:343–351.

QUESTIONS

26. Which patient presentation is most consistent with the diagnosis of depression?
    A. recurrent diarrhea and cramping
    B. difficulty initiating sleep
    C. diminished cognitive ability
    D. consistent early morning wakening

27. Of the following individuals in need of an antidepressant, who is the best candidate for fluoxetine (Prozac) therapy?
    A. an 80-year-old woman with depressed mood 1 year after the death of her husband
    B. a 45-year-old man with mild hepatic dysfunction
    C. a 28-year-old woman who occasionally "skips a dose" of her prescribed medication
    D. a 44-year-old woman with decreased appetite

28. In caring for elderly patients, the NP considers that all of the following is true except:
    A. many older patients with dementia have a component of depression.
    B. dementia signs and symptoms usually evolve over months, but depression usually has a more rapid onset.
    C. with dementia, a patient is aware of difficulties with cognitive ability.
    D. treating concurrent depression can help improve symptoms of dementia.

29. Which of the following is most consistent with the diagnosis of dysthymia?
    A. a 23-year-old man with a 2-month episode of depressed mood after a job loss
    B. a 45-year-old woman with "jitteriness" and difficulty initiating sleep for the past 6 months
    C. a 38-year-old woman with fatigue and anhedonia for the past 2 years
    D. a 15-year-old boy with a school adjustment problem and weekend marijuana use for the past year

30. Drug treatment options for a patient with bipolar disorder often include all of the following except:
    A. methylphenidate (Ritalin).
    B. lithium carbonate.
    C. risperidone (Risperdal).
    D. valproic acid (Depakote).

31. Which of the following drugs is likely to be the most dangerous when taken in overdose?
    A. a 4-week supply of fluoxetine
    B. a 2-week supply of nortriptyline
    C. a 3-week supply of nefazodone
    D. a 3-day supply of diazepam

32. One week into sertraline (Zoloft) therapy, a patient complains of a recurrent dull frontal headache that is relieved with acetaminophen. Which of the following is true in this situation?

   A. This is a common, transient side effect of selective serotonin reuptake inhibitor (SSRI) therapy.
   B. She should discontinue the medication.
   C. Fluoxetine should be substituted.
   D. Desipramine should be added.

33. A patient has been taking fluoxetine for 1 week and complains of mild nausea and diarrhea. You advise that:

   A. this is a common, long-lasting side effect of SSRI therapy.
   B. he should discontinue the medication.
   C. another antidepressant should be substituted.
   D. he should be taking the medication with food.

34. Which of the following medications is most likely to cause sexual dysfunction?

   A. nefazodone (Serzone)
   B. fluoxetine (Prozac)
   C. nortriptyline (Pamelor)
   D. bupropion (Wellbutrin)

35. SSRI withdrawal syndrome is best characterized as:

   A. bothersome but not life-threatening.
   B. potentially life-threatening.
   C. most often seen with agents that have a long half-life.
   D. associated with seizure risk.

36. Which of the following is most consistent with the presentation of a patient with bipolar I disorder?

   A. increased need for sleep
   B. impulsive behavior
   C. fatigue
   D. anhedonia

37. In general, pharmacological intervention for patients with depression should:

   A. be given for about 4 to 6 months.
   B. continue for at least 6 months after remission is achieved.
   C. be continued indefinitely with a first episode of depression.
   D. be titrated to a lower dose after symptom relief is achieved.

38. Depression often manifests with all of the following except:

   A. psychomotor retardation.
   B. irritability.
   C. palpitations.
   D. increased feelings of guilt.

39. A 44-year-old man is taking an SSRI and complains of new onset of sexual dysfunction and difficulty achieving orgasm. You advise him that:

   A. this is a transient side effect often seen in the first weeks of therapy.
   B. switching to another SSRI would likely be helpful.
   C. this is a common adverse effect of SSRI therapy that is unlikely to resolve without adjustment in his therapy.
   D. he should see an urologist for further evaluation.

40. Which of the following agents has the longest $T\frac{1}{2}$?

   A. fluoxetine
   B. paroxetine
   C. citalopram
   D. sertraline

41. Patient presentation possibly common to anxiety and depression includes:

   A. feeling of worthlessness.
   B. psychomotor agitation.
   C. dry mouth.
   D. appetite disturbance.

42. Which of the following describes prescriptions for antidepressant medications written by primary care providers?

   A. dose too high
   B. dose too low
   C. excessive length of therapy
   D. appropriate length of therapy

ANSWERS

26.	D	27.	C	28.	C
29.	C	30.	A	31.	B
32.	A	33.	D	34.	B
35.	A	36.	B	37.	B
38.	C	39.	C	40.	A
41.	B	42.	B		

DISCUSSION

Depression is a common health problem with at least a 15% lifetime occurrence rate. DSM-IV-R criteria for depression include the presence of particular symptoms and findings for at least 2 weeks. The person has had five or more of the following symptoms, which are a definite change from usual functioning. Either depressed mood or decreased interest or pleasure must be one of the five, with findings reported by the patient or noted by others, or both.

- Mood, often with a marked diurnal variation in mood, with morning mood being more depressed than later in the day.
- Interests, with lack of interest or pleasure in activities normally or formerly found to be pleasurable.
- Eating, with a marked increase or decrease in appetite noted with corresponding change in weight.
- Sleep, with reports of excessive or insufficient amounts. Reports of early morning wakening, such as 3 or 4 a.m., with inability to fall back to sleep, are common.
- Motor activity, with reports of activity being agitated or retarded. Agitated mood and irritability are commonly noted together.
- Fatigue, with report of lack of energy.
- Self-worth, with report of worthlessness or inappropriate guilt.
- Concentration, with report of difficulty concentrating, trouble thinking clearly, or indecisiveness.
- Thoughts of death. The patient has had repeated thoughts about death and dying (other than the fear of dying), has had thoughts of suicide (with or without a plan), or has made a suicide attempt.

The symptoms cause clinically important distress or impair work, social, or personal functioning and cannot be attributed to another health condition. Other symptoms of depression are often reported. Hypochondriasis is found in about 30% of patients; such a patient is unable to process objective information that he or she has no particular health problem. Alternatively, a person with hypochondriasis perceives that an existing health problem is far more serious than it is in reality. Suicidal thoughts are often present, most often passive ideas without a plan. The patient often agrees with the statement, "If I could just die in my sleep, that would be all right." As with anyone with suicidal ideation, a thorough safety evaluation should be completed.

In an older adult, depression is sometimes mistaken for new-onset or worsening dementia. A patient with dementia typically has cognitive changes that are slowly progressive over months to years, however. The cognitive changes reported by patients with depression usually have evolved over a much shorter period with the patient often accurately reporting what changes have occurred.

Anxiety is often reported by a depressed person and is a common comorbid condition. In individuals with depression, the mood disturbance occurs first, followed in several weeks by the addition of anxiety-related symptoms. Depression should be considered as the diagnosis rather than anxiety if the patient reports feeling worse while taking benzodiazepines. The concept that a person has either depression or anxiety has been largely replaced with the realization that mood disorders occur on a continuum, with most individuals with mood disorders showing features of depression and anxiety.

Psychomotor agitation with fidgeting and irritability is often found in patients with depression, especially in children and adolescents. In these age groups, this presentation is more likely than psychomotor retardation. This type of increased activity is also found in type A adults with depression.

Intervention for patients with depression includes a combination of support, counseling, and medication. Interpersonal therapy, including counseling and support, alone has a 40% to 60% efficacy with a high relapse rate. As a single therapeutic modality, this is most effective for individuals with reactive depression. Combined therapy of pharmacological intervention and interpersonal therapy allows the patient to have effective therapy for what is now recognized as a biochemical disorder, while acquiring the cognitive skills that are helpful in dealing with what is often a chronic, relapsing condition.

Dysthymia is found in approximately 3% of the general population and is characterized by low-level daily depression with at least two of the previously identified depressive symptoms for at least 2 years in adults and 1 year in children. As with people who are depressed, patients with dysthymia respond well to a combination of interpersonal and pharmacological intervention. A patient who reports a life-changing feeling with antidepressant use, often described as "feeling good to be alive for the first time," is likely dysthymic. The person's underlying personality emerges after being suppressed or altered by the debilitating effects of the low-level depression that characterizes dysthymia.

Depressed mood may follow a significant life stressor, such as death of a loved one or loss of a job; normal sadness or grief is often inappropriately labeled as depression. An important difference is that the person who is sad, as might be reported in an individual who was recently laid off from work, or the person who is grieving, such as an individual whose loved one recently died, can identify the reason for the altered mood. With time and support, most people with normative sadness or grief find that the altered mood improves. If criteria for depression last longer than 3 months after the precipitating event, the diagnosis of major depression should be considered. Treatment for adjustment disorder with depressed mood lasting beyond 3 months is the same as treatment for major depression, recognizing that interpersonal therapy can be highly effective in assisting patients in dealing with loss. Although treating a reactive depression is helpful in lifting mood and restoring function, such treatment would not relieve the normal sadness associated with loss.

Primary care providers write 80% of all antidepressant prescriptions, making the acquisition of skill in prescribing these helpful medications crucial to practice. All prescription antidepressants are about equally effective if taken in therapeutic doses for sufficient lengths of time. Primary care providers tend to underdose antidepressants, however, and prescribe them for an insufficient length of therapy. Current treatment guidelines offer recommendations for length of therapy (Box 12–2). Long-term antidepressant therapy should be considered when there is a high risk of depression relapse (Box 12–3).

When prescribing an antidepressant, the provider should encourage psychotherapy to work on building skills needed to help manage this usually long-term health problem. In

---

BOX 12–2

Length of Pharmacological Intervention in Depression

Minimum of 9–12 months therapy
■ Acute phase treatment to bring symptoms under control and into remission lasts up to 3 months
■ Continue medication for a minimum of 6 months after depression remission achieved
■ Relapse highest in first 2 months after discontinuation of therapy
With >2 episodes, 80% relapse in 1 year without treatment
■ Consider maintenance therapy as with any chronic illness

Source: University of Michigan Health System. http://www.guidelines.gov/summary/summary.aspx?doc_id=8330, Depression, 2005, accessed 10/1/09.

BOX 12–3

Risks in Depression Relapse

Dysthymia preceding episode
Poor recovery between episodes
Current episode >2 years
Onset depression <20 y.o., >50 y.o.
Family history of depression
Severe symptoms such as suicide and psychosis

---

particular, the provider should convey the message to the patient that the use of antidepressants can help facilitate therapy.

When choosing an antidepressant, the prescriber should ask the following questions:

• What has worked in the past? Unless now contraindicated, this should be the agent of choice.
• What has worked for relatives? Certain medications seem to have greater activity at given serotonin receptor sites. Besides having heard positive comments about the medication from family members, relatives often have similar serotonin receptor site activity and response to a given medication.
• What are the most bothersome signs and symptoms of the depression? An antidepressant with activity against these or at least one that will not make these worse should be chosen. If insomnia and anxiety bother a depressed person, using a highly energizing medication is a poor choice (Tables 12–3 and 12–4).
• What are the potential drug-drug interactions? As with all medication use, a careful inventory should be taken so that potential drug-drug interactions can be avoided (Box 12–4).

When choosing an antidepressant, the side-effect profile is critical. Often a given agent has a desirable side effect, such as sedation in a patient having difficulty with sleep or anxiety. In addition, the drug's half-life influences the therapeutic choice, with products with a shorter T½ being desirable in elderly patients and patients with hepatic disease. A younger adult could benefit from the use of a drug with a longer T½ if he or she skips a dose from time to time.

Another consideration in choosing an antidepressant is its toxicity when taken in overdose. A suicidal patient clearly needs hospitalization to ensure safety and appropriate treatment. As with many conditions, however, depression is a disease with episodes of improvement and deterioration. The prescriber should consider the risk of an intentional overdose.

A 2-week supply of a tricyclic antidepressant (TCA) in full therapeutic dose would likely be lethal, with significantly smaller amounts capable of causing seizures and dysrhythmias. SSRIs and atypical antidepressants have a significantly better safety profile when taken in overdose; usually more than a 2-month supply of a full therapeutic dose is needed to cause life-threatening effects.

Antidepressants generally work by causing an increase in availability of certain neurotransmitters, such as serotonin, norepinephrine, and dopamine. This increased availability allows for greater activity at the neurotransmitter's respective receptor sites. There is evidence that interpersonal therapy also increases serotonin availability.

SSRIs are a heterogeneous group of drugs with a common mechanism of action: blocking reuptake of serotonin in the central nervous system and increasing amounts of serotonin available to postsynaptic neurons. The end effect is that more serotonin is available for action at selected receptors. Serotonin is active at numerous receptor sites (Table 12–5).

With all antidepressants, a receptor site–induced effect is immediate when therapy is initiated. The length of onset of therapeutic action is usually several weeks, however. This length of onset is likely associated with time needed for change in receptor site activity.

When a patient who is depressed takes antidepressants while undergoing an ongoing significant life stressor, such as family or marital discord or abuse, depressive symptoms usually subside as the medication takes effect. If the stressor continues, however, the antidepressant may seem to lose its initial effectiveness. Ongoing interpersonal therapy can be highly effective in augmenting pharmacological treatment in such situations.

In early SSRI therapy, the patient often complains of drug-related side effects, including headache, nausea, and diarrhea; these resolve within 2 to 6 weeks. Advising the patient that these side effects are expected, easily treatable, and transient helps avoid the problem of the patient discontinuing this important therapeutic agent. The headache is usually frontal in location and resolves with acetaminophen. Using a nonsteroidal anti-inflammatory drug may contribute further to the gastrointestinal upset often found in the first weeks of SSRI use. Taking the medication with food can minimize

TABLE 12–3
Selective Serotonin Reuptake Inhibitors (SSRIs)

SSRI	Half-life	Labeled Indications	Adverse Reaction Profile	Comments
Paroxetine (Paxil)	T½ 26 hr, no active metabolites	Major depressive disorder Panic disorder with or without agoraphobia Obsessive-compulsive disorder Social anxiety disorder Generalized anxiety disorder Post-traumatic stress disorder Premenstrual dysphoric disorder	Sedating (hs dosing likely best) Some anticholinergic effect. More constipation (13%) than diarrhea (11%) Antihistamine-like activity may increase appetite	Helpful in depression with anxiety Elimination via renal and hepatic routes Fewer problems with limited renal/hepatic function Low mania induction in bipolar. With relatively short T½ and lack of active metabolites, helpful in the treatment of depression in elderly patients. Because of short T½, slow tapering dose when discontinuing medication is recommended to avoid significant withdrawal syndrome
Fluvoxamine (Luvox)	T½ 16 hr No active metabolites	Obsessive-compulsive disorder Social anxiety disorder	High rate of gastrointestinal upset and sleep disturbance compared with other SSRIs	Adverse-effect profile can limit utility
Sertraline (Zoloft)	T½ 25–65 hr Metabolite T½ 52–102 hr	Major depression, obsessive-compulsive disorder, panic disorder, post-traumatic stress disorder, premenstrual dysphoric disorder, social anxiety disorder	Equal numbers find it sedating and energizing Low rate of nervousness, anorexia	Take with food to enhance absorption
Citalopram (Celexa) Escitalopram (Lexapro)	Citalopram: Racemic compound T½ 24–48 hr for parent compound, metabolite T½ 2 days for one, 4 days for another Escitalopram: Single isomer of citalopram with shorter T½ 33 hr	Major depression, generalized anxiety disorders	Equal numbers reporting somnolence and insomnia. Favorable gastrointestinal profile Low rates of agitation and anorexia	Escitalopram 10 mg is therapeutically equivalent to citalopram 20–40 mg with a possibly superior adverse-effect profile
Prozac (Fluoxetine)	T½ 24–72 hr Metabolite T½ 4–16 days	Major depressive disorder Bulimia nervosa Obsessive-compulsive disorder Premenstrual dysphoric disorder Panic disorder with or without agoraphobia	Energizing, anorexia common	Morning dosing recommended. Protracted T½ can present problem in elderly patients Missed doses less of a problem because of protracted T½ Weight loss of ~3–5 lb common in early months of use, but usually not sustained long-term

Source: Posternak M, Zimmerman M. Antidepressants. In: Goldberg R, ed. *Practical Guide to the Care of the Psychiatric Patient*. 3rd ed. Philadelphia, PA: Mosby; 2007:108–136.

TABLE 12–4
Atypical, Tricyclic, and Tetracyclic Antidepressants

Agent	Half-life	Adverse Reactions	Comments
Nefazodone (Serzone)	4 hr	Low anxiety, insomnia rate Excellent gastrointestinal side-effect profile Low rate nausea, diarrhea Problems with somnolence, dry mouth, dizziness Take with food for slower absorption and less drowsiness Excellent sexual function profile	Inhibits neuron reuptake of serotonin and norepinephrine 5-HT₂ antagonist Antidepressant/anxiolytic agent Good alternative for SSRI nonresponder or when SSRI sexual dysfunction an issue. Concerns about hepatotoxicity led FDA to add product warning, resulting in infrequent use of this agent
Venlafaxine (Effexor)	5 hr (4–24 hr)	Stimulating in larger amounts Patients often need trazodone or other agent to help with sleep Significant nausea with rapid onset of high dose Dose-dependent increases in diastolic blood pressure Average 5 mm Hg response	SSRI-like effect only in low doses, with norepinephrine uptake blockade at medium to high doses, similar to TCA effect, but with fewer adverse effects. Dopamine effect at very high doses, similar to bupropion. Withdrawal syndrome similar to SSRIs
Duloxetine (Cymbalta)	8–17 hr	Rare liver toxicity risk, most often noted in presence of other hepatic risk factors. Few anticholinergic adverse effects	Serotonin norepinephrine reuptake inhibitor. Indicated for treatment of mood disorders and neuropathic pain
Bupropion (Wellbutrin)	9.8 hr (3.9–24 hr) Extended-release 29 hr (20–38 hr)	Few anticholinergic effects Energizing Possible increased libido, agitation (25%) Avoid with significant manifestation of anxiety, agitation, insomnia	Blocks reuptake of dopamine at presynaptic neuron, especially in high doses, some increase in norepinephrine transmission. Dopamine receptor sites likely stimulated in substance abuse, making bupropion a helpful antidepressant for a person with a history of substance abuse. Nonaddicting and nonintoxicating Avoid use in presence of eating disorder or if anorexia is a major component of depression. Weight loss often seen (28% >5 lb) after initiation of therapy Do not give if history of or risk for seizure, closed head injury history, history of quiescent epilepsy Seizure risk worsens if dose increased rapidly
Mirtazapine (Remeron)	20–40 hr	Potent H₁ inhibitor Weight gain common Major side effect is sedation that is worse in lower doses. Little sexual dysfunction or gastrointestinal side effect	Effect likely due to increase in central noradrenergic and serotoninergic activity Selectively stimulates 5HT₁A while blocking 5HT₂ and 5HT₃ Higher doses more receptor site-selective and associated with fewer side effects

Continued

TABLE 12-4

Atypical, Tricyclic, and Tetracyclic Antidepressants —cont'd

Agent	Half-life	Adverse Reactions	Comments
Tricyclic antidepressants ("-tyline" or "-ine" suffix; includes nortriptyline [Pamelor, active precursor of amitriptyline], desipramine [Norpramin], active metabolic of imipramine)	24–32 hr	Weight gain Anticholinergic activity (blurred vision, dry mouth, memory loss, sweating, anxiety, postural hypotension, dizziness, and tachycardia) Constipation a problem, but infrequent nausea. Little sexual dysfunction	Inexpensive, more effective than SSRI in more severe depression, likely owing to its norepinephrine and serotonin activity More bothersome side-effect profile leads to high dropout rate Primary care providers seldom prescribe sufficient doses to relieve depression Wean off over 2–4 weeks to avoid TCA withdrawal symptoms; sleep disturbance, nightmares, gastrointestinal upset, malaise, irritability
Trazodone	5 hr (3–9 hr)	Highly sedating, dizziness, favorable gastrointestinal side-effect profile. Priapism risk found in 1 in 6000 men using drug. Patient should be informed to go to emergency department promptly for painful erection lasting >30 min	Anxiolytic and antidepressant activity 5-HT$_2$ antagonist Clinical use limited by marked sedation Effective hypnotic with little morning drowsiness at doses 25–100 mg taken 1 hr before sleep May use in low, frequent doses as benzodiazepine alternative for generalized anxiety

Source: Posternak M, Zimmerman M. Antidepressants. In: Goldberg R, ed. *Practical Guide to the Care of the Psychiatric Patient.* 3rd ed. Philadelphia, PA: Mosby; 2007:108–136.

BOX 12–4

Cytochrome P450 Isoenzyme Inhibition by Selective Serotonin Reuptake Inhibitors

CYP ISOENZYMES

	1A2	2C9	2C19	2D6	3A4
Escitalopram	0	0	0	0	0
Citalopram	+	0	0	+	0
Fluoxetine	+	++	+ to ++	+++	++
Paroxetine	+	+	+	+++	+
Sertraline	+	+	+ to ++	+	+

0 = minimal or weak inhibition; +, ++, +++ = mild, moderate, or strong inhibition.

nausea and diarrhea. Because potential chelation effect and impact of altered stomach pH on drug absorptions, taking many medications with an antacid can potentially limit the drug's effectiveness.

Use of SSRIs is often associated with sexual function problems. Decreased libido, anorgasmia, and erectile dysfunction are often reported. If this is a problem, switching the patient to an atypical antidepressant or TCA may be indicated because the use of these products is associated much less often with sexual dysfunction. These medications can carry their own adverse effect, however. In particular, TCAs are seldom well tolerated in a dose that is therapeutic for depression therapy. Additional options for SSRI sexual dysfunction include adding bupropion to the therapeutic regimen; support for this

TABLE 12–5

Serotonin Activity

Serotonin Receptor Site	Activity When Stimulated	Comments
5-HT$_{1A}$	Antidepressant, anti–obsessive-compulsive behavior, antipanic, anti–social phobia action, antibulimia effect	Action at this site basis of most antidepressant, antipanic therapy Reason that shyness often lifts with SSRI use
5-HT$_{1C}$, 5-HT$_{2C}$	Influence cerebrospinal fluid production, cerebral circulation Regulation of sleep Perception of pain Cardiovascular function	Reason tachycardia, dizziness, alteration of sleep patterns and change in pain perception occur with SSRI use
5-HT$_{1D}$	Antimigraine activity	Triptan preparations work by stimulating this receptor site TCAs also work at this site and are helpful in preventing migraine
5-HT$_2$	Agitation, akathisia, anxiety, panic, insomnia, sexual dysfunction Excessively upregulated in those with depression	Receptor site highly stimulated in activating SSRI such as fluoxetine. Activity at this receptor site causes sexual dysfunction associated with SSRI use Nefazodone (Serzone) and trazodone (Desyrel) antagonize action at this site and helpful in treatment of anxious depression and have a more favorable sexual function profile
5-HT$_3$	When stimulated, nausea, gastrointestinal distress, diarrhea, headache	Particularly stimulated with antidepressants with poor gastrointestinal side-effect profile Products such as ondansetron (Zofran, a 5-HT$_3$ antagonist) block activity at this site

Source: Maxmen J, Ward N. *Psychotropic Drug Facts Fast*. 3rd ed. New York, NY: Norton; 2002.

common practice is largely based on anecdotal reports. Taking a 1-day "drug holiday" from SSRI use, with sexual activity planned for the end of the drug-free period offers a reasonable option for a person with relatively infrequent sexual activity. This practice can lead to SSRI-withdrawal symptoms toward the end of the drug-free period, however, with all products except fluoxetine. Given its long T½, this practice is unlikely to be helpful for a person taking fluoxetine.

A withdrawal syndrome may be seen with SSRI use longer than 5 weeks when the product is rapidly discontinued. In SSRI-withdrawal syndrome, there is a sudden change in the amount of serotonin available and an alteration in receptor site action. Its onset is related to the T½ of the drug, with three to five half-lives before the drug clears fully. Symptoms occur more rapidly after SSRI discontinuation with a drug with a short T½ and may not occur at all in a drug with a protracted T½ (e.g., fluoxetine).

Symptoms of SSRI-withdrawal syndrome include dizziness, paresthesia, anxiety, nausea, sleep disturbance, and insomnia. Although disturbing and uncomfortable, this syndrome, in contrast to benzodiazepine withdrawal, is not dangerous or life-threatening and generally resolves within days to a few weeks.

TCAs are helpful but often misunderstood and underused medications. TCAs have a more problematic side-effect profile compared with SSRIs. In addition, they require considerable prescriber skill and patient cooperation. These medications are likely superior to SSRIs when depression is moderate to severe and characterized by emotional withdrawal, guilt, anorexia, and middle to late insomnia. In addition, they are effective in depressed patients who also have chronic pain, fibromyalgia, migraine, or the need for sedative or hypnotic agents. Choosing a TCA (e.g., nortriptyline [Pamelor]) with less anticholinergic effect and slowly increasing the dose helps enhance patient adherence.

If a patient with depression also has episodes of mania, bipolar I disorder is present. Bipolar disorders occur in approximately 1% of the general population. Characteristics of mania include the following. For at least 1 week, or less if hospitalized, the person's mood is persistently high, irritable, or expansive, coupled with three or more of these symptoms:
- Grandiosity or exaggerated self-esteem
- Reduced need for sleep
- Increased talkativeness
- Flight of ideas or racing thoughts
- Easy distractibility
- Psychomotor agitation or increased goal-directed activity (social, sexual, work, or school)
- Poor judgment (as shown by spending sprees, sexual misadventures, poor investments)

The severity of the symptoms is such that there is at least one of the following: material distress impairs work, social, or personal functioning; psychotic features; and need for hospitalization to protect the person or others.

In bipolar I disorder, the patient usually presents with cycles of elevated or irritated mood lasting longer than 1 week. Bipolar I disorder is most common in women, with an onset around puberty. If a patient with depression has episodes of mania lasting fewer than 4 days with little social incapacitation, the diagnosis of bipolar II disorder is made. In patients with bipolar II disorder, the episodes of mania are relatively mild (hypomania) and may be productive in contrast to the low point of depression.

Further descriptors of bipolar disease include rapid cycling and cyclothymic disorder. In rapid-cycle bipolar disorder, there are four or more hypomanic, manic, mixed, or major depressive episodes in a 1-year period. In cyclothymic disorder, the mood disorder has been present for at least 2 years with episodes of mania lasting fewer than 4 days, too brief to fit standard criteria of mania or hypomania. If a TCA is given to a person with bipolar disorder, approximately 15% develop mania. This also happens when an energizing SSRI such as fluoxetine is given. Ongoing evaluation and treatment of a person with bipolar disorder requires significant expertise; expert advice should be sought. Treatment usually includes the use of mood-stabilizing medications, such as lithium carbonate, valproic acid, carbamazepine, and second generation antipsychotics such as risperidone.

Discussion Sources

Posternak M, Zimmerman M. Depression: identification and diagnosis. In: Goldberg R, ed. *Practical Guide to the Care of the Psychiatric Patient*. 3rd ed. Philadelphia, PA: Elsevier Mosby; 2007:86–106.

Posternak M, Zimmerman M. Antidepressants. In: Goldberg R, ed. *Practical Guide to the Care of the Psychiatric Patient*. 3rd ed. Philadelphia, PA: Elsevier Mosby; 2007:108–136.

Truman C. Antidepressants. In: Goldberg R, ed. *Practical Guide to the Care of the Psychiatric Patient*. 3rd ed. Philadelphia, PA: Elsevier Mosby; 2007:137–157.

University of Michigan Health System. http://www.guidelines.gov/summary/summary.aspx?doc_id= 8330, Depression, 2005, accessed 9/30/09.

QUESTIONS

43. Which of the following is most consistent with the diagnosis of anxiety?

    A. nausea
    B. difficulty initiating sleep
    C. diminished cognitive ability
    D. consistent early morning wakening

44. When prescribing a benzodiazepine, the NP considers that:

    A. the drugs are virtually interchangeable, with similar durations of action and therapeutic effect.
    B. the onset of therapeutic effect is usually rapid.
    C. these drugs have a low abuse potential in substance abusers.
    D. elderly adults may use doses similar to those needed by younger adults.

45. The drug buspirone (Buspar) has:
   A. low abuse potential.
   B. significant antidepressant action.
   C. a withdrawal syndrome when discontinued, similar to benzodiazepines.
   D. rapid onset of action.

46. A 24-year-old woman has a new onset of panic disorder. As part of her clinical presentation, you expect to find all of following except:
   A. peak symptoms at 10 minutes into the panic attack.
   B. history of agoraphobia.
   C. report of chest pain during panic attack.
   D. history of thought disorder.

47. As you develop the initial treatment plan for a woman with panic disorder, you consider prescribing:
   A. carbamazepine (Tegretol).
   B. risperidone (Risperdal).
   C. citalopram (Celexa).
   D. bupropion (Wellbutrin).

48. Diagnostic criteria for generalized anxiety disorder include all of the following except:
   A. difficulty concentrating.
   B. consistent early morning wakening.
   C. apprehension
   D. irritability.

49. Which of the following is often reported by anxious patients?
   A. constipation
   B. muscle tension
   C. hive-form rash
   D. somnolence

50. Pharmacological intervention in an anxiety disorder should be:
   A. generally given for about 4 to 6 months.
   B. continued for at least 6 months after remission is achieved.
   C. continued indefinitely with a first diagnosis of the condition.
   D. titrated to a highest dose recommended after symptom relief is achieved.

51. The use of which of the following drugs often mimics generalized anxiety disorder?
   A. sympathomimetics
   B. benzodiazepines
   C. anticholinergics
   D. alpha-beta antagonists

52. When prescribing a benzodiazepine, the NP should consider that:
   A. the ingestion of 3 to 4 days' therapeutic dose can be life-threatening.
   B. the medication must be taken at the same hour every day.
   C. concomitant use of alcohol should be avoided.
   D. onset of therapeutic effect takes many days.

53. A middle-aged woman who has taken therapeutic dose of lorazepam for the past 6 years wishes to stop taking the medication. You advise her that:
   A. she can discontinue the drug immediately if she thinks it no longer helps with her symptoms.
   B. rapid withdrawal in this situation can lead to tremors and hallucinations.
   C. she should taper down the dose of the medication over the next week.
   D. gastrointestinal upset is typically reported during the first week of benzodiazepine withdrawal.

54. Risk of benzodiazepine misuse is minimized by use of:
   A. agents with a shorter T½.
   B. the drug as an as-needed rescue medication for acute anxiety.
   C. more lipophilic products.
   D. products with long duration of action.

55. Concomitant health problems found in a patient with panic disorder often include:
   A. irritable bowel syndrome.
   B. thought disorders.
   C. hypothyroidism.
   D. *Helicobacter pylori* colonization.

56. In providing primary care for a patient with post-traumatic stress disorder (PTSD), you consider that all of the following are likely to be reported except:
   A. agoraphobia.
   B. feeling of detachment.
   C. hyperarousal.
   D. poor recall of the precipitating event.

57. Preferred pharmacological treatment options for patients with PTSD include:
   A. methylphenidate (Ritalin).
   B. oxazepam (Serax).
   C. lithium carbonate.
   D. buspirone (Buspar).

58. Which of the following medications is used to assist in treating irritability and impulsivity often found in patients with PTSD?

    A. carbamazepine

    B. trazodone

    C. kava kava

    D. diazepam

59. Which of the following is an over-the-counter herbal preparation used to relieve symptoms of depression?

    A. valerian root

    B. melatonin

    C. kava kava

    D. St. John's wort

60. Patients with treatment-resistant panic disorder often respond to:

    A. imipramine.

    B. bupropion.

    C. clonidine.

    D. a monoamine oxidase inhibitor.

61. In treating a person with panic disorder using an SSRI, the NP should consider that there is:

    A. considerable abuse potential with these medications.

    B. no significant therapeutic advantage over TCAs.

    C. a reduction in number and severity of panic attacks.

    D. significant toxicity in overdose.

ANSWERS

43.	B	**44.**	B	**45.**	A
46.	D	**47.**	C	**48.**	B
49.	B	**50.**	B	**51.**	A
52.	C	**53.**	B	**54.**	D
55.	A	**56.**	D	**57.**	D
58.	A	**59.**	D	**60.**	C
61.	C				

DISCUSSION

Anxiety is a normal human emotion that is an important part of fear response. It helps a person focus on the issue at hand, such as anxiety associated with taking an important examination or making a presentation. Anxiety can also be protective, heightening senses when an individual encounters a dangerous situation. This is a rational, expected emotion when present for an appropriate reason and should dissipate with the cessation of the stressor. Anxiety becomes problematic, however, when it is exaggerated, is prolonged, or interferes with daily function.

Generalized anxiety disorder (GAD) is present in approximately 2% to 4% of the population. The typical age of onset is usually in the teen to young adult years; 15% have a first-degree relative with GAD. DMS-IV criteria for GAD include the following:

• Excessive anxiety or worry, despite information to the contrary. This must be present on most days for at least 6 months.

• A report of difficulty controlling worry, with physical or mental distress causing impairment in social or occupational function.

• These problems cannot be attributed to use of medications or alcohol, disease, or other conditions.

• The above-mentioned criteria are associated with three or more of the following: muscle tension, restlessness, fatigue, difficulty concentrating, irritability, and difficulty initiating sleep.

Anxiety often occurs in patients with depression, making the differentiation between these two common disorders problematic. A patient with depression that has an anxious component usually reports nervous feelings after the onset of depressed mood. Also in depression, the patient has feelings of worthlessness and the feeling that situations are hopeless; patients with anxiety often report feeling "worried sick" and helpless.

The cardinal presenting signs of anxiety disorder are related to the hypersympathetic state. Physical manifestations include tachycardia, hyperventilation, palpitations, tremors, and sweating. When establishing the diagnosis of GAD, it is important to rule out many clinical conditions that can mimic the disorder, including thyrotoxicosis; alcohol withdrawal; or abuse of sympathomimetic drugs such as caffeine, amphetamines, and cocaine.

Treatment recommendations for pharmacological intervention in anxiety disorders are similar to the guidelines for depression therapy. Treatment should begin with a 3-month trial period of working with the patient to find the correct medication and dose that help abate symptoms. The practitioner should encourage psychotherapy to work on building skills needed to help manage a long-term health problem. In particular, the practitioner should convey the message to the patient that the use of anxiolytic agents can help facilitate therapy. This acute care phase should be followed with a 6- to 12-month maintenance period, yielding a minimal treatment period of 9 months, although longer term therapy should be considered, especially if symptoms recur.

Choice of a therapeutic agent is guided by numerous factors, including asking about what has worked in the past and what has worked in the treatment of relatives with similar conditions. Neurotransmitters implicated in anxiety include γ-aminobutyric acid (GABA), the brain's major inhibitory chemical, and serotonin (5-HT). Norepinephrine, dopamine, and epinephrine likely play a role as well. Drug therapy for patients with anxiety disorders includes agents that enhance GABA function, such as benzodiazepines, and products that enhance the availability of serotonin, such as SSRIs.

The mechanism of action of benzodiazepines is as a mediator of GABA, enhancing its activity. Benzodiazepines are highly effective in the treatment of anxiety disorders. Because numerous benzodiazepines are available, choosing the appropriate agent can seem daunting. Critical differences can be found in these agents, however. Some agents, such as diazepam (Valium), are more lipophilic, entering the brain more rapidly and igniting an effect promptly. Although this may seem to be a desired therapeutic effect for severely anxious patients, this rapid ignition can also be intoxicating. More hydrophilic benzodiazepines, such as lorazepam, give reasonable therapeutic effect while having a slower onset of action and tend to be less intoxicating. In addition, with a highly lipophilic agent, excess is stored in body fat; this leaves a large repository for the drug resulting in a longer $T\frac{1}{2}$.

As with any drug, the $T\frac{1}{2}$ should be considered. Products such as diazepam and clonazepam (Klonopin) with a long $T\frac{1}{2}$ give sustained effect without periods of withdrawal. With drugs with a shorter $T\frac{1}{2}$, such as oxazepam (Serax), therapeutic gaps can occur. The use of drugs with a shorter $T\frac{1}{2}$ without active metabolites should be considered, however, when treating elderly persons.

One issue that needs to be considered when prescribing benzodiazepines is their abuse and misuse. Prescribers often hesitate to use these highly effective agents because of fear of providing the patient with a potentially habituating drug with the possibility of needing increasing doses. In reality, psychological dependence does occur occasionally, but careful prescribing can help avoid this.

Psychological benzodiazepine dependence is usually associated with a rapid-onset agent, possibly giving a sensation of intoxication. In addition, prescribing at dosing intervals beyond the duration of action of the drug gives alternating periods of drug effect and withdrawal. The perception of difference is significant and possibly perceived as a buildup of unpleasant anxiety followed by a period of relief or rescue provided by the patient, with the cycle repeated with each drug dose. Using a benzodiazepine as an as-needed product increases the likelihood of abuse because this heightens the patient's awareness of drug versus no-drug state. Psychological benzodiazepine dependency can be avoided by using a slow-onset product such as clonazepam that has a long $T\frac{1}{2}$. If using short-acting products, the prescriber must give adequate number of doses per day. If using on an as-needed basis, the prescriber should advise a maximal number of available or prescribed doses per week such as three or four times per week, rather than once or twice a day. Increasing tolerance to high therapeutic dose, usually at a level two to four times the prescribed level, creates physical dependence on benzodiazepines.

When taken alone in overdose, benzodiazepines have a favorable toxicity profile. Sedation is enhanced, however, when benzodiazepines are combined with alcohol and barbiturates, leading to a potentially life-threatening condition. As a result, accidental and intentional fatalities can occur.

Physical benzodiazepine dependence is a significant problem. When working with the patient to discontinue benzodiazepine use, reducing the dose by 25% per week should be considered. Rapid withdrawal can lead to tremors, hallucinations, seizures, and a delirium tremens–like state. Onset occurs a few days after the last dose in a benzodiazepine with a shorter $T\frac{1}{2}$ (e.g., lorazepam) to up to 3 weeks in one with a longer $T\frac{1}{2}$ (e.g., clonazepam).

Panic disorder affects 2% to 4% of the general population. Average age of onset is 27 years; new onset is rare after age 45 years. There is a strong comorbidity with depression. The female-to-male ratio for panic disorder is approximately 1:1 if seen without agoraphobia. Panic disorder with agoraphobia is more common in women, however, with a ratio of 2:1. A strong family history of agoraphobia is often also reported.

Diagnostic criteria for panic disorder include a history of at least one attack followed by at least 1 month of worry about an additional attack, pondering implications of attacks or significant change of behavior related to attack.

Panic attack is central to panic disorder. This is a period of intense fear or discomfort developing abruptly and peaking within 10 minutes with at least four characteristic symptoms present. Panic attack symptoms include palpitations, tachycardia, sweating, trembling, shortness of breath, choking, chest pain, chills, nausea, dizziness, and a sensation of de-realization and depersonalization. Additional symptoms include fear of losing control or dying, paresthesia, and hot flashes. In addition to the characteristics mentioned, many individuals with panic disorder have problems with alcohol abuse, depression, dizziness, and chronic fatigue. Irritable bowel syndrome is often found in patients with panic disorder.

Because of the low abuse potential and favorable side-effect profile, SSRIs have become the initial treatment of choice for persons with panic disorder. SSRI use helps decrease the number and severity of panic attacks and, to a lesser degree, phobia and anxiety related to the attacks. This class of medication is significantly more effective against panic disorders than TCAs.

When using an SSRI for treating a patient with panic disorder, "start low, go slow" should guide therapy. Individuals with panic disorder usually do not tolerate a rapid induction or change in any therapy because of their heightened sympathetic state. An agent with an early side-effect profile that the patient is likely to tolerate should be chosen, such as a product that is less rather than more energizing with a lower rate of insomnia, nervousness, and akathisia, such as paroxetine (Paxil) or citalopram (Celexa); a more energizing SSRI such as fluoxetine (Prozac) is unlikely to be well tolerated. Also, SSRI use can precipitate panic attacks with early use, but prevent them after the full therapeutic effect is realized.

TCAs can also be used in treating patients with panic disorder. Because patients with panic disorder are sensitive to the sensation of tachycardia, a product with serotoninergic rather than norepinephrine activity should be chosen, such as clomipramine (Anafranil) or nortriptyline (Pamelor). As with SSRIs, the prescriber should start with a low dose and increase it slowly. TCAs carry a much more problematic adverse effect-profile than the SSRIs and are not well tolerated in a therapeutic dose. The safety issues associated with TCA use, such as cardiotoxicity and neurotoxicity in overdose, also need to be considered.

Monoamine oxidase inhibitors are the most potent drugs available for treating patients with panic disorder. Because of side effects and the need for dietary restriction while patients take the medications, their use is generally limited to individuals with treatment-resistant panic disorder. Consultation and care by a psychopharmacology team with experience in prescribing these medications is recommended.

Post-traumatic stress disorder (PTSD) is an anxiety disorder that occurs after a significant single event, such as a natural disaster, being the victim of a crime, or exposure to combat conditions. It may also be precipitated by recurrent trauma, such as serving in combat, living in a war-torn area, or domestic abuse. Horror and helplessness are expected emotions in response to a traumatic life event for at least 1 month afterward. These emotions last significantly longer in patients with PTSD, however, and are coupled with intrusive recall of the event, numbing of emotions, detachment, hyperarousal, and impaired social and occupational function.

Treatment of patients with PTSD requires an interdisciplinary approach of expert providers. Pharmacological intervention often includes the use of an SSRI or a TCA.

Benzodiazepines should be used with caution because substance abuse is a common comorbid condition in patients with PTSD. Buspirone (Buspar), with its anxiolytic action and low abuse potential, provides a reasonable therapeutic option for the anxiety usually associated with this condition. Carbamazepine (Tegretol) and valproic acid (Depakote) have been used with some success in treating irritability, aggression, and impulsiveness. Clonidine (Catapres) and propranolol (Inderal) can be helpful in minimizing hyperarousal. Trazodone (Desyrel) offers a nonaddicting option to enhance sleep.

Patients often choose to treat anxiety and depression with herbal products, which are available over-the-counter in unlimited supply. Although encouraging and facilitating patient self-care is an important part of the role of the NP, the use of herbal products should be approached with caution. Herbal medications are considered nutritional supplements and are not subject to the regulatory process common to prescription and over-the-counter medications. As a result, quality control in their production may be lacking, leading to inconsistent amounts of herbs per dose. In addition, when a patient takes an herbal product to treat symptoms of anxiety and depression, he or she is self-medicating a potentially life-threatening disease. Using herbs with prescription medications may lead to problems with drug interactions or additive effects, such as when St. John's wort is used concurrently with an SSRI. The NP and patient need to be aware of the effects, efficacy, and side-effect profiles of these products (Table 12–6).

TABLE 12–6

Over-the-Counter Herbal Products for Anxiety and Depression

Agent	Mechanism of Action	Comments
St. John's Wort	Like MAOI, SSRI, TCA >10 active compounds	Compared with TCA, less anticholinergic effect, weight gain, less efficacy in more severe depression. Compared with SSRI, similar potential for energizing such as fluoxetine, similar efficacy in mild to moderate depression with limited study TID–QID dosing needed; 6–8 weeks before clinical effect. Little information on drug interactions; likely prudent to avoid concurrent use of SSRI, TCA, MAOI. Potentially photosensitizing, peripheral neuropathy in high doses
Kava kava	Action at GABA receptors similar to benzodiazepines	Satisfactory response compared with placebo, low-dose oxazepam (Serax) Sedating, can potentiate effects of alcohol Cross-allergenic with pepper
Valerian root	Action similar to benzodiazepines	5%–10% with paradoxical stimulating effect Available in aromatic tea, but weaker, with shorter duration of action. Less drug hangover than with benzodiazepines

GABA, γ-aminobutyric acid; MAOI, monoamine oxidase inhibitor; SSRI, selective serotonin reuptake inhibitor; TCA, tricyclic antidepressant.

Discussion Source

Goldberg R, Posner D. Anxiety disorders: diagnosis and management. In: Goldberg R, ed. *Practical Guide to the Care of the Psychiatric Patient*. 3rd ed. Philadelphia, PA: Elsevier Mosby; 2007:158–177.

QUESTIONS

62. You note that a 25-year-old woman has bruises on her right shoulder. She states: "I fell up against the wall." The bruises appear finger-shaped. She denies that another person injured her. What is your best choice of statement in response to this?

    A. "Your bruises really look as if they were caused by someone grabbing you."
    B. "Was this really an accident?"
    C. "I notice the bruises are in the shape of a hand."
    D. "How did you fall?"

63. Which of the following statements is true concerning domestic violence?

    A. It is found largely among people of lower socioeconomic status.
    B. The person in an abusive relationship usually seeks help.
    C. Routine screening is indicated during pregnancy.
    D. A predictable cycle of violent activity followed by a period of calm is the norm.

64. to 68. The following questions should be answered true or false.

____ 64. Access to a firearm by a male perpetrator is associated with increased risk of abuse toward women only in lower socioeconomic income households.

____ 65. The NP is in an ideal position to provide counseling to both members of a couple involved in domestic violence, particularly if both members of the couple are members of the NP's practice panel.

____ 66. Women's violence against male partners is as likely to result in serious injury as men's violence toward women.

____ 67. Interpersonal violence is uncommon in same-sex relationships.

____ 68. Child abuse is present in about half of all homes where partner mistreatment occurs.

ANSWERS

62.	C	63.	C	64.	False
65.	False	66.	False	67.	False
68.	True				

DISCUSSION

Interpersonal violence among family members (i.e., domestic violence) is found in all socioeconomic and ethnic groups. Because providers working with lower income and certain ethnic groups are perhaps more vigilant about domestic violence, however, it often appears that this abuse is more of a problem in certain groups.

Abuse can take numerous forms: psychological, financial, emotional, and physical. Acts of violence are typically thought to be against the victim, but often include destruction of property, intimidation, and threats. A cycle of tension building including criticism, yelling, and threats followed by violence and then a quieter period of apologies and promises to change is often seen. This cycle usually accelerates over time, however, with the violence being less predictable. Love for the perpetrator, hope that things will change, and fear of the consequences of leaving the relationship help to keep the victim in the relationship. These items also usually prevent victims from coming forth and asking for help.

As with counseling and screening for other health problems, using objective statements beginning with "I" is helpful. When a patient denies that finger-shaped bruises are caused by intentional injury by another person, the NP can simply state what is seen. This statement reinforces the assessment of abuse and allows the patient to offer more information. In a situation in which a patient is verbally abused in the NP's presence, the NP should reinforce his or her role as patient advocate by stating that the behavior is unacceptable in the NP's presence. Some providers fear that this statement can possibly precipitate another episode of abuse; however, this is unlikely.

Applying the BATHE model is helpful in framing the problem and forming a therapeutic relationship and directing intervention. Developed by Stuart and Lieberman, this model provides a guide for gathering information while helping the patient reflect on the issues at hand. The components of the model are as follows.

• BATHE
  • B—Background:
    • How are things at home? At work? Has anything changed? Good or bad? Anything you wish would change?
  • A—Affect, anxiety
    • How do you feel about home life? Work? School? Life in general?
  • T—Trouble
    • What worries you the most? How stressed are you about this problem?
  • H—Handling
    • How are you handling the problems in your life? How much support do you get at home or work? Who gives you support in dealing with problems?
  • E—Empathy
    • "That sounds difficult."

- You might want to add SOAP to the BATHE:
  - *S*—Support
    - Normalize problems, but do not minimize.
    - "Many people struggle with the same (similar) problem."
    - "What supports or resources can you use to help deal with this?"
      - Some providers may use selected self-disclosure for this. Self-disclosure usually works best in crises that are common and not of unusually tragic proportions, such as timely death or job change.
  - *O*—Objectivity
    - Watch your reactions to the story. Maintain your professional composure without acting stonelike, but be mindful of "recoiling" gestures.
    - Help client with objectivity.
      - "What is the worst thing that can happen?"
      - "How likely is that?"
      - "Then what would happen?"
  - Acceptance
    - Coach the client to personal acceptance.
      - "That is an understandable way to feel."
      - "I think you have done well considering the stress."
      - "I wonder if you are not being too hard on yourself."
  - *A*—Acknowledge client priorities.
    - "It sounds like family is more important to you than your work."
  - Acknowledge readiness or difficulty in making a change.
    - "Change is hard and sometimes very scary."
    - "It sounds to me like you are (not) ready to make a change."
  - *P*—Present focus
    - Assist client in focusing on the present, without minimizing concerns of the past and future.
      - "How could you cope better?"
      - "What could you do differently?"
- What to do after you have gathered this information
  - Negotiate a problem-focused contract for behavioral change.
    - Repeat after me, "I promise not to harm myself or anyone else in any way between now and my next visit with _____."

- Homework assignment with "I" messages.
  - "I would like more help with the children."
  - "I feel really unimportant to you when _____."
  - "I feel angry when _____."
- How do you keep this to 15 minutes?
  - Focus the client, using open and close-ended questions. Tell the client how much time you have, particularly with revisit.
    - "We have ___ (fill in the blank) minutes to chat. What would you like to focus on?"
    - If client cannot focus, ask, "If one problem in your life could just disappear, what would you choose?"

Interpersonal violence is likely as common in same-sex relationships as in opposite-sex relationships, but it is not as well studied. Violent behavior by a woman against a male partner is unlikely to result in injury as serious as a man's violence toward a woman, in part because of the usual disparity in body size and lower likelihood of weapon use. In all socioeconomic groups, access to a firearm by a perpetrator is associated with increased risk of abuse for serious or fatal injury; this is also a risk for completed suicide. The NP is in an ideal position to direct the couple to the appropriate resources for help in domestic violence, but should not attempt to provide this counseling because of the complexity of this type of care. Individual treatment is the rule as long as the violent behavior continues. Child abuse is present in about half of all households where there is partner abuse.

Discussion Sources

American Psychiatric Association. *Diagnostic and Statistical Manual of Mental Disorders*. 4th ed. Arlington, VA: American Psychiatric Publishing, Inc; 2000.

Stuart M, Lieberman J. *The 15-Minute Hour: Practical Therapeutic Intervention in Primary Care*. 3rd ed. Philadelphia, PA: Saunders; 2002.

U.S. Department of Agriculture, Safety, Health and Employee Welfare Division. www.da.usda.gov/shmd/aware.htm, Domestic violence awareness handbook, accessed 9/30/09.

13

Female Reproductive and Genitourinary Systems

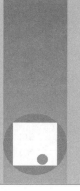

QUESTIONS

1. Which of the following is a contraindication to combined oral contraception (COC)?

   A. mother with a history of breast cancer
   B. personal history of hepatitis A at age 10 years
   C. presence of factor V Leiden mutation
   D. cigarette smoking

2. A 22-year-old woman taking a 35-mcg ethinyl estradiol COC calls after forgetting to take her pills for 2 consecutive days. She is 2 weeks into the pack. You advise her to:

   A. take two pills today and two pills tomorrow.
   B. discard two pills and take two pills today.
   C. discard the rest of the pack and start a new pack with the first day of her next menses.
   D. continue taking the pills for the rest of the cycle.

3. When counseling a woman about COC use, you advise that:

   A. long-term use of COC is discouraged because the body needs a "rest" from birth control pills from time to time.
   B. fertility is often delayed for many months after discontinuation of COC.
   C. there is an increase in the rate of breast cancer after protracted use of COC.
   D. premenstrual syndrome symptoms are often improved with use of COC.

4. Noncontraceptive benefits of COC use include a decrease in all of the following except:

   A. iron-deficiency anemia.
   B. pelvic inflammatory disease (PID).
   C. cervicitis.
   D. ovarian cancer.

5. Which of the following women is the best candidate for progestin-only pill (POP) use?

   A. an 18-year-old woman who frequently forgets to take prescribed medications
   B. a 28-year-old woman with multiple sexual partners
   C. a 32-year-old woman who is breastfeeding a 4-week-old infant
   D. a 26-year-old woman who wants to use the pill to help "regulate" her menstrual cycle

6. A 38-year-old nulliparous woman who smokes two and a half packs a day is in an "on-and-off" relationship. The woman presents seeking contraception. Which of the following represents the most appropriate method?

   A. contraceptive ring (NuvaRing)
   B. COC
   C. contraceptive patch (Ortho Evra)
   D. vaginal diaphragm

7. Which of the following statements is true concerning vaginal diaphragm use?

   A. When in place, the woman is aware that the diaphragm fits snugly against the vaginal walls.
   B. This is a suitable form of contraception for women with recurrent urinary tract infection.
   C. After insertion, the cervix should be smoothly covered.
   D. The device should be removed within 2 hours of coitus to minimize the risk of infection.

8. According to the World Health Organization (WHO) guidelines, which of the following is a clinical condition where use of a copper-containing IUD should be approached with caution?

   A. uncomplicated valvular heart disease
   B. AIDS-defining illness
   C. hypertension
   D. dysmenorrhea

See full color images of this topic on DavisPlus at http://davisplus.fadavis.com | Keyword: Fitzgerald

9. Which of the following is the most appropriate response to a 27-year-old woman who is taking phenytoin (Dilantin) for the treatment of a seizure disorder and is requesting hormonal contraception?

    A. "A barrier method would be the preferable choice."
    B. "COC is the best option."
    C. "Depo-Provera (medroxyprogesterone acetate in a depot injection [DMPA]) use will likely not interact with your seizure medication."
    D. "Copper-containing IUD use is contraindicated."

10. Which of the following is commonly found after 1 year of using DMPA (Depo-Provera)?

    A. weight gain
    B. hypermenorrhea
    C. acne
    D. rapid return of fertility when discontinued

11 to 19. The following questions should be answered by responding yes or no.

According to WHO guidelines, who is a COC candidate?

____ 11. a 22-year-old who smokes one pack per day

____ 12. a 29-year-old with PID

____ 13. a 45-year-old with tension-type headache

____ 14. a 32-year-old breastfeeding a 6-month-old infant

____ 15. a 28-year-old with type 1 diabetes mellitus

According to WHO guidelines, who is a candidate for a copper-containing IUD?

____ 16. a 45-year-old with fibroids with uterine cavity distortion

____ 17. a 33-year-old who smokes two packs per day

____ 18. a 25-year-old with hypertension

____ 19. a 33-year-old with low-grade squamous intraepithelial lesions noted on Pap test

20. As you prescribe COC containing the progestin drospirenone (Yasmin, Yaz), you offer the following advice:

    A. "Always take this pill on a full stomach."
    B. "You should not take acetaminophen when using this birth control pill."
    C. "Avoid using potassium-containing salt substitutes."
    D. "You will likely notice that premenstrual syndrome symptoms might become worse."

21. With genitourinary tract exposure to the spermicide nonoxynol-9, a woman is likely at increased risk for:

    A. cervical stenosis.
    B. urinary tract infection.
    C. increased perivaginal lactobacilli colonization.
    D. ovarian malignancy.

22. With the use of a levonorgestrel intrauterine system (Mirena), which one of the following is normally noted?

    A. endometrial hyperplasia
    B. hypermenorrhea
    C. increase in PID rates
    D. reduction in menstrual flow

23. The reduction in free androgens noted in a woman using COC can yield an improvement in:

    A. cycle control.
    B. acne vulgaris.
    C. breast tenderness.
    D. rheumatoid arthritis.

24. With DMPA in depot injection (Depo-Provera), the recommended length of use is usually:

    A. less than 1 year.
    B. no more than 2 years.
    C. as long as the woman desires this form of contraception.
    D. as determined by her lipid response to the medication.

25. When can a woman safely conceive after discontinuing COC?

    A. immediately
    B. after 1 to 2 months
    C. after 3 to 4 months
    D. after 5 to 6 months

26. When prescribing the contraceptive patch (Ortho Evra) or vaginal ring (NuvaRing), the NP considers that:

    A. these are progestin-only products.
    B. candidates include women who have difficulty remembering to take a daily pill.
    C. there is significant drug interactions with both products.
    D. contraceptive efficacy is less than with COC.

ANSWERS

1.	C	2.	A	3.	D
4.	C	5.	C	6.	D
7.	C	8.	B	9.	C
10.	A	11.	Yes	12.	Yes
13.	Yes	14.	Yes		

15. Yes, in the absence of advanced vascular disease

16.	No	17.	Yes	18.	Yes
19.	Yes	20.	C	21.	B
22.	D	23.	B	24.	B
25.	A	26.	B		

DISCUSSION

Despite the availability of numerous methods of highly reliable contraception, nearly half of all pregnancies in the United States are unplanned. Rates of continued contraception use vary greatly according to the method. Helping a woman choose an effective and acceptable form of family planning is an important part of providing health care.

Available for more than four decades, COC has been used by millions of women. This highly reliable form of contraception usually results in 1 pregnancy per 1000 women with perfect use and 50 pregnancies per 1000 women with typical use. The patch (Ortho Evra) and ring (NuvaRing) are also highly effective forms of contraception containing estrogen and progestin with reported rates of 99% efficacy when used as directed.

Contraceptive effect is achieved through the action of the COC, patch, and ring progestin and estrogen components. Progestational effects help to inhibit ovulation by suppressing luteinizing hormone (LH), thickening endocervical mucus, and hampering implantation by endometrial atrophy. Through estrogenic effects, ovulation is inhibited by suppression of follicle-stimulating hormone (FSH) and LH and by alteration of endometrial cellular structure.

When COC, ring, or patch is discontinued, fertility usually returns promptly. Contrary to common belief, there is no need to delay conception after discontinuing these contraceptive forms; prolonged combined hormonal contraceptive use is not associated with future infertility or other health problems.

Noncontraceptive benefits of combined hormonal contraception include lower rates of benign breast tumors and dysmenorrhea. Menstrual volume is reduced by about 60%, resulting in decreased rates of iron deficiency anemia. Decreased rates of endometrial, ovarian, and colon cancers are particularly noted among long-term users (>5 years). Owing in part to the endometrial thinning, COC can be safely used for an extended time without withdrawal, which is an attractive option for a woman who does not wish to menstruate or who has a health problem that is exacerbated by menstruation. Although COC is not protective against sexually transmitted infections (STIs), COC users have decreased frequency of pelvic inflammatory disease (PID), which results from thickened endocervical mucus; this results in a lower rate of future ectopic pregnancy. Decreased rates of acne, hirsutism, and ovarian cyst; reduction in premenstrual syndrome; and improvement in rheumatoid arthritis symptoms are also noted among COC users. Improvement in acne is usually noted after about 3 months of use, whereas improvement in hirsutism usually takes about 6 months; these improvements persist while the woman is taking COC and are usually reversible when COC is discontinued. COC is also a highly effective family planning option for a wide variety of women with chronic health problems (Table 13–1).

The highest dropout rates with COC and progestin-only pill (POP) use are in the first 3 months of use. The most frequently mentioned reasons are breakthrough bleeding (BTB) and inconvenience of use. Although BTB is bothersome, it is not harmful and does not indicate lesser contraceptive benefit. BTB can be minimized by taking COC or POP within the same 4-hour period every day. Cigarette smoking increases the likelihood of BTB and should be discouraged. BTB rate increases dramatically when pills are missed. Advice about what to do in the event of missed pills is an important part of providing contraceptive care (Table 13–2). Compared with COC use, BTB rates with the use of the contraceptive ring and patch are usually lower after the first few weeks of use. This difference is largely due to the fact that the patch and ring do not require a daily action on the user's part, and adherence is significantly better.

Nausea with COC, patch, ring, and hormone therapy is a commonly reported adverse effect. Nausea is usually a transient problem noted in the first months of use and can be minimized by taking the medication with food or at bedtime. If vomiting occurs within 2 hours of taking COC, the dose should be retaken.

COC hormones interact with a few drugs. Interaction is noted, however, with many antiepileptic drugs (AEDs), including phenytoin, carbamazepine, phenobarbital, and primidone, potentially causing a reduction in therapeutic levels of these important medications. The BTB rate is greater in women using COC, patch, and ring and AEDs partly because of more rapid metabolism of estrogen. A woman with a seizure disorder who wishes to use hormonal contraception is likely to have a reduction in frequency and severity of seizures while using DMPA (Depo-Provera) because progestin use has long been noted to be protective against seizures. In addition, DMPA does not seem to interact with AEDs. Levonorgestrel implants might have the same effect. Use of barrier methods, IUDs, or levonorgestrel-containing intrauterine systems (Mirena) does not interfere with AEDs and has no effect on seizure threshold.

The progestins used in most COC, patch, and ring formulations are testosterone derivatives. Drospirenone, found in the COC products Yasmin and Yaz, is an analogue of an aldosterone antagonist and has potassium-sparing qualities. Drospirenone should be used with caution in hepatic or renal dysfunction or with concomitant use of angiotensin receptor blocker, angiotensin-converting enzyme inhibitor, salt substitute, or potassium-sparing diuretic. A potential benefit of a drospirenone-containing COC is improvement in premenstrual syndrome symptoms.

Although POP inconsistently suppresses ovulation, this form of contraception likely works through thickening of endocervical mucus and through the alteration of the endometrium. POP use offers certain advantages and disadvantages compared with COC. With failure rates of 1% to 4%, POP is a less effective contraceptive than COC. The nausea rate with its use is significantly lower than with COC use, owing to the lack of estrogen. POPs are taken daily, a

TABLE 13–1

World Health Organization Precautions for Use of Combined Oral Contraceptive Pills

Category 4: Refrain From Use	Category 3: Exercise Caution	Category 2: Advantages Outweigh Risk	Category 1: No Restriction
• Venous thromboembolism • CHD, CVA • Structural heart disease • Breast cancer • Pregnancy • Lactation (<6 wk postpartum) • Acute hepatitis • Hepatic adenoma • Headache with focal neurological symptoms • Major surgery with prolonged mobilization • Age >35, smoking ≥20 cigarettes/day • Hypertension (>160/>100 mm Hg or with vascular disease) • Known thrombotic mutations (factor V Leiden, prothrombin mutations, protein S, C, or antithrombin deficiency)	• Postpartum <21 days • Lactation (6 wk–5 mo) • Undiagnosed vaginal bleeding • Age ≥35 and smoking <20 cigarettes/day • History breast cancer but no recurrence in past 5 yr • Interacting drugs (select antiepileptics such as phenytoin, carbamazepine, valproate) • Gallbladder disease • DM type 1 or type 2 >20 years' duration or with vascular disease • Past history breast cancer, no current disease for 5 yr • Hypertension adequately controlled without vascular disease	• Age ≥40 • Severe headache with oral contraceptive use • DM type 1 or type 2 without vascular disease • Major surgery without immobilization • Sickle cell disease • Hypertension (140/100–159/109 mm Hg) • Undiagnosed breast mass • Cervical cancer • Age >50 • Nonadherence factors • Family history lipid disorders • Family history premature MI • BMI ≥30 • Lactation ≥6 mo	• Age menarche to 40 • Postpartum ≥21 days without breastfeeding • Smoking age <35 • Post therapeutic or spontaneous abortion • History gestational DM • Varicose veins • Mild headache • PID, STI history • HIV • Benign breast disease • Family history breast, cervical, ovarian cancer • Cervical ectropion • Uterine fibroids • Past history ectopic pregnancy • Obesity • Thyroid disease • Depression • Minor surgery without mobilization • Menorrhagia • Irregular menses • History gestational DM • Ovarian or endometrial cancer

BMI, body mass index; CHD, congestive heart disease; CVA, cerebrovascular disease; DM, diabetes mellitus; MI, myocardial infarction.
Source: www.who.int/reproductive-health/publications/mec, accessed 10/3/09.

schedule many women find more convenient than the typically 3-weeks-on, 1-week-off schedule with COC. POP must be used daily, however, for maximal efficacy. For lactating women who wish to use an oral hormonal contraceptive, POP is highly effective and does not alter the quality or quantity of breast milk. One significant disadvantage with POP use is bleeding irregularity, ranging from prolonged flow to amenorrhea.

The contraceptive patch (Ortho Evra) and contraceptive intravaginal ring (NuvaRing) contain estrogen and progestin as a birth control method in a nonoral form. Both of these methods have the advantage of infrequent dosing, with a new patch needed once a week and a new ring needed

every 3 weeks. With proper use, contraceptive efficacy is similar to that of COC. Observed contraceptive failure rates are usually lower with the patch and ring, likely because of greater ease of use. Adverse effects and contraindications to patch and ring use are similar to those of COC use. Women who dislike or forget to take a daily pill often welcome the opportunity to use the patch or ring.

DMPA (Depo-Provera), given every 90 days, is a highly reliable form of contraception (99.7% efficacy). DMPA is best suited for women who do not wish a pregnancy for at least 18 months because resumption of fertility is frequently delayed 6 to 12 months. When the injection is given within the first few days of menses, the contraceptive effect is

TABLE 13–2
Missed Combined Oral Contraceptive Pill Advice

Missed Pill	Action	Comment
With use of ≥30-mcg ethinyl estradiol pills, with 1 or 2 active pills missed	Take active pill as soon as possible and then continue taking pills daily, 1 each day	No additional contraceptive protection needed. If pills missed in first week of use and unprotected intercourse, use EC
With use of ≥30-mcg ethinyl estradiol pills, missed ≥3 active pills in first 2 weeks of the pack	Take an active pill as soon as possible and then continue taking pills daily, 1 each day	Use condoms or abstain from sex until she has taken active pills for 7 days in a row. Consider EC use if pills were missed during the first week with unprotected intercourse
With use of ≥30-mcg ethinyl estradiol pills, missed ≥3 active pills in third week of a traditional 4-week pack	Finish the pack of active pills and start new pack of active pills without withdrawal period	No additional contraceptive method required
With use of <30-mcg ethinyl estradiol pills, with 1 active pill missed	Take active pill as soon as possible and then continue taking pills daily, 1 each day.	No additional contraceptive method required. Consider EC if pills were missed during the first week of use with unprotected intercourse
With use of <30-mcg ethinyl estradiol pills, with ≥2 active pills missed	Take active pill as soon as possible and then continue taking pills daily, 1 each day	Use condoms or abstain from sex until she has taken active pills for 7 days in a row. Consider EC use if pills were missed during the first week with unprotected intercourse

EC, emergency contraception.

Source: Nelson A. Combined oral contraceptives. In: Hatcher R, Trussell J, Nelson A, Cates W, Stewart F, Kowal D, eds. *Contraceptive Technology*. 19th ed. New York, NY: Ardent Media, Inc; 2007:193–270.

immediate. When it is started 5 days after the onset of menses, a backup method of contraception should be used for 1 week. Depo-Provera may be started immediately postpartum if the woman is not breastfeeding and initiated 3 to 6 weeks postpartum if she is breastfeeding. Earlier use can diminish quantity but not quality of breast milk. Irregular bleeding, a common problem during the first few months of DMPA injection use, can be minimized by the use of a prostaglandin inhibitor such as ibuprofen, 400 mg tid, or naproxen sodium, 375 to 540 mg bid, for 3 to 5 days. Estrogen supplements, such as a 0.1-mg estrogen patch used for 7 to 10 days, can also be helpful, but are seldom needed to manage this bothersome but not dangerous adverse effect. After 1 year of DMPA use, 30% to 50% of women have amenorrhea. According to observations from limited study, bone density is occasionally noted to be reduced in women using DMPA. This condition is largely reversible, however, when the medication is discontinued. The U.S. Food and Drug Administration (FDA) has assigned a boxed warning to DMPA, highlighting that prolonged use can result in the loss of bone density and recommending that the medication not be used for more than 2 years unless other methods cannot be used; bone density seems to normalize quickly with discontinuation of the medication. Calcium supplementation, at 1000 to 1500 mg/d, weight-bearing exercise, and vitamin D supplementation should be recommended; this advice is helpful for general bone health.

Standard IUDs, such as the copper-containing ParaGard (Copper T 380A), are an effective form of contraception with a failure rate of 0.5% to 2.9%. The mechanism of contraceptive action is not entirely understood, but it is unlikely that these are abortifacients. There is often an increase in menstrual bleeding and upper reproductive tract infection with their use, and IUDs are not widely used, in part because of the incorrect health-care provider perception that few women can safely use this highly effective contraceptive method (Table 10–3). Mirena is a levonorgestrel-containing intrauterine system of drug delivery that produces marked endometrial atrophy. As a result, about 50% of Mirena users are amenorrheic at the end of 1 year of use. Thickened endocervical mucus is also noted, which limits the ascent of infection into the upper reproductive tract and minimizes PID risk. This is a particularly helpful method of contraception for women with menorrhagia.

TABLE 13–3

World Health Organization Precautions for the Use of Copper-containing IUD

Category 4: Refrain from Use	Category 3: Exercise Caution	Category 2: Advantages Outweigh Risk	Category 1: No Restriction
• Current PID (within 3 mo) • Current purulent cervicitis or chlamydial infection or gonorrhea • Unexplained vaginal bleeding • Cervical cancer, awaiting treatment • Uterine fibroids with distortion of uterine cavity	• AIDS-defining illness • Cirrhosis with severe decompensation • Postpartum <4 wk	• High risk for HIV • HIV infection • Age <20 • Immediately post first-trimester therapeutic abortion • Nulliparous • Complicated valvular heart disease • Severe dysmenorrhea	• Immediately post first-trimester therapeutic abortion • Parous • Hypertension • Vascular disease • Uncomplicated valvular heart disease • Cervical intraepithelial neoplasia • Uterine fibroids without distortion of uterine cavity • Postpartum >4 weeks

Source: www.who.int/reproductive-health/publications/mec, accessed 10/30/09

The diaphragm, a barrier method of contraception, is placed in the vagina before intercourse. This device, which has an effectiveness rate of 80% to 95%, should be used in conjunction with a spermicide and removed no sooner than 6 hours after coitus. When properly fitted and in the appropriate position, the woman and her partner should be unaware of the diaphragm's presence. If either partner can feel the diaphragm, the device is either the wrong size or not properly inserted. Because a diaphragm should always be used with a spermicide, a woman with a history of recurrent urinary tract infection (UTI) is not an ideal candidate for diaphragm use. Although the thought behind this long-held advice is that the diaphragm increases UTI risk as a result of potential pressure on the woman's lower urinary tract, the risk more likely arises from the concurrent use of a spermicide. A woman who is exposed to the spermicide nonoxynol-9, either through vaginal use or with a male partner who uses condoms with this spermicide, is likely at increased risk of UTI. The proposed mechanism of this risk is the antibacterial effect of the spermicide, which is to reduce lactobacilli, a normal component of the periurethral flora. Lactobacilli produce hydrogen peroxide and lactic acid, providing the periurethral area and vagina with a pH that inhibits bacterial growth and blocks potential sites of attachment and is toxic to uropathogens.

Discussion Source

Nelson A. Combined oral contraceptives. In: Hatcher R, Trussell J, Nelson A, Cates W, Stewart F, Kowal D, eds. *Contraceptive Technology*. 19th ed. New York, NY: Ardent Media, Inc; 2007:193–270.

QUESTIONS

27. An 18-year-old woman requests emergency contraception after having unprotected vaginal intercourse approximately 18 hours ago. Today is day 12 of her normally 27- to 29-day menstrual cycle. You advise her that:

    A. emergency hormonal contraception use reduces the risk of pregnancy by approximately 33%.

    B. all forms of emergency contraception must be used within 12 hours after unprotected intercourse.

    C. the likelihood of conception is minimal.

    D. taking emergency hormonal contraceptive offers an effective emergency contraceptive option.

28. Which of the following is likely not among the proposed mechanisms of action of emergency contraception pills?

    A. inhibits ovulation

    B. acts as an abortifacient

    C. slows sperm transport

    D. slows ovum transport

29. A 24-year-old woman who requests emergency contraception pills wants to know the effects if pregnancy does occur. You respond that there is the risk of increased rate of:

    A. spontaneous abortion.

    B. birth defects.

    C. placental abruption.

    D. none of the above.

30. A woman who has used emergency contraception pills should be advised that if she does not have a normal menstrual period within _____ weeks, a pregnancy test should be obtained.

    A. 1–2
    B. 2–3
    C. 3–4
    D. 4–5

ANSWERS

27.	D	28.	B
29.	D	30.	C

DISCUSSION

As previously mentioned, nearly half of all pregnancies are unplanned. Emergency contraception, used after coitus to minimize the risk of unintended pregnancy when a contraceptive method fails or is not used, is an effective method of minimizing the number of unintended pregnancies (Box 13–1). An estimated 800,000 annual pregnancy terminations could be avoided if knowledge of and access to emergency contraception were widely available.

Numerous methods are available, including the use of COC, POP, and copper-containing IUDs. Emergency contraception with oral hormonal agents is highly effective, reducing the risk of pregnancy by 75% or more, according to the following model: If 100 fertile women have unprotected heterosexual intercourse in the second to third weeks of their cycles, eight typically become pregnant. One or two typically become pregnant when using emergency contraception. The mechanism of action is not established, but it likely helps reduce pregnancy risk by multiple methods, including inhibiting or delaying ovulation or impairing ovum or sperm transport. Emergency contraception is unlikely to prevent pregnancy by preventing implantation of a fertilized ovum because the resulting minor endometrial changes would likely be insufficient to yield this result. Use of oral hormonal emergency contraception would not interrupt an established pregnancy or increase risk of early pregnancy loss. If pregnancy does occur, use of emergency contraception does not seem to be teratogenic. Because of slowed tubal motility, a theoretical but not observed risk of ectopic pregnancy exists.

A copper-containing IUD such as the ParaGard (Copper T 380A) can be inserted within 5 days after intercourse as a form of emergency contraception. Because of the risk of upper reproductive tract infections, use of a copper-containing IUD is contraindicated in the presence of STI. In addition to providing ongoing contraception, IUD insertion provides a hormone-free emergency contraception option.

Menstrual bleeding should be expected within 3 to 4 weeks of using emergency contraception. If none occurs, a pregnancy test should be done.

Discussion Sources

Stewart F, Trussell J, Van Look P. Emergency contraception. In: Hatcher R, Trussell J, Nelson A, Cates W, Stewart F, Kowal D, eds. *Contraceptive Technology*. 19th ed. New York, NY: Ardent Media, Inc; 2007:87–116.

The Emergency Contraception Website. http://ec.princeton.edu/, accessed 10/3/09.

BOX 13–1

Emergency Hormonal Contraception: Indications and Mechanism of Action

CANDIDATES FOR EMERGENCY CONTRACEPTION

Any time unprotected sexual intercourse occurs including potential method failure (e.g., late for or missed pills, late for Depo-Provera, dislodged or misplaced diaphragm, condom break or slippage, expelled IUD)

EMERGENCY CONTRACEPTION MECHANISM OF ACTION

Depending on time taken during menstrual cycle
■ Inhibit or delay ovulation (most likely effect)
■ Inhibit tubal transport of egg or sperm
■ Interfere with fertilization
Unlikely mechanism of action
■ *Emergency hormonal contraception use results in minimal to no alteration to endometrium and is unlikely to inhibit implantation of a fertilized egg*

Source: Stewart F, Trussell J, Van Look P. Emergency contraception. In: Hatcher R, Trussell J, Nelson A, Cates W, Stewart F, Kowal D, eds. *Contraceptive Technology*. 19th ed. New York, NY: Ardent Media, Inc; 2007:87–116.

QUESTIONS

31. In advising a woman about menopause, the NP considers that:

- **A.** the average age at last menstrual period for a North American woman is 47 to 48 years.
- **B.** hot flashes and night sweats occur in about 80% of women.
- **C.** women with surgical menopause usually have milder symptoms.
- **D.** follicle-stimulating hormone (FSH) and luteinizing hormone (LH) levels are suppressed.

32. Findings in estrogen deficiency (atrophic) vaginitis include:

- **A.** a malodorous vaginal discharge.
- **B.** an increased number of lactobacilli.
- **C.** a reduced number of white blood cells.
- **D.** a pH greater than 5.0.

33. A 53-year-old woman who is taking hormone therapy (HT) with conjugated equine estrogen, 0.625 mg/d, with MPA, 2.5 mg, has bothersome atrophic vaginitis symptoms. You advise that:

- **A.** her oral estrogen dose should be increased.
- **B.** topical estrogen may be helpful.
- **C.** the MPA component should be discontinued.
- **D.** baking soda douche should be tried.

34. For a woman with bothersome hot flashes who cannot take HT, alternative options with demonstrated efficacy include the use of all of the following except:

- **A.** venlafaxine.
- **B.** sertraline.
- **C.** gabapentin.
- **D.** clonidine.

35. Absolute contraindications to postmenopausal HT include:

- **A.** unexplained vaginal bleeding.
- **B.** seizure disorder.
- **C.** dyslipidemia.
- **D.** migraine headache.

36. In advising a perimenopausal woman about HT, you consider that it may:

- **A.** reduce the risk of venous thrombotic events.
- **B.** significantly reduce serum triglyceride levels.
- **C.** worsen hypertension in most women.
- **D.** help preserve bone density.

37. Postmenopausal HT use can result in:

- **A.** a reduction in the rate of cardiovascular disease.
- **B.** an increase in the rate of rheumatoid arthritis.
- **C.** a reduction in the frequency and severity of vasomotor symptoms.
- **D.** a disturbance in sleep patterns.

38. The progestin component of HT is given to:

- **A.** counteract the negative lipid effects of estrogen.
- **B.** minimize endometrial hyperplasia.
- **C.** help with vaginal atrophy symptoms.
- **D.** prolong ovarian activity.

39. Concerning selective estrogen receptor modulator therapy such as raloxifene (Evista), which of the following statements is correct?

- **A.** Concurrent progestin opposition is needed.
- **B.** Hot flashes are reduced in frequency and severity.
- **C.** Use is contraindicated when a woman has a history of breast cancer.
- **D.** Osteoporosis risk is reduced with use.

40. During perimenopause, which of the following is likely to be noted?

- **A.** Symptoms are most likely in the week before the onset of the menses.
- **B.** The length of the perimenopausal period is predictable.
- **C.** Symptoms are less severe in women who smoke.
- **D.** Hot flashes are uncommon.

41. Which of the following is likely to be noted with short-term (less than 1 to 2 years) HT use in a postmenopausal woman?

- **A.** reduction in dementia risk
- **B.** significant increase in breast cancer risk
- **C.** minimized menopausal symptoms
- **D.** increase in cardiovascular risk

42. Which body area has the greatest concentration of estrogen receptors?

- **A.** vulva
- **B.** vascular bed
- **C.** heart
- **D.** brain

43. Examples of phytoestrogens include all of the following except:

- **A.** black cohosh.
- **B.** ginseng.
- **C.** vitamin E.
- **D.** soy products.

44. Adding an androgen to HT may be well suited for a woman with:

   A. late-onset menopause.
   B. severe hot flashes despite maximized estrogen therapy.
   C. low osteoporosis risk.
   D. alopecia.

45. The typical HT regimen contains _____ of the estrogen dose of COC.

   A. one-eighth
   B. one-fourth
   C. one-half
   D. three-fourths

46. When reviewing the use of nutritional supplements for the management of menopausal symptoms, the NP considers that:

   A. few high-quality studies support the use of these products.
   B. the use of these products is consistently reported to be helpful.
   C. the products can be safely used as long as blood hormone levels are carefully evaluated.
   D. the use of these products is associated with a greater reduction in menopausal symptoms than with prescription HT.

47. Which of the following statements is true?

   A. Many over-the-counter progesterone creams contain sterols that the human body is unable to use.
   B. All progesterones are easily absorbed via the skin.
   C. Soy is an example of a phytoprogesterone.
   D. Progesterones, whether synthetic or plant-based, should not be used by a woman who has undergone a hysterectomy.

ANSWERS

31.	B	**32.**	D	**33.**	B
34.	D	**35.**	A	**36.**	D
37.	C	**38.**	B	**39.**	D
40.	A	**41.**	C	**42.**	A
43.	C	**44.**	B	**45.**	B
46.	A	**47.**	A		

DISCUSSION

A woman's life is characterized by a series of shifts: first, a woman transitions to the reproductive years, then to the premenopausal period, and then to the menopausal and post-menopausal years. Each transition is normal, expected, and not a disease state. Perimenopause and menopause are often symptom-producing events, however.

Perimenopause is the time surrounding menopause; its onset is marked by the beginning symptoms of menopause and ends with the cessation of menses. The average onset of perimenopause is 40 to 45 years; it occurs earlier in cigarette smokers. Perimenopause lasts an average of 4 years, but can range from a few months to 10 years. Menopause, when the final menstrual period occurs, marks another transition in a woman's reproductive life. By definition, a woman is in menopause when she has had no naturally occurring menstrual period for 12 months. The average age for a North American woman at menopause is 51.3 years, with some women living one-third of their lives after this time.

During perimenopause, menstrual irregularity is common, with the interval between periods becoming longer or shorter, and flow can become heavier or lighter. Ovulation becomes more erratic, but pregnancy is still possible. Hot flashes and sleep problems are usually worse in the week before the menses and are reported by approximately 65% to 75% of women during perimenopause. During this stage, estrogen levels are usually normal, but FSH levels are elevated. As mentioned, the woman often notes hot flashes or flushes during the week before the onset of the menses, a time when hormonal shifts are most dramatic. Because most women associate menopause symptoms with irregular or absent menstrual bleeding, these perimenopausal symptoms can be confusing as the woman is menstruating on a regular basis. Although low estrogen levels have often been implicated as the cause of perimenopausal symptoms, likely the shifting levels of multiple biological substances is implicated.

As the menopausal period progresses, LH and FSH levels increase dramatically as the anterior lobe of the pituitary sends out an abundance of these substances in an attempt to induce ovulation; the ovaries fail to respond with ovulation, sometimes leading to heavy, anovulatory menstrual bleeding. Levels of estrogen forms (estradiol, estrogen) and androgens (testosterone, progesterone, androsterone, and dehydroepiandrosterone) are reduced. Hot flashes now usually become more frequent and severe, in part induced by the FSH surge. About 80% of woman going through menopause have hot flashes, ranging in severity from mildly bothersome to debilitating. Compared with naturally occurring menopause, women with surgical menopause usually have more severe symptoms, likely because the hormonal shifts are more rapid and dramatic.

Estrogen receptors are found in high concentrations in the vulva, vagina, urethra, and trigone of the bladder. As a result, symptoms of urogenital atrophy from estrogen shifts are a common perimenopausal and menopausal problem. These receptors are found in lower concentrations in the vascular bed, heart, brain, bone, and eye, areas of the body that also exhibit changes during perimenopause and menopause.

Vasomotor symptoms can be debilitating, causing disturbed sleep, avoidance of social situations where hot flashes occur, and numerous other problems. Women often seek advice from their health-care provider about minimizing these symptoms. Numerous lifestyle modifications can be quite helpful (Table 13–4). When these measures are inadequate, pharmacological intervention is often appropriate.

HT, usually in the form of an estrogen supplement prescription, is likely the most commonly used and most effective therapy that has been extensively studied for hot flash management. When given during the first years after menopause, reduction of hot flashes by 80% to 95% is expected. All types and routes of administration of estrogen are effective. Although the benefit seems to be dose-related, even low doses of estrogen are often effective. Higher doses (equivalent of 1 mg of oral estradiol) usually provide relief in about 4 weeks, whereas lower doses usually take about 8 to 12 weeks to provide similar hot flash effect. Lower-dose HT is usually better tolerated with less breast tenderness and uterine bleeding. The FDA and the American College of Obstetrics and Gynecology recommend using the lowest dose of HT that is effective; the length of therapy should be dictated by clinical response and kept as short as possible (Table 13–5).

As with all medication use, HT comes with the possibility for adverse effects. Endometrial cancer risk with unopposed estrogen use is considerable, with the rate of 4 to 5 per 1000 users per year, with a 5-year use risk of 2% and a 10-year use risk of 4%. As a result, unless a woman taking HT has undergone a hysterectomy, she must also take a progestin to minimize this risk. An observed increased risk of breast cancer in women who use HT has also been noted, particularly with long-term use. Supplemental estrogen use should be avoided in women who have a history of or are at high risk

TABLE 13–5

What Estrogen Form? What Dose? How Much Relief?

The three most commonly used prescription hormone therapy agents include oral conjugated equine estrogen and oral and transdermal estradiol-17β. The amount of hot flash relief women get from each form and dose differs

Estrogen Form	Dose (mg)	Reported Hot Flash Relief (%)
Oral conjugated equine estrogen	0.625	94
	0.4	78
	0.3	78
Oral estradiol-17β	2	96
	1	89
	0.5	79
	0.25	55
Transdermal estradiol-17β	0.1	96
	0.05	96
	0.025	86

for cardiovascular disease, breast cancer, uterine cancer, or venous thromboembolic events and in women with active liver disease. Compared with the oral form, transdermal estrogen use is associated with a lower thromboembolic risk in short-term studies.

TABLE 13–4

Lifestyle Modification to Minimize Hot Flash Triggers

Hot flashes can often be reduced in number and minimized in severity with simple lifestyle changes

Hot Flash Trigger	Intervention
Spicy foods, chocolate, other foods	Keep food diary to track triggers. Avoid triggers or eat in small amounts
Alcohol use	Note if certain amounts of types of alcohol trigger hot flashes. Restrict or avoid use
Elevated ambient temperature and humidity	Control room temperature and humidity. Using climate control to achieve a cool room with low humidity is particularly helpful in improving sleep quality
Tight, restrictive clothing	Dress in layers that can be removed and replaced in response to hot flashes
Cigarette smoking	Tobacco use is associated with a marked increase in hot flashes. Smoking cessation improves overall health and reduces hot flash frequency and severity
Hot baths or showers	Well-known hot flash trigger. Also tends to worsen dry skin, a common complaint during perimenopause and menopause. Taking a cool shower or bath minimizes hot flash risk
Relaxation techniques, self-hypnosis	In many smaller studies, shown to be helpful in reducing hot flash severity and frequency

Source: Nelson A, Stewart F. Menopause and perimenopausal health. In Hatcher R, Trussell J, Nelson A, Cates W, Stewart F, Kowal D, eds. *Contraceptive Technology.* 19th ed. New York, NY: Ardent Media, Inc; 2007:699–745.

Many women who use oral HT continue to have symptoms of atrophic vaginitis; the addition of topical estrogen via an estrogen-containing vaginal cream, ring, or tablet can be helpful. Increasing the dose of oral estrogen is seldom helpful and likely increases HT adverse effects. The use of over-the-counter vaginal lubricants and moisturizers can also afford great relief for vaginal dryness that interferes with sexual activity.

Occasionally, a woman with significant vasomotor symptoms does not or cannot use HT for relief. Low-dose antidepressant (selective serotonin reuptake inhibitors [SSRIs] and selective serotonin and norepinephrine reuptake inhibitors [SNRIs]) therapy can reduce the frequency and severity of hot flashes by 35%. Examples of options include the SNRI venlafaxine (Effexor) and the SSRIs sertraline (Zoloft) and paroxetine (Paxil). Typically, the doses given to minimize vasomotor symptoms are less than the doses used for the treatment of depression. The usual adverse effects associated with the use of these medications can be anticipated; sexual dysfunction including anorgasmia is common with SSRI and SNRI use. Gabapentin (Neurontin) has also demonstrated efficacy in reducing vasomotor symptoms. Older antihypertensives, such as methyldopa (Aldomet) and clonidine (Catapres), have been used for this purpose with little effect.

In a woman who continues to menstruate but is having significant perimenopausal symptoms, low-dose oral contraceptives can be helpful for symptom relief and for cycle regulation. Oral contraceptives contain approximately three to four times the estrogen dose of usual-dose HT.

After menopause, androgen levels also decrease, leading to loss of lean muscle mass, attenuated libido, and additional bone loss. Androgen supplementation, usually in the form of low-dose testosterone, can be helpful in women with postmenopausal low libido and in women with continued hot flashes despite HT, a particularly common problem in younger women who have undergone surgical menopause. The prescriber and the patient need to be aware of the risks of estrogen supplementation and the risks of specific androgens, such as acne and hirsutism (common) and alopecia, vocal changes, and clitoral enlargement (less common); as with all medications, the use of HT should be approached with caution and is contraindicated in some women (Table 13–6).

Estrogen deficiency is a potent risk factor in the development of osteoporosis, which is most common in postmenopausal woman. By age 80, the average woman has lost greater than 30% of her premenopausal bone density. When taken with calcium supplements, postmenopausal HT can help reduce the risk of postmenopausal fracture by 50% by minimizing further bone loss. Because of the greater observed rate of venous thrombotic events with short-term and long-term HT use and invasive breast cancer with longer term use, however, and the availability of other medications to treat bone thinning such as bisphosphonates and salmon calcitonin (Miacalcin), HT should not be used solely for this purpose.

Because the vaginal introitus remains colonized with protective flora when HT is used, there are lower rates of

TABLE 13–6

Contraindications to and Caution With Postmenopausal Estrogen Therapy

Absolute contraindication
- Unexplained vaginal bleeding
- Acute liver disease
- Chronic impaired liver function
- Thrombotic disease
- Neuro-ophthalmologic vascular disease
- Endometrial cancer (controversial—short-term use for management of severe menopausal symptoms occasionally acceptable)
- Breast cancer (controversial—short-term use for management of severe menopausal symptoms occasionally acceptable)

Use with caution, considering if benefit outweighs risk
- Seizure disorder (owing to potential drug-drug interaction)
- Dyslipidemia, particularly hypertriglyceridemia (transdermal, intravaginal hormone therapy has limited lipid impact)

Source: National Guideline Clearinghouse. http://www.guideline.gov/summary/summary.aspx?ss=15&doc_id=10038, Menopause and hormone therapy (HT): collaborative decision-making and management, accessed 10/3/09.

urogenital atrophy and UTIs in women using this therapy. Some women using HT continue to need topical estrogen, however, in the form of a vaginal cream, tablet, or estrogen-impregnated ring (Estring) to help minimize urogenital atrophy symptoms.

Phytoestrogens are chemical substances similar to estrogen, in particular estradiol, that are found in more than 300 plants, including apples, carrots, coffee, potatoes, yams, soy products, flaxseed, ginseng, bean sprouts, red clover sprouts, sunflower seeds, rye, wheat, sesame seeds, linseed, black cohosh, and bourbon. These are active substances that bind to estrogen receptor sites and have mild estrogenic effects and some antiestrogenic activity in some areas by binding and blocking to sites in the breast, colon, and rectum. Over-the-counter topical creams made of wild yam, a phytoprogesterone, are available and commonly used by women seeking relief from hot flashes. Because of poor bioavailability, however, little of the product actually reaches circulation. In limited study of women who were breast cancer survivors, high-dose vitamin E, 800 IU/d, modestly reduced the number of hot flashes. Few high-quality studies support the use of nutritional supplements for management of menopausal symptoms. Women often view these supplements as a safe alternative to drug therapy, however.

Discussion Sources

Estrogen and progestogen use in postmenopausal women: July 2008 position statement of The North American Menopause Society. http://www.menopause.org/PSHT08.pdf, *Menopause,* 2008, accessed 10/3/09.

Grady D. Clinical practice: management of menopausal symptoms. *N Engl J Med.* 2006;355:2338–2347.

Nelson A, Stewart F. Menopause and perimenopausal health. In: Hatcher R, Trussell J, Nelson A, Cates W, Stewart F, Kowal D, eds. *Contraceptive Technology.* 19th ed. New York, NY: Ardent Media, Inc; 2007:699–745.

QUESTIONS

48. Patients with urge incontinence often report urine loss:
    A. with exercise.
    B. at night.
    C. associated with a strong sensation of needing to void.
    D. as dribbling after voiding.

49. Patients with urethral stricture often report urine loss:
    A. with exercise.
    B. during the day.
    C. associated with urgency.
    D. as dribbling after voiding.

50. Patients with stress incontinence often report urine loss:
    A. with lifting.
    B. at night.
    C. associated with a strong sensation of needing to void.
    D. as dribbling after voiding.

51. Factors that contribute to stress incontinence include:
    A. detrusor overactivity.
    B. pelvic floor weakness.
    C. urethral stricture.
    D. urinary tract infection (UTI).

52. Factors that contribute to urge incontinence include:
    A. detrusor overactivity.
    B. pelvic floor weakness.
    C. urethral stricture.
    D. UTI.

53. Pharmacological intervention for patients with urge incontinence includes:
    A. doxazosin (Cardura).
    B. tolterodine (Detrol).
    C. finasteride (Proscar).
    D. pseudoephedrine.

54. Intervention for patients with stress incontinence includes:
    A. establishing a voiding schedule.
    B. gentle bladder-stretching exercises.
    C. periurethral bulking agent injection.
    D. restricting fluid intake.

55. Which form of urinary incontinence is most common in elderly persons?
    A. stress
    B. urge
    C. iatrogenic
    D. overflow

ANSWERS

48.	C	49.	D	50.	A
51.	B	52.	A	53.	B
54.	C	55.	B			

DISCUSSION

Urinary incontinence (UI) is the involuntary loss of urine in sufficient amounts to be a problem. This condition is often thought by many women to be a normal part of aging. In reality, numerous treatment options are available after the cause of urinary incontinence is established (Table 13–7). In all cases, urinalysis and urine culture and sensitivity should be obtained. Further diagnostic testing should be directed by patient presentation. If UTI is present, treatment with the appropriate antimicrobial is indicated.

Urge incontinence is the most common form of urinary incontinence in elderly persons. Behavioral therapy, including a voiding schedule and gentle bladder stretching, are helpful. Pharmacological intervention is indicated in conjunction with behavioral therapy (Table 13–8). Tolterodine (Detrol) and solifenacin succinate (VESIcare) are selective muscarinic receptor antagonists that block bladder receptors and limit bladder contraction. Helpful in the treatment of urge incontinence, the use of these products is associated with a decrease in the numbers of micturitions and of incontinent episodes, along with an increase in voiding volume. Oxybutynin is a nonselective muscarinic receptor antagonist that blocks receptors in the bladder and oral cavity, with activity similar to that of tolterodine; adverse effects include dry mouth and constipation.

Discussion Sources

Ogundele O, Silverberg MD. http://emedicine.medscape.com/article/778772, Urinary incontinence, accessed 10/3/09.

Weiss B. http://www.aafp.org/afp/20050115/315.html, Selecting medications for the treatment of urinary incontinence, *American Family Physician,* 2005, accessed 10/3.09.

TABLE 13–7

Clinical Issues in Urinary Incontinence

Type of Urinary Incontinence	Etiology and Population Most Often Affected	Clinical Presentation	Treatment Options
Urge incontinence	Detrusor overactivity causing uninhibited bladder contractions Most common form of incontinence in elderly women	Strong sensation of needing to empty the bladder that cannot be suppressed, often coupled with involuntary loss of urine	Avoiding stimulants, gentle bladder stretching by increasing voiding interval by 15–30 min after establishing a half-hour voiding schedule Add agent to reduce bladder contraction such as an anticholinergic; options include tolterodine (Detrol), oxybutynin (Ditropan), solifenacin succinate (VESIcare)
Stress incontinence	Weakness of pelvic floor and urethral muscles Most common form of incontinence in women; rare in men	Loss of urine with activity that causes increase in intra-abdominal pressure such as coughing, sneezing, exercise	Support to the area through the use of a vaginal tampon, urethral stents, periurethral bulking agent injections, and pessary use. Kegel and other similar exercises most helpful in younger patients. Pelvic floor rehabilitation with biofeedback, electrical stimulation and bladder training Surgical intervention can be helpful in 75%–80% Topical and systemic estrogen therapy, formerly recommended for this condition, now recognized as not helpful and perhaps contributing to stress incontinence symptoms
Urethral obstruction	Obstruction of bladder outflow through urethral obstruction (prostatic, stricture, tumor) resulting in urinary retention with overflow and detrusor instability Most commonly found in older men	Dribbling postvoid coupled with urge incontinence on presentation	Treatment of urethral obstruction
Transient incontinence	Associated with acute event such as delirium, UTI, medication use, restricted activity	Presentation consistent with underlying process	Treatment of underlying process, discontinuation of offending medication

TABLE 13–8

Select Medications and Their Effect on Urinary Continence

Type of Medication	Effect on Urinary Continence
Diuretics	Increase in volume and frequency of voiding
Drugs with anticholinergic activity such as first-generation antihista-mines, tricyclic antide-pressants, antipsychotics	Urinary retention, overflow incontinence, alteration in sensorium, fecal impaction
Opioids	Urinary retention, overflow, alteration in sensorium, fecal impaction
Alcohol	Increase in volume, frequency, and urgency of voiding alteration in sensorium
Sedatives, hypnotics, benzodiazepines	Alteration in sensorium, reduced mobility
Alpha-adrenergic antagonists (prazosin, doxazosin, terazosin)	Relaxing internal urethral sphincter
	This may be a desired effect in a man with BPH, likely less helpful in a woman with bladder-emptying issues

BPH, benign prostatic hyperplasia.

QUESTIONS

56. Which of the following is not a normal finding in a woman during the reproductive years?

    A. vaginal pH of 4.5 or less
    B. *Lactobacillus* as the predominant vaginal organism
    C. thick, white vaginal secretions during the luteal phase
    D. vaginal epithelial cells with adherent bacteria

57. Which of the following findings is most consistent with vaginal discharge during ovulation?

    A. dry and sticky
    B. milky and mucoid
    C. stringy and clear
    D. tenacious and odorless

58. Physical examination of a 19-year-old woman with a 3-day history of vaginal itch reveals moderate perineal excoria-tion; vaginal erythema; and a white, clumping discharge. Expected microscopic examination findings include:

    A. a pH greater than 6.0.
    B. an increased number of lactobacilli.
    C. hyphae.
    D. an abundance of white blood cells.

59. Women with bacterial vaginosis typically present with:

    A. vulvitis.
    B. pruritus.
    C. dysuria.
    D. malodorous discharge.

60. Treatment of vulvovaginitis caused by *Candida albicans* includes:

    A. metronidazole gel.
    B. clotrimazole cream.
    C. hydrocortisone ointment.
    D. clindamycin cream.

61. A 24-year-old woman presents with a 1-week history of thin, green-yellow vaginal discharge with perivaginal irrita-tion. Physical examination findings include vaginal erythema with petechial hemorrhages on the cervix, numerous white blood cells, and motile organisms on microscopic exami-nation. These findings most likely represent:

    A. motile sperm with irritative vaginitis.
    B. trichomoniasis.
    C. bacterial vaginosis.
    D. condyloma acuminatum.

62. A preferred treatment option for trichomoniasis is:

    A. metronidazole.
    B. clindamycin.
    C. acyclovir.
    D. azithromycin.

63. Treatment options for bacterial vaginosis include all of the following except:

    A. oral metronidazole.
    B. clindamycin cream.
    C. oral clindamycin.
    D. oral azithromycin.

64. A 30-year-old woman presents without symptoms, but states that her male partner has dysuria without penile discharge. Examination reveals a friable cervix covered with thick yellow discharge. This description is most consistent with an infection caused by:

    A. *Chlamydia trachomatis.*
    B. *Neisseria gonorrhoeae.*
    C. human papillomavirus (HPV).
    D. *Trichomonas vaginalis.*

65. Which of the following agents is active against *N. gonorrhoeae*?

   A. cefixime

   B. metronidazole

   C. ketoconazole

   D. amoxicillin

66. Which of the following agents is active against *C. trachomatis*?

   A. amoxicillin

   B. metronidazole

   C. azithromycin

   D. ceftriaxone

67. Which of the following statements is true of gonococcal infection?

   A. The risk of transmission from an infected woman to a male sexual partner is about 80%.

   B. Most men have asymptomatic infection.

   C. The incubation period is about 2 to 3 weeks.

   D. The organism rarely produces beta-lactamase.

68. Complications of gonococcal and chlamydial genitourinary infection in women include all of the following except:

   A. pelvic inflammatory disease (PID).

   B. tubal scarring.

   C. acute pyelonephritis.

   D. acute peritoneal inflammation.

69. What percentage of sexually active adults has serological evidence of human herpesvirus 2 (HHV-2) (herpes simplex type 2)?

   A. 5

   B. 15

   C. 25

   D. 35

70. All of the following are likely reported in a woman with an initial episode of genital HHV-2 infection except:

   A. painful ulcer.

   B. inguinal lymphadenopathy.

   C. thin vaginal discharge.

   D. pustular lesions.

71. Treatment options for HHV-2 genital infection include:

   A. ribavirin.

   B. indinavir.

   C. famciclovir.

   D. cyclosporine.

ANSWERS

56.	D	**57.**	C	**58.**	C
59.	D	**60.**	B	**61.**	B
62.	A	**63.**	D	**64.**	A
65.	A	**66.**	C	**67.**	B
68.	C	**69.**	C	**70.**	D
71.	C				

DISCUSSION

Vulvovaginitis is one of the most common gynecological problems. Treatment is guided by presentation and causative organism (Table 13–9). Chlamydial infection ♂ is one of the most common STIs, affecting primarily adolescents and adults younger than 25 years. The causative organism, *C. trachomatis* immunotype D–K, is an obligate intracellular parasite closely related to gram-negative bacteria. This infection causes cervicitis in most infected women. About one-half have urethral infection, and one-third have endometrial involvement; despite this, many women are asymptomatic, although mucopurulent vaginal discharge, dysuria, dyspareunia, and postcoital bleeding may be reported.

Clinical presentation of *C. trachomatis* genitourinary infection in women typically includes the presence of mucopurulent discharge, often adherent to a friable cervix. Cervical motion and adnexal tenderness is usually present when there is endometrial involvement and PID. Diagnostic testing includes DNA probe endocervical testing or urinalysis for ligase chain reaction.

Treatment options for uncomplicated *C. trachomatis* infection include antimicrobials that act against intracellular organisms, such as doxycycline, erythromycin, and azithromycin. Azithromycin is given in a highly efficacious, well-tolerated, single-dose oral therapy.

Gonorrhea, ♂ caused by the gram-negative diplococcus *N. gonorrhoeae,* is also a common STI. This organism has a short incubation period of 1 to 5 days and is likely to cause infection in approximately 20% of men who have sexual contact with infected women and approximately 80% of women who have sexual contact with infected men.

Most men with gonococcal infection have no symptoms. In women, presentation typically includes dysuria with a milky to purulent, occasionally blood-tinged, vaginal discharge. With anal-insertive sex, rectal infection leading to proctitis is often seen. Because the organism frequently produces beta-lactamase, the choice of a therapeutic agent should include agents with beta-lactamase stability, such as ceftriaxone and cefixime. Because of increasing rates of resistance, the use of the fluoroquinolones to treat this infection is no longer recommended.

Genital herpes ♂ is a result of infection with a HHV. Most often, HHV-2 is the causative organism; HHV-1, the

TABLE 13–9

Female Genitourinary Infection

Conditions	Causative Organism	Clinical Presentation	Treatment Options
Chancroid	*H. ducreyi*	Painful genital ulcer, multiple lesions common, inguinal lymphadenitis	Primary: azithromycin 1 g orally in a single dose, or ceftriaxone 250 mg intramuscularly (IM) in a single dose Alternative: ciprofloxacin 500 mg orally twice a day for 3 days, or erythromycin base 500 mg orally three times a day for 7 days
Genital herpes	HHV-2, also known as herpes simplex type 2 (rarely human herpesvirus 1)	Painful ulcerated lesions, lymphadenopathy, particularly with primary outbreak. Subsequent outbreaks often less severe	For primary infection (initial episode): acyclovir 400 mg PO tid × 7–10 days or famciclovir 250 mg PO tid × 7–10 days or valacyclovir 1 g PO bid × 7–10 days For episodic recurrent infection: acyclovir 800 mg tid × 2 days or 400 mg PO tid × 5 days or famciclovir 1000 mg bid × 1 day or 125 mg PO bid × 5 days or valacyclovir 1g PO qd × 5 days or valacyclovir 500 mg PO bid × 5 days For suppression of recurrent infection: acyclovir 400 mg PO bid or famciclovir 250 mg PO bid or valacyclovir 1 g PO qd For patient with <9 recurrences per year, another treatment option is valacyclovir 500 mg qd with an increase to 1 g qd if breakthrough
Lymphogranuloma venereum	Invasive serovar L1, L2, L3 of *C. trachomatis*	Vesicular or ulcerative lesion on external genitalia with inguinal lymphadenitis or buboes	Primary therapy: doxycycline 100 mg PO bid × 21 days Alternative therapy: erythromycin 500 mg qid × 21 days
Nongonococcal urethritis and cervicitis	*C. trachomatis* (50%), *Mycoplasma hominis*, *Mycoplasma genitalium* Assume concomitant infection with *N. gonorrhoeae*, unless ruled out by accurate diagnostic testing	Irritative voiding symptoms, rarely mucopurulent vaginal discharge, cervicitis, often asymptomatic	Primary therapy: azithromycin 1 g PO as a single dose or doxycycline 100 mg PO bid × 7 days Alternative therapy: erythromycin base 500 mg PO qid × 7 days or ofloxacin 300 mg bid × 7 days or levofloxacin 500 mg qd × 7 days

TABLE 13–9
Female Genitourinary Infection—cont'd

Conditions	Causative Organism	Clinical Presentation	Treatment Options
Gonococcal urethritis and cervicitis	*N. gonorrhoeae* Assume concomitant infection with *N. gonorrhoeae*, unless ruled out by accurate diagnostic testing	Irritative voiding symptoms, occasional purulent vaginal discharge, cervicitis	Recommended therapy: single-dose therapy for uncomplicated infection Cefixime 400 mg po or ceftriaxone 125 mg IM Concurrently treat with azithromycin 1 g as a single dose or doxycycline 100 mg bid × 7 days if chlamydial infection has not been ruled out Alternative therapy in the presence of severe beta-lactam allergy: spectinomycin 2 g IM as single dose
Genital warts (condyloma acuminata)	Human papillomavirus	Verruca-form lesions or can be subclinical or unrecognized	Patient-applied therapy: podofilox 0.5% solution or imiquimod 5% cream Provider-applied therapy: liquid nitrogen or cryoprobe, trichloroacetic acid, podophyllin resin, or surgical removal
Bacterial vaginosis	Overgrowth of anaerobes including *Gardnerella* species and *Mycoplasma hominis*	Increased volume of vaginal secretions; thin, gray, homogeneous discharge; burning; pruritus. On microscopic examination: vaginal pH >4.5, clue cells, positive whiff test, few white blood cells	First-line therapies: metronidazole 500 mg bid × 7 days or metronidazole gel 0.75%, 1 applicator (5 g) intravaginally qd × 5 days or clindamycin cream 2%, 1 applicator (5 g) intravaginally at hs × 7 days Alternative regimens: metronidazole 2 g as single dose or clindamycin 300 mg bid × 7 days or clindamycin ovules 100 g intravaginally at bedtime × 3 days, or tinidazole 2 g PO daily × 2 days or 1 g PO daily × 5 days
Candidiasis	*Candida albicans, Candida glabrata, Candida tropicalis*	Itching, burning, thick white-to-yellow adherent, curdlike discharge, vulvovaginal excoriation, erythema, excoriation. On microscopic examination: hyphae, pseudohyphae, pH <5, few white blood cells	Single-day therapy options: fluconazole (Diflucan) 150 mg PO as single dose), butoconazole 2% SR cream (Gynazole-1), tioconazole 6.5% (Vagistat-1), miconazole (Monistat) 1200 mg, as single dose vaginally

Continued

TABLE 13–9

Female Genitourinary Infection—cont'd

Conditions	Causative Organism	Clinical Presentation	Treatment Options
Pelvic inflammatory disease	*N. gonorrhoeae, C. trachomatis, E. coli, Mycoplasma* and *Ureaplasma* species, others	Irritative voiding symptoms, fever, abdominal pain, cervical motion tenderness, vaginal discharge	Various 3- and 7-day therapies with azole antifungal vaginal creams, suppositories, tablets (miconazole, butoconazole, terconazole [Terazol], tioconazole) Recommended therapy for outpatient treatment: ceftriaxone 250 mg IM as a single dose plus doxycycline 100 mg bid × 14 days with or without metronidazole 500 mg bid × 14 days Alternate oral regimens: ofloxacin 400 mg PO bid or levofloxacin 500 mg PO qd with or without metronidazole 500 mg PO bid × 14 days. Alternate regimen should be used only with awareness of quinolone-resistant *N. gonorrhoeae,* but may be the primary treatment alternative in the presence of significant penicillin or cephalosporin allergy
Trichomoniasis	*T. vaginalis*	Dysuria, itching, vulvovaginal irritation, dyspareunia, yellow-green vaginal discharge, cervical petechial hemorrhages ("strawberry spots") in about 30% On microscopic examination: motile organisms and white blood cells	Recommended therapy: metronidazole (Flagyl) or tinidazole (Tindamax) 2 g as a one-time dose. Alternative therapy: metronidazole 500 mg PO bid × 7 days

Sources: Gilbert D, Moellering R, Eliopoulus G, Sande M. *The Sanford Guide to Antimicrobial Therapy*. 38th ed. Sperryville, VA: Antimicrobial Therapy, Inc; 2008; and Workowski KA, Berman SM. Sexually transmitted disease treatment guidelines, 2006. *MMWR Morb Mortal Wkly Rep.* 2006;55(No. RR-11):1–94.

virus form that causes cold sores, is rarely implicated. HHV-2 can infect the perioral area, however. The clinical presentation usually includes a painful ulcerated genital lesion, often accompanied by inguinal lymphadenopathy. If lesions involve the vagina or its introitus, a thin, sometimes profuse discharge accompanies the infection. Treatment with an antiviral such as acyclovir, famciclovir, or valacyclovir for acute infection, recurrence, or suppression is highly effective.

As with all STIs, a critical part of care is discussion of preventive strategies, including condom use and limiting the number of sexual partners. NPs should offer and encourage testing for other STIs, including HIV, hepatitis B, and syphilis.

Discussion Sources

Gilbert D, Moerlling R, Eliopoulos G, Chambers H, Saag M. *The Sanford Guide to Antimicrobial Therapy*. 39th ed. Sperryville, VA: Antimicrobial Therapy, Inc; 2009:21–25.

Workowski KA, Berman SM. Sexually transmitted disease treatment guidelines, 2006. *MMWR Morb Mortal Wkly Rep.* 2006;55(No. RR-11):1–94.

QUESTIONS

72. Women with PID typically present with all of the following except:

    A. dysuria.
    B. leukopenia.
    C. cervical motion tenderness.
    D. abdominal pain.

73. The most likely causative pathogen in a 26-year-old woman with PID is:

    A. *Escherichia coli.*
    B. Enterobacteriaceae.
    C. *C. trachomatis.*
    D. *Pseudomonas.*

74. Which of the following is a treatment option for a 30-year-old woman with PID and a history of severe hive-form reaction when taking a penicillin or cephalosporin?

    A. ofloxacin with metronidazole
    B. amoxicillin with gentamicin
    C. cefixime with vancomycin
    D. clindamycin with azithromycin

ANSWERS

72. B   73. C   74. A

DISCUSSION

PID is an infectious disease consisting of endometritis, salpingitis, and oophoritis. It is caused by various pathogens, including *C. trachomatis, N. gonorrhoeae, Haemophilus influenzae, Streptococcus* species, select anaerobes, *Mycoplasma* species, and *Ureaplasma* species; approximately 60% of infections are acquired through sexual transmission. Clinical presentation usually includes lower abdominal pain, abnormal vaginal discharge, dyspareunia, fever, gastrointestinal upset, or abnormal vaginal bleeding. An adnexal mass may be palpable when tubo-ovarian abscess is present. Supporting laboratory findings include elevated erythrocyte sedimentation rate or C-reactive protein level and leukocytosis with neutrophilia. Although diagnosis can usually be made from clinical findings, transvaginal ultrasound may show tubal thickening with or without free pelvic fluid or tubo-ovarian abscess.

Treatment options differ according to patient presentation. When a woman with PID is severely ill, is pregnant, or has tubo-ovarian abscess, hospitalization for hydration and parenteral antibiotic therapy is indicated. In most situations, outpatient therapy with oral or parenteral antibiotics is sufficient. Ceftriaxone, 250 mg intramuscularly as a one-time dose, followed by doxycycline, 100 mg bid for 2 weeks, is likely the most commonly used treatment regimen and is highly effective. A fluoroquinolone with or without metronidazole offers an effective oral treatment option that is a reasonable alternative in the presence of severe penicillin or cephalosporin allergy; when considering this combination, the practitioner must realize that *N. gonorrhoeae* is often quinolone-resistant.

As with all STIs, a critical part of care is discussion of preventive strategies, including condom use and limiting the number of sexual partners. NPs should offer and encourage testing for other STIs, including HIV, hepatitis B, and syphilis.

Discussion Sources

Gilbert D, Moerlling R, Eliopoulos G, Chambers H, Saag M. *The Sanford Guide to Antimicrobial Therapy.* 39th ed. Sperryville, VA: Antimicrobial Therapy, Inc; 2009:21–25.

Workowski KA, Berman SM. Sexually transmitted disease treatment guidelines, 2006. *MMWR Morb Mortal Wkly Rep.* 2006;55(No. RR-11):1–94.

QUESTIONS

75. A concomitant health problem occasionally seen with genital condyloma acuminatum is:

    A. cervical carcinoma.
    B. PID.
    C. vaginal fistula.
    D. reactive arthritis (Reiter syndrome).

76. Which of the following best describes lesions associated with condyloma acuminatum?

    A. verruciform
    B. plaquelike
    C. vesicular-form
    D. bullous

77. Treatment options for patients with condyloma acuminatum include:

    A. imiquimod (Aldara).
    B. azithromycin.
    C. acyclovir.
    D. metronidazole.

78. Which HPV types are most likely to cause condyloma acuminatum?

    A. 1, 2, and 3
    B. 6 and 11
    C. 16 and 18
    D. 22 and 24

79. Which HPV types are most often associated with cervical cancer?

A. 1, 2, and 3
B. 6 and 11
C. 16 and 18
D. 22 and 24

80. What percentage of anogenital and cervical cancers can be attributed to HPV infection?

A. less than 30
B. 30 to 50
C. 50 to 80
D. 95 or greater

81. Which of the following terms describes the mechanism of action of imiquimod (Aldara)?

A. keratolytic
B. immune modulator
C. cryogenic
D. cytolytic

ANSWERS

75.	A	**76.**	A	**77.**	A
78.	B	**79.**	C	**80.**	D
81.	B				

DISCUSSION

Condyloma acuminatum is a verruciform lesion seen in genital warts and is an STI. The causative agent is human papillomavirus (HPV), and infection with multiple HPV types is usually seen with genital infection. Anal, penile, and cervical carcinomas can be consequences of HPV infection. Not all HPV types are correlated with malignancy, however. HPV types with high malignancy risks include types 16, 18, 31, 33, 35, 39, and 45, whereas low malignancy risks are seen with infection with types 6, 11, 40, 42, 43, 44, 54, 61, 70, 72, and 81. HPV types 6 and 11 most often cause genital warts. About 50% of patients have spontaneous regression of warts without intervention. Treatment options include podofilox, imiquimod, trichloroacetic acid, or cryotherapy. Prescribing patient-administered therapies such as imiquimod (Aldara) or podofilox saves the cost and inconvenience of office visits. Surgical intervention is typically reserved for complicated, recalcitrant lesions.

As with all STIs, a critical part of care is discussion of preventive strategies, including condom use and limiting the number of sexual partners. NPs should offer and encourage testing for other STIs, including HIV, hepatitis B, and syphilis.

Discussion Sources

Gilbert D, Moerlling R, Eliopoulos G, Chambers H, Saag M. *The Sanford Guide to Antimicrobial Therapy*. 39th ed. Sperryville, VA: Antimicrobial Therapy, Inc; 2009:21–25.

Workowski KA, Berman SM. Sexually transmitted disease treatment guidelines, 2006. *MMWR Morb Mortal Wkly Rep*. 2006;55(No. RR-11):1–94.

QUESTIONS

82. How long after contact do clinical manifestations of syphilis typically occur?

A. less than 1 week
B. 1 to 3 weeks
C. 2 to 4 weeks
D. 4 to 6 weeks

83. Which of the following is not representative of the presentation of primary syphilis?

A. painless ulcer
B. palpable inguinal nodes
C. flu-like symptoms
D. spontaneously healing lesion

84. Which of the following is not representative of the presentation of secondary syphilis?

A. generalized rash
B. chancre
C. arthralgia
D. lymphadenopathy

85. Which of the following is found in tertiary syphilis?

A. arthralgia
B. lymphadenopathy
C. macular or papular lesions involving the palms and soles
D. gumma

86. Syphilis is most contagious during which of the following?

A. before onset of signs and symptoms
B. at the primary stage
C. at the secondary stage
D. at the tertiary stage

87. First-line treatment options for primary syphilis include:

A. penicillin.
B. ciprofloxacin.
C. erythromycin.
D. ceftriaxone.

ANSWERS

82.	C	83.	C	84.	B
85.	D	86.	C	87.	A

DISCUSSION

Caused by the spirochete *Treponema pallidum*, syphilis ♂ is a complex, multiorgan disease. ♂ Sexual contact is the usual route of transmission. The initial lesion forms about 2 to 4 weeks after contact; contagion is greatest during the secondary stage. Treatment is guided by the stage of disease and clinical manifestations (Table 13–10).

As with all STIs, a critical part of care is discussion of preventive strategies, including condom use and limiting the number of sexual partners. The NP should offer and encourage testing for other STIs, including HIV and hepatitis B.

Discussion Source

Workowski KA, Berman SM. Sexually transmitted disease treatment guidelines, 2006. *MMWR Morb Mortal Wkly Rep.* 2006;55(No. RR-11):1–94.

TABLE 13–10

Stages of Syphilis, Clinical Manifestations, and Recommended Treatment

Stage of Syphilis	Clinical Manifestations	Treatment Options	Comment
Primary syphilis	Painless genital ulcer with clean base and indurated margins, localized lymphadenopathy	Recommended therapy: • Benzathine penicillin G 2.4 million U IM as a 1-time dose Alternative therapy in penicillin allergy: • Doxycycline 100 mg PO bid × 2 weeks or • Tetracycline 500 mg PO qid × 2 weeks or • Ceftriaxone 1 g IM or IV q 24 h × 8–10 days	Azithromycin 2 g as a 1-time dose has been suggested, although issues of emerging resistance are concerning
Secondary syphilis	Diffuse maculopapular rash involving palms and soles, generalized lymphadenopathy, low-grade fever, malaise, arthralgias and myalgia, headache	Recommended therapy: • Benzathine penicillin G 2.4 million U IM as a 1-time dose Alternative therapy in penicillin allergy: • Doxycycline 100 mg PO bid × 2 weeks or • Tetracycline 500 mg PO qid × 2 weeks	Also treatment for latent syphilis of <1 year's duration
Late or tertiary syphilis	Gumma (granulomatous lesions involving skin, mucous membranes, bone), aortic insufficiency, aortic aneurysm, Argyll Robertson pupil, seizures	Recommended therapy: • Benzathine penicillin G 2.4 million U IM × 3 weekly doses Alternative therapy in penicillin allergy: • Doxycycline 100 mg PO bid × 4 weeks or • Tetracycline 500 mg PO qid × 4 weeks Expert consultation advisable, especially in the face of neurosyphilis	Also treatment for latent syphilis of >1 year's or unknown duration

Source: Workowski KA, Berman SM. Sexually transmitted disease treatment guidelines, 2006. *MMWR Morb Mortal Wkly Rep.* 2006;55 (No. RR-11):1–94.

14

Older Adults

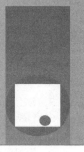

QUESTIONS

1. In the elderly population, the current fastest growing group is the age range:
   A. 71 to 75 years.
   B. 76 to 80 years.
   C. 81 to 84 years.
   D. 85 years and older.

2. The age range referred to as "young old" is:
   A. 60 to 65 years.
   B. 66 to 70 years.
   C. 65 to 74 years.
   D. 70 to 80 years.

3. Which of the following is most commonly reported as the largest single source of income for elderly people?
   A. Social Security
   B. public/private pension earnings
   C. asset income
   D. family financial support

4. The poverty rate among elderly people residing in the United States can best be described as:
   A. at approximately the same level across ethnic and age groups.
   B. highest among the old old.
   C. greatest among married couples.
   D. highest among older adults depending on investment income as a substantial part of their finances.

DISCUSSION

The older adult population is usually classified into four groups: the young old, 65 to 74 years old; the old old, 75 to 84 years old; the oldest old, 85 to 100 years old; and the elite old, more than 100 years old. Significant increase in the population group older than 65 years is projected to occur from 2010 to 2030. This increase is largely attributable to the aging of the "Baby Boomers," the demographic born from 1946 to 1964, and to a sharp decline in mortality at older ages. Currently, the fastest growing group of older adults is those older than age 85 years.

Among elderly people residing in the United States, Social Security is mentioned as the most important source of income. Private or public pension and income from other financial investments together are mentioned as most important at less than half the frequency. In the early 1970s, the poverty rate for elderly adults was approximately 20%. Currently, the older adult demographic has an overall poverty rate of approximately 11%, which is a significant improvement. Certain groups, including the old-old, women living alone, and select ethnic groups, have poverty rates double the overall rate.

Discussion Source

Centers for Disease Control and Prevention. http://www.cdc.gov/nchs/data/nvsr/nvsr54/nvsr54_14.pdf, National Vital Statistics Reports, United States Life Tables vol 54(13), 2007, accessed 10/1/09.

ANSWERS

| 1. | D | 2. | C |
| 3. | A | 4. | B |

See full color images of this topic on DavisPlus at http://davisplus.fadavis.com | Keyword: Fitzgerald

QUESTIONS

5 to 9.   Match the following age-related changes in the senses with the problem reported by the older adult.

_____ **5.** Difficulty with appreciating the content of conversation in noisy environment
_____ **6.** Decline in sense of smell
_____ **7.** Painless vision change that includes central vision distortion
_____ **8.** Results in near vision blurriness
_____ **9.** Can result in peripheral vision loss

A. Hyposmia
B. Presbycusis
C. Presbyopia
D. Age-related maculopathy
E. Chronic glaucoma

ANSWERS

5.   B   **6.**   A   **7.**   D   **8.**   C   **9.**   E

DISCUSSION

Normative aging results in changes in the senses. In addition, certain diseases that result in changes in the senses are more common in older adults (Table 14–1).

Discussion Source

Merck Manual of Geriatrics. www.merck.com/mrkshared/mmg/contents.jsp, accessed 10/1/09.

QUESTIONS

10. Age-related changes in an elderly adult include all of the following except:
   A. total body water decreases by 10% to 15% between ages 20 and 80 years.
   B. body weight as fat increases from 18% to 36% in men and from 33% to 45% in women.
   C. increase in serum albumin.
   D. increase in gastric pH.

11. A general principle of drug absorption in an elderly adult is best described as:
   A. amount of absorption is decreased.
   B. rate of absorption is changed.
   C. drug absorption is altered but predictable.
   D. bioavailability is altered.

12. When evaluating serum creatinine in an elderly adult, the clinician considers that:
   A. this value is influenced by glomerular filtration rate.
   B. age-related physiological changes do not influence this laboratory value.
   C. male and female norms are equivalent.
   D. an increase is an expected age-related change.

13. Anticipated age-related changes that can result in less drug effect include:
   A. loss of beta-2 receptor sites.
   B. lower gastrointestinal (GI) pH.
   C. increased renin-angiotensin production.
   D. increased GI motility.

14. When prescribing a diuretic, the NP considers that elderly people:
   A. have diminished ability to conserve sodium.
   B. have increased ability to excrete potassium.
   C. have continued response to a thiazide despite increasing creatinine.
   D. often develop allergic reaction to these products.

15. In an older adult with impaired renal function, the clinician anticipates that there is usually no need to adjust the antimicrobial dose with the use of:
   A. ceftriaxone.
   B. tobramycin.
   C. levofloxacin.
   D. vancomycin.

16. Which of the following medications has little anti-cholinergic effect?
   A. diphenhydramine
   B. amitriptyline
   C. chlorpheniramine
   D. loratadine

17. The process of absorption, distribution, metabolism, and elimination of a drug is known as:
   A. pharmacodynamics.
   B. drug interactions study.
   C. pharmacokinetics.
   D. therapeutic transformation.

TABLE 14–1

Age-Related Changes and Conditions That Result in Changes of the Senses

Condition	Etiology	Result	Comment
Presbyopia	Hardening of lens	Close vision problems	Nearly all adults ≥45 y.o. need reading glasses
Senile cataracts	Lens clouding	Progressive vision dimming, distance vision problems, close vision usually retained and may initially improve	Risk factors: Tobacco use, poor nutrition, sun exposure, corticosteroid therapy Potentially correctable with surgery, lens implant
Open-angle glaucoma	Painless, gradual onset of increased intraocular pressure leading to optic atrophy	Loss of peripheral vision	≥80% of all glaucoma. Periodic screening with tonometry, assessment of visual fields. Treatment with topical miotics, beta blockers, other drugs, or surgery effective in vision preservation
Angle-closure glaucoma	Sudden increase in intraocular pressure	Usually unilateral, acutely red, painful eye with vision change including halos around lights; eyeball firm compared with other eyeball	Immediate referral to ophthalmologist for rapid pressure reduction via medication, possible surgery
Age-related maculopathy (MD)	Thickening, sclerotic changes in retinal basement membrane complex	Painless vision changes including distortion of central vision	Besides aging, risk factors include tobacco use, sun exposure, family history. Dry form: No treatment available except to minimize risk factors that worsen the condition. Wet form: Laser treatment and other therapies to obliterate neovascular membrane
Hyposmia	Neural degeneration	Decline in sense of smell, usually gradual, resulting in fine taste discrimination (largely a function of smell)	Accelerated by tobacco use
Presbycusis	Multifactorial including loss of eighth cranial nerve sensitivity	Difficult with appreciating the content of conversation in noisy environment. Person can hear, but cannot understand	Accelerated by excessive noise exposure. Hearing aids helpful
Cerumen impaction	Conductive hearing loss	General diminution of hearing	Cerumen removal

Source: Merck Manual of Geriatrics. www.merck.com/mrkshared/mmg/contents.jsp, accessed 7/29/09.

18. When prescribing a medication, the clinician considers that half-life is the amount of time needed to decrease the serum concentration of a drug by:

    A. 25%.
    B. 50%.
    C. 75%.
    D. 100%.

19. Under ordinary circumstances, how many half-lives are usually needed for a drug to reach steady state?

    A. 0.5 to 1
    B. 1 to 3
    C. 3 to 5
    D. 5 to 7

20. Compared with a healthy 40-year-old adult, CYP 450 isoenzyme levels can decrease by ___% in elderly adults after age 70.

    A. 10
    B. 20
    C. 30
    D. 40

TABLE 14–2

Age-Related Changes Important to Medication Use

	Age 20–30 Years	Age 60–80 Years
Percent body weight as water	60%	53%
Lean muscle mass	Baseline	≥20% reduction
Serum albumin (average)	4.7 g	3.8 g
Relative kidney weight	100%	80%
Relative hepatic blood flow	100%	55%–60%

Source: Katzung B. Special aspects in geriatric pharmacology. In: Katzung B. *Basic and Clinical Pharmacology*. 10th ed. New York, NY: McGraw Medical; 2007:983–990.

ANSWERS

10.	C	11.	B	12.	A
13.	A	14.	A	15.	A
16.	D	17.	C	18.	B
19.	C	20.	C		

DISCUSSION

"Start low, go slow" is geriatric prescribing advice all clinicians likely learned. Although there is wisdom in this adage, a more complete understanding of numerous age-related factors is needed for safe prescribing for elderly adults.

Elderly people are a heterogeneous group who constitute a small portion of the North American population, yet uses approximately one-third of prescription medications and nearly three-fourths of all over-the-counter medications. Because advancing age is often accompanied by various health problems, elderly adults often have multiple health-care providers and multiple prescribers and medications. In addition, normative age-related physiological changes can influence pharmacological responses; these changes are often accentuated by illness (Table 14–2). Financial constraints commonly cause elderly adults to use a medication less often than prescribed or to attempt to substitute. The clinician must be aware of these factors to prescribe for older adults safely and effectively.

Because the term "elder" or "elderly adult" is typically used to describe any person age 65 or older, this could imply that aging occurs only after this milestone. In reality, normal age-related changes influencing drug therapy occur gradually over decades. These changes often lead to altered pharmacokinetics; components of pharmacokinetics include drug absorption, distribution, biotransformation (metabolism), and excretion. A simple way of remembering pharmacokinetics principles is that this is what the body does to the drug. At the same time, pharmacodynamics, the study of biochemical and physiological effects of drugs, or what the drug does to the body or disease does not change over the life span. Normative age-related changes, such as the loss of the beta-2-receptor sites, result in less of a clinical effect with beta-2-agonist use, however.

Although age alone likely does not alter the amount of the drug absorbed, age-related changes can significantly influence the rate of absorption. A drug's half-life ($T\frac{1}{2}$), defined as the time required for the amount of drug in the body to be reduced by one-half, is often increased in older adults. As gastric acid production decreases, stomach pH increases, potentially prolonging the initial breakdown of medication made to dissolve in low pH. In addition, age-related decreases in GI blood flow, gastric motility, and gastric emptying mean that medication stays in the gut longer, whereas decreased GI surface area can lead to erratic absorption. The use of antacids in the elderly population complicates this situation by increasing stomach pH further, potentially allowing the formation of an inactive drug-antacid compound, and delivering drug to absorption sites in the intestines at a variable rate; proton pump inhibitors and histamine-2 receptor antagonists also increase stomach pH.

Drug distribution can be altered by age-related changes. Serum albumin, an important plasma protein used to bind and distribute various medications including warfarin

(Coumadin) and phenytoin (Dilantin), decreases with aging. With less albumin available for drug binding, potentially more free drug is available. These changes, coupled with altered drug elimination, often lead to a decrease in the dose needed in an aging adult. The amount of the plasma protein alpha-1-acid glycoprotein, with an affinity for binding with certain medications including propranolol, quinidine, and lidocaine, increases; as a result, less free drug is in circulation.

Age-related hepatic changes include decreased hepatic, blood flow, mass, and functioning hepatocytes and diminished activity of hepatic enzymes responsible for drug metabolism. These changes contribute to a prolonged drug $T\frac{1}{2}$ and longer duration of action than found in younger adults. In addition, ability to recover from alcohol-induced, medication-induced, or viral-induced hepatic damage is lessened.

Renal changes noted in aging are numerous. Glomerular filtration rate (GFR), the rate plasma is filtered through the glomeruli, continues at the maximal adult rate through age 50. GFR then begins a gradual decline, with approximately 80% of maximal adult rate at age 60, 70% by age 70, and 55% by age 80. GFR, coupled with reduced renal mass, loss of functional nephrons, and diminished renal blood flow, can lead to problems with drug elimination. Health problems such as diabetes mellitus and hypertension can compromise renal function further. As a result, having an accurate measure of renal function before prescribing is important. Formed from lean muscle, creatinine production and excretion rate are equal in health. Lean muscle mass decreases in aging; this decline parallels age-related renal function changes; this can lead to a normal serum creatinine in elderly adults when renal function is significantly impaired.

Compared with serum creatinine, creatinine clearance and GFR provide a more accurate measure of renal function, especially in an older adult. Many medications that are excreted via the renal route carry a notice of needed dose adjustment in the presence of impaired renal function, using creatinine clearance or GFR levels as the guide for appropriate dose. Creatinine clearance is most accurately measured by obtaining a 24-hour urine specimen. Given that a medication that requires dose adjustment in the presence of renal impairment often needs to be started urgently, waiting for the results of a 24-hour urine test to be collected and analyzed is often impractical. Using the Cockcroft-Gault equation provides a reasonable estimate of creatinine clearance. As creatinine clearance is reduced, dose or dosing interval adjustment of numerous medications, including angiotensin-converting enzyme inhibitors and certain antibiotics, is required. GFR can be calculated using the formula found at the National Kidney Foundation's website at http://www.kidney.org/professionals/kdoqi/gfr_calculator.cfm. The dosing interval of trimethoprim-sulfamethoxazole (Bactrim) needs to be adjusted in the presence of renal impairment with abnormal creatinine clearance or GFR. In contrast, ceftriaxone (Rocephin) can be used without dose or dosing interval adjustment in the presence of altered GFR or creatinine clearance.

Medications with significant systemic anticholinergic effect should be avoided in older adults because of risk of confusion, urinary retention, constipation, visual disturbance, and hypotension. If anticholinergic effect is unavoidable, a product in the class with the least amount of this effect should be chosen. A tricyclic antidepressant can be a helpful and inexpensive treatment option for the management of chronic neuropathic pain, but can have significant anticholinergic effect. Compared with amitriptyline, nortriptyline has significantly less of this effect, however, and is likely a better treatment option. If an antihistamine is needed, loratadine offers an option with little anticholinergic effect, whereas diphenhydramine is a less attractive option, owing to its strong anticholinergic effect.

The adage, "start low, go slow" in prescribing for elderly adults has an often forgotten third part: "but get to goal." Clinicians, in their zeal to provide safe pharmacotherapeutic care for older adult patients, often prescribe enough of a medication to give anticipated adverse effects, but not enough to provide the desired therapeutic effect. Knowledge of the safe and appropriate medication doses in older adults, keeping in mind the age-related effects on pharmacokinetics, is a critical part to safe prescriptive practice.

Discussion Sources

Fick DM. http://archinte.ama-assn.org/cgi/content/full/163/22/2716, Updating the Beers criteria for potentially inappropriate medication use in older adults, 2002, accessed 10/1/09.

Katzung B. Special aspects in geriatric pharmacology. In: Katzung B. *Basic and Clinical Pharmacology*. 10th ed. New York, NY: McGraw Medical; 2007:983–990.

QUESTIONS

21. While making a home visit to a bedridden 89-year-old man, you note that he is cachectic, dehydrated, but cognitively intact. He states he is not receiving his medications regularly, and that his granddaughter is supposed to take care of him, but mentions, "She seems more interested in my Social Security check." The patient is unhappy, but asks that you not "tell anybody" because he wants to remain in his home. The most appropriate action would be to:

    A. talk with the patient's granddaughter and evaluate her ability to care for the patient.
    B. visit the patient more frequently to ensure that his condition does not deteriorate.
    C. report the situation to the appropriate state agency.
    D. honor the patient's wishes because a competent patient has the right to determine care.

22. Which of the following statements is true concerning elder maltreatment?

    A. This problem is found mainly in families of lower socioeconomic status.

    B. An elderly adult who is being mistreated usually seeks help.

    C. Routine screening is indicated as part of the care of an older adult.

    D. In most instances of elder maltreatment, a predictable cycle of physical violence directed at the older adult followed by a period of remorse on the part of the perpetrator is the norm.

23. Risk factors for becoming a perpetrator of elder maltreatment include all of the following except:

    A. a high level of hostility about the caregiver role.

    B. poor coping skills.

    C. assumption of caregiving responsibilities at a later stage of life.

    D. maltreatment as a child.

24. Elder maltreatment is considered to be underreported, with an estimated ___ cases going unreported to each one case that is reported.

    A. three

    B. four

    C. five

    D. six

25. The most commonly reported form of elder maltreatment form:

    A. physical abuse.

    B. sexual exploitation.

    C. financial exploitation.

    D. neglect.

ANSWERS

21.	C	22.	C	23.	C
24.	C	25.	D		

DISCUSSION

The Centers for Disease Control and Prevention (CDC) defines elder maltreatment as any abuse and neglect of persons age 60 and older by a caregiver or another person in a relationship involving an expectation of trust. Elder maltreatment can take various forms (Table 14–3). Every state in the United States and many Canadian provinces have enacted legislation to protect vulnerable older adults from abuse, with a requirement for health-care workers and others who come in contact with older adults to report this abuse to the appropriate protective authorities. Elder maltreatment is significantly underreported; for every one case reported, an estimated five other cases go unreported. Neglect is the most commonly encountered type of elder maltreatment. In times of economic difficulty, the rate of financial exploitation usually increases.

A combination of individual, relational, community, and societal factors contribute to the risk of an individual becoming a perpetrator of elder maltreatment. Understanding these factors can help identify various opportunities for prevention.

Risk factors for perpetration of elder maltreatment include a current diagnosis of mental illness or alcohol abuse, a high level of hostility about the caregiver role, poor coping skills, inadequate preparation for caregiving responsibilities, assumption of caregiving responsibilities at an early age, and maltreatment as a child. At the relationship level, additional risk factors emerge, including a high level of financial and emotional dependence on a vulnerable elder, a past experience of disruptive behavior, and lack of social support. Elder mistreatment is likely to be more prevalent in a cultural and community milieu where tolerance of aggressive behavior and negative beliefs about aging and elderly adults exist; formal services such as respite care for individuals providing care to elderly adults are limited, inaccessible, or unavailable; family members are expected to care for elderly adults without seeking help from others; and individuals are encouraged to endure suffering or remain silent regarding their pain. At the institutional level, such as in a long-term care or assisted living facility, unsympathetic or negative attitudes toward residents, chronic staffing problems, lack of administrative oversight, staff burnout, and stressful working conditions are considered risk factors for elder maltreatment.

Certain factors have been identified as being protective against elder mistreatment, including strong personal relationships, community support for the caregiver role, and coordinated resources to help serve elderly adults and caregivers. Factors within institutional settings that can be protective include effective monitoring systems in place; clear, understandable institutional policies and procedures regarding patient care; ongoing education on elder abuse and neglect for employees; education about and clear guidance on how durable power of attorney is to be used; and regular visits by family members, volunteers, and social workers.

Discussion Sources

Centers for Disease Control and Prevention. http://www.cdc.gov/violenceprevention/eldermaltreatment/, Elder mistreatment, accessed 10/1/09.

Elder Maltreatment Alliance. http://www.eldermaltreatment.com/asp/information.asp, Information, accessed 10/1/09.

TABLE 14–3
Forms of Elder Maltreatment

Form of Elder Maltreatment	Descriptions
Physical abuse	Elderly adult is injured by another individual including being scratched, bitten, slapped, pushed, hit, or burned; assaulted or threatened with a weapon including a knife, gun, or other object; or inappropriately restrained
Sexual abuse or abusive sexual contact	Any sexual contact against elderly adult's will, including acts in which elderly adult is unable to understand the act or is unable to communicate consent. Abusive sexual contact is defined as intentional touching, either directly or through the clothing, of the genitalia, anus, groin, breast, mouth, inner thigh, or buttocks
Psychological or emotional abuse	Any event in which elderly adult experiences trauma after exposure to threatening acts or coercive tactics. Examples include humiliation or embarrassment; controlling behavior such as prohibiting or limiting access to transportation, telephone, money, or other resources; social isolation; disregarding or trivializing needs; or damaging or destroying property
Neglect	Failure or refusal of a caregiver or other responsible person to provide for elderly adult's basic physical, emotional, or social needs, or failure to protect elderly adult from harm. Examples include not providing adequate nutrition, hygiene, clothing, shelter, or access to necessary health care, or failure to prevent exposure to unsafe activities and environments
Abandonment	Willful desertion of elderly adult by caregiver or other responsible person
Financial abuse or exploitation	Unauthorized or improper use of resources of elderly adult for monetary or personal benefit, profit, or gain by another individual. Examples include forgery, misuse or theft of money or possessions, use of coercion or deception to surrender finances or property, or improper use of guardianship or power of attorney
Self-neglect	This form of elder maltreatment is, as defined, instituted by the elderly adult, not another individual, and is the failure or refusal of elderly adult to address his or her own basic physical, emotional, or social needs. Examples include self-care tasks such as nourishment, clothing, hygiene, and shelter; proper or appropriate use of medications; and managing or administering one's finances. This is also characterized by the lack of intervention to halt or modify the behavior by another individual who is often in the position to recognize the problem

QUESTIONS

26. Orthostatic (postural) hypotension is defined as an excessive decrease in blood pressure (BP) with position, usually greater than _____ mm Hg systolic and _____ mm Hg diastolic.

    A. 10, 5
    B. 15, 7
    C. 20, 10
    D. 30, 15

27. Orthostatic hypotension is present in about _____% of older adults.

    A. 10
    B. 20
    C. 30
    D. 40

28. The use of all of the following medications is commonly recognized as a risk for postural hypotension except:

    A. nifedipine.
    B. furosemide.
    C. clonidine.
    D. atenolol.

29. Lifestyle interventions for an older adult with orthostatic hypotension should include counseling about:

    A. avoiding the use of compression stockings.
    B. minimizing salt intake.
    C. flexing the feet multiple times before changing position.
    D. restricting fluids.

30. In assessing a person with or at risk for orthostatic hypotension, the BP should be measured after 5 minutes in the supine position and then ___ and ___ minutes after standing.

   A. 1, 3
   B. 2, 4
   C. 3, 5
   D. 5, 10

ANSWERS

26.	C	**27.**	B	**28.**	D
29.	C	**30.**	A		

DISCUSSION

Although not a specific disease state, orthostatic (postural) hypotension is a manifestation of abnormal BP regulation. Normal BP is usually maintained by the sympathetic system causing an increase in heart rate and contractility in response to the pooling of blood in the lower extremity and trunk veins because of position change. Simultaneous parasympathetic (vagal) inhibition also increases heart rate. With continued standing, activation of the renin-angiotensin-aldosterone system and antidiuretic hormone secretion cause sodium and water retention and increase circulating blood volume. When these mechanisms do not work properly, BP control is not maintained with position change. The end result is a transient decrease in venous return, reduced cardiac output, and a decrease in BP; usually the first patient-reported effects from the decrease in BP are light-headedness, dizziness, or blurred vision that occur within seconds of changing position, most often from sitting to standing. Orthostatic hypotension is defined as an excessive decrease in BP when an upright position is assumed; the change in BP is usually greater than 20 mm Hg systolic and greater than 10 mm Hg diastolic with resulting symptoms that occur within seconds changing position from supine or sit to standing. This condition is present in about 20% of older adults and is a potent risk factor for falls.

Although age-related changes in the cardiovascular and cerebrovascular systems contribute to orthostatic hypotension, the use of certain medications can cause or worsen the condition. The medications most often implicated typically cause a decrease in circulating volume or peripheral vasodilation; these medications include loop diuretics, tricyclic antidepressants, calcium channel blockers, alpha-adrenergic blockers, centrally acting antihypertensives such as clonidine, and nitrates. Certain disease states that alter baseline cardiac output and vascular capacity, increasing orthostatic risk, are common in older adults; these include aortic stenosis, dehydration, peripheral vascular insufficiency, and electrolyte disturbances. Alcohol use is also a potent contributor, as is prolonged bedrest; beta blocker use is seldom implicated. Cardiac rhythm disturbances usually occur with regularity, which results in more consistent symptoms, not simply with position change, and are not a significant orthostatic hypotension contributor.

In assessing a person with or at risk for orthostatic hypotension, BP should be measured after the patient has been in a supine position for 5 minutes and then at 1 and 3 minutes after standing. Patient symptoms should be recorded. If the patient is too symptomatic or ill to stand, the maneuvers should be performed with supine to sit position change. If hypotension is accompanied by an increase of heart rate to greater than 100 bpm, altered circulating volume is the likely cause.

When orthostatic hypotension is documented, possible contributing factors, such as medications implicated in the condition, should be modified. Fluid and electrolyte imbalance, if a contributor, should be corrected. In addition, instruction about lifestyle modification to minimize risk is a critical and often overlooked intervention. This instruction includes information about moving slowly and deliberately with position change from supine to sit or supine to stand, dorsiflexing the feet multiple times before position change, and avoiding standing in one position for an excessive length of time; the use of compression stockings to enhance venous return can also be helpful. If not contraindicated by cardiac or other health issues, an increase in sodium and fluid intake usually helps increase circulating volume and minimizes orthostatic risk.

Discussion Sources

Katzung B. Special aspects in geriatric pharmacology. In: Katzung B. *Basic and Clinical Pharmacology*. 10th ed. New York, NY: McGraw Medical; 2007:983–990.

Merck Manual of Geriatrics. http://www.merck.com/mmpe/sec07/ch069/ch069d.html, Orthostatic hypotension, accessed 10/1/09.

QUESTIONS

31. Most falls in older adults occur in:

   A. a health-care institution.
   B. a public place.
   C. the patient's home.
   D. an outdoor setting.

32. The NP is asked to evaluate a 77-year-old woman who recently had an unexpected fall. The patient is normally healthy and has no mobility limitations or other obvious risk factors. During the history, the NP learns that the patient did not attempt to break the fall, "I just suddenly found myself on the floor." This statement suggests:

    A. a previously undiagnosed cognitive impairment that requires further evaluation.

    B. that underlying sensory deficits (visual, hearing) are the most likely cause of the fall and require physical assessment.

    C. that a history of alcohol use or abuse should be explored.

    D. a syncopal episode requiring a cardiovascular and neurological evaluation.

33. In an older adult, the greatest risk of long-term complication is associated with fracture of the:

    A. forearm.
    B. spine.
    C. ankle.
    D. hip.

34. Fall risk in an older adult is decreased with the use of which of the following footwear?

    A. sandal
    B. jogging shoe
    C. slipper
    D. semirigid sole shoe

35. With the use of insulin, fall risk in an older adult is most likely to occur _____ of the medication.

    A. at the onset of action
    B. at the peak of action
    C. at the middle point of duration of action
    D. toward the end of anticipated duration of action

36. An older adult who has recently fallen has a(n) _____ times increased risk of falling again within the next year.

    A. 1 to 2
    B. 2 to 3
    C. 3 to 4
    D. 4 to 5

37. With the use of a benzodiazepine in an older adult, the risk of fall is most likely to occur _____ of the medication.

    A. at the onset of action
    B. at the peak of action
    C. at the middle point of duration of action
    D. toward the end of anticipated duration of action

ANSWERS

31.	C	**32.**	D	**33.**	D
34.	D	**35.**	B	**36.**	B
37.	B				

DISCUSSION

Falls are a significant source of morbidity and mortality in the elderly population; multiple falls are associated with increased risk of death. Approximately one-third of community-dwelling elderly adults and two-thirds of long-term care residents experience falls each year. Of elderly adults who fall, 20% to 30% sustain moderate to severe injuries that reduce mobility and independence and increase the risk of premature death. Older adults are hospitalized for fall-related injuries five times more often than they are for injuries from other causes. For adults 65 years old or older, 60% of fatal falls happen at home, 30% occur in public places, and 10% occur in health-care institutions.

Risk factors for falls are numerous and are modifiable and nonmodifiable (Table 14–4). Polypharmacy, in particular the use of medications associated with postural hypotension, increases fall risk. Additional risks include personal history of a stroke or fall; a person who has fallen is two to three times more likely to fall within the next year. Environmental hazards in the home, including poorly placed furnishings and inadequate lighting, often contribute to falls. Wearing thick, soft-soled shoes, such as a jogging shoe, also increases fall risk.

TABLE 14–4
Fall and Fracture Risk Factors in Older Adults

Postural hypotension
Sensory impairment including altered vision and hearing
Parkinsonism
Osteoporosis
Osteoarthritis
Altered gait and balance including decreased proprioception, increased postural sway, slower righting reflexes, peripheral neuropathy, stroke
Psychotropic medication use, especially products with sedating effect
Cardiac drug use, especially products with properties that cause or contribute to postural hypotension
Environmental hazards

Source: Wachel T. Falls. In: Wachel T. *Geriatric Clinical Advisor.* Philadelphia, PA: Mosby; 2007:77–78.

Comprehensive elder care should focus on minimizing modifiable fall risks. When a fall does occur, the patient should be promptly and appropriately assessed. Questions should be asked to investigate for an underlying condition that could have contributed to the fall and is amenable to intervention and often subtle age-related changes that can contribute to increased fall risk (see Table 14–4). These questions are as follows:

- What was the patient doing when he or she fell?
- Was there an aura or warning that the fall was impending?
- Was there a vision loss?
- Did the patient experience dizziness?
- Was there a loss of consciousness?
- Did the patient break the fall?
- Is this an isolated incident, or are falls occurring more frequently?
- What medications is the patient taking? In particular, notation should be made of newly added medications or increased dose of existing medications.
- Was the patient drinking alcohol or taking other potentially intoxicating medications?

The assessment of an older adult after a fall should focus on identification of possible correctable fall risk factors and fall-related injury and should include, at minimum, the following:

- Vital signs and evaluation of orthostasis.
- Cardiovascular assessment.
- Sensory assessment.
- Assessment of gait and balance, including the use of the "Get Up and Go" test, in which the elderly adult is asked to rise from a straight-backed chair, walk 10 feet using usual walking aid such as a cane if applicable, turn, and return to the chair and sit down, with the clinician observing balance with sitting and on standing, pace and stability with walking, ability to turn without staggering, and time to complete the task.
- Survey for fall-related injuries.

The most common fall-related injuries are osteoporotic fractures of the hip, spine, or forearm. Of all fall-related fractures, hip fractures are the most serious and lead to the greatest number of health problems and deaths.

Nonpharmacological interventions to prevent falls include the following:

- Review medications; assess doses, and eliminate high-risk drugs that can contribute to falls (Table 14–5).
- Evaluate for postural hypotension.
- Provide prevention and treatment interventions for osteoporosis.
- Recommend proper footwear, avoiding slippers, sandals, and soft-soled jogging shoes in favor of an enclosed toe, tie shoe with a semirigid sole.
- Provide an obstacle free, well-lit environment.
- Raise chair heights and seat heights; add arm rests.
- Prescribe physical therapy as indicated.
- Counsel avoidance of quick position change and to perform multiple foot flex maneuvers before trying to move from supine to stand or sit to stand.
- Treat for any concomitant conditions associated with increased fall risk.

Discussion Sources

Merck Manual of Geriatrics. http://www.merck.com/mmpe/sec07/ch069/ch069d.html, Orthostatic hypotension, accessed 8/4/09.

Patient Safety Authority. http://www.patientsafetyauthority.org/ADVISORIES/AdvisoryLibrary/2008/Mar5(1)/Pages/16.aspx, Medication assessment: one determinant of falls risk, accessed 8/18/09.

Wachel T. Falls. In: Wachel T. *Geriatric Clinical Advisor.* Philadelphia, PA: Mosby Elsevier; 2007:77–78.

QUESTIONS

38. Factors that contribute to stress incontinence include:
    A. detrusor overactivity.
    B. pelvic floor weakness.
    C. urethral stricture.
    D. urinary tract infection (UTI).

39. Factors that contribute to urge incontinence include:
    A. detrusor overactivity.
    B. pelvic floor weakness.
    C. urethral stricture.
    D. UTI.

40. Pharmacological intervention for patients with urge incontinence includes:
    A. doxazosin (Cardura).
    B. tolterodine (Detrol).
    C. finasteride (Proscar).
    D. pseudoephedrine.

41. Intervention for patients with stress incontinence includes:
    A. establishing a voiding schedule.
    B. gentle bladder-stretching exercises.
    C. periurethral bulking agent injection.
    D. restricting fluid intake.

42. Which form of urinary incontinence is most common in older adults?
    A. stress
    B. urge
    C. iatrogenic
    D. overflow

43. Medications used to treat urge incontinence and overactive bladder usually have anticholinergic and antimuscarinic effects that can lead to problems in older adults including:
    A. tachycardia and hypertension.
    B. sedation and dry mouth.
    C. agitation and excessive saliva production.
    D. loose stools and loss of appetite.

TABLE 14–5

Medication Use Associated With Increased Fall Risk in Older Adults

Medication Class	Example	Comment
Anxiolytics and hypnotics	Benzodiazepines, long-acting and shorter acting, including lorazepam, oxazepam, alprazolam, temazepam, triazolam Nonbenzodiazepines including zolpidem	In particular, gait issues most likely to arise with onset and peak of medication's action, usually ½–2 hr after benzodiazepine or hypnotic is taken
Antidepressants	Tricyclic antidepressants (TCAs) such as amitriptyline, selective serotonin reuptake inhibitors (SSRIs) such as sertraline, citalopram	Orthostatic hypotension risk, typically worse with TCA compared with SSRI use
Neuroleptics and antipsychotics including atypical or second-generation antipsychotics (SGA)	Neuroleptics including haloperidol, SGA including risperidone	Orthostatic hypotension and dizziness risk significant and extrapyramidal movement risk
Opioid analgesics/antagonists	Meperidine, morphine, codeine	Risk of sedation. Meperidine particularly problematic. Pain should be appropriately and adequately treated and opioids used if benefit outweighs risk and with careful monitoring.
Insulin, oral hypoglycemics	Insulins, short-acting and longer acting, sulfonylureas such as glyburide, glipizide	Fall risk most often seen in presence of drug-induced hypoglycemia. If this occurs, it is most likely noted at drug's peak of action
Cardiac medications	Antihypertensives including diuretics, calcium channel blockers (CCBs), high-dose beta blockers, and nitrates	Fall risk increases with excessive diuretic use because of circulating volume constriction or peripheral vasodilation related to CCB or nitrate use. With high-dose beta blocker use, normative heart rate increase with position change can be blunted, resulting in dizziness

Note: This list is not intended to include all medications associated with increased fall risk in older adults, but rather to highlight products with well-documented risk.

Source: Patient Safety Authority. http://www.patientsafetyauthority.org/ADVISORIES/AdvisoryLibrary/2008/Mar5(1)/Pages/16.aspx, Medication assessment: one determinant of falls risk, accessed 8/18/09.

---

44. Poorly controlled diabetes mellitus is a potential cause of reversible urinary incontinence primarily caused by which of the following mechanisms?

    A. increased urinary volume
    B. increased UTI risk
    C. irritating effect of increased glucose in the urine
    D. decreased ability to perceive need to void

45. A 78-year-old woman who has osteoarthritis affecting both knees but no current problems with urinary incontinence is placed on a loop diuretic. She is now at increased risk for _____ urinary incontinence.

    A. overflow
    B. urge
    C. functional
    D. idiopathic

46. The diagnosis of _____ should be considered in an older adult with new-onset urinary incontinence coupled with an acute change in mental status.
    A. dementia
    B. spinal cord compression
    C. bladder stone
    D. delirium

ANSWERS

38.	B		**39.**	A		**40.**	B
41.	C		**42.**	B		**43.**	B
44.	A		**45.**	C		**46.**	D

DISCUSSION

Urinary incontinence is the involuntary loss of urine in sufficient amounts to be a problem. This condition is often thought by many elderly adults, women in particular, to be a normal part of aging. In reality, numerous treatment options are available after the cause of urinary incontinence is established (Table 14–6). In all cases, urinalysis and urine culture and sensitivity should be obtained. If UTI is present, treatment with an appropriate antimicrobial is indicated. Further diagnostic testing should be directed by patient presentation.

Urge incontinence is the most common form of urinary incontinence in elderly persons. Behavioral therapy, including a voiding schedule and gentle bladder stretching, are helpful. Pharmacological intervention is indicated in conjunction with behavioral therapy (see Table 14–6). Tolterodine (Detrol) and solifenacin succinate (VESIcare) are selective muscarinic receptor antagonists that block bladder receptors and limit bladder contraction. Helpful in the treatment of urge incontinence, the use of these products is associated with a decrease in the numbers of micturitions and of incontinent episodes, along with an increase in voiding volume. Oxybutynin (Ditropan) is a nonselective muscarinic receptor antagonist that blocks receptors in the bladder and oral cavity, with activity similar to that of tolterodine; adverse effects include dry mouth and constipation with increased risk for fecal impaction. Common to virtually all medications with systemic anticholinergic effect is the risk of sedation and alteration in sensorium (Table 14–7).

Numerous conditions can contribute to urinary incontinence transiently or permanently. Potentially treatable causes of urinary incontinence are represented in the *DIAPPERS* mnemonic.

*D*elirium
*I*nfection (urinary tract)
*A*trophic urethritis and vaginitis
*P*harmaceuticals (diuretics, others)
*P*sychological disorders (depression)
*E*xcessive urine output (heart failure, hyperglycemia)
*R*estricted mobility
*S*tool impaction

Discussion Sources

Katzung B. Special aspects in geriatric pharmacology. In: Katzung B. *Basic and Clinical Pharmacology*. 10th ed. New York, NY: McGraw Medical; 2007:983–990.

Ogundele O, Silverberg MD. http://emedicine.medscape.com/article/778772, Urinary incontinence, accessed 8/19/09.

Resnick NM. Urinary incontinence in the elderly. *Medical Grand Rounds*. 3:281–290, 1984.

Weiss B. http://www.aafp.org/afp/20050115/315.html, Selecting medications for the treatment of urinary incontinence, *American Family Physician*, accessed 8/19/09.

AUTHOR'S NOTE

Please see Index for information on commonly encountered problems in older adults, including delirium, dementia, depression, urinary tract infection, male and female genitourinary problems, endocrine disorders, pneumonia, chronic obstructive pulmonary disease, heart failure, and others.

Dr. Sally Miller's assistance in the development of this chapter is gratefully acknowledged.

TABLE 14–6

Clinical Issues in Urinary Incontinence

Type of Urinary Incontinence	Etiology and Population Most Often Affected	Clinical Presentation	Treatment Options
Urge incontinence	Detrusor overactivity causing uninhibited bladder contractions Most common form of incontinence in elderly adults	Strong sensation of needing to empty bladder that cannot be suppressed, often coupled with involuntary loss of urine	Avoiding stimulants, gentle bladder stretching by increasing voiding interval by 15–30 min after establishing a half-hour voiding schedule Add agent to reduce bladder contraction such as an anticholinergic; options include tolterodine (Detrol), oxybutynin (Ditropan), solifenacin succinate (VESIcare)
Stress incontinence	Weakness of pelvic floor and urethral muscles Most common form of incontinence in women; rare in men	Loss of urine with activity that causes increase in intra-abdominal pressure such as coughing, sneezing, exercise	Support to the area through the use of a vaginal tampon, urethral stents, periurethral bulking agent injections, and pessary use. Kegel and other similar exercises most helpful in younger patients. Pelvic floor rehabilitation with biofeedback, electrical stimulation, and bladder training Surgical intervention can be helpful in 75%–80%. Topical and systemic estrogen therapy formerly recommended for this condition, now recognized as not helpful and perhaps contributing to stress incontinence symptoms When urge and stress incontinence are present, the term mixed urinary incontinence is often used
Urethral obstruction	Obstruction of bladder outflow through urethral obstruction (prostatic, stricture, tumor) resulting in urinary retention with overflow and detrusor instability Most commonly found in older men	Postvoid dribbling coupled with urge incontinence on presentation	Treatment of urethral obstruction
Functional incontinence	Associated with inability to get to the toilet or lack of awareness of need to void	Usually in person with mobility issues or altered cognition. Worsened by unavailability of a helper to assist in toileting activities	Ameliorated by having assistant who is aware of voiding cue available to help with toileting activities
Transient incontinence	Associated with acute event such as delirium, UTI, medication use, restricted activity	Presentation consistent with underlying process	Treatment of underlying process, discontinuation of offending medication

TABLE 14–7

Select Medications and Their Effect on Urinary Continence

Type of Medication	Effect on Urinary Continence
Diuretics	Increase in volume and frequency of voiding. Use in older adult with limited mobility can result in functional urinary incontinence
Drugs with anticholinergic/antimuscarinic activity such as first-generation antihistamines, tricyclic antidepressants, antipsychotics, many medications specifically used to treat urge incontinence such as tolterodine (Detrol), oxybutynin (Ditropan), solifenacin succinate (VESIcare)	Urinary retention, overflow incontinence, alteration in sensorium, sedation, dry mouth, constipation with increased risk for fecal impaction. Use in older adult with limited mobility can result in functional urinary incontinence
Opioids	Urinary retention, overflow, alteration in sensorium, sedation, constipation with increased risk for fecal impaction. These effects can lead to functional urinary incontinence
Alcohol	Increase in volume, frequency, and urgency of voiding alteration in sensorium
Sedatives, hypnotics, benzodiazepines	Alteration in sensorium, sedation, reduced mobility. This can lead to functional urinary incontinence
Alpha-adrenergic antagonists (prazosin, doxazosin, terazosin), all also used to treat hypertension and medications in this class specific for BPH treatment such as tamsulosin	Relaxing internal urethral sphincter. This can be a desired effect in a man with BPH, but is likely less helpful in a woman with bladder emptying issues. Use of these medications potentially increases risk of postural hypotension in older adult

BPH, benign prostatic hyperplasia.

15
Pediatrics

QUESTIONS

1. Which of the following is appropriate advice to give to a mother who is breastfeeding her 10-day-old infant?

    A. "Your milk will come in today."
    B. "To minimize breast tenderness, the baby should not be kept on each breast for more than 5 to 10 minutes."
    C. "A pacifier should be offered between feedings."
    D. "The baby's urine should be light or colorless."

2. Which of the following is appropriate advice to give to a mother who is breastfeeding her 12-hour-old infant?

    A. "You will likely have enough milk to feed the baby within a few hours of birth."
    B. "The baby might need to be awakened to be fed."
    C. "Supplemental feeding is needed unless the baby has at least four wet diapers in the first day of life."
    D. "The baby will likely have a seedy yellow bowel movement today."

3. Compared with the use of infant formula, advantages of breastfeeding include all of the following except:

    A. lower incidence of diarrheal illness.
    B. greater weight gain in the first few weeks of life.
    C. reduced risk of allergic disorders.
    D. lower occurrence of constipation.

4. At 3 weeks of age, the average-weight formula-fed infant should be expected to take:

    A. 2 to 3 oz every 2 to 3 hours.
    B. 2 to 3 oz every 3 to 4 hours.
    C. 3 to 4 oz every 2 to 3 hours.
    D. 3 to 4 oz every 3 to 4 hours.

5. In infants, solid foods are best introduced no earlier than:

    A. 1 to 3 months.
    B. 3 to 5 months.
    C. 4 to 6 months.
    D. 6 to 8 months.

6. Nursing infants generally maximally receive about which percentage of the maternal dose of a drug?

    A. 1%
    B. 3%
    C. 5%
    D. 10%

7. Most drugs pass into breast milk through:

    A. active transport.
    B. facilitated transfer.
    C. simple diffusion.
    D. creation of a pH gradient.

8. To remove a drug from breast milk through "pump and dump," the process must be continued for:

    A. two infant feeding cycles.
    B. approximately 8 hours.
    C. three to five half-lives of drug.
    D. a period of time that is highly unpredictable.

9. When counseling a breastfeeding woman about alcohol use during lactation, you relate that:

    A. drinking a glass of wine or beer will enhance the let-down reflex.
    B. because of its high molecular weight, relatively little alcohol is passed into breast milk.
    C. maternal alcohol use causes a reduction in the amount of milk ingested by the infant.
    D. infant intoxication may be seen with as little as one to two maternal drinks.

See full color images of this topic on DavisPlus at http://davisplus.fadavis.com | Keyword: Fitzgerald

10. A 23-year-old woman is breastfeeding her healthy newborn. She wishes to use hormonal contraception. Which of the following represents the best regimen?

- **A.** combined oral contraception initiated at 2 weeks
- **B.** progesterone-only oral contraception initiated at 3 weeks
- **C.** medroxyprogesterone acetate (Depo-Provera) given day 1 postpartum
- **D.** All forms of hormonal contraception are contraindicated during lactation.

11. The anticipated average daily weight gain during the first 3 months of life is approximately:

- **A.** 15 g.
- **B.** 20 g.
- **C.** 25 g.
- **D.** 30 g.

12. The average required caloric intake in an infant from age 0 to 3 months is usually:

- **A.** 40 to 60 kcal/kg/d.
- **B.** 60 to 80 kcal/kg/d.
- **C.** 80 to 100 kcal/kg/d.
- **D.** 100 to 120 kcal/kg/d.

ANSWERS

1.	D	**2.**	B	**3.**	B
4.	A	**5.**	C	**6.**	A
7.	C	**8.**	C	**9.**	C
10.	B	**11.**	D	**12.**	D

DISCUSSION

Breastfeeding provides the ideal form of nutrition during infancy. In the United States, approximately 60% of all infants are breastfed at birth, with only about 25% continuing by 6 months. Health-care providers can help influence successful breastfeeding. The content of commercially prepared formula available in the developed world continues to be improved with composition closer to breast milk. Infant formula continues to lack critically important components, however. Breast milk contains immunoactive factors that help protect infants against infectious disease and may reduce the frequency of allergic disorders. Human milk transfers to the infant the mother's antibodies to disease. About 80% of the cells in breast milk are macrophages, cells that kill bacteria, fungi, and viruses. In contrast to formula-fed infants, a breastfed infant's digestive tract contains large amounts of *Lactobacillus bifidus,* beneficial bacteria that prevent the growth of harmful organisms.

If an infant is formula-fed, the parents and caregivers should be encouraged to hold the infant during feeding to have the interaction inherent in breastfeeding. Questions about frequency, amount, and type of feedings are often asked during well-baby visits. Counseling should be offered to help ensure optimal nutrition (Box 15–1 and Table 15–1).

If a nursing mother becomes ill or has a chronic health problem, she is often erroneously advised to discontinue breastfeeding on the basis of the incorrect assumption by the

---

BOX 15–1

Guidelines for Nutrition in the First Months of Life

- ■ Frequency of feeding during months 1 and 2
  - ■ Breastfed infants: A minimum of 10 minutes at each breast every 1½ to 3 hours; bottle-fed infants: 2–3 oz every 2 to 3 hours
- ■ Fluoride supplementation is advisable for breastfed infants and if formula is not mixed with fluoridated water
- ■ Solid foods are best introduced at age 4 to 6 months
- ■ Signs that an infant is ready for solid food
  - ■ Doubled birth weight and at least 4 to 6 months of age
  - ■ More than 32 oz formula per day or more than 8 to 10 feedings (breast or bottle) per day

Sources: Nemours Foundation. http://kidshealth.org/parent/nutrition_fit/nutrition/feednewborn.html, Feeding your newborn, accessed 10/3/09.

Nemours Foundation. http://kidshealth.org/parent/nutrition_fit/nutrition/feed13m.html, Feeding your 1–3 month-old, accessed 10/3/09.

Nemours Foundation. http://kidshealth.org/parent/nutrition_fit/nutrition/feed47m.html, Feeding your 4–7 month-old, accessed 10/3/09.

TABLE 15–1

Anticipated Weight Gain and Caloric Requirements in the First 3 Years of Life

Age	Anticipated Average Weight Gain per Day (g)	Required Kilocalorie per Kilogram per Day
0–3 mo	26–31	100–120 kcal
3–6 mo	17–18	105–115 kcal
6–9 mo	12–13	100–105 kcal
9–12 mo	9	100–105 kcal
1–3 yr	7–9	100 kcal

health-care provider that most medications are not safe to use. Most medications can be used during lactation, but the benefit of improved maternal health should be balanced against the risk of exposing an infant to medication.

Postpartum contraception is usually an important concern of new mothers. Some women may opt not to breastfeed, fearing an inability to access reliable hormonal contraception while lactating. Many options are available, however, including the use of the progestin-only pill (POP) and medroxyprogesterone acetate (Depo-Provera, Depo-SubQ Provera 104). For lactating women who wish to use an oral hormonal contraceptive, POP is highly effective and does not alter the quality or quantity of breast milk. One significant disadvantage of POP use is bleeding irregularity, ranging from prolonged flow to amenorrhea. Medroxyprogesterone acetate in a depot injection given every 90 days is a highly reliable form of contraception with 99.7% efficacy. progestin-only contraceptive options can be started immediately postpartum if the woman is not breastfeeding and started at 3 to 6 weeks postpartum if she is breastfeeding. Earlier use could diminish the quantity, but not quality, of breast milk. Nonsystemic contraceptive methods, such as barrier methods, intrauterine devices, and levonorgestrel intrauterine systems, are also acceptable.

Nearly all breastfeeding mothers use some type of medication (most often analgesic agents such as nonsteroidal anti-inflammatory drugs, acetaminophen, opioids, and antibiotics) in the first 2 weeks after giving birth. About 25% need to use medication intermittently to manage episodic disease. Such medications usually include analgesics, antihistamines, decongestants, and antibiotics.

About 5% of breastfeeding women have a chronic health problem necessitating daily use of a medication; the most common long-term medications used are for treating asthma, mental health problems, seizure disorder, and hypertension. Nursing infants usually get about 1%, often less, of the maternal dose, and only a few drugs are contraindicated.

The "pump-and-dump" procedure is a less-than-helpful way to reduce drug levels in a mother's milk because it creates an area of lower drug concentration in the empty breast. This enables the drug to diffuse from the area of high concentration (maternal serum) to the area of low concentration (breast milk). If the mother takes a medication that may be problematic for the nursing infant, pumping and discarding the milk needs to continue for three to five half-lives of the medication.

Alcohol has a low molecular weight and is highly lipid soluble; both of these characteristics allow it to have easy passage into breast milk. Even in small amounts, alcohol ingestion by a nursing mother can cause a smaller amount of milk produced and reduction in the let-down reflex and less rhythmic and frequent sucking by the infant, resulting in a smaller volume of milk ingested. Cigarette smoking is similarly problematic. Nicotine, a highly lipid-soluble substance with a low molecular weight, passes easily into breast milk. Maternal cigarette smoking can reduce milk supply

and expose an infant to passive smoke. Infant crankiness, diarrhea, tachycardia, and vomiting have been reported with high maternal nicotine intake.

Discussion Sources

Briggs G, Freeman R, Yaffe S. *Drugs in Pregnancy and Lactation*. 8th ed. Philadelphia, PA: Lippincott Williams & Wilkins; 2008.

Hale T. *Medications and Mothers' Milk*. 16th ed. Amarillo, TX: Pharmasoft Medical Publishers; 2008.

QUESTIONS

13. Which of the following is most consistent with a normal developmental examination for a 3-month-old infant born at 40 weeks' gestation?

    A. sitting briefly with support
    B. experimenting with sound
    C. rolling over
    D. having a social smile

14. Which of the following is most consistent with a normal developmental examination for a thriving 5-month-old infant born at 32 weeks' gestation?

    A. sitting briefly with support
    B. experimenting with sound
    C. rolling over
    D. performing hand-to-hand transfers

15. A healthy full-term infant at age 3 to 5 months should be able to:

    A. gesture to an object.
    B. bring hands together.
    C. reach for an object with one hand.
    D. feed self biscuit.

16. A healthy infant at age 9 to 11 months is expected to:

    A. roll back to stomach.
    B. imitate "bye-bye."
    C. play peek-a-boo.
    D. hand toy on request.

17. A healthy 2-year-old child is able to:

    A. speak in phrases of two or more words.
    B. throw a ball.
    C. scribble spontaneously.
    D. ride a tricycle.

18. At which age would a child likely start to imitate housework?

    A. 15 months
    B. 18 months
    C. 24 months
    D. 30 months

19. A healthy 3-year-old child is expected to:

   A. give his or her first and last names.
   B. use pronouns.
   C. kick a ball.
   D. name a best friend.

20. A healthy 6- to 7-month-old infant is able to:

   A. roll back to stomach.
   B. feed self cracker.
   C. reach for an object.
   D. crawl on abdomen.

21. You examine a healthy 9-month-old infant from a full-term pregnancy and expect to find that the infant:

   A. sits without support.
   B. cruises.
   C. has the ability to recognize his or her own name.
   D. imitates a razzing noise.

22. A healthy 3-year-old child is in your office for well-child care. You expect this child to be able to:

   A. name three colors.
   B. alternate feet when climbing stairs.
   C. speak in two-word phrases.
   D. tie shoelaces.

23. Which of the following would not be found in newborns?

   A. best vision at a range of 8 to 12 inches
   B. presence of red reflex
   C. light-sensitive eyes
   D. lack of defensive blink

24. Which of the following do you expect to find in an examination of a 2-week-old infant?

   A. a visual preference for the human face
   B. a preference for low-pitched voices
   C. indifference to the cry of other neonates
   D. poorly developed sense of smell

25. Which of the following is the most appropriate response in a developmental examination of a healthy 5-year-old child?

   A. the ability to name a best friend
   B. giving gender appropriately
   C. naming an intended career
   D. hopping on one foot

DISCUSSION

Performing a developmental assessment is one of the most important parts of providing pediatric primary care. Besides providing a marker for evaluating the child, the assessment also affords an important learning tool for the parents. Pointing out milestones to be achieved in the near future and their impact on safety can help the family prepare appropriately (Table 15–2).

Discussion Source

Engel J. Development. In: Engel J. *Pediatric Assessment*. 5th ed. St. Louis, MO: Mosby Elsevier; 2006.

QUESTIONS

26. At which of the following ages in an infant's life is parental anticipatory guidance about teething most helpful?

   A. 1 to 2 months
   B. 2 to 4 months
   C. 4 to 6 months
   D. 8 to 10 months

27. At which of the following ages in a young child's life is parental anticipatory guidance about temper tantrums most helpful?

   A. 8 to 10 months
   B. 10 to 12 months
   C. 12 to 14 months
   D. 14 to 16 months

28. At which of the following ages in a young child's life is parental anticipatory guidance about using "time out" as a discipline method most helpful?

   A. 12 to 18 months
   B. 18 to 24 months
   C. 24 to 30 months
   D. 30 to 36 months

29. At which of the following ages in a young child's life is parental anticipatory guidance about protection from falls most helpful?

   A. at birth
   B. 2 months
   C. 4 months
   D. 6 months

ANSWERS

13.	B	**14.**	B	**15.**	B
16.	C	**17.**	A	**18.**	A
19.	A	**20.**	A	**21.**	C
22.	B	**23.**	D	**24.**	A
25.	A				

TABLE 15–2

Anticipated Early Childhood Developmental Milestones

Age	Able to Be Observed During Office Visit	Reported by Parent or Caregiver
Newborn	• Moves all extremities • Spontaneous stepping • Reacts to sound by blinking, turning • Responds to cries of other neonates • Well-developed sense of smell • Cries when uncomfortable • Preference for higher pitched voices Reflexes • Tonic neck • Palmar grasp • Babinski response • Rooting awake and asleep • Sucking	• Able to be calmed by feeding, cuddling • Reinforces presence of developmental tasks seen in examination room
1–2 mo	• Lifts head • Holds head erect • Regards face • Follows objects through visual field • Moro and palmar grasp reflexes fading	• Spontaneous smile • Recognizes parents
3–4 mo	• Grasps cube • Reaches for objects • Brings objects to mouth • Raspberry sound	• Laughs, squeals, vocalizes in response to others • Recognizes food by sight • Rolls back to side
5 mo	• Back straight when pulled to sitting • Bears weight on legs when standing • Plays with feet • Sits with support	• Imitates others • Repeats interesting actions
6–8 mo	• Sits without support • Scoops small object with rake grip; some thumb use • Hand-to-hand transfer • Imitates "bye-bye" • Stranger and separation anxiety begins (6 mo) and increases during this time period • Pulls feet into mouth	• Coughs, snorts to attract attention • Closes lips in response to dislike of food • Rolls back to stomach and stomach to back • Recognizes "no" • Chains together syllables (dada, papa, mama) but does have meaning
9–11 mo	• Crawls, pulling self forward by hands, then creeps with abdomen off floor • Stands initially by holding onto furniture, later stands solo • Imitates peek-a-boo and pat-a-cake • Picks up small object with thumb and index finger	• Cruises • Follows simple command, such as "Come here." Assigns meaning to words such as "mama, papa, dada"
12–15 mo	• Initially walks with help, progresses to walking solo • Neat pincer grasp • Places cube in cup • Hands over objects on request • Builds tower of two bricks	• Says one to two words • Indicates wants by pointing • Scribbles spontaneously • Imitates animal sounds

Continued

TABLE 15–2

Anticipated Early Childhood Developmental Milestones—cont'd

Age	Able to Be Observed During Office Visit	Reported by Parent or Caregiver
15–20 mo	• Points to several body parts • Throws a ball overhand • Seats self in chair • Climbs	• Uses a spoon with little spilling • Walks up and down steps with help • Understands two-step commands • Feeds self • Carries and hugs doll • Imitates housework • Speech: 4–6 words by 15 mo, increases to ≥10 words by 18 mo • Scribbles vigorously • Builds tower of ≥3 cubes
24 mo	• Speaks in sentences of ≥2 words • Kicks ball on request • Jumps with both feet • Uses pronouns • Developing handedness	• Runs • Copies vertical and horizontal lines • Has up to a 300-word vocabulary • Washes and dries hands • Parallel play • Puts on simple clothing
30 mo	• Walks backward • Hops on one foot • Copies circle	• Gives first and last name • Uses plurals • Usually separates easily from parents
36 mo	• Holds crayons with fingers • Nearly all speech intelligible to people not in daily contact with child • Three-word sentences	• Walks down stairs alternating steps • Rides tricycle • Copies circles • Dresses with supervision
3–4 yr	• Responds to command to place object in, on, or under a table • Knows gender • Draws circle when one is shown	• Takes off jacket and shoes • Washes and dries face • Cooperative play • Speech includes plurals, personal pronouns, verbs • Skips • Asks many questions
4–5 yr	• Runs and turns while maintaining balance • Stands on one foot for at least 10 seconds • Counts to 4 • Draws a person without torso • Copies (1) by imitation • Verbalizes activities to do when cold, hungry, tired	• Buttons clothes • Dresses self (not including tying shoelaces) • Can play without adult input for about 30 min
5–6 yr	• Catches ball • Knows age • Knows right from left hand • Draws person with six to eight parts, including torso • Identifies best friend • Likes teacher	• Able to complete simple chores • Understands concept of 10 items; likely counts higher by rote • Has sense of gender
6–7 yr	• Copies triangle shape • Draws person with at least 12 parts • Prints name • Reads multiple single-syllable words	• Ties shoelaces • Counts to ≥30 • Able to differentiate morning from later in day • Generally plays well with peers • No significant behavioral problems in school • Can name intended career

TABLE 15–2

Anticipated Early Childhood Developmental Milestones—cont'd

Age	Able to Be Observed During Office Visit	Reported by Parent or Caregiver
7–8 yr	• Copies diamond shape • Reads simple sentences • Draws person with at least 16 parts	• Ties shoes • Knows day of the week
8–9 yr	• Able to give response to question such as what to do if an object is accidentally broken	• Able to add, subtract, borrow, carry • Understands concept of working as a team
9–10 yr	• Knows month, day, year • Gives months of the year in sequence	• Able to multiply and do complex subtraction • Has increased reading fluency
10–12 yr	• Beginning of pubertal changes for many girls	• Able to perform simple division • Has complex reading skills

Source: Engel J. Development. In: Engel J. *Pediatric Assessment*. 5th ed. St. Louis, MO: Mosby; 2006.

30. At which of the following ages in a young child's life is parental anticipatory guidance about toilet training readiness most helpful?

A. 12 months
B. 15 months
C. 18 months
D. 24 months

31. At which of the following ages in a young child's life is parental anticipatory guidance about infant sleep position most helpful?

A. birth
B. 2 weeks
C. 2 months
D. 4 months

ANSWERS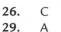

| 26. | C | 27. | B | 28. | B |
| 29. | A | 30. | C | 31. | A |

DISCUSSION

Providing health advice to the growing family is a critical part of the NP's role. During anticipatory guidance counseling, the NP should review the normal developmental landmarks that the child is expected to reach in the near future and offer advice about how parents can cope with, adapt to, and avoid problems with these changes. This guidance is tailored to meet the needs of the family, but typically follows a developmental framework.

Discussion Source

American Academy of Pediatrics. http://pediatrics.aappublications. org/cgi/data/120/6/1376/DC1/1, Recommendations for pediatric preventive care, accessed 10/3/09.

QUESTIONS

32. When considering a person's risk for measles, mumps, and rubella, the NP considers the following:

A. Children should have two doses of the measles, mumps, and rubella (MMR) vaccine before the sixth birthday.
B. Considerable mortality and morbidity occur with all three diseases.
C. Most cases in the United States occur in infants.
D. The use of the vaccine is often associated with protracted arthralgia.

33. Which of the following is true about the MMR vaccine?

A. This vaccine contains live virus.
B. Its use is contraindicated in persons with a history of egg allergy.
C. Revaccination of an immune person is associated with risk of allergic reaction.
D. One dose is recommended for young adults who have not been previously immunized.

ANSWERS

| 32. | A | 33. | A |

DISCUSSION

The MMR vaccine is a live, attenuated vaccine. The recommended schedule for early childhood immunization is two doses of MMR vaccine given between 12 and 15 months and between 4 and 6 years (Fig. 15–1). Two immunizations 1 month apart are recommended for older children who were not immunized earlier in life. As with other immunizations, giving additional doses to individuals with an unclear immunization history is safe.

Rubella, also known as German measles, ♂ typically causes a relatively mild, 3- to 5-day illness with little risk of complication for the person infected. When rubella is contracted during pregnancy, however, the effects on the fetus can be devastating. Immunizing the entire population against rubella protects unborn children from the risk of congenital rubella syndrome. Measles can cause severe illness with serious sequelae, including encephalitis and pneumonia. Sequelae of mumps include orchitis.

The MMR vaccine is safe to use during lactation, but its use in pregnant women is discouraged because of the possible risk of passing the virus on to the unborn child; this risk exists in theory but has not been noted in ongoing observation. The MMR vaccine is well tolerated, with rare reports of mild, transient adverse reaction such as rash and sore throat. Systemic reaction to the MMR vaccine is rare.

Discussion Source

Centers for Disease Control and Prevention. Recommended Childhood Immunization Schedule—United States, 2008, 2009, http://www.cdc.gov/Vaccines/recs/schedules/child-schedule.htm, accessed 10/3/09.

QUESTIONS

34. When advising parents about injectable influenza immunization, the clinician considers the following about the vaccine:

    A. The vaccine is contraindicated with a personal history of an anaphylactic reaction to eggs.
    B. Its use is limited to children older than 2 years.
    C. The vaccine contains live virus.
    D. Its use is not recommended for members of households of high-risk patients.

35. A 7-year-old child with type 1 diabetes mellitus is about to receive injectable influenza vaccine. His parents and he should be advised that:

    A. the vaccine is more than 90% effective in preventing influenza.
    B. use of the vaccine is contraindicated during antibiotic therapy.
    C. localized immunization reactions are common.
    D. a short, intense, flu-like syndrome typically occurs after immunization.

36. When giving influenza vaccine to a 7-year-old who has not received this immunization in the past, the NP considers that:

    A. two doses 4 weeks or more apart should be given.
    B. a single dose is adequate.
    C. children in this age group have the highest rate of influenza-related hospitalization.
    D. the vaccine should not be given to a child with shellfish allergy.

37. With regard to seasonal influenza prevention in well children, the NP considers that:

    A. compared with school-aged children, younger children (<24 months old) have an increased risk of seasonal influenza-related hospitalization.
    B. a full adult dose of seasonal influenza vaccine should be given starting at age 4 years.
    C. the use of the seasonal influenza vaccine in well children is discouraged.
    D. widespread use of the vaccine is likely to increase risk of eczema and antibiotic allergies.

38. When advising a patient about immunization with the nasal spray flu vaccine, the NP considers the following:

    A. Its use is acceptable during pregnancy.
    B. Its use is limited to children younger than age 6 years.
    C. It contains live virus.
    D. It is recommended for household members of high-risk patients.

ANSWERS

34.	A	35.	C	36.	A
37.	A	38.	C		

DISCUSSION

Influenza is a viral illness that typically causes many days of incapacitation and suffering and the risk of hospitalization and death. Immunization is about 70% to 80% effective in preventing or reducing the severity of the influenza A and B viruses.

Having a mild illness or taking an antibiotic is not a contraindication to any immunization, including influenza. The injectable vaccine does not contain live virus and is not shed; there is no risk of shedding an infectious agent to household contacts. Injectable influenza vaccine is recommended for household members of high-risk patients to avoid transmission of infection.

The nasal-spray flu vaccine, also known as live attenuated influenza vaccine (LAIV), differs from the injectable influenza

Recommended immunization schedule for persons aged 0 through 6 years — United States, 2010
(for those who fall behind or start late, see the catch-up schedule)

Vaccine ▼ Age ▶	Birth	1 month	2 months	4 months	6 months	12 months	15 months	18 months	19–23 months	2–3 years	4–6 years
Hepatitis B[1]	HepB	HepB			HepB						
Rotavirus[2]			RV	RV	RV[2]						
Diphtheria, Tetanus, Pertussis[3]			DTaP	DTaP	DTaP	see footnote3	DTaP				DTaP
Haemophilus influenzae type b[4]			Hib	Hib	Hib[4]	Hib					
Pneumococcal[5]			PCV	PCV	PCV	PCV					PPSV
Inactivated Poliovirus			IPV	IPV	IPV						IPV
Influenza[6]					Influenza (Yearly)						
Measles, Mumps, Rubella[7]						MMR		see footnote8			MMR
Varicella[8]						Varicella		see footnote9			Varicella
Hepatitis A[9]						HepA (2 doses)				HepA Series	
Meningococcal[10]										MCV	

Range of recommended ages for all children except certain high-risk groups

Range of recommended ages for certain high-risk groups

This schedule includes recommendations in effect as of December 15, 2009. Any dose not administered at the recommended age should be administered at a subsequent visit, when indicated and feasible. The use of a combination vaccine generally is preferred over separate injections of its equivalent component vaccines. Considerations should include provider assessment, patient preference, and the potential for adverse events. Providers should consult the relevant Advisory Committee on Immunization Practices statement for detailed recommendations: http://www.cdc.gov/vaccines/pubs/acip-list.htm. Clinically significant adverse events that follow immunization should be reported to the Vaccine Adverse Event Reporting System (VAERS) at http://www.vaers.hhs.gov or by telephone, 800-822-7967.

1. **Hepatitis B vaccine (HepB).** (Minimum age: birth)
   At birth:
   * Administer monovalent HepB to all newborns before hospital discharge.
   * If mother is hepatitis B surface antigen (HBsAg)-positive, administer HepB and 0.5 mL of hepatitis B immune globulin (HBIG) within 12 hours of birth.
   * If mother's HBsAg status is unknown, administer HepB within 12 hours of birth. Determine mother's HBsAg status as soon as possible and, if HBsAg-positive, administer HBIG (no later than age 1 week).
   After the birth dose:
   * The HepB series should be completed with either monovalent HepB or a combination vaccine containing HepB. The second dose should be administered at age 1 or 2 months. Monovalent HepB vaccine should be used for doses administered before age 6 weeks. The final dose should be administered no earlier than age 24 weeks.
   * Infants born to HBsAg-positive mothers should be tested for HBsAg and antibody to HBsAg 1 to 2 months after completion of at least 3 doses of the HepB series, at age 9 through 18 months (generally at the next well-child visit).
   * Administration of 4 doses of HepB to infants is permissible when a combination vaccine containing HepB is administered after the birth dose. The fourth dose should be administered no earlier than age 24 weeks.
2. **Rotavirus vaccine (RV).** (Minimum age: 6 weeks)
   * Administer the first dose at age 6 through 14 weeks (maximum age: 14 weeks 6 days). Vaccination should not be initiated for infants aged 15 weeks 0 days or older.
   * The maximum age for the final dose in the series is 8 months 0 days
   * If Rotarix is administered at ages 2 and 4 months, a dose at 6 months is not indicated.
3. **Diphtheria and tetanus toxoids and acellular pertussis vaccine (DTaP).** (Minimum age: 6 weeks)
   * The fourth dose may be administered as early as age 12 months, provided at least 6 months have elapsed since the third dose.
   * Administer the final dose in the series at age 4 through 6 years.
4. **Haemophilus influenzae type b conjugate vaccine (Hib).** (Minimum age: 6 weeks)
   * If PRP-OMP (PedvaxHIB or Comvax [HepB-Hib]) is administered at ages 2 and 4 months, a dose at age 6 months is not indicated.
   * TriHiBit (DTaP/Hib) and Hiberix (PRP-T) should not be used for doses at ages 2, 4, or 6 months for the primary series but can be used as the final dose in children aged 12 months through 4 years.
5. **Pneumococcal vaccine.** (Minimum age: 6 weeks for pneumococcal conjugate vaccine [PCV]; 2 years for pneumococcal polysaccharide vaccine [PPSV])
   * PCV is recommended for all children aged younger than 5 years. Administer 1 dose of PCV to all healthy children aged 24 through 59 months who are not completely vaccinated for their age.
   * Administer PPSV 2 or more months after last dose of PCV to children aged 2 years or older with certain underlying medical conditions, including a cochlear implant. See MMWR 1997;46(No. RR-8).

6. **Inactivated poliovirus vaccine (IPV)** (Minimum age: 6 weeks)
   * The final dose in the series should be administered on or after the fourth birthday and at least 6 months following the previous dose.
   * If 4 doses are administered prior to age 4 years a fifth dose should be administered at age 4 through 6 years. See MMWR 2009;58(30):829–30.
7. **Influenza vaccine (seasonal).** (Minimum age: 6 months for trivalent inactivated influenza vaccine [TIV]; 2 years for live, attenuated influenza vaccine [LAIV])
   * Administer annually to children aged 6 months through 18 years
   * For healthy children aged 2 through 6 years (i.e., those who do not have underlying medical conditions that predispose them to influenza complications), either LAIV or TIV may be used, except LAIV should not be given to children aged 2 through 4 years who have had wheezing in the past 12 months.
   * Children receiving TIV should receive 0.25 mL if aged 6 through 35 months or 0.5 mL if aged 3 years or older.
   * Administer 2 doses (separated by at least 4 weeks) to children aged younger than 9 years who are receiving influenza vaccine for the first time or who were vaccinated for the first time during the previous influenza season but only received 1 dose.
   * For recommendations for use of influenza A (H1N1) 2009 monovalent vaccine see MMWR 2009;58(No. RR-10).
8. **Measles, mumps, and rubella vaccine (MMR).** (Minimum age: 12 months)
   * Administer the second dose routinely at age 4 through 6 years. However, the second dose may be administered before age 4, provided at least 28 days have elapsed since the first dose.
9. **Varicella vaccine.** (Minimum age: 12 months)
   * Administer the second dose routinely at age 4 through 6 years. However, the second dose may be administered before age 4, provided at least 3 months have elapsed since the first dose.
   * For children aged 12 months through 12 years the minimum interval between doses is 3 months. However, if the second dose was administered at least 28 days after the first dose, it can be accepted as valid.
10. **Hepatitis A vaccine (HepA).** (Minimum age: 12 months)
   * Administer to all children aged 1 year (i.e., aged 12 through 23 months). Administer 2 doses at least 6 months apart.
   * Children not fully vaccinated by age 2 years can be vaccinated at subsequent visits
   * HepA also is recommended for older children who live in areas where vaccination programs target older children, who are at increased risk for infection, or for whom immunity against hepatitis A is desired.
11. **Meningococcal vaccine.** (Minimum age: 2 years for meningococcal conjugate vaccine [MCV4] and for meningococcal polysaccharide vaccine [MPSV4])
   * Administer MCV4 to children aged 2 through 10 years with persistent complement component deficiency, anatomic or functional asplenia, and certain other conditions placing them at high risk.
   * Administer MCV4 to children previously vaccinated with MCV4 or MPSV4 after 3 years if first dose administered at age 2 through 6 years. See MMWR 2009; 58:1042–3.

The Recommended Immunization Schedules for Persons Aged 0 through 18 Years are approved by the **Advisory Committee on Immunization Practices** (http://www.cdc.gov/vaccines/recs/acip), the **American Academy of Pediatrics** (http://www.aap.org), and the **American Academy of Family Physicians** (http://www.aafp.org). Department of Health and Human Services • Centers for Disease Control and Prevention

Figure 15–1 *Recommendations and Guidelines: 2009 Child & Adolescent Immunization Schedules. Available at http://www.cdc.gov/ vaccines/recs/schedules/child-schedule.htm. Accessed 12/28/09.*

Recommended immunization schedule for persons aged 7 through 18 years — United States, 2010 (for those who fall behind or start late, see the catch-up schedule)

Vaccine ▼ Age ►	7–10 years	11–12 years	13–18 years
Tetanus, Diphtheria, Pertussis[1]		Tdap	Tdap
Human Papillomavirus[2]	see footnote 2	HPV (3 doses)	HPV Series
Meningococcal[3]	MCV	MCV	MCV
Influenza[4]	Influenza (Yearly)		
Pneumococcal[5]	PPSV		
Hepatitis A[6]	HepA Series		
Hepatitis B[7]	HepB Series		
Inactivated Poliovirus[8]	IPV Series		
Measles, Mumps, Rubella[9]	MMR Series		
Varicella[10]	Varicella Series		

Range of recommended ages for all children except certain high-risk groups

Range of recommended ages for catch-up immunization

Range of recommended ages for certain high-risk groups

This schedule includes recommendations in effect as of December 15, 2009. Any dose not administered at the recommended age should be administered at a subsequent visit, when indicated and feasible. The use of a combination vaccine generally is preferred over separate injections of its equivalent component vaccines. Considerations should include provider assessment, patient preference, and the potential for adverse events. Providers should consult the relevant Advisory Committee on Immunization Practices statement for detailed recommendations: **http://www.cdc.gov/vaccines/pubs/acip-list.htm**. Clinically significant adverse events that follow immunization should be reported to the Vaccine Adverse Event Reporting System (VAERS) at **http://www.vaers.hhs.gov** or by telephone, 800-822-7967.

1. **Tetanus and diphtheria toxoids and acellular pertussis vaccine (Tdap).**
   (Minimum age: 10 years for Boostrix and 11 years for Adacel)
   • Administer at age 11 or 12 years for those who have completed the recommended childhood DTP/DTaP vaccination series and have not received a tetanus and diphtheria toxoid (Td) booster dose.
   • Persons aged 13 through 18 years who have not received Tdap should receive a dose.
   • A 5-year interval from the last Td dose is encouraged when Tdap is used as a booster dose; however, a shorter interval may be used if pertussis immunity is needed.
2. **Human papillomavirus vaccine (HPV).** (Minimum age: 9 years)
   • Two HPV vaccines are licensed: a quadrivalent vaccine (HPV4) for the prevention of cervical, vaginal and vulvar cancers (in females) and genital warts (in females and males), and a bivalent vaccine (HPV2) for the prevention of cervical cancers in females.
   • HPV vaccines are most effective for both males and females when given before exposure to HPV through sexual contact.
   • HPV4 or HPV2 is recommended for the prevention of cervical precancers and cancers in females.
   • HPV4 is recommended for the prevention of cervical, vaginal and vulvar precancers and cancers and genital warts in females.
   • Administer the first dose to females at age 11 or 12 years.
   • Administer the second dose 1 to 2 months after the first dose and the third dose 6 months after the first dose (at least 24 weeks after the first dose).
   • Administer the series to females at age 13 through 18 years if not previously vaccinated.
   • HPV4 may be administered in a 3-dose series to males aged 9 through 18 years to reduce their likelihood of acquiring genital warts.
3. **Meningococcal conjugate vaccine (MCV4).**
   • Administer at age 11 or 12 years, or at age 13 through 18 years if not previously vaccinated.
   • Administer to previously unvaccinated college freshmen living in a dormitory.
   • Administer MCV4 to children aged 2 through 10 years with persistent complement component deficiency, anatomic or functional asplenia, or certain other conditions placing them at high risk.
   • Administer to children previously vaccinated with MCV4 or MPSV4 who remain at increased risk after 3 years (if first dose administered at age 2 through 6 years) or after 5 years (if first dose administered at age 7 years or older). Persons whose only risk factor is living in on-campus housing are not recommended to receive an additional dose. See *MMWR* 2009;58:1042–3.
4. **Influenza vaccine (seasonal).**
   • Administer annually to children aged 6 months through 18 years.

   • For healthy nonpregnant persons aged 7 through 18 years (i.e., those who do not have underlying medical conditions that predispose them to influenza complications), either LAIV or TIV may be used.
   • Administer 2 doses (separated by at least 4 weeks) to children aged younger than 9 years who are receiving influenza vaccine for the first time or who were vaccinated for the first time during the previous influenza season but only received 1 dose.
   • For recommendations for use of influenza A (H1N1) 2009 monovalent vaccine. See *MMWR* 2009;58(No. RR-10)
5. **Pneumococcal polysaccharide vaccine (PPSV).**
   • Administer to children with certain underlying medical conditions, including a cochlear implant. A single revaccination should be administered after 5 years to children with functional or anatomic asplenia or an immunocompromising condition. See *MMWR* 1997;46(No. RR-8).
6. **Hepatitis A vaccine (HepA).**
   • Administer 2 doses at least 6 months apart.
   • HepA is recommended for children aged older than 23 months who live in areas where vaccination programs target older children, who are at increased risk for infection, or for whom immunity against hepatitis A is desired.
7. **Hepatitis B vaccine (HepB).**
   • Administer the 3-dose series to those not previously vaccinated.
   • A 2-dose series (separated by at least 4 months) of adult formulation Recombivax HB is licensed for children aged 11 through 15 years.
8. **Inactivated poliovirus vaccine (IPV).**
   • The final dose in the series should be administered on or after the fourth birthday and at least 6 months following the previous dose.
   • If both OPV and IPV were administered as part of a series, a total of 4 doses should be administered, regardless of the child's current age.
9. **Measles, mumps, and rubella vaccine (MMR).**
   • If not previously vaccinated, administer 2 doses or the second dose for those who have received only 1 dose, with at least 28 days between doses.
10. **Varicella vaccine.**
   • For persons aged 7 through 18 years without evidence of immunity (see *MMWR* 2007;56[No. RR-4]), administer 2 doses if not previously vaccinated or the second dose if only 1 dose has been administered.
   • For persons aged 7 through 12 years, the minimum interval between doses is 3 months. However, if the second dose was administered at least 28 days after the first dose, it can be accepted as valid.
   • For persons aged 13 years and older, the minimum interval between doses is 28 days.

The Recommended Immunization Schedules for Persons Aged 0 through 18 Years are approved by the **Advisory Committee on Immunization Practices** (**http://www.cdc.gov/vaccines/recs/acip**), **the American Academy of Pediatrics (http://www.aap.org)**, and **the American Academy of Family Physicians (http://www.aafp.org)**. Department of Health and Human Services • Centers for Disease Control and Prevention

Figure 15–1 cont'd

Catch-up immunization schedule for persons aged 4 months through 18 years who start late or who are more than 1 month behind — United States, 2010

The table below provides catch-up schedules and minimum intervals between doses for children whose vaccinations have been delayed. A vaccine series does not need to be restarted, regardless of the time that has elapsed between doses. Use the section appropriate for the child's age.

Vaccine	Minimum Age for Dose 1	Minimum Interval Between Doses			
		Dose 1 to Dose 2		Dose 3 to Dose 4	Dose 4 to Dose 5
PERSONS AGED 4 MONTHS THROUGH 6 YEARS					
Hepatitis B[1]	Birth	4 weeks	8 weeks (and at least 16 weeks after first dose)		
Rotavirus[2]	6 wks	4 weeks	4 weeks[2]		
Diphtheria, Tetanus, Pertussis[3]	6 wks	4 weeks	4 weeks	6 months	6 months[3]
Haemophilus influenzae type b[4]	6 wks	4 weeks if first dose administered at younger than age 12 months / 8 weeks (as final dose) if first dose administered at age 12-14 months / No further doses needed if first dose administered at age 15 months or older	4 weeks[4] if current age is younger than 12 months / 8 weeks (as final dose)[4] if current age is 12 months or older and first dose administered at younger than age 12 months and second dose administered at younger than age 15 / No further doses needed if previous dose administered at age 15 months or older	8 weeks (as final dose) This dose only necessary for children aged 12 months through 59 months who received 3 doses before age 12 months	
Pneumococcal[5]	6 wks	4 weeks if first dose administered at younger than age 12 months / 8 weeks (as final dose for healthy children) if first dose administered at age 12 months or older or current age 24 through 59 months / No further doses needed for healthy children if first dose administered at age 24 months or older	4 weeks if current age is younger than 12 months / 8 weeks (as final dose for healthy children) if current age is 12 months or older / No further doses needed for healthy children if previous dose administered at age 24 months or older	8 weeks (as final dose) This dose only necessary for children aged 12 months through 59 months who received 3 doses before age 12 months or for high-risk children who received 3 doses at any age	
Inactivated Poliovirus[6]	6 wks	4 weeks	4 weeks	4 weeks[6]	
Measles, Mumps, Rubella[7]	12 mos	4 weeks			
Varicella[8]	12 mos	3 months			
Hepatitis A[9]	12 mos	6 months			
PERSONS AGED 7 THROUGH 18 YEARS					
Tetanus, Diphtheria/ Tetanus, Diphtheria, Pertussis[10]	7 yrs[10]	4 weeks	4 weeks if first dose administered at younger than age 12 months / 6 months if first dose administered at age 12 months or older	6 months if first dose administered at younger than age 12 months	
Human Papillomavirus[11]	9 yrs	Routine dosing intervals are recommended[11]			
Hepatitis A[9]	12 mos	6 months			
Hepatitis B[1]	Birth	4 weeks	8 weeks (and at least 16 weeks after first dose)		
Inactivated Poliovirus[6]	6 wks	4 weeks	4 weeks	6 months	
Measles, Mumps, Rubella[7]	12 mos	4 weeks			
Varicella[8]	12 mos	3 months if the person is younger than age 13 years / 4 weeks if the person is aged 13 years or older			

1. **Hepatitis B vaccine (HepB).**
   - Administer the 3-dose series to those not previously vaccinated.
   - A 2-dose series (separated by at least 4 months) of adult formulation Recombivax HB is licensed for children aged 11 through 15 years.
2. **Rotavirus vaccine (RV).**
   - The maximum age for the first dose is 14 weeks 6 days. Vaccination should not be initiated for infants aged 15 weeks 0 days or older.
   - The maximum age for the final dose in the series is 8 months 0 days.
   - If Rotarix was administered for the first and second doses, a third dose is not indicated.
3. **Diphtheria and tetanus toxoids and acellular pertussis vaccine (DTaP).**
   - The fifth dose is not necessary if the fourth dose was administered at age 4 years or older.
4. ***Haemophilus influenzae* type b conjugate vaccine (Hib).**
   - Hib vaccine is not generally recommended for persons aged 5 years or older. No efficacy data are available on which to base a recommendation concerning use of Hib vaccine for older children and adults. However, studies suggest good immunogenicity in persons who have sickle cell disease, leukemia, or HIV infection, or who have had a splenectomy; administering 1 dose of Hib vaccine to these persons who have not previously received Hib vaccine is not contraindicated.
   - If the first 2 doses were PRP-OMP (PedvaxHIB or Comvax), and administered at age 11 months or younger, the third (and final) dose should be administered at age 12 through 15 months and at least 8 weeks after the second dose.
   - If the first dose was administered at age 7 through 11 months, administer the second dose at least 4 weeks later and a final dose at age 12 through 15 months.
5. **Pneumococcal vaccine.**
   - Administer 1 dose of pneumococcal conjugate vaccine (PCV) to all healthy children aged 24 through 59 months who have not received at least 1 dose of PCV on or after age 12 months.
   - For children aged 24 through 59 months with underlying medical conditions, administer 1 dose of PCV if 3 doses were received previously or administer 2 doses of PCV at least 8 weeks apart if fewer than 3 doses were received previously.
   - Administer pneumococcal polysaccharide vaccine (PPSV) to children aged 2 years or older with certain underlying medical conditions, including a cochlear implant, at least 8 weeks after the last dose of PCV. See *MMWR* 1997;46(No. RR-8).
6. **Inactivated poliovirus vaccine (IPV).**
   - The final dose in the series should be administered on or after the fourth birthday and at least 6 months following the previous dose.

- A fourth dose is not necessary if the third dose was administered at age 4 years or older and at least 6 months following the previous dose.
- In the first 6 months of life, minimum age and minimum intervals are only recommended if the person is at risk for imminent exposure to circulating poliovirus (i.e., travel to a polio-endemic region or during an outbreak).

7. **Measles, mumps, and rubella vaccine (MMR).**
   - Administer the second dose routinely at age 4 through 6 years. However, the second dose may be administered before age 4, provided at least 28 days have elapsed since the first dose.
   - If not previously vaccinated, administer 2 doses with at least 28 days between doses.
8. **Varicella vaccine.**
   - Administer the second dose routinely at age 4 through 6 years. However, the second dose may be administered before age 4, provided at least 3 months have elapsed since the first dose.
   - For persons aged 12 months through 12 years, the minimum interval between doses is 3 months. However, if the second dose was administered at least 28 days after the first dose, it can be accepted as valid.
   - For persons aged 13 years and older, the minimum interval between doses is 28 days.
9. **Hepatitis A vaccine (HepA).**
   - HepA is recommended for children aged older than 23 months who live in areas where vaccination programs target older children, who are at increased risk for infection, or for whom immunity against hepatitis A is desired.
10. **Tetanus and diphtheria toxoids vaccine (Td) and tetanus and diphtheria toxoids and acellular pertussis vaccine (Tdap).**
    - Doses of DTaP are counted as part of the Td/Tdap series
    - Tdap should be substituted for a single dose of Td in the catch-up series or as a booster for children aged 10 through 18 years; use Td for other doses.
11. **Human papillomavirus vaccine (HPV).**
    - Administer the series to females at age 13 through 18 years if not previously vaccinated.
    - Use recommended routine dosing intervals for series catch-up (i.e., the second and third doses should be administered at 1 to 2 and 6 months after the first dose). The minimum interval between the first and second doses is 4 weeks. The minimum interval between the second and third doses is 12 weeks, and the third dose should be administered at least 24 weeks after the first dose.

Information about reporting reactions after immunization is available online at http://www.vaers.hhs.gov or by telephone, 800-822-7967. Suspected cases of vaccine-preventable diseases should be reported to the state or local health department. Additional information, including precautions and contraindications for immunization, is available from the National Center for Immunization and Respiratory Diseases at http://www.cdc.gov/vaccines or telephone, 800-CDC-INFO (800-232-4636). Department of Health and Human Services • Centers for Disease Control and Prevention

Figure 15–1 cont'd

vaccine or "flu shot" because it contains weakened live influenza viruses instead of killed viruses and is administered by nasal spray instead of injection. The nasal-spray flu vaccine contains three different influenza viruses that are sufficiently weakened as to be incapable of causing disease, but that have sufficient strength to stimulate a protective immune response. The viruses in the LAIV are cold adapted and temperature sensitive. As a result, the viruses can grow in the nose and throat, but not in the lower respiratory tract where the temperature is higher. LAIV is currently approved for use in healthy people 2 to 49 years old. The licensed indications for the LAIV vaccine continue to expand; practitioners should keep abreast of these expanded indications. Aside from the age restrictions, individuals who should not receive LAIV include those with a health condition that places them at high risk for complications from influenza, including patients with chronic heart or lung disease, such as asthma or reactive airways disease, patients with immunosuppression, children or adolescents receiving long-term aspirin therapy, people with a history of Guillain-Barré syndrome, pregnant women, and people with a history of allergy to any of the components of LAIV or to eggs. In addition, there is a potential but seldom noted risk of transmission of the vaccine viruses and subsequent illness to close contacts. Adverse effects include nasal irritation and discharge, muscle aches, sore throat, and fever.

The optimal time to receive seasonal influenza vaccine is usually in October or November, about 1 month before the anticipated onset of the flu season. When a child younger than 8 years receives influenza vaccine for the first time, two doses 4 or more weeks apart should be given. Annual influenza vaccine is recommended for children 6 months old or older with chronic health problems.

The Centers for Disease Control and Prevention more recently announced that virtually all children younger than 18 years should be immunized against seasonal influenza. This recommendation recognizes that children are often the first to introduce influenza into the community and then transmit the disease to adults. Children 5 to 18 years old get the flu at rates higher than any other age group. Although they tend not to become seriously ill with the disease, children with the flu typically miss many days of school. Their parents and caregivers are usually out of the workforce for an equal number of days providing care for the sick child, and often then come down with the flu a few days later. Influenza strains such as novel H1N1, an influenza A virus also known as swine flu, and H5N1, an influenza A virus also know as avian flu, seem to cause greater disease burden in younger adults.

Discussion Sources

Centers for Disease Control and Prevention. http://www.cdc.gov/Vaccines/recs/schedules/child-schedule.htm, Recommended childhood immunization schedule—United States, 2008, 2009, accessed 10/3/09.

Centers for Disease Control and Prevention. http://www.cdc.gov/flu/, Seasonal influenza, 2009, accessed 10/3/09.

QUESTIONS

39. Which of the following statements is true about the hepatitis B virus (HBV) vaccine?
    - **A.** The vaccine contains live HBV.
    - **B.** Children should have hepatitis B surface antibody (HBsAb, anti-HBs) titers drawn after three doses of vaccine.
    - **C.** Hepatitis B immunization should be offered to all children.
    - **D.** Serological testing for hepatitis B surface antigen (HBsAg) should be checked before HBV vaccination is initiated in children.

40. You are making rounds in the nursery and examine the neonate of a mother who is HBsAg-positive. Your most appropriate action is to:
    - **A.** administer hepatitis B immune globulin (HBIG).
    - **B.** isolate the infant.
    - **C.** administer hepatitis B immunization.
    - **D.** give hepatitis B immunization and HBIG.

41. Hepatitis B vaccine should not be given to a child with a history of anaphylactic reaction to:
    - **A.** egg.
    - **B.** baker's yeast.
    - **C.** neomycin.
    - **D.** streptomycin.

42. Infants who have been infected perinatally with HBV have an estimated ___% lifetime chance of developing hepatocellular carcinoma or cirrhosis.
    - **A.** 10
    - **B.** 25
    - **C.** 50
    - **D.** 75

ANSWERS

39.	C	**40.**	D
41.	B	**42.**	B

DISCUSSION

A small, double-stranded DNA virus that contains the inner protein of hepatitis B core antigen and an outer surface of hepatitis B surface antigen causes hepatitis B. The virus is transmitted through exchange of body fluids. Hepatitis B infection can be prevented by limiting exposure to blood and body fluids and through immunization. Recombinant hepatitis B vaccine, which does not contain live virus, is well tolerated, but is contraindicated in a person who has a history of anaphylactic reaction to baker's yeast. Children should be immunized in early childhood, preferably in the first year of life. The well-child visit at age 11 to 12 years offers an opportunity to update hepatitis B and other immunizations before adolescence.

Infants who have been infected perinatally with HBV have an estimated 25% lifetime chance of developing hepatocellular carcinoma or cirrhosis. As a result, all pregnant women should undergo screening for HBsAg at the first prenatal visit, regardless of HBV vaccine history. The HBV vaccine is not 100% effective, and a woman could have carried HbsAg since before pregnancy. During the first 24 hours of life, a neonate born to a mother with HBsAg should receive HBV immunization and HBIG to minimize the risk of perinatal transmission and subsequent development of chronic hepatitis B.

About 90% to 95% of people who receive the vaccine develop HBsAb after three doses, which implies protection from the virus. Routine testing for the presence of HBsAb after immunization is not generally recommended.

Administration of HBIG after exposure with a repeat dose in 1 month is about 75% effective in protecting from hepatitis B after percutaneous, sexual, or mucosal exposure to HBV. Along with postexposure HBIG, HBV vaccine series should be started.

Discussion Source

National Center for HIV/AIDS, Viral Hepatitis, STD, and TB Prevention. http://www.cdc.gov/NCIDOD/DISEASES/hepatitis/b, Viral hepatitis B, accessed 10/3/09.

QUESTIONS

43. Which of the following statements is correct about the varicella vaccine?
   A. This vaccine contains killed varicella-zoster virus (VZV).
   B. A short febrile illness is common during the first days after vaccination.
   C. Children should have a varicella titer drawn before receiving the vaccine.
   D. Mild cases of chickenpox have been reported in immunized patients.

44. Expected outcomes with the use of varicella vaccine include a reduction in the rate of all of the following except:
   A. shingles.
   B. Reye syndrome.
   C. aspirin allergy.
   D. invasive varicella.

45. A parent asks about varicella-zoster immune globulin, and you reply that it is a:
   A. synthetic product that is well tolerated.
   B. derived blood product that has been known to transmit infectious disease.
   C. blood product obtained from a single donor.
   D. pooled blood product with an excellent safety profile.

ANSWERS

43. D   **44.** C   **45.** D

DISCUSSION

VZV causes the highly contagious, systemic disease commonly known as chickenpox. Varicella infection usually confers lifetime immunity. Reinfection may be seen, however, in immunocompromised patients. More often, re-exposure causes an increase in antibody titers without causing disease.

VZV can lie dormant in sensory nerve ganglion. Later reactivation causes shingles, a painful, vesicular-form rash in a dermatomal pattern. About 15% of people who have had chickenpox develop shingles at least once during their lifetime. Shingles rates are markedly reduced in people who have received varicella vaccine compared with people who have had chickenpox.

A patient-reported history of varicella is considered a valid measurement of immunity, with 97% to 99% of persons having serological evidence of immunity. Among older children and adults with an unclear or negative varicella history, most are also seropositive. Varicella immunity should be confirmed through varicella titers, even in the presence of a positive varicella history, in health-care workers because of their risk of exposure and potential transmission of the disease.

The varicella vaccine contains attenuated virus. The vaccine is administered in two doses, one at age 1 year and the second at age 4 to 6 years. Older children and adults with no history of varicella infection or previous immunization should receive two immunizations 4 to 8 weeks apart. In particular, health-care workers, family contacts of immunocompromised patients, and day-care workers without evidence of varicella immunity should be targeted for varicella vaccine. In addition, adults who are in environments with high risk of varicella transmission (e.g., college dormitories, military barracks, long-term care facilities) should receive the immunization if there is no evidence of varicella immunity.

The vaccine is highly protective against severe, invasive varicella. Mild forms of chickenpox are occasionally reported after immunization, however. Varicella immune globulin, as with all forms of immune globulin, provides temporary, passive immunity to infection. Immune globulin is a pooled blood product with an excellent safety profile. Although most cases are seen in children younger than 18 years, the greatest varicella mortality is found in persons 30 to 49 years old.

Discussion Source

Centers for Disease Control and Prevention. Available at http://www.cdc.gov/vaccines/vpd-vac/child-vpd.htm, Vaccine preventable disease: varicella, 2009, accessed 10/3/09.

QUESTIONS

46. An 11-year-old child presents with no documented primary tetanus immunization series. Which of the following represents the immunization needed?

    A. three doses of diphtheria, tetanus, and acellular pertussis vaccine 2 months apart

    B. tetanus immune globulin now and two doses of tetanus-diphtheria (Td) 1 month apart

    C. tetanus, diphtheria, and acellular pertussis vaccine (Tdap) × 1 dose, with doses of Td vaccine in 1 and 6 months

    D. Td as a single dose

47. Problems after tetanus immunization typically include:

    A. localized reaction at site of injection.

    B. myalgia and malaise.

    C. low-grade fever.

    D. diffuse rash.

48. Which wound presents the greatest risk for tetanus infection?

    A. a puncture wound obtained while playing in a garden

    B. a laceration obtained from a knife used to trim raw beef

    C. a human bite

    D. an abrasion obtained by falling on a sidewalk

49. Infection with *Corynebacterium diphtheriae* usually causes:

    A. a diffuse rash.

    B. meningitis.

    C. pseudomembranous pharyngitis.

    D. a gastroenteritis-like illness.

ANSWERS

46.	C	47.	A	48.	A
49.	C				

DISCUSSION

Tetanus infection is caused by *Clostridium tetani*, an anaerobic, gram-positive, spore-forming rod. This organism, which is found in soil, particularly if it contains manure, enters the body through a contaminated wound and causes a life-threatening systemic disease characterized by painful muscle weakness and spasm ("lockjaw"). Diphtheria, the "d" part of the DTaP and Tdap vaccines, is caused by *C. diphtheriae*, a gram-negative bacillus. This disease is typically transmitted person to person or through contaminated liquids such as milk. Diphtheria is characterized by severe respiratory tract infection, including the appearance of pseudomembranous pharyngitis.

Tetanus and diphtheria are uncommon infections because of widespread immunization. A primary series of three diphtheria, tetanus, and acellular pertussis vaccine injections given in early childhood provides long-term immunity. A booster tetanus dose every 10 years is recommended, but protection is likely for 20 to 30 years after a primary series. Using Td rather than tetanus toxoid for the primary series and booster doses in adults assists in keeping diphtheria immunity as well; the use of a single dose of Tdap during adulthood provides additional protection from pertussis, whereas older children (≥7 years old) undergoing a "catch-up" immunization schedule should receive one Tdap and two Td doses at the appropriate interval. At the time of a wound-producing injury, tetanus immune globulin provides temporary protection for individuals who have not received tetanus immunization.

Tetanus and diphtheria with or without acellular pertussis immunizations are well tolerated and produce few adverse reactions. A short-term, localized area of redness and warmth is common and is not predictive of future problems with tetanus immunization.

Discussion Sources

Centers for Disease Control and Prevention. http://www.cdc.gov/ncidod/dbmd/diseaseinfo/diptheria_t.htm, Vaccine preventable disease: diphtheria, 2009, accessed 10/3/09.

Centers for Disease Control and Prevention. http://www.cdc.gov/vaccines/vpd-vac/tetanus/default.htm, Vaccine preventable disease: tetanus, 2009, accessed 10/3/09.

Centers for Disease Control and Prevention. http://www.cdc.gov/vaccines/vpd-vac/child-vpd.htm, Vaccine preventable disease: pertussis, 2009, accessed 10/3/09.

QUESTIONS

50. Which of the following is the primary source of hepatitis A infection?

    A. blood products

    B. shellfish

    C. contaminated drinking water

    D. intimate person-to-person contact

51. When answering questions about hepatitis A vaccine, you consider that it:

   A. contains live virus.
   B. should be given to all children, unless contraindicated.
   C. frequently causes systemic postimmunization reaction.
   D. is nearly 100% protective after a single injected dose.

52. Usual treatment options for a child with hepatitis A include:

   A. interferon alfa.
   B. ribavirin.
   C. acyclovir.
   D. supportive care.

ANSWERS

| 50. | C | 51. | B | 52. | D |

DISCUSSION

Hepatitis A infection is caused by hepatitis A virus (HAV), a small RNA virus. Transmitted primarily by fecally contaminated drinking water and food supplies, hepatitis A is typically a self-limited infection that responds well to supportive care with a very low mortality rate. Although raw shellfish growing in contaminated water can be problematic, fecally contaminated water supplies are the most common source of infection. In developing countries with limited pure water, most children contract this disease by age 5 years. In North America, adults 20 to 39 years old account for nearly 50% of the reported cases; children are often affected more than adults and account for virtually all the remaining infections. The local public health department should be consulted for advice when an outbreak of hepatitis A infection occurs.

All children and select high-risk groups should be immunized against HAV. Two doses of HAV vaccine are recommended to ensure an enhanced immunological response. HAV vaccine, which does not contain live virus, is usually well tolerated without systemic reaction.

Discussion Source

National Center for HIV/AIDS, Viral Hepatitis, STD, and TB Prevention. http://www.cdc.gov/NCIDOD/DISEASES/ hepatitis/a, Viral hepatitis A, accessed 10/4/09.

QUESTIONS

53. Which of the following statements is true about oral poliovirus vaccine (OPV)?

   A. It contains killed virus.
   B. It is the preferred method of immunization in North America.
   C. Two doses should be administered by a child's fourth birthday.
   D. After administration of OPV, poliovirus can be shed from the stool.

54. Which of the following statements is true about inactivated poliovirus vaccine (IPV)?

   A. It contains live virus.
   B. It is the preferred method of immunization in North America.
   C. Two doses should be administered by a child's fourth birthday.
   D. After administration of IPV, poliovirus may be shed from the stool.

55. Which of the following is the route of transmission of the poliovirus?

   A. fecal-oral
   B. droplet
   C. blood and body fluids
   D. skin-to-skin contact

ANSWERS

| 53. | D | 54. | B | 55. | A |

DISCUSSION

Polioviruses are highly contagious and capable of causing paralytic, life-threatening infection. The infection is transmitted by the fecal-oral route. Rates of infection among household contacts may be 96%. Since 1994, North and South America have been declared free of indigenous poliomyelitis, largely because of the efficacy of poliovirus immunization. The vaccine is available in two forms: a live-virus vaccine that is given orally and an injectable vaccine that contains inactivated virus. When OPV is used, a small amount of weakened virus is shed via the stool. This shedding presents household members with possible exposure to poliovirus, resulting in a rare risk of paralytic poliomyelitis, known as vaccine-associated paralytic poliomyelitis (VAPP). Because of VAPP risk, OPV is no longer used in the United States and Canada, but it is used in other countries.

Discussion Source

Centers for Disease Control and Prevention.
    http://www.cdc.gov/vaccines/vpd-vac/polio/default.htm#vacc,
    Vaccine preventable disease: polio, 2009, accessed 10/4/09.

QUESTIONS

56. Which of the following is most likely to have lead poisoning?

   A. a developmentally disabled 5-year-old child who lives in a 15-year-old house in poor repair

   B. an infant who lives in a 5-year-old home with copper plumbing

   C. a toddler who lives in an 85-year-old home

   D. a preschooler who lives nears an electric generating plant

57. You are devising a program to screen preschoolers for lead poisoning. The most sensitive component of this campaign is:

   A. environmental history.

   B. physical examination.

   C. hematocrit level.

   D. hemoglobin level.

58. Patients with plumbism present with which kind of anemia?

   A. macrocytic, hyperchromic

   B. normocytic, normochromic

   C. hemolytic

   D. microcytic, hypochromic

59. At which of the following ages should screening begin for a child who has significant risk of lead poisoning?

   A. 3 months

   B. 6 months

   C. 1 year

   D. 2 years

60. Intervention for a child with a lead level of 10 to 20 mcg/dL usually includes all of the following except:

   A. removal from the lead source.

   B. iron supplementation.

   C. chelation therapy.

   D. encouraging a diet high in vitamin C.

61. Intervention for a child with a lead level of 40 to 50 mcg/dL usually includes:

   A. chelation therapy.

   B. calcium supplementation.

   C. exchange transfusion.

   D. iron depletion therapy.

ANSWERS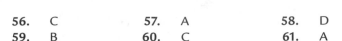

56.	C	**57.**	A	**58.**	D
59.	B	**60.**	C	**61.**	A

DISCUSSION

Lead poisoning, or plumbism, remains a significant public health problem. It is a reportable disease found in more than 2 million children and adults in the United States and is caused by exposure to lead in the environment. Ingested lead inactivates heme synthesis by inhibiting the insertion of iron into the protoporphyrin ring. This leads to the development of a microcytic, hypochromic anemia; basophilic stippling is often noted on red blood cell morphology. In addition, lead is significantly toxic to the solid organs, bones, and nervous system.

The major source of lead poisoning in children is lead-based paint. This paint has not been available in the United States for more than 30 years. Unless deleading procedures have been performed, however, most homes built before 1957 contain lead-based paint. A diet low in calcium, iron, zinc, magnesium, and copper, and high in fat, which is a typical diet for children living in poverty, enhances oral lead absorption.

For lead poisoning to occur, there must be an intersection between the environmental hazard and the child. In older homes, the point of greatest risk is the window because the windowsills and putty have high lead concentration. Because toddlers are the ideal height to reach windowsills and are often drawn to open windows, the age of greatest risk is 2 to 3 years. Summer is the season of greatest risk. Children can acquire lead through two major sources, inhaled paint powder and ingested paint chips. Inhalation of paint dust is a potent lead source for infants and for children with lead levels less than 45 mcg/dL, although toddlers and children with lead levels of more than 45 mcg/dL are typically poisoned by also eating paint chips. The question often arises as to why children would eat a nonfood substance such as a paint chip; these chips are reported to have a slightly sweet taste.

Besides paint, other lead hazards may be encountered. Lead-glazed pottery used to store and serve acidic beverages, soft water delivered by lead-lined pipes, lead-soldered vessels used for cooking, and fumes from burnt casings of batteries can contribute to lead burden. In addition, soil around the base of the home often contains lead-based paint, and soil around highways often contains lead residual from automotive fuel; although the practice of adding lead to gasoline was discontinued many years ago in North America, this practice persists in other countries. In addition, the lead found in the soil can persist for decades. Certain folk medicines from the Middle East and Mexico have been found to contain lead.

Clinical manifestation of lead poisoning is usually not apparent until a child's lead level is markedly elevated.

Because most children have low-level, chronic lead exposure with few or no symptoms, periodic screening of all children is recommended. Primary prevention of lead poisoning should be the goal, to reduce risk for all children. After lead risk is identified, removing the child or limiting exposure is vital. Most children with lead levels of 10 to 35 mcg/dL are treated with removal from the source, improved nutrition, and iron therapy. With lead levels of 36 to 50 mcg/dL, chelation with an agent such as succimer in addition to the previously listed interventions is indicated. With lead levels greater than 51 mcg/dL, hospital admission with expert evaluation is likely the most prudent course to avoid serious problems (including encephalopathy) associated with markedly elevated lead levels.

Discussion Sources

Centers for Disease Control and Prevention. http://www.cdc.gov/nceh/lead/, Lead paint poisoning prevention program, 2009, accessed 10/4/09.

Marcus S. http://www.emedicine.com/EMERG/topic293.htm, eMedicine: lead toxicity, accessed 10/4/09.

QUESTIONS

62. The most likely causative organism of bronchiolitis is:
    A. *Haemophilus influenzae.*
    B. parainfluenza virus.
    C. respiratory syncytial virus.
    D. coxsackievirus.

63. One of the most prominent clinical features of bronchiolitis is:
    A. fever.
    B. vomiting.
    C. wheezing.
    D. conjunctival inflammation.

64. In most children with bronchiolitis, intervention includes:
    A. aerosolized ribavirin therapy.
    B. supportive care.
    C. oral theophylline therapy.
    D. ibuprofen therapy.

65. Common clinical findings in a young child with bronchiolitis include all of the following except:
    A. pharyngitis.
    B. tachypnea.
    C. bradycardia.
    D. conjunctivitis.

ANSWERS

| 62. | C | 63. | C | 64. | B | 65. | C |

DISCUSSION

Bronchiolitis is a common illness in early childhood; the peak incidence is in children younger than 2 years with more than 90% of episodes occurring between November and April. The most likely causative organism is respiratory syncytial virus (RSV); it is less often caused by parainfluenza, influenza, and adenovirus. During the acute stage of infection, bronchiolar respiratory and ciliated epithelial cell function is altered, producing increased mucus secretion, cell death, and sloughing. This stage is followed by peribronchiolar lymphocytic infiltrate and submucosal edema; the end result is narrowing and obstruction of small airways with resulting cough and wheezing. Additional findings include tachypnea, mild fever, conjunctivitis, and pharyngitis. Bronchiolitis is usually diagnosed by clinical findings; antigen tests of nasal washings provide rapid, accurate RSV detection. This information can be particularly helpful in the setting of an outbreak in a day-care or other similar setting.

In most children, bronchiolitis runs a course of 2 to 3 weeks of the above-mentioned mild upper respiratory symptoms with expiratory wheezing; these findings resolve as ciliary function returns. Supportive therapy is usually sufficient. In infants younger than 3 months and in children with chronic health problems, hypoxemia and hypercapnia with occasional apnea are more common, necessitating hospital admission for hydration and oxygenation. The use of corticosteroids, ribavirin, and bronchodilators including beta$_2$-agonists remains controversial with little evidence of efficacy, although standard asthma therapies are effective in children who also have underlying reactive airway disease. Long-term sequelae of bronchiolitis often include recurrent airway reactivity.

Discussion Source

Louden M. http://www.emedicine.com/emerg/topic365.htm, eMedicine: bronchiolitis, accessed 10/4/09.

QUESTIONS

66. You examine a newborn with a capillary hemangioma on her thigh. You advise her parents that this lesion:
    A. is likely to increase in size over the first year of life.
    B. should be treated to avoid malignancy.
    C. usually resolves within the first months of life.
    D. is likely to develop a superimposed lichenification.

67. You examine a 2-month-old infant with a port-wine lesion over her right cheek. You advise the parents that this lesion:

    A. needs to be surgically excised.

    B. grows proportionally with the child.

    C. becomes lighter over time.

    D. may become malignant.

68. A 10-day-old child presents with multiple raised lesions resembling flea bites over the trunk and nape of the neck. The infant is nursing well and has no fever or exposure to animals. These lesions likely represent:

    A. erythema toxicum neonatorum.

    B. milia.

    C. neonatal acne.

    D. staphylococcal skin infection.

69. An Asian couple comes in with their 4-week-old infant, who has blue-black macules scattered over the buttocks. These most likely represent:

    A. mottling.

    B. mongolian spots.

    C. ecchymosis.

    D. hemangioma.

70. The most important aspect of skin care for patients with eczema is:

    A. frequent bathing with antibacterial soap.

    B. consistent use of medium- to high-potency topical steroids.

    C. application of lubricants.

    D. treatment of dermatophytes.

71. A common site for eczema in infants is the:

    A. dorsum of the hand.

    B. face.

    C. neck.

    D. flexor surfaces.

ANSWERS

66.	A	**67.**	B	**68.**	A
69.	B	**70.**	C	**71.**	B

DISCUSSION

Numerous dermatologic conditions are found in early infancy. Parents understandably have concerns about these lesions. It is important for the NP to have a thorough knowledge of common conditions.

Capillary or strawberry hemangioma ♂ is a congenital vascular malformation. Such lesions are rarely present at birth and become evident in the first weeks of life, growing rapidly in the first year, then plateauing in size, and eventually regressing. About 90% disappear by age 9, usually leaving bluish vascularity over the area. If the lesion is large or involves a vital organ such as the eye or extremity, treatment by an expert in the condition is indicated. Treatment can include the use of products to alter vascularity, such as injectable corticosteroids, laser therapy, or interferon alfa injection.

A port-wine stain ♂ is a flat hemangioma with a stable course. These lesions usually appear on the face and are usually present at birth. Port-wine stains tend to deepen in color as time goes on and grow proportionally with the child. Although not malignant, the lesions are often disfiguring and can be minimized or occasionally eliminated through the use of laser therapy.

The typical presentation of milia is as white pinpoint papular lesions caused by sebaceous hyperplasia. The usual distribution is over the nose, cheeks, and other areas with an abundance of sebaceous glands. The cause is likely the maternal androgenic effect on the sebaceous glands. Benign in nature, milia resolve without special therapy by 4 weeks to 6 months of life.

Erythema toxicum neonatorum ♂ is a benign rash of unknown etiology that occurs in about 50% of full-term infants. Usually beginning in the first 10 days of life, the lesions look like flea bites and are widely distributed; the palms and soles are spared. The lesions usually fade by 5 to 7 days after eruption without specific treatment and do not seem to bother the infant.

Mongolian spots ♂ occur in about 90% of children of African and Asian ancestries and in less than 10% of children of European ancestry. The distribution is usually over the lower back and buttocks, but can occur over a wider area. Caused by an accumulation of melanocytes, these are benign lesions that typically fade by age 7 without special therapy. Uninformed providers can misinterprate this normal finding as an ecchymotic area, raising the suspicion of child abuse.

Acne neonatorum consists of open and closed comedones and pustules over the forehead and cheeks, similar to the adolescent version of the condition. The etiology is likely the effect of maternal androgens on the infant's skin. It usually resolves in about 4 to 8 weeks, but occasionally persists up to age 1 year. Low-dose benzoyl peroxide can be used as therapy, although the lesions typically resolve without intervention.

Eczema or atopic dermatitis is a manifestation of a type I hypersensitivity reaction. This type of reaction is caused when immunoglobulin E antibodies occupy receptor sites on mast cells, causing a degradation of the mast cells and subsequent release of histamine, vasodilation, mucous gland stimulation, and tissue swelling. There are two subgroups of type I hypersensitivity reactions: atopy and anaphylaxis.

The atopy subgroup comprises numerous common clinical conditions, such as allergic rhinitis, atopic dermatitis, allergic gastroenteropathy, and allergy-based asthma. Atopic diseases have a strong familial component and tend to cause localized rather than systemic reactions. Individuals with atopic disease are often able to identify allergy-inducing agents. Treatment for atopic disease of eczema includes avoidance of offending agents, minimizing skin dryness by limiting soap and water exposure, and consistent use of lubricants. The NP should explain to the patient that the skin tends to be sensitive and needs to be treated with some care. When flares occur, the skin eruption is largely caused by histamine release. Antihistamines and topical corticosteroids should be used to control eczema flares. With an acute flare of eczema or with contact dermatitis, a topical corticosteroid with intermediate to high potency is likely needed to control acute symptoms. After this control is achieved, the lowest potency topical corticosteroid that yields the desired effect should be used.

Discussion Source

Morelli J, Weston W. Skin. In: Hay W, Levin M, Sondheimer J, eds. *Current Pediatric Diagnosis and Treatment.* 18th ed. Columbus, OH: McGraw-Hill Medical; 2007.

QUESTIONS

72. Which of the following is the most prudent first-line treatment choice for a toddler with acute otitis media (AOM) who requires antimicrobial therapy?

    A. ceftibuten
    B. amoxicillin
    C. cefuroxime
    D. azithromycin

73. Most AOM is caused by:

    A. certain gram-positive and gram-negative bacteria and respiratory viruses.
    B. gram-negative bacteria and pathogenic viruses.
    C. rhinovirus and *Staphylococcus aureus.*
    D. predominately beta-lactamase–producing organisms.

74. Which of the following represents the best choice of clinical agents for a child who has severe type 1 penicillin allergy who requires antimicrobial therapy?

    A. ciprofloxacin
    B. clarithromycin
    C. amoxicillin
    D. cefixime

75. Which of the following does not represent a risk factor for recurrent AOM in younger children?

    A. pacifier use after age 10 months
    B. history of first episode of AOM before age 3 months
    C. exposure to second-hand smoke
    D. penicillin allergy

76. Which of the following antimicrobial agents affords the most effective activity against *Streptococcus pneumoniae*?

    A. ciprofloxacin
    B. cefixime
    C. trimethoprim-sulfamethoxazole (TMP-SMX)
    D. cefuroxime

77. A 3-year-old boy with AOM continues to have otalgia and fever (>39°C [>102.2°F]) after 3 days of amoxicillin 80 mg/kg/d with an appropriate dose of clavulanate (Augmentin) therapy. Which of the following is recommended?

    A. Watch and wait while using analgesics.
    B. Start antimicrobial therapy with oral azithromycin.
    C. Initiate therapy with oral clindamycin.
    D. Administer intramuscular ceftriaxone.

78. Which of the following is most consistent with the diagnosis of AOM?

    A. ear pulling in the infant
    B. tympanic membrane (TM) retraction
    C. TM immobility to insufflation
    D. anterior cervical lymphadenopathy

79. Which of the following is absent in otitis media with effusion (OME)?

    A. fluid in the middle ear
    B. otalgia
    C. fever
    D. itch

80. Treatment of OME usually includes:

    A. symptomatic therapy.
    B. antimicrobial therapy.
    C. an antihistamine.
    D. a mucolytic.

81. Clindamycin is most effective against:

    A. *S. pneumoniae.*
    B. *H. influenzae.*
    C. *Moraxella catarrhalis.*
    D. Adenovirus.

82. Characteristics of *M. catarrhalis* include:

    A. high rate of beta-lactamase production.
    B. antimicrobial resistance because of altered protein binding sites.
    C. often being found in middle ear exudate on recurrent otitis media.
    D. gram-positive organism.

83. Characteristics of *H. influenzae* include:

    A. rare beta-lactamase production.

    B. antimicrobial resistance because of altered protein binding sites.

    C. organism most commonly isolated from mucoid middle ear effusion.

    D. gram-positive organism.

84. Characteristics of *S. pneumoniae* include:

    A. beta-lactamase production common.

    B. antimicrobial resistance because of altered protein binding sites.

    C. organism most commonly isolated from mucoid middle ear effusion.

    D. gram-negative organism.

ANSWERS

72.	B	**73.**	A	**74.**	B
75.	D	**76.**	D	**77.**	D
78.	C	**79.**	C	**80.**	A
81.	A	**82.**	A	**83.**	C
84.	B				

DISCUSSION

In children, acute otitis media (AOM) 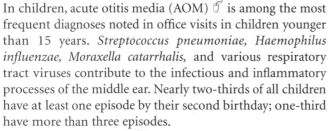 is among the most frequent diagnoses noted in office visits in children younger than 15 years. *Streptococcus pneumoniae, Haemophilus influenzae, Moraxella catarrhalis,* and various respiratory tract viruses contribute to the infectious and inflammatory processes of the middle ear. Nearly two-thirds of all children have at least one episode by their second birthday; one-third have more than three episodes.

The eustachian tubes provide drainage of middle ear secretions and protection of the middle ear from pharyngeal secretions and bacterial contaminants. As a result, conditions that cause eustachian tube dysfunction or eustachian tube obstruction, such as allergic rhinitis, upper respiratory infection, and craniofacial abnormalities, encourage status of secretions and allow aspiration of pharyngeal flora into the middle ear, resulting in AOM. Passive cigarette smoke exposure, feeding in a supine position, and pacifier use beyond age 10 months likely also predispose a child to AOM secondary to eustachian tube dysfunction or eustachian tube obstruction. Because children in day-care settings typically have more upper respiratory infections, attendance at group child care is also a risk factor for nasopharyngeal carriage of bacteria implicated in AOM. Bottle feeding is a risk factor for AOM, with rates significantly lower among infants who were breastfed for the first 6 to 12 months of life; boys and children of Native American ancestry are also noted to be at increased risk. An additional intervention to reduce AOM risk includes universal childhood influenza immunization.

S. pneumoniae causes 40% to 50% of AOM; it is the least likely of the three major causative bacteria to resolve without antimicrobial intervention and causes the most significant symptoms. This organism has exhibited resistance more recently to numerous antibiotic agents, including amoxicillin, cephalosporins, and macrolides. The mechanism of resistance is an alteration of intracellular protein-binding sites, which can typically be overcome by using higher doses of amoxicillin, certain cephalosporins, and, rarely, clindamycin. The pneumococcal conjugate vaccine is effective in reducing risk of invasive pneumococcal disease and in minimizing AOM risk when caused by serotypes included in the vaccine.

H. influenzae and *M. catarrhalis* are gram-negative organisms capable of producing beta-lactamase. Although these two organisms have relatively high rates of spontaneous resolution (50% and 90%), without antimicrobial intervention, *H. influenzae* is the organism most commonly isolated from mucoid and serious middle ear effusion, conditions often noted in recurrent AOM. Beta-lactamase production by organisms probably contributes less to AOM treatment failure than to prescribing an inadequate dosing of amoxicillin needed to eradicate drug-resistant *S. pneumoniae*. Respiratory syncytial virus is commonly isolated from the middle ear fluid in children with AOM. Other common viral agents include human rhinovirus and coronavirus. AOM caused by these viral agents usually resolves in 7 to 10 days with supportive care alone.

Appropriate assessment is critical to the diagnosis of AOM (Table 15–3). Ear pulling in preverbal children is often noted, but is not considered diagnostic for the condition. The TM can be retracted or bulging and is typically reddened with loss of translucency and mobility on insufflation. The components of AOM include objective findings such as a bulging, erythematous TM with limited or absent mobility and distinct otalgia with discomfort clearly referable to the ear that results in interference with or precludes normal activity or sleep. Additional components include an air-fluid level behind the TM and otorrhea. With recovery, TM mobility returns in about 1 to 2 weeks, but middle ear effusion typically persists for 4 to 6 weeks, often up to 3 months.

AOM is a common clinical problem. The American Academy of Pediatrics (AAP) has developed treatment recommendations for children with AOM. These recommendations apply only to otherwise healthy children without underlying conditions that could alter the natural course of AOM, including anatomic abnormalities such as cleft palate, certain genetic conditions such as Down syndrome, immunodeficiencies, presence of cochlear implants, and recurrent AOM.

One important point made in the American Academy of Pediatrics AOM treatment guidelines is that "watch and wait" can be an appropriate approach to treating AOM. Placebo-controlled trials of AOM during the past 30 years have shown consistently that most children do well, without adverse sequelae, without antibacterial therapy. As a result, observation without use of antibacterial agents in a child

TABLE 15–3

Diagnosis of Acute Otitis Media (AOM)

COMPONENTS OF AOM	Objective findings • Bulging TM • TM erythema • Limited or absent TM mobility • Air-fluid level behind TM • Otorrhea Distinct otalgia • Discomfort clearly referable to the ear that results in interference with or precludes normal activity or sleep
RATIONALE FOR OBSERV-ATION AS TREATMENT OPTION IN AOM	In otherwise well child • Low risk for adverse outcome without antimicrobial therapy • High rate of spontaneous AOM resolution without antimicrobial therapy Appropriate option only if • Illness meets "nonsevere" definition • Follow-up can be ensured • Antibacterial agents started if symptoms persist or worsen
NONSEVERE VERSUS SEVERE ILLNESS	Nonsevere illness • Mild otalgia and fever <39°C (<102.2°F) in the past 24 hours Severe illness • Moderate to severe otalgia or fever ≥39°C (≥102.2°F)

Source: Subcommittee on Management of Acute Otitis Media: Diagnosis and management of acute otitis media. *Pediatrics*. 2004;113:1451–1465.

with uncomplicated AOM is an option for selected children based on diagnostic certainty, age, illness severity, and assurance of follow-up. Appropriate analgesia should be provided for all children with AOM.

Amoxicillin remains the first-line antimicrobial for the treatment of AOM in children with less severe illness. Given the wide therapeutic index of this medication and the prevalence of drug-resistant *S. pneumoniae*, 80 to 90 mg/kg/d is the recommended dose. Amoxicillin/clavulanate (Augmentin), 80 to 90 mg/kg/d, is recommended as first-line therapy for a child with AOM and severe illness or in the case of treatment failure with amoxicillin (Tables 15–4 and 15–5).

Children younger than 3 months old with AOM should be routinely seen in 1 to 2 days because of increased risk of treatment failure. In a child older than 3 months, otalgia, fever, and other symptoms that persist beyond 3 days of therapy can indicate treatment failure, and repeat evaluation is in order and a change in therapy is recommended (see Table 15–5). If the child seems to be recovering, follow-up at 4 to 8 weeks is often advised, in part to evaluate for otitis media with effusion (OME). OME, also known as serous otitis media, 𝒯 is defined as the presence of fluid in the middle ear in the absence of signs or symptoms of acute infection. With OME, 80% of children clear the middle ear by 8 weeks. If OME persists beyond 8 weeks, the presence of communication problems and other symptoms dictates the need for further evaluation and treatment. Routine retreatment with an antimicrobial is not indicated for OME

(Table 15–6). When a child is seen at follow-up, measures to reduce AOM risk should be reviewed and reinforced.

Discussion Source

Subcommittee on Management of Acute Otitis Media. Diagnosis and management of acute otitis media. *Pediatrics*. 2004;113:1451–1465.

TABLE 15–4

Criteria for Initial Antibacterial Agent Treatment or Observation in Acute Otitis Media

Age	Certain Diagnosis	Uncertain Diagnosis
<6 mo	Antibacterial therapy	Antibacterial therapy
6 mo–2 yr	Antibacterial therapy	Antibacterial therapy if severe illness; observation option if nonsevere illness
≥2 y	Antibacterial therapy if severe illness; observation option if nonsevere illness	Observation option

TABLE 15–5

Antimicrobial Treatment in Acute Otitis Media

Clinically Defined Treatment Failure at 48–72 Hours after Initial Management with Observation Option or at Diagnosis for Patients Being Treated Initially with Antibacterial Agents

Temperature ≥39°C (≥102.2°F) or Severe Otalgia

	Recommended	Alternative for Penicillin Allergy
No	Amoxicillin 80–90 mg/kg/d	Non–type I: Cefdinir, cefuroxime, or cefpodoxime Type I: Azithromycin, clarithromycin
Yes	Amoxicillin-clavulanate 90 mg/kg/d of amoxicillin with 6.4 mg/kg/d of clavulanate	Ceftriaxone 1 or 3 days

Clinically Defined Treatment Failure at 48–72 Hours after Initial Management with Antibacterial Agents

Temperature ≥39°C (≥102.2°F) or Severe Otalgia

	Recommended	Alternative for Penicillin Allergy
No	Amoxicillin-clavulanate 90 mg/kg/d of amoxicillin component with 6.4 mg/kg/d of clavulanate	Non–type I: Ceftriaxone 3 days Type I: Clindamycin
Yes	Ceftriaxone 3 days	Tympanocentesis, clindamycin

Source: Subcommittee on Management of Acute Otitis Media: Diagnosis and management of acute otitis media. *Pediatrics.* 2004;113:1451–1465.

TABLE 15–6

Otitis Media with Effusion

DEFINED	Fluid in middle ear without signs or symptoms of ear infection
FIRST-LINE INTERVENTION	Watchful waiting in most 75%–90% resolve within 3 mo without specific treatment
SELECT INTERVENTION IN AT-RISK CHILDREN	With persistent effusion accompanied by language delay or suspected or documented hearing loss: Tympanostomy best studied intervention

Source: aappolicy.aappublications.org/cgi/content/full/pediatrics;113/5/1412#SEC7, accessed 10/6/09.

QUESTIONS

85. Which of the following is most likely to be part of the clinical presentation of urinary tract infection (UTI) in a 20-month-old child?

   A. urinary frequency and urgency
   B. fever
   C. suprapubic tenderness
   D. nausea and vomiting

86. Which of the following is the most common UTI organism in children?

   A. *Pseudomonas aeruginosa*
   B. *Escherichia coli*
   C. *Klebsiella pneumoniae*
   D. *Proteus mirabilis*

87. All of the following uropathogens are capable of reducing urinary nitrates to nitrites except:

    A. *E. coli.*
    B. *Proteus* species.
    C. *K. pneumoniae.*
    D. *Staphylococcus saprophyticus.*

88. Which of the following is considered the ideal method for obtaining a urine sample for culture and sensitivity in an 18-month-old-old girl with suspected UTI?

    A. suprapubic aspiration
    B. transurethral bladder catheterization
    C. bag collection
    D. diaper sample

89. When choosing an antimicrobial agent for the treatment of UTI in a febrile child, the NP considers that:

    A. gram-positive organisms are the most likely cause of infection.
    B. a parenteral aminoglycoside is the preferred treatment choice.
    C. the use of an oral third generation cephalosporin is acceptable if gastrointestinal function is intact.
    D. nitrofurantoin use is considered first-line therapy.

90. When evaluating the urinalysis of a 10 month old infant with UTI, the NP considers that:

    A. leukocytes would be consistently noted.
    B. proteinuria is usually absent.
    C. urobilinogen can be present.
    D. 20% of urinalyses can be normal.

91. In children 2 months to 2 years old with UTI, antimicrobial therapy should be prescribed for:

    A. 3 to 5 days.
    B. 5 to 10 days.
    C. 7 to 14 days.
    D. 14 to 21 days.

92. The preferred urinary tract imaging study for a 22-month-old girl with first-time UTI is:

    A. renal ultrasound.
    B. renal scan.
    C. cystogram.
    D. none unless a second UTI occurs.

93. The urinary tract abnormality most often associated with UTI in younger children is:

    A. bladder neck stricture.
    B. ureteral stenosis.
    C. renal scarring.
    D. vesicoureteral reflux.

ANSWERS

85.	B	**86.**	B	**87.**	D
88.	A	**89.**	C	**90.**	D
91.	C	**92.**	C	**93.**	D

DISCUSSION

Although often thought of as a problem primarily of women, UTIs do occur in early childhood. Rates in girls younger than 1 year are about 6.5% and at 1 to 2 years are 8.1%. The rates are lower in boys: 3.3% at younger than 1 year and 1.9% at 1 to 2 years. Uncircumcised boys can have rates of UTI 20 times higher than that in circumcised boys, but this difference decreases dramatically when normal penile growth loosens the foreskin, usually occurring by the time the boy is 1 to 2 years old.

The clinical presentation of UTI in children can be without the classic symptoms such as frequency, dysuria, or flank pain. In younger children, UTI often manifests as irritability, lethargy, and fever with no obvious focal infectious source. Older children often present with abdominal pain or unexplained fever or both; as children approach puberty, flank pain becomes more common. UTI should be considered in infants and young children 2 months to 2 years old with unexplained fever, particularly in boys younger than 6 months and girls younger than 2 years who have a temperature greater than or equal to 39°C (≥102.2°F).

A urinalysis should be obtained in a child with unexplained fever or symptoms that suggest a UTI; however, the urinalysis may be negative in 20% of cases. Any of the following findings are suggestive, although not diagnostic, of UTI: positive leukocyte esterase, positive nitrite, more than five white blood cells (WBCs) per high-power field in spun specimen, and bacteria present in unspun Gram-stained specimen. An evaluation for sepsis should also be initiated if clinical presentation warrants.

The method of obtaining a urinalysis in younger children has been long debated. Suprapubic bladder aspiration yields the specimen that is least likely to be contaminated; for the parent and child, this method can be fraught with fear, and it requires special provider skill. Next best is transurethral bladder catheterization. Less acceptable because of the high rate of skin and fecal contamination is a urine specimen collection via bag.

UTIs in children can be associated with anatomic abnormalities, with vesicoureteral reflux the most commonly associated problem. Reflux nephropathy causes scarring and is a risk factor for renal failure, but is largely avoidable with early reflux recognition and proper treatment. Little difference is usually found in the clinical presentation and laboratory findings of cystitis or pyelonephritis in a febrile child, and determining whether a UTI is limited to the lower urinary tract or involves the soft tissue of the kidney is not clinically significant. The management of a child with UTI is dictated by the clinical severity of the illness, rather than by the specific site of infection in the urinary tract. As a result, a single documented UTI in a child must be taken seriously.

If an infant or young child 2 months to 2 years old with suspected UTI is assessed as toxic, dehydrated, or unable to retain oral intake, hospitalization should be considered. Initial antimicrobial therapy should be administered parenterally, usually with a second or third generation cephalosporin. An aminoglycoside such as gentamicin is a second-line choice and can be used if there is a history of severe penicillin allergy. For a child who is well hydrated and able to take an antimicrobial and fluids orally, home-based care is reasonable. An oral second or third generation cephalosporin is a reasonable initial therapy; there is a small risk of treatment failure with the use of TMP-SMX. The optimal length of antimicrobial therapy in pediatric UTI has not been established, although little evidence exists to support the clinical superiority of longer (7 to 10 days) versus shorter (3 to 5 days) therapy. If the child responds to therapy, antimicrobial prophylaxis with an oral cephalosporin or TMP-SMX should be continued until imaging and urological evaluations are complete. Although fluoroquinolone antibiotics have not been widely used in children, ciprofloxacin is approved by the U.S. Food and Drug Administration (FDA) for use in pediatric patients for the treatment of UTI; this use is approved starting at age 1 year.

Urinary tract abnormality is a major risk factor for pediatric UTI, with vesicoureteral reflux noted in 30% to 50% of cases. Reflux increases the risk of ascending infection, which leads to pyelonephritis and renal scarring. Urinary tract imaging should be considered for all children with UTI, particularly if this occurs before toilet training. Renal ultrasound is an easily obtained, noninvasive test, but when used as the sole study, reflux often is missed. The preferred test for vesicoureteral reflux is cystogram. A renal scan is the best study for detecting renal scarring, a finding present only after infection, but misses reflux. If reflux or other urinary tract abnormality is noted on imaging, antimicrobial prophylaxis should continue until the abnormality is corrected.

Discussion Sources

Alper B, Curry S. available at www.aafp.org/afp/20051215/2483. html, Urinary tract infection in children. *American Family Physician*, 2005, accessed 10/3/09.

Ferri F. Ferri's Best Test: *A Practical Guide to Clinical Laboratory Medicine and Diagnostic Imaging.* 2nd ed. Philadelphia, PA: Elsevier Mosby; 2009.

QUESTIONS

94. You examine a 10-year-old boy with suspected streptococcal pharyngitis. His mother asks if he can get a "shot of penicillin." You consider the following when counseling her about the use of intramuscular (IM) penicillin:

    A. There is nearly a 100% cure rate in streptococcal pharyngitis when IM penicillin is used.
    B. Treatment failure rates with IM penicillin approach 20%.
    C. The risk of severe allergic reaction with IM products is similar to that of oral preparations.
    D. Injectable penicillin has a superior spectrum of antimicrobial coverage compared with the oral form of the drug.

95. You examine a 15-year-old presenting with a 1-day history of sore throat, low-grade fever, maculopapular rash, and cervical and occipital lymphadenopathy. The most likely diagnosis is:

    A. scarlet fever.
    B. roseola.
    C. rubella.
    D. rubeola.

96. A 4-year-old child presents with fever; exudative pharyngitis; anterior cervical lymphadenopathy; and a fine, raised, pink rash. The most likely diagnosis is:

    A. scarlet fever.
    B. roseola.
    C. rubella.
    D. rubeola.

97. An 18-year-old woman has a chief complaint of "a sore throat and swollen glands" for the past 3 days. Her physical examination reveals exudative pharyngitis, minimally tender anterior and posterior cervical lymphadenopathy, and maculopapular rash. Abdominal examination reveals right and left upper quadrant abdominal tenderness. The most likely diagnosis is:

    A. group A beta-hemolytic streptococcal pharyngitis.
    B. infectious mononucleosis.
    C. rubella.
    D. scarlet fever.

98. Which of the following is most likely to be found in the laboratory data of a child who has infectious mononucleosis?

    A. neutrophilia
    B. lymphocytosis with atypical lymphocytes
    C. positive antinuclear antibody
    D. macrocytic anemia

99. You examine a 15-year-old boy who has infectious mononucleosis with marked tonsillar hypertrophy, exudative pharyngitis, difficulty swallowing, and a patent airway. You consider prescribing:

- **A.** amoxicillin.
- **B.** prednisone.
- **C.** ibuprofen.
- **D.** acyclovir.

100. A 2-year-old girl presents with pustular, ulcerating lesions on the hands and feet and oral ulcers. The child is cranky, well hydrated, and afebrile. The most likely diagnosis is:

- **A.** hand-foot-and-mouth disease.
- **B.** aphthous stomatitis.
- **C.** herpetic gingivostomatitis.
- **D.** Vincent angina.

101. A 6-year-old boy presents with a 1-day history of fiery red, maculopapular facial rash concentrated on the cheeks. He has had mild headache and myalgia for the past week. The most likely diagnosis is:

- **A.** erythema infectiosum.
- **B.** roseola.
- **C.** rubella.
- **D.** scarlet fever.

ANSWERS

94.	B	95.	C	96.	A
97.	B	98.	B	99.	B
100.	A	101.	A		

DISCUSSION

Developing an accurate diagnosis of an acute febrile illness with associated rash or skin lesion can be a daunting task. Knowledge of the infectious agent, its incubation period, its mode of transmission, and its common clinical presentation can be helpful (Table 15–7). ♂

Discussion Sources

Habif T, Campbell J, Chapman MS, Dinulous J, Zug K. *Atopic Dermatology*. Philadelphia, PA: Mosby Elsevier; 2006.

McKinnon H, Howard T. http://www.aafp.org/afp/20000815/804.html, Evaluating the febrile patient with a rash, accessed 10/4/09.

QUESTIONS

102. Which of the following best describes asthma?

- **A.** intermittent airway inflammation with occasional bronchospasm
- **B.** a disease of bronchospasm leading to airway inflammation
- **C.** chronic airway inflammation with superimposed bronchospasm
- **D.** relatively fixed airway constriction

103. A 5-year-old boy has a 1-year history of moderate persistent asthma that is normally well controlled with budesonide via nebulizer twice a day and the use of albuterol once or twice a week as needed for wheezing. Three days ago, he developed a sore throat, clear nasal discharge, and a dry cough. In the past 24 hours, he has had intermittent wheezing, necessitating the use of albuterol, 2 puffs with use of an age-appropriate spacer every 3 hours, with partial relief. Your next most appropriate action is to obtain:

- **A.** a chest radiograph.
- **B.** an oxygen saturation measurement.
- **C.** a peak expiratory flow (PEF) measurement.
- **D.** a sputum smear for WBCs.

104. You examine a 4-year-old girl who has an acute asthma flare. She is using budesonide and albuterol as directed and continues to have difficulty with coughing and wheezing. Respiratory rate is within 50% of upper limits of normal for her age. Her medication regimen should be adjusted to include:

- **A.** theophylline.
- **B.** salmeterol (Serevent).
- **C.** prednisolone.
- **D.** montelukast (Singulair).

105. Which of the following is inconsistent with the diagnosis of asthma?

- **A.** a troublesome nocturnal cough
- **B.** cough or wheeze after exercise
- **C.** morning sputum production
- **D.** colds "go to the chest" or take more than 10 days to clear

TABLE 15–7
Rash-Producing Febrile Illness

Clinical Condition With Causative Agent	Presentation	Comments
Scarlet fever Agent: *S. pyogenes* (group A beta-hemolytic streptococci)	Scarlatina form or sandpaper-like rash with exudative pharyngitis, fever, headache, tender, localized anterior cervical lymphadenopathy. Rash usually erupts on day 2 of pharyngitis and often peels a few days later	Presence of rash does not imply more severe or serious disease or greater risk of contagion Treatment: Identical to streptococcus pharyngitis
Roseola Agent: Human herpes virus-6 (HHV-6)	Discrete rosy-pink macular or maculopapular rash lasting hours to 3 days that follows a 3- to 7-day period of fever, often quite high	90% of cases seen in children <2 yr. Febrile seizures in 10% of children affected Supportive treatment
Rubella Agent: Rubella virus	Mild symptoms; fever, sore throat, malaise, nasal discharge, diffuse maculopapular rash lasting ~3 days Posterior cervical and postauricular lymphadenopathy 5–10 days before onset of rash Arthralgia in ~25% (most common in women)	Incubation period ~14–21 days with disease transmissible for ~1 week before onset of rash to ~2 weeks after rash appears Generally a mild self-limiting illness. Greatest risk is effect of virus on unborn child, especially with first-trimester exposure (~80% rate congenital rubella syndrome) Prevent by immunization.
Measles Agent: Rubeola virus	Usually acute presentation with fever, nasal discharge, cough, generalized lymphadenopathy, conjunctivitis (copious clear discharge), photophobia, Koplik spots (appear ~2 days before onset of rash as white spots with blue rings held within red spots in oral mucosa) Pharyngitis is usually mild without exudate Maculopapular rash onset 3–4 days after onset of symptoms, may coalesce to generalized erythema	Incubation period ~10–14 days with disease transmissible for ~1 week before onset of rash to ~2–3 weeks after rash appears Central nervous system and respiratory tract complications common. Permanent neurological impairment or death possible. Supportive treatment and intervention for complications Prevent by immunization
Hand-foot-and-mouth disease Agent: Coxsackievirus A16	Fever, malaise, sore mouth anorexia; 1–2 days later, lesions. Also can cause conjunctivitis, pharyngitis. Duration of disease 2–7 days	Transmission via oral-fecal or droplet. Highly contagious with incubation periods of 2–6 weeks. Supportive treatment
Fifth disease Agent: Human parvovirus B19	3–4 days of mild flu-like illness followed by 7–10 days of red rash that begins on face with slapped cheek appearance, spreads to trunk and extremities. Rash onset corresponds with disease immunity with patient. Viremic and contagious before but not after onset of rash	Droplet transmission. Leukopenia common. Risk of hydrops fetalis when contracted by woman during pregnancy. Supportive treatment
Infectious mononucleosis Agent: Epstein-Barr virus (human herpesvirus 4)	Rash: Maculopapular rash in ~20%, rare petechial rash. Fever, "shaggy" purple-white exudative pharyngitis, malaise, marked diffuse lymphadenopathy, hepatic and splenic tenderness and occasional enlargement.	Incubation period 20–50 days. >90% develop a rash if given amoxicillin or ampicillin. Potential for respiratory distress when enlarged tonsils and lymphoid tissue impinge on upper airway; using systemic corticosteroids may be helpful,

TABLE 15–7

Rash-Producing Febrile Illness—cont'd

Clinical Condition With Causative Agent	Presentation	Comments
	Diagnostic testing: Heterophil antibody test (Monospot). Leukopenia with lymphocytosis with atypical lymphocytes	although use is not strongly evidence based. Avoid contact sports for ≥1 mo because of risk of splenic rupture.
Acute HIV infection Agent: human immunodeficiency virus	Maculopapular rash, fever, mild pharyngitis, ulcerating oral lesions, diarrhea, diffuse lymphadenopathy	Most likely to occur in response to infection with large viral load. Consult with HIV specialist concerning initiation of antiretroviral therapy
Kawasaki disease Agent: Unknown	For acute phase illness (usually lasts ~11 days), fever ≥104°F lasting ≥5 days, polymorphous exanthem on trunk, flexor regions, and perineum, erythema of oral cavity ("strawberry tongue") with extensively chapped lips, bilateral conjunctivitis usually without eye discharge, cervical lymphadenopathy, edema and erythema of hands and feet with peeling skin (late finding, usually 1–2 weeks after onset of fever), no other illness accountable for findings	Usually in children age 1–8 yr. Treatment with IV immunoglobulin and PO aspirin during acute phase is associated with reduction in rate of coronary abnormalities such as coronary artery dilation and coronary aneurysm. Expert consultation and treatment advise about aspirin use and ongoing monitoring warranted

106. Celeste is a 9-year-old with moderate intermittent asthma. She is not using a prescribed inhaled corticosteroid but is using albuterol prn to relieve her cough and wheeze. According to her mother, she currently uses about six albuterol doses per day. You consider that:

   A. albuterol use can continue.
   B. excessive albuterol use is a risk factor for asthma death.
   C. she should also use salmeterol (Serevent) to reduce her albuterol use.
   D. theophylline should be added to her treatment plan.

107. In the treatment of asthma, leukotriene modifiers should be used as:

   A. long-acting bronchodilators.
   B. inflammatory inhibitors.
   C. rescue drugs.
   D. intervention in acute inflammation.

108. According to the National Asthma Education and Prevention Program Expert Panel Report 3 (NAEPP EPR-3) guidelines, which of the following is not a risk factor for asthma death?

   A. hospitalization or an emergency department visit for asthma in the past month
   B. current use of systemic corticosteroids or recent withdrawal from systemic corticosteroids
   C. difficulty perceiving airflow obstruction or its severity
   D. rural residence

109. A middle-school student presents, asking for a letter stating that he should not participate in gym class because he has asthma. The most appropriate response is to:

   A. write the note because gym class participation could trigger an asthma flare.
   B. excuse him from outdoor activities only to avoid pollen exposure.
   C. remind him that with appropriate asthma care, he should be capable of participating in gym class.
   D. excuse him from indoor activities only to avoid dust mite exposure.

110. After inhaled corticosteroid or leukotriene modifier therapy is initiated, clinical effects are seen:

    A. immediately.
    B. within the first week.
    C. in about 1 to 2 weeks.
    D. in about 1 to 2 months.

111. Compared with albuterol, levalbuterol (Xopenex):

    A. has a different mechanism of action.
    B. has the ability to provide greater bronchodilation with a lower dose.
    C. has an anti-inflammatory effect similar to an inhaled corticosteroid.
    D. is contraindicated for use in children.

112. In caring for a child with an acute asthma flare, the NP considers that, according to the NAEPP EPR-3 guidelines, antibiotic use is recommended:

    A. routinely.
    B. with evidence of infection.
    C. when asthma flares are frequent.
    D. with sputum production.

ANSWERS

102.	C	103.	C	104.	C
105.	C	106.	B	107.	B
108.	D	109.	C	110.	C
111.	B	112.	B		

DISCUSSION

Asthma is a common chronic disorder of the airways that is complex and characterized by variable and recurring symptoms, airflow obstruction, bronchial hyperresponsiveness, underlying inflammation, and a resulting decrease in the ratio of forced expiratory volume in 1 second to forced vital capacity. Although the condition ranks second after allergic rhinitis as the most common chronic respiratory disease in North America, many persons with asthma continue to be undiagnosed and are untreated.

The goals of asthma care according to the NAEPP EPR-3 are presented as follows, with a brief explanation of the rationale for each objective:

• Minimal or, ideally, no chronic symptoms such as cough and wheeze

Asthma symptoms typically follow a circadian rhythm in which bronchospasm is worse during the night sleep hours. A marker of effective airway inflammation control is minimal nocturnal symptoms. With young children, parents often report awakening to the child's repeated cough while the child continues to sleep. Conversely, asthma flares are often harder to control during the nighttime hours.

• Minimize emergency department or other emergency visits

When airway inflammatory control is poor, children with asthma typically use emergency services for treatment of frequent acute flares. With appropriate asthma family teaching to help with management of acute and chronic airway inflammation and its resulting symptoms, emergency visits can be minimized or eliminated.

• Minimal (ideally no) use of prn short-acting beta$_2$-agonist (no more than 1 or 2 days of beta$_2$-agonist use per week)

Asthma is a disease of airway inflammation with superimposed bronchospasm. The need for a short-acting beta$_2$-agonist as a rescue drug should be viewed as failure to provide adequate airway inflammatory control. Excessive beta$_2$-agonist use is a risk factor for asthma death.

• No limitations on activities, including physical activity

When airway inflammation is inadequate, asthma symptoms such as cough or wheeze can accompany or immediately follow physical activity. A child with well-controlled asthma should be able and encouraged to participate in fitness and leisure activities.

• Maintain normal or near-normal pulmonary function testing

With asthma treatment that focuses on the prevention of airway inflammation and bronchospasm, the PEF can be normal or near normal. The body's normal circadian rhythm provides a variation of awakening to late evening PEF of 10% to 15%. With asthma, this variation increases to more than 15%, reflecting the nocturnal bronchospasm that is a part of the disease. Usually a child younger than 4 or 5 has some difficulty with obtaining a peak flow.

• No or minimal side effects while optimal medications are given

Because of the wide range of asthma medications currently available, the NP, patient, and family can work together to find a lifestyle and treatment regimen that provides optimal care with minimal to few adverse medication effects.

• Prevent progressive loss of lung function

The formerly held concept in asthma was that no matter how severe the airway obstruction, the process was fully reversible. The newer disease model acknowledges that continued airway inflammation contributes to significant and potentially permanent airway remodeling and fixed obstruction. In addition, there is evidence that poorly controlled asthma can contribute to overall attenuated lung development in children.

The backbone of therapy for mild persistent, moderate persistent, or severe persistent asthma is the use of an inflammatory controller drug, such as an inhaled corticosteroid; additional options include mast cell stabilizers such as nedocromil or cromolyn and leukotriene modifiers such as montelukast or zafirlukast. Although all these products have anti-inflammatory capability, inhaled corticosteroids have proved to be the most effective in preventing airway inflammation and are recognized as the preferred asthma controller drug. Adding a leukotriene modifier to an inhaled corticosteroid or increasing the dosage of the inhaled corticosteroid also improves asthma outcome. The clinical effects of inhaled corticosteroid and leukotriene modifier take at least 1 to 2 weeks to be seen. Adding a long-acting beta$_2$-agonist such as salmeterol or formoterol is also an option when inhaled corticosteroid therapy is insufficient, but should be prescribed only with the understanding of the boxed warning related to the small but significant increased asthma death risk with use. Theophylline remains helpful in preventing bronchospasm; because it has a narrow therapeutic index, the theophylline dose must be closely titrated and monitored with serial serum drug levels, which significantly limit the drug's usefulness.

Rescue medications that relieve acute superimposed bronchospasm include short-acting beta$_2$-agonists, such as albuterol, levalbuterol, and pirbuterol. Compared with albuterol and pirbuterol, some of the therapeutic advantages of levalbuterol include greater bronchodilation with fewer side effects and at a lower dosage.

When acute asthma flare is present with increased symptoms and objective measurement of airflow obstruction, rapidly acting higher potency anti-inflammatory therapy with an oral corticosteroid is needed. Adding more bronchodilators, such as theophylline and salmeterol, does not reverse the cause of the bronchospasm, which is significant airway inflammation. Leukotriene modifiers are helpful in preventing, but not acutely treating, inflammation (Table 15–8 and Fig. 15–2).

Because asthma is a lower airway disease, a child with asthma has more of a problem with expiration, or getting air out, than with inspiration, or getting air in. This condition leads to findings characteristic of air trapping, such as decreased PEF rate, prolonged expiratory phase, thoracic hyperresonance on percussion, and hyperinflation seen on chest radiographs. Oxygen desaturation is a late finding in an acute asthma flare.

Discussion Source

National Asthma Education and Prevention Program, Expert Panel Report 3. http://www.nhlbi.nih.gov/guidelines/asthma/asthsumm.pdf, Guidelines for the diagnosis and management of asthma, accessed 10/4/09.

QUESTIONS

113. What advice should you give to a breastfeeding mother whose infant has gastroenteritis?

    A. Discontinue breastfeeding.
    B. Give the infant oral rehydration solution.
    C. Continue breastfeeding.
    D. Supplement with flat ginger ale.

114. What advice should you give to the parents of a toddler with gastroenteritis?

    A. Try sips of cola.
    B. Give the child sips of an oral rehydration solution.
    C. Give the child sips of Gatorade.
    D. Try sips of apple juice.

115. The onset of symptoms of food poisoning caused by *Staphylococcus* species is typically how many hours after the ingestion of the offending substance?

    A. 0.5 to 1
    B. 1 to 4
    C. 4 to 8
    D. 8 to 12

116. The onset of symptoms in food poisoning caused by *Salmonella* species is typically how many hours after the ingestion of the offending substance?

    A. 2 to 8
    B. 8 to 12
    C. 12 to more than 24
    D. 24 to 36

117. To obtain the most accurate hydration status in a child with acute gastroenteritis, the NP should ask about:

    A. the time of last urination.
    B. thirst.
    C. quantity of liquids taken.
    D. number of episodes of vomiting and diarrhea.

118. What percentage of body weight is typically lost in a child with moderate dehydration?

    A. 2% to 3%
    B. 3% to 5%
    C. 6% to 10%
    D. 11% to 15%

119. Clinical features of shigellosis include all of the following except:

    A. bloody diarrhea.
    B. high fever.
    C. malaise.
    D. vomiting.

ANSWERS

113.	C	**114.**	B	**115.**	B
116.	C	**117.**	A	**118.**	C
119.	D				

DISCUSSION

Acute gastroenteritis is a common episodic disease of childhood, usually viral in nature. A child presents with short-duration vomiting and diarrhea; the vomitus and stool are free of blood, and the stool is free of pus. In addition, the child usually does not have a fever. Given that these viral illnesses are highly contagious and easily transmitted person to person, usually there is a history of contacts with children or

TABLE 15–8

Pediatric Asthma Medications

Medication	Mechanism of Action	Indication	Comment
Inhaled corticosteroids	Inhibit eosinophilic action and other inflammatory mediators, potentate effects of beta$_2$-agonists	Controller drug, prevention of inflammation	Need consistent use to be helpful
Mast cell stabilizer Cromolyn sodium (Intal), nedocromil (Tilade)	Halts degradation of mast cells and release of histamine and other inflammatory mediators (mast cell stabilizer)	Controller drug, prevention of inflammation	• Need consistent use to be helpful • Less clinical effect compared with inhaled corticosteroids
Leukotriene modifier Leukotriene antagonists (montelukast [Singulair], zafirlukast [Accolate])	Inhibits action of inflammatory mediator, leukotriene, by blocking select receptor sites	Controller drug, prevention of inflammation	Likely less effective than inhaled corticosteroids. Particularly effective add-on medication when disease control inadequate with inhaled corticosteroid, when asthma complicated by allergic rhinitis
Oral corticosteroids	Inhibit eosinophilic action and other inflammatory mediators	Treatment of acute inflammation such as in asthma flare	• Indicated in treatment of acute asthma flare to reduce inflammation • In higher dose and with longer therapy (>2 weeks), adrenal suppression may occur • No taper needed if use is short-term (<10 days) and at lower dose • Potential for causing gastropathy, particularly gastric ulcer and gastritis
Beta$_2$-agonist Albuterol (Ventolin, Proventil), pirbuterol (Maxair), levalbuterol (Xopenex)	Bronchodilation via stimulation of beta-2 receptor site	Rescue drugs for treatment of acute bronchospasm	• Onset of action 15 min • Duration of action 4–6 hr
Long-acting beta$_2$-agonists (salmeterol [Serevent], formoterol [Foradil])	Beta$_2$-agonist; bronchodilation via stimulation of beta-2 receptor site	Prevention of bronchospasm	Salmeterol • Onset of action 1 hr • Duration of action 12 hr • Indicated for prevention rather than treatment of bronchospasm • Patient should also have short-acting beta$_2$-agonist as rescue drug Formoterol • Onset of action 15–30 hr • Duration of action 12 hr • Indicated for prevention rather than treatment of bronchospasm • Patient should also have short-acting beta$_2$-agonist as rescue drug

TABLE 15–8
Pediatric Asthma Medications—cont'd

Medication	Mechanism of Action	Indication	Comment
Anticholinergics (ipratropium bromide [Atrovent], tiotropium bromide [Spiriva])	Anticholinergic and muscarinic antagonist, yielding bronchodilation	Treatment and prevention of bronchospasm	• Onset of action ≥1 hr • Best used to avoid rather than treat bronchospasm associated with COPD and asthma • Well tolerated
Theophylline	Mild bronchodilator, helps with diaphragmatic contraction	Prevention of bronchospasm, mild anti-inflammatory	• Narrow therapeutic index drug with numerous drug interactions • Monitor carefully for toxicity by checking drug levels and clinical presentation

Stepwise Approach for Managing Asthma in Children Aged 0 to 4 years: NAEPP Guidelines

Moderate to Severe Persistent

Intermittent

Step 1
Preferred:
SABA prn

Mild Persistent

Step 2
Preferred:
Low-dose ICS

Alternative:
Montelukast or cromolyn

Step 3
Preferred:
Medium-dose ICS

Step 4
Preferred:
Medium-dose ICS
and either
montelukast or LABA

Step 5
Preferred:
High-dose ICS
and either
montelukast or LABA

Step 6
Preferred:
High-dose ICS
and either
montelukast or LABA
and
oral corticosteroids

ICS = Inhaled corticosteroids; LABA = long-acting β₂-agonist; SABA = short-acting β₂-agonist

Stepwise Approach for Managing Asthma in Children Aged 5 to 11 years: NAEPP Guidelines

Severe Persistent

Intermittent

Step 1
Preferred:
SABA prn

Mild Persistent

Step 2
Preferred:
Low-dose ICS

Alternative:
LTRA, cromolyn, nedocromil, or theophylline

Moderate Persistent

Step 3
Preferred:
Medium-dose ICS
or
Low-dose ICS
and either
LABA, LTRA, or theophylline

Step 4
Preferred:
Medium-dose ICS + LABA
Alternative:
Medium-dose ICS
and either
LTRA or theophylline

Step 5
Preferred:
High-dose ICS + LABA
Alternative:
High-dose ICS
and either
LTRA or theophylline

Step 6
Preferred:
High-dose ICS + LABA + oral corticosteroids
Alternative:
High-dose ICS
and either
LTRA or theophylline **and** oral corticosteroids

LTRA = leukotriene receptor antagonist

Figure 15–2 Stepwise approach for managing asthma in children 0–4 years old. (NAEPP Guidelines). *Available at http://www.nhlbi.nih.gov/guidelines/asthma/asthsumm.pdf. Accessed 12/28/09.*

adults who have similar symptoms. The duration of illness is usually short (< 4 days with no sequelae).

An important part of the assessment of a child with acute gastroenteritis is determining hydration status. Asking about the last urination is a helpful way of evaluating this. If the child has voided within the previous few hours, the degree of dehydration is minimal. Many other clinical parameters are helpful in assessing for dehydration (Table 15–9). Although mild dehydration can usually be managed with frequent small-volume feedings of commercially prepared oral rehydration solutions such as Pedialyte, a child with moderate to severe dehydration likely needs parenteral fluids in addition to small amounts of fluids orally as tolerated. Because of inappropriate glucose and electrolyte composition, sports drinks such as Gatorade and soda are inappropriate for rehydration. The use of antidiarrheal agents is usually discouraged because of the risk of increasing the severity of illness if toxin-producing bacteria are the causative agent.

Warning signs during acute gastroenteritis include fever coupled with bloody or pus-filled stools. If these are present, a bacterial source of infection such as shigellosis should be considered. Stool culture should be obtained, and appropriate antimicrobial therapy should be initiated.

Improperly handled food is a common source of the gastrointestinal infection commonly known as food poisoning. A child typically presents, often along with family members and caregivers who ate the same food, with a history of sudden onset of abdominal pain, nausea, and vomiting. Knowledge of the timing of the onset of symptoms is helpful when attempting to discern the offending organism. Most food poisoning episodes are short and self-limiting, resolving over a few hours to days without special intervention.

Discussion Sources

Diskin A. http://www.emedicine.com/emerg/topic213.htm, eMedicine: gastroenteritis, accessed 10/4/09.
Engel J. Abdomen. In: Engel J. *Pediatric Assessment.* 5th ed. St. Louis, MO: Mosby Elsevier; 2006.

QUESTIONS

120. The most common reason for precocious puberty in girls is:
   A. ovarian tumor.
   B. adrenal tumor.
   C. exogenous estrogen.
   D. early onset of normal puberty.

121. The most common reason for precocious puberty in boys is:
   A. testicular tumor.
   B. a select number of relatively uncommon health problems.
   C. exogenous testosterone.
   D. early onset of normal puberty.

122. Which of the following is noted in a child with premature thelarche?
   A. breast enlargement
   B. accelerated linear growth
   C. pubic hair
   D. body odor

123. Which of the following is noted in a child with premature adrenarche?
   A. breast development
   B. accelerated linear growth
   C. pubic hair
   D. menstruation

ANSWERS

120.	D	**121.**	B	**122.**	A
123.	C				

TABLE 15–9

Clinical Presentation of Child With Dehydration

Clinical Presentation	Mild Dehydration	Moderate Dehydration	Severe Dehydration
Skin turgor	Normal	Slightly to moderately decreased	Markedly decreased with tenting possible
Capillary refill	2 sec	2–4 sec	>4 sec
Tears	Normal to slightly decreased	Slightly decreased	Markedly decreased to absent
Pulse	Normal	Slightly increased	Tachycardia
Blood pressure	Normal	Normal	Low
Mucous membranes	Normal to slightly dry	Dry	Parched
Urine output	Mildly decreased	Decreased	Anuria

Source: Engel J. Abdomen. In: Engel J. *Pediatric Assessment.* 5th ed. St. Louis, MO: Mosby; 2006.

DISCUSSION

Precocious puberty in girls has long been defined as the onset of secondary sexual characteristics before the child's eighth birthday. More recent study reveals that there is likely a group of girls who have the onset of slowly developing secondary sexual characteristics between ages 6 and 8 years as a benign normal variant. Consequently, the most common reason for precocious puberty in girls is early onset of normal puberty. A subset of girls, particularly girls with pubertal changes noted before the sixth birthday, often have significant health problems, however, such as ovarian or adrenal tumors. Expert evaluation and referral is indicated in these children. Evaluation typically includes measuring bone age, level of follicle-stimulating hormone, and level of luteinizing hormone; abdominal ultrasound; and other studies warranted by clinical presentation. Treatment depends on the cause. In the absence of an adrenal or ovarian tumor or other secondary cause, counseling about the nature of the process of early puberty should be discussed with the child and family.

Because girls typically achieve nearly all of their adult height 1 year after the first menstrual period, a girl achieving menarche at a premature age often has short stature. If the child and family wish to attempt to halt the onset of puberty, a gonadotropin-releasing hormone analogue can be given by injection to counteract the effects of endogenous hormones. Study is ongoing on the long-term effect of this therapy on the child's health.

Premature thelarche is a relatively common, benign process in which breast development is noted in female toddlers. Usually present unilaterally or bilaterally, the child has no other signs of puberty including accelerated linear growth. Reassurance and ongoing monitoring are the typical course of treatment. In premature adrenarche, a parent usually reports that a child 5 to 6 years old has body odor, pubic hair, and, rarely, axillary hair. There are no other signs of puberty, including accelerated linear growth. Reassurance and ongoing monitoring constitute the typical course of treatment.

In boys, precocious puberty is defined as the onset of secondary sexual characteristics before the ninth birthday. Overall, this condition is less common in boys than in girls and is unlikely to be a benign normal variation. Gonadal and adrenal tumors and a select number of genetically based diseases are the most likely causes. Prompt referral to expert care is indicated.

Discussion Source

Kaplowitz P. http://www.emedicine.com/ped/TOPIC1882.HTM, eMedicine: precocious puberty, accessed 10/4/09.

QUESTIONS

124. An innocent murmur has which of the following characteristics?
    A. occurs late in systole
    B. has localized area of auscultation
    C. becomes softer when the patient moves from supine to standing position
    D. frequently obliterates the second heart sound (S_2)

125. The murmur of atrial septal defect is usually:
    A. found in children with symptoms of cardiac disease.
    B. first found on a 2- to 6-month well-baby examination.
    C. found with mitral valve prolapse.
    D. presystolic in timing.

126. A Still murmur:
    A. is heard in the presence of cardiac pathology.
    B. has a humming or vibratory quality.
    C. is a reason for denying sports participation clearance.
    D. can become louder when the patient is standing.

ANSWERS

124. C   125. B   126. B

DISCUSSION

The ability to assess appropriately children with a heart murmur is an important part of the role of an NP. Knowledge of the most common murmurs, the clinical presentation of the murmurs, and the impact on a child's health is critical to appropriate assessment. It is also necessary to be able to determine the need for specialty referral (Table 15–10).

QUESTIONS

127. When assessing a febrile child, the NP considers that:
    A. even minor temperature elevation is potentially harmful.
    B. nuchal rigidity is usually not found in early childhood meningitis.
    C. fever-related seizures usually occur at the peak of the temperature.
    D. most children with temperatures of 38.3°C to 40°C (101°F to 104°F) have a potentially serious bacterial infection.

TABLE 15–10

Differential Diagnosis of Common Heart Murmurs in Children

When evaluating a child with cardiac murmur:

- Ask about major symptoms of heart disease: chest pain, congestive heart failure symptoms, palpitations, syncope, activity intolerance, poor growth and development
- The bell of the stethoscope is most helpful for auscultating lower pitched sounds, and the diaphragm is better for higher pitched sounds
- Systolic murmurs are graded on a 1-to-6 scale, from barely audible to audible with stethoscope off the chest. Diastolic murmurs are usually graded on the same scale, but abbreviated to grades 1 to 4 because these murmurs are not loud enough to reach grades 5 and 6.
- A critical part of the evaluation of a child with a heart murmur is the decision to offer antimicrobial prophylaxis. No prophylaxis is needed with benign murmurs. Refer to the American Heart Association's Guidelines for the latest advice

Murmur	Important Cardiac Examination Findings	Additional Findings	Comments
Newborn	Grade 1–2/6 early systolic, vibratory, heard best at left lower sternal border (LLSB) with little radiation Pulses intact, otherwise well neonate	Subsides or disappears when pressure applied to abdomen	Heard in first few days of life; disappears in 2–3 weeks Benign condition
Still (vibratory innocent murmur)	Grade 1–3/6 early systolic ejection, musical or vibratory, short, often buzzing, heard best midway between apex and LLSB	Softens or disappears when sitting, standing, or with Valsalva maneuver Louder when supine or with fever or tachycardia	Usual onset age 2–6 y.o.; may persist through adolescence Benign condition
Hemic	Grade 1–2/6 systolic ejection, high-pitched, heard best in pulmonic and aortic areas	Heard only in presence of increased cardiac output, such as fever, anemia, stress	Disappears when underlying condition resolves Usually seen without cardiac disease Most often heard in children and younger adults with thin chest walls
Venous hum	Grade 1–2/6 continuous musical hum heard best at upper right sternal border (URSB) and upper left sternal border (ULS) and the lower neck	Disappears in supine position, when jugular vein is compressed Common after 3 y.o.	Believed to be produced by turbulence in subclavian and jugular veins Benign condition
Pulmonary outflow ejection murmur	Grade 1–2/6 soft, short, systolic ejection murmur, heard best at LLSB, usually localized	Softens or disappears when sitting, standing, or with Valsalva maneuver Louder when supine	Heard throughout childhood Benign condition but has qualities similar to murmurs caused by pathological condition such as atrial septal defect (ASD), coarctation of the aorta (COA), pulmonic stenosis (PS)
Patent ductus arteriosus	Grade 2–4/6 continuous murmur heard best at ULSB and left infraclavicular area	In premature newborns, seen with active precordium. In older children, seen with full pulses	Normal ductus closure occurs by day 4 of life Often isolated finding but may be seen with COA, ventricular septal defect (VSD) Accounts for ±12% of all congenital heart disease Twice as common in girls In preterm infants <1500 g, rate 20%–60%

TABLE 15–10

Differential Diagnosis of Common Heart Murmurs in Children—cont'd

Murmur	Important Cardiac Examination Findings	Additional Findings	Comments
Atrial septal defect	Grade 1–3/6 systolic ejection murmur heard best at ULSB with widely split fixed S_2	Accompanying mid-diastolic murmur heard at fourth intercostal space (ICS) left sternal border (LSB) commonly caused by increased flow across tricuspid valve	Two times as common in girls Child may be entirely well or present with heart failure Often missed in the first few months of life or even entire childhood Watch for children with easy fatigability Cyanosis rare
Ventricular septal defect	Grade 2–5/6 regurgitant systolic murmur heard best at LLSB Occasionally holosystolic, usually localized	Thrill may be present and a loud P_2 with large left-to-right shunt	Usually without cyanosis Children with small- to moderate-sized left-to-right shunt without pulmonary hypertension likely to have minimal symptoms Larger shunts may result in CHF with onset in infancy
Aortic stenosis	Grade 2–5/6 systolic ejection murmur heard best in upper left sternal border (ULSB) or a second right ICS, possibly with paradoxically split S_2	Ejection click at apex, third left ICS, second right ICS Radiation or thrill to the carotid arteries	More common in boys than girls In children, usually caused by unicuspid (if noted in infancy) or bicuspid (if noted in childhood) valve Mild exercise intolerance common
Coarctation of aorta (COA)	Grade 1–5/6 systolic ejection murmur heard best at ULSB and left interscapular area (on back)	Weak or absent femoral pulses, hypertension in arms	Often seen with aortic stenosis (AS), mitral regurgitation (MR) Presence of dorsalis pedis pulse in child essentially rules out this condition
Mitral valve prolapse	Grade 1–3/6 mid-systolic click followed by late systolic murmur heard best at the apex	Murmur heard earlier in systole and often louder with standing or squatting	Often with pectus excavatum, straight back (>85%)
Pulmonic valve stenosis	Grade 2–5/6 heard best at ULSB, ejection click at second left ICS	Radiates to back S_2 may be widely split	No symptoms with mild to moderate disease Usually a fusion of valvular cusps

Source: Park M. *Pediatric Cardiology for Practitioners*. 5th ed. St. Louis, MO: Mosby; 2007.

128. Which of the following is not seen during body temperature increase found in fever?

    A. lower rate of viral replication
    B. toxic effect on select bacteria
    C. negative effect on *S. pneumoniae* growth
    D. increased rate of atypical pneumonia pathogen replication

129. When providing care for a febrile patient, the NP bears in mind that all of the following are true except that:

    A. the use of antipyretics has been associated with prolonged illness.
    B. antipyretics shorten the course of viral and bacterial illness.
    C. fever increases metabolic demand.
    D. in a pregnant woman, increased body temperature is a potential first-trimester teratogen.

130. Concerning the use of antipyretics in a febrile young child, which of the following statements is true?

    A. A child with a serious bacterial infection does not have fever reduction with an antipyretic.
    B. The degree of temperature reduction in response to antipyretic therapy is not predictive of presence or absence of bacteremia.
    C. Compared with ibuprofen, acetaminophen is more effective in reducing higher fevers.
    D. Ibuprofen should not be used if a child is also taking a macrolide.

131. When evaluating a child who has bacterial meningitis, the NP expects to find cerebrospinal fluid (CSF) results of:

    A. low protein.
    B. predominance of lymphocytes.
    C. glucose at about 30% of serum levels.
    D. low opening pressure.

132. When evaluating a child who has aseptic or viral meningitis, the NP expects to find CSF results of:

    A. low protein.
    B. predominance of lymphocytes.
    C. glucose at about 30% of serum levels.
    D. low opening pressure.

133. Sepsis is defined as the:

    A. clinical manifestation of systemic infection.
    B. presence of bacteria in the blood.
    C. circulation of pathogens.
    D. allergenic response to infection.

134. Gina is 2 years old and presents with a 3-day history of fever, crankiness, and congested cough. Her respiratory rate is more than 50% of the upper limits of normal for age. Tubular breath sounds are noted at the right lung base. Skin turgor is normal, and she is wearing a wet diaper. She is alert, is resisting the examination as age appropriate, and engages in eye contact. Temperature is 38.3°C (101°F). Gina's diagnostic evaluation should include:

    A. chest x-ray.
    B. urine culture and sensitivity measurement.
    C. lumbar puncture.
    D. sputum culture.

135. As part of the evaluation in a febrile 3-year-old boy, the following WBC count with differential is obtained:
WBCs 22,100/mm³
Neutrophils 75% (normal 40% to 70%) with toxic granulation
Bands 15% (normal 0% to 4%)
Lymphocytes 4% (normal 30% to 40%)
These results increase the likelihood that the cause of this child's infection is:

    A. viral.
    B. parasitic.
    C. fungal.
    D. bacterial.

136. As part of the evaluation in a febrile 18-month-old girl, the following WBC count with differential is obtained:
WBCs 6100/mm³
Neutrophils 35% (normal 40% to 70%)
Bands 3% (normal 0% to 4%)
Lymphocytes 52% (normal 30% to 40%)
Reactive lymphocytes 10%
These results increase the likelihood that the cause of this child's infection is:

    A. viral.
    B. parasitic.
    C. fungal.
    D. bacterial.

137. Which of the following is the most appropriate way of relieving discomfort in a child with varicella?

    A. ibuprofen
    B. aspirin
    C. acetaminophen
    D. alcohol rub

138. Which of the following is the most effective way to reduce fever in an 18-month-old with a temperature of 39.7°C (103.5°F) and AOM?

    A. ibuprofen

    B. aspirin

    C. acetaminophen

    D. cool water bath

139. Which of the following medications can be given at the onset of a febrile illness to minimize the risk of recurrence in a child with a history of febrile seizure?

    A. ibuprofen

    B. phenytoin

    C. phenobarbital

    D. diazepam

ANSWERS

127.	B	**128.**	D	**129.**	B
130.	B	**131.**	C	**132.**	B
133.	A	**134.**	A	**135.**	D
136.	A	**137.**	C	**138.**	A
139.	D				

DISCUSSION

Most young children with an acute febrile illness do not have a serious bacterial infection and recover fully without sequelae. Historically, about 4% of febrile young children with no obvious source of infection have serious sequelae, however, including death; the risk of serious illness in the presence of fever is now significantly reduced in the advent of immunization against *H. influenzae* type B and *S. pneumoniae*. Nonetheless, the evaluation and treatment of a febrile child are an important part of providing pediatric health care.

Fever is a complex physiological reaction that occurs when exogenous pyrogens (microorganisms and their products, drugs, incompatible blood products) are introduced to the body. This triggers the production of endogenous pyrogens (polypeptides produced by host cells such as monocytes, macrophages, interleukin-1α, interferon-α, interferon-β, tumor necrosis factor), which increase prostaglandin synthesis. Prostaglandins activate thermoregulatory neurons and alter the hypothalamic set-point. Vasomotor center reactions increase heat conservation and heat production.

Although parents and health-care providers usually treat fever with antipyretics and other options, an increase in body temperature has benefits. During fever, viral replication rate is reduced. Increased body temperature is toxic to encapsulated bacteria, particularly *S. pneumoniae*. In animal models and clinical trials in humans, the presence of fever has been associated with improvement in the morbidity and mortality associated with infectious diseases. The use of antipyretics including acetaminophen and ibuprofen has also been associated with prolonged illness. Conversely, a child with fever is often uncomfortable and cranky, which reinforces the perception that this is a condition that warrants treatment. Fever also increases metabolic demands, a potential problem in a child or adult with a chronic health problem; in pregnancy, fever is potentially teratogenic in the first trimester and increases metabolic demands throughout pregnancy.

Fear of febrile seizure also contributes to the propensity to treat fever aggressively, with the thought that if the body temperature is reduced, seizure risk is reduced. A simple febrile seizure actually is most likely to occur as fever is increasing rather than at its peak. A familial tendency has been noted with febrile seizure, but the condition is not predictive of the development of epilepsy. A simple febrile seizure is a benign and common event in children 6 months to 5 years old; a child who has had one seizure is at increased risk for a recurrence. Although there are effective therapies, which need to be daily, that reduce risk and could prevent the occurrence of additional simple febrile seizures, including phenobarbital and phenytoin (Dilantin), the potential adverse effects of these therapies outweigh the potential benefit in this self-limiting condition. In situations in which parental anxiety about febrile seizures is severe, intermittent oral diazepam (Valium) at the onset of febrile illness can be effective in preventing recurrence. Although use of antipyretics may improve the comfort of the child, these agents do not prevent febrile seizures.

In the first 2 years of life, most children average four to six acute febrile episodes per year, with health care sought in about two-thirds of cases. Of these younger children with temperatures less than 39°C (<102.2°F), 80% to 90% have a viral or obvious bacterial source, and 10% to 20% have no obvious source for fever. The most common causes of fever in young children are viruses and bacteria, with fungi, parasites, neoplasms, collagen vascular disease, and factitious disease being important, but less common. Before pneumococcal conjugate vaccine (PCV7 [Prevnar]) was available, *S. pneumoniae* was implicated in approximately 90% of cases of occult bacteremia in febrile infants and young children. This vaccine provides activity against the seven most common pneumococcal serotypes implicated in invasive pneumococcal disease and dramatically reduces, but does not eliminate, the risk of invasive pneumococcal disease.

In a previously well, nontoxic febrile child 3 months to 3 years old without identifiable source of fever and temperature less than 39°C (<102.2°F), the evaluation for the source of fever should start with a careful history and physical examination. If the child is alert and has a nontoxic appearance, no tests or antibiotics are usually needed. The child's caregivers should be advised about the appropriate use of antipyretics, increased fluid intake, and signs of deteriorating condition. Follow-up in 48 hours is prudent if fever persists; follow-up should be sooner if the child's condition worsens.

Advising the child's caregivers about the appropriate choice and use of antipyretics is an important part of providing care for a child with non–life-threatening illness and fever. As previously mentioned, fever plays an important role in controlling infection. If a child with fever appears fairly comfortable, no treatment is needed. Even a cranky child usually is not harmed and may be helped by allowing the fever to run its course. If the child is uncomfortable with fever, commonsense measures include dressing the child lightly and increasing fluid intake. A cooling bath should not be used because the resulting shivering would drive up body temperature.

The choice of an antipyretic is dictated by numerous factors, including the length of time for onset of action of the product (ideally, less than half an hour) and the duration of action (ideally, 4 to 8 hours), with no or few major reported adverse effects. Ibuprofen and acetaminophen are the most commonly prescribed antipyretics; both have onset of action within half an hour of the dose. The duration of action of acetaminophen is about 4 hours, whereas the duration of ibuprofen is around 6 hours. The antipyretic potential of acetaminophen is equal to that of ibuprofen for lower grade fevers ($<39°C$ [$<102.5°F$]); with fever greater than this level, ibuprofen has greater antipyretic potential. Acetaminophen has an excellent gastrointestinal adverse event profile, but can be hepatotoxic with excessive use and high dose. Ibuprofen is usually well tolerated, but does have the potential to cause gastric ulcer and gastritis, albeit usually with long-term high-dose use. Aspirin should not be prescribed to a child with a febrile illness because of its association with Reye syndrome. Ibuprofen should not be prescribed for varicella because its use is implicated in necrotizing fasciitis.

A young child with high fever ($≥40.9°C$ [$≥105.6°F$]) is three times more likely to be bacteremic than a child with a temperature equal to or less than $39°C$ ($≤102.5°F$). The degree of temperature reduction in response to antipyretic therapy is not predictive of presence or absence of bacteremia. In one major study, among infants with bacteremia, but without meningitis, differences from nonbacteremic children were detected in clinical appearance before fever reduction, but not after defervescence. All children with meningitis appeared seriously ill before and after defervescence.

When sepsis is suspected, a septic work-up should be initiated (Table 15–11). Empirical antimicrobial therapy with ceftriaxone, usually at a dose of 50 mg/kg IM up to a maximum dose of 1 g, every 24 hours, with supportive care is prudent, pending the outcome of evaluation. The child can be managed at home if the following conditions are met: The child is intact neurologically, adequate hydration can be maintained via the oral route, the caregiver is willing and able to provide the needed close attention to the child, and follow-up and emergency care are easily accessible.

A total WBC count with differential is obtained as part of the evaluation of a child with suspected sepsis. The most typical WBC pattern found in severe bacterial infection is the "left shift." A "left shift" is usually seen in the presence of

TABLE 15–11

Evaluation of Young Child With Suspected Sepsis

Evaluation	Rationale
Complete blood count with white blood cell differential	Identify viral versus bacterial shifts, general leukocytic response
Blood culture	Potentially identify causative organism in sepsis
Urinalysis and urine culture via transurethral catheter or suprapubic tap	Evaluate for urinary tract infection including pyelonephritis, particularly important in child <2 y.o.
Lumbar puncture with cerebrospinal fluid analysis	Evaluate for bacterial or viral meningitis, particularly important if alterations in neurological examination
Chest x-ray	Rule in or out pneumonia or other respiratory tract condition that can contribute to sepsis, particularly important if dyspnea, tachypnea, decreased breath sounds, WBC >20,000 mm^3, or other findings suggestive of lower respiratory tract infection
Stool culture, fecal WBC count	Only if diarrhea present, to evaluate for possible focus of infection

Source: Egland A. http://www.emedicine.com/PED/topic2698.htm, eMedicine: Fever in the young infant, accessed 10/6/09.

severe bacterial infection, such as appendicitis and pneumonia. The following is typically noted:

- Leukocytosis: An elevation in the total WBC count.
- Neutrophilia: An elevation in the number of neutrophils in circulation, defined as more than 10,000 neutrophils/mm³. Neutrophils are also known as polys or segs, both referring to the polymorph shape of the segmented nucleus of this WBC.
- Bandemia: An elevation in the number of bands or young neutrophils in circulation. Usually, less than 4% of the total WBCs in circulation are bands. When this percentage is exceeded, and the absolute band counts exceed 500/mm³, bandemia is present. This finding indicates that the body has called up as many mature neutrophils that were available in storage pool and is now accessing less mature forms. Bandemia reinforces further the potential seriousness of the infection.
- Toxic granulation: Often reported on WBC morphologic study.

Other neutrophil forms do not belong in circulation even with severe infection; these include myelocytes and metamyelocytes, immature neutrophil forms that are typically found in granulopoiesis pool. The presence of these cells in the circulation is an ominous marker for life-threatening bacterial infection.

In viral infection, the total WBC count can be elevated, but is often normal or slightly depressed (leukopenia). Lymphocytes, the leukocytes most active in viral infection, predominate. Atypical or reactive lymphocytes are often reported on WBC morphology.

To eliminate or support the diagnosis of meningitis, lumbar puncture with cerebrospinal fluid (CSF) evaluation should be part of the evaluation of a febrile younger child who has an altered neurological examination. Pleocytosis, defined as a CSF WBC count of more than 5 cells/mm³, is an expected finding in meningitis caused by bacterial, viral, tubercular, fungal, or protozoan infection. An elevated CSF opening pressure is also a nearly universal finding. Typical CSF response in bacterial meningitis includes a median WBC count of 1200 cells/mm³ with 90% to 95% neutrophils; additional findings are a reduction in CSF glucose below the normal level of about 60% of the plasma level and an elevated CSF protein level. CSF results in viral or aseptic meningitis include normal glucose level, normal to slightly elevated protein level, and lymphocytosis. Further testing to ascertain the causative organism is warranted.

Treatment of a child with meningitis includes supportive care and use of the appropriate anti-infective agent. Acyclovir is an option in aseptic meningitis, pending identification of the offending virus. Ceftriaxone with vancomycin is usually the treatment of choice in suspected bacterial meningitis, pending bacterial sensitivity results. Treatment of other forms of sepsis in a younger child depends on its cause. Prudent practitioners should seek expert help in evaluating and treating a child with suspected or documented sepsis.

Discussion Sources

Graneto J. http://www.emedicine.com/EMERG/topic377.htm, eMedicine: pediatrics, fever, accessed 10/6/09.
Tejani N. http://www.emedicine.com/EMERG/topic376.htm, eMedicine: febrile seizures, accessed 10/6/09.

QUESTIONS

140. When treating a 3-year-old well child with community-acquired pneumonia (CAP), the NP realizes that the most likely causative pathogen is:
    A. *Mycoplasma pneumoniae.*
    B. a respiratory virus.
    C. *H. influenzae.*
    D. *S. pneumoniae.*

141. Which of the following is the most appropriate antimicrobial for treatment of CAP in a 2-year-old who is clinically stable and able to be treated in the outpatient setting?
    A. azithromycin
    B. doxycycline
    C. TMP-SMX
    D. levofloxacin

142. Which of the following is most likely to be noted in a 3-year-old with CAP?
    A. complaint of pleuritic chest pain
    B. sputum production
    C. report of dyspnea
    D. tachypnea

143. What percentage of children have an episode of pneumonia by age 5?
    A. less than 10%
    B. about 10%
    C. about 20%
    D. about 30%

144. Which of the following antimicrobials provides effective activity against atypical pathogens?
    A. amoxicillin
    B. cefprozil
    C. ceftriaxone
    D. clarithromycin

ANSWERS

140.　B　　　　141.　A　　　　142.　D
143.　C　　　　144.　D

DISCUSSION

Pneumonia is the most common cause of death from infectious disease and the eighth leading cause of overall mortality in the United States. Although pneumonia is often considered to be a disease primarily of older adults and chronically ill individuals, about 20% of children develop pneumonia by age 5 years. Most often caused by bacteria or viruses, pneumonia is an acute lower respiratory tract infection involving lung parenchyma, interstitial tissues, and alveolar spaces. The term community-acquired pneumonia (CAP) is used to describe the onset of the disease in an individual who resides within the community, not in a nursing home or other care facility, with no recent (within 2 weeks) hospitalization.

Most children with pneumonia present with cough. Tachypnea is the most sensitive, although not specific, finding. In particular, the diagnosis of lower respiratory tract disease should be considered with a respiratory rate exceeding 50/min in children younger than 1 year and a rate exceeding 40/min in children older than 1 year. Pulse oximetry is also informative, but less so than respiratory rate. Compared with an adult with pneumonia, a child is less likely to complain of dyspnea, produce sputum, or report pleuritic chest pain. Diagnostic evaluation of a child with CAP usually includes a chest x-ray; further evaluation for invasive disease (sepsis) should be dictated by clinical presentation.

Although numerous organisms are implicated in CAP in children, few are seen with significant frequency. Respiratory viruses are the causes in most; *S. pneumoniae* and the atypical pathogens including *M. pneumoniae* and *C. pneumoniae* are also implicated. As with adults with CAP, sputum specimens are usually unobtainable and the results are unreliable in children with CAP; the choice of an antimicrobial is largely empirically based.

Successful community-based care of a child with CAP requires many factors. The child must have intact gastrointestinal function and be able to take and tolerate oral medications and adequate amounts of fluids. A competent caregiver must be available. Also, the child should be able to return for follow-up examination and evaluation.

As previously mentioned and consistent with CAP treatment in adults, antimicrobial therapy in children with pneumonia is chosen empirically. In adequate dosages, amoxicillin or a cephalosporin provides activity against *S. pneumoniae,* but is ineffective against the atypical pathogens. A macrolide such as azithromycin or clarithromycin provides activity against nonresistant *S. pneumoniae* and the atypical pathogens. Treatment failure is possible when a macrolide is used and drug-resistant *S. pneumoniae* is the causative organism, in which case ceftriaxone, vancomycin, or linezolide can be used. Although respiratory fluoroquinolones such as levofloxacin and moxifloxacin are effective in the presence of drug-resistant *S. pneumoniae,* these products are not labeled for use in children younger than 18 years. Although tetracyclines including doxycycline are used in treating CAP in adults, these medications should not be

prescribed to children younger than 11 years because of the risk of tooth staining. Because most childhood CAP is viral in origin, watchful waiting can also be used, whereby the child is not placed on an antimicrobial regimen, but rather is observed to see whether the illness improves over a few days.

NPs are ideally positioned to help minimize risk for pneumonia through immunization and hygienic measures. Nearly two-thirds of all fatal pneumonia is caused by *S. pneumoniae,* the pneumococcal organism. Pneumococcal conjugate vaccine is recommended for all children, starting in infancy to minimize the risk of invasive pneumococcal disease. The use of influenza vaccine can help minimize the risk of postinfluenza pneumonia. Ensuring adequate ventilation, reinforcing cough hygiene, and proper hand washing can help minimize pneumonia risk.

Discussion Sources

Gilbert D, Moerlling R, Eliopoulos G, Chambers H, Saag M. *The Sanford Guide to Antimicrobial Therapy*. 39th ed. Sperryville, VA: Antimicrobial Therapy, Inc; 2009:35–36.

Ostapchuk M, Roberts D, Haddy R. http://www.aafp.org/afp/20040901/899.html, Community-acquired pneumonia in infants and children, American Family Physician, 2004, accessed 10/6/09.

QUESTIONS

145. Sam is a 4-year-old boy who presents with a 1-week history of intermittent fever, rash, and "watery red eyes." Clinical presentation is of an alert child who is cooperative with examination but irritable, with temperature of 37°C, pulse rate of 132 bpm, and respiratory rate of 38/min. Physical examination findings include nasal crusting; dry, erythematous, cracked lips; red, enlarged tonsils without exudate; and elevated tongue papillae. The diagnosis of Kawasaki disease is being considered. Additional findings are likely to include:

    A. vesicular-form rash.
    B. exudative conjunctivitis.
    C. peeling hands.
    D. occipital lymphadenopathy.

146. Laboratory findings in Kawasaki disease include all of the following except:

    A. sterile pyuria.
    B. elevated liver enzyme levels.
    C. blood cultures positive for offending bacterial pathogen.
    D. elevated erythrocyte sedimentation rate.

147. Long-term consequences of Kawasaki disease include:

    A. renal insufficiency.
    B. coronary artery obstruction.
    C. hepatic failure.
    D. hypothyroidism.

148. The cause of Kawasaki disease is:

    A. fungal.

    B. viral.

    C. bacterial.

    D. unknown.

149. An important part of the treatment of Kawasaki disease includes:

    A. antibiotics.

    B. antivirals.

    C. immune globulin.

    D. antifungals.

ANSWERS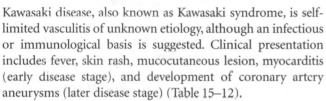

145.	C	146.	C	147.	B
148.	D	149.	C		

DISCUSSION

Kawasaki disease, also known as Kawasaki syndrome, is self-limited vasculitis of unknown etiology, although an infectious or immunological basis is suggested. Clinical presentation includes fever, skin rash, mucocutaneous lesion, myocarditis (early disease stage), and development of coronary artery aneurysms (later disease stage) (Table 15–12).

Occurring primarily in the late winter and spring at 3-year intervals, Kawasaki disease now surpasses rheumatic fever as the leading cause of acquired heart disease in the United States among children younger than 5 years. The development of coronary artery aneurysms can lead to coronary artery obstruction, myocarditis, heart failure, pericarditis, mitral or aortic insufficiency, and dysrhythmias. Risk of aneurysm is increased in patients who have fever for more than 16 days, have recurrence of fever after an afebrile period of at least 48 hours, are male, are younger than 1 year, and have cardiomegaly at the time of diagnosis. Some patients who do not fulfill the criteria for Kawasaki disease have been diagnosed as having "incomplete" or "atypical" Kawasaki disease, a diagnosis that often is based on echocardiographic findings of coronary artery abnormalities.

Although no specific laboratory test for Kawasaki disease exists, the presence of certain laboratory findings can support the diagnosis when coupled with clinical presentation. In the acute stage (days 1 to 11), leukocytosis with a left shift and elevated erythrocyte sedimentation rate are found; both are neither sensitive nor specific for the condition. Blood and urine cultures fail to identify an offending organism. In the subacute stage (days 11 to 21), the platelet count is often markedly elevated, with a measurement of more than 1 million/mm³ being common. These values begin to normalize

TABLE 15–12

Diagnostic Criteria for Kawasaki Disease

- Fever ≥5 days in duration, usually abrupt in onset, symptoms with no response to antibiotic therapy, if given, usually with irritability out of proportion to degree of fever or other signs
- In addition to fever of at least 5 days' duration, ≥4 of the following should be present:
  - Changes in extremities (erythema, edema, desquamation), usually with discomfort so that child may refuse to bear weight
  - Desquamation of fingers and toes begins in the periungual region, may also involve the palms and soles, usually noted at 1–2 weeks after onset of fever
  - Bilateral, nonexudative conjunctivitis
  - Polymorphous rash
  - Cervical lymphadenopathy
  - Changes in lips and oral cavity (pharyngeal edema, dry/fissured or swollen lips, strawberry tongue)

Note: If fever is present with fewer than four of the above symptoms, the diagnosis is established with echocardiogram to evaluate the coronary arteries to support or exclude the disease.

during the convalescent stage (days 21 to 60), but may not reach baseline values for 8 weeks.

During the acute stage of Kawasaki disease, or if the diagnosis is in question, an echocardiogram should be obtained. The study should be repeated in the second or third week of disease and repeated 1 month after laboratory tests have resolved. Treatment of Kawasaki disease includes consultation with experts in managing this condition and the use of immune globulin and aspirin. Confirmation of the diagnosis and treatment are likely to involve consultation with a specialist in this disease. Long-term prognosis is generally related to the degree of permanent cardiac involvement.

Discussion Source

American Heart Association. http://www.americanheart.org/presenter.jhtml?identifier=3004559, Diagnosis, treatment, and long-term management of Kawasaki disease, 2004, accessed 10.9.09.

QUESTIONS

150. A young child should use a rear-facing car seat until at least age _____ and weight of _____.

    A. 6 months, 15 lb

    B. 9 months, 18 lb

    C. 12 months, 20 lb

    D. 15 months, 25 lb

151. You anticipate that adult car seat belts fit correctly when a child is approximately _____ tall and is _____ old.

  A. 51 inches, 6 to 8 years
  B. 53 inches, 5 to 7 years
  C. 57 inches, 8 to 12 years
  D. 59 inches, 12 to 14 years

152. In general, children should ride in the back seat of the car until age:

  A. 10 years.
  B. 11 years.
  C. 12 years.
  D. 13 years.

ANSWERS

150. C   **151.** C   **152.** D

DISCUSSION

Knowledge of appropriate child car seat restraint is an important part of providing pediatric primary care (Table 15–13).

TABLE 15–13
Types of Car Safety Seats

Age	Type of Seat	General Guideline
Infants	Infant-only and rear-facing convertible	All infants should always ride rear-facing until they are at least 1 y.o. and weigh at least 20 lb
Toddlers and preschoolers	Convertible, combination, and forward-facing	Children 1 y.o. and weighing at least 20 lb can ride forward-facing. It is best to ride rear-facing as long as possible
School-aged children	Booster	Booster seats are for older children who have outgrown their forward-facing car safety seats. Children should stay in a booster seat until the adult seat belts fit correctly (usually when a child reaches about 4 feet 9 inches in height and is 8–12 y.o.)
Older children	Seat belts	Children who have outgrown their booster seats should ride in a lap and shoulder belt; they should ride in the back seat until 13 y.o.

Source: Car safety seats: a parents' guide, www.aap.org/family/Carseatguide.htm, accessed 10/6/09.

16
Childbearing

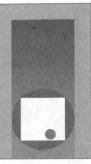

QUESTIONS

1. to 4. Match the stage of pregnancy with the appropriate term.

____ **1.** Fertilization ovum	**A.** Embryo
____ **2.** Up to 2 weeks postconception	**B.** Fetus
____ **3.** 8 to 12 weeks	**C.** Blastocyst
____ **4.** 13 weeks to term	**D.** Zygote

ANSWERS

1. D	**2.** C	**3.** A	**4.** B

DISCUSSION

Knowledge of appropriate terminology is a critical component to providing prenatal care
(Table 16–1).

QUESTIONS

5 to 10. Match uterine size with stage of pregnancy.

____ **5.** Nongravid	**A.** Size of a baseball
____ **6.** 8 weeks	**B.** Softball or grapefruit
____ **7.** 10 weeks	**C.** Size of a large lemon
____ **8.** 12 weeks	**D.** Size of a tennis ball or orange
____ **9.** 16 weeks	**E.** Uterine fundus at umbilicus
____ **10.** 20 weeks	**F.** Uterine fundus halfway between symphysis pubis and umbilicus

ANSWERS

5. C	**6.** D	**7.** A
8. B	**9.** F	**10.** E

See full color images of this topic on DavisPlus at http://davisplus.fadavis.com | Keyword: Fitzgerald

TABLE 16–1

Stages of Human Pregnancy

Period	Stage
At fertilization	Zygote
Up to 2 weeks	Blastocyst
2–8 weeks	Embryo
8–12 weeks to term	Fetus
Born before 37 weeks	Preterm infant
Born at 37–42 weeks	Term infant
Born after 42 weeks	Post-term infant

DISCUSSION

Knowledge of normal pregnancy development is a critical component to providing prenatal care (Table 16–2).

QUESTIONS

11. Approximately ___% of fetuses are in vertex position by the 36th week of pregnancy.
    A. 30
    B. 50
    C. 75
    D. 95

12. Recommended weight gain during pregnancy for a woman with a desirable or healthy body mass index (BMI) is:
    A. 15 to 20 lb
    B. 20 to 30 lb
    C. 25 to 35 lb
    D. 35 to 45 lb

13. For a healthy woman with a desirable or healthy prepregnancy BMI, daily caloric requirements during pregnancy are typical baseline caloric needs plus ___ kcal.
    A. 100
    B. 300
    C. 600
    D. 1000

14. For a healthy woman with a healthy or desirable prepregnancy BMI, daily caloric requirements during lactation are typical baseline caloric needs plus ___ kcal.
    A. 250
    B. 500
    C. 750
    D. 1000

TABLE 16–2

Uterine Size During Pregnancy

Stage of Pregnancy	Uterine Size	Comment
Nongravid	Lemon	Mobile, firm, nontender
8 weeks	Tennis ball or orange	Hegar's sign (softening of uterine isthmus), Goodell's sign (softening of vaginal portion of the cervix), and Chadwick's sign (blue-violet vaginal color) often present by this time
10 weeks	Baseball	First fetal heart tone via abdominal Doppler at 10–12 weeks
12 weeks	Softball or grapefruit	Rising above symphysis pubis, uterine fundus palpable through abdominal wall
16 weeks	Halfway between symphysis pubis and umbilicus	Quickening first noted in woman who has been pregnant before (≥2nd trimester) during 16–17 weeks, at ~18 weeks with first pregnancy
20–36 weeks	~1 cm gain in fundal height per week	Uterine fundus at the umbilicus at 20 weeks. Usually concordant with gestational age, ±1 cm
At term	Uterus dips into pelvis with fetal head engagement, fundal height decreases	Vertex position (cephalic) in 95% by 36 weeks

Source: McFee J. Comprehensive prenatal care. In: Bader T, ed. *OB/GYN Secrets*. Philadelphia, PA: Elsevier; 2005.

15. Recommended calcium intake for a woman during pregnancy is _____ mg of elemental calcium per day.
    A. 500 to 750
    B. 750 to 1000
    C. 1000 to 1200
    D. 1200 to 1500

16. Increased folic acid intake before conception is likely to reduce the risk of which of the following birth defects?

    A. congenital cataract
    B. pyloric stenosis
    C. clubfoot
    D. open neural tube defect

17. Maternal iron requirements are greatest during what part of pregnancy?

    A. first trimester
    B. second and third trimesters
    C. equal throughout pregnancy
    D. preconception

18. The most common form of acquired anemia during pregnancy is:

    A. iron deficiency.
    B. folate deficiency.
    C. vitamin B_{12} deficiency.
    D. hypoproliferative.

19. Concerning the use of alcohol during pregnancy, which of the following statements is most accurate?

    A. Although potentially problematic, maternal alcohol intake does not increase the risk of miscarriage.
    B. Risk to the fetus from alcohol exposure is greatest in the third trimester.
    C. No level or time of exposure is considered to be safe.
    D. Risk of fetal alcohol syndrome is present only if alcohol exposure has occurred throughout the pregnancy.

20. Pica (ingestion of nonfood substances) during pregnancy should be considered:

    A. a harmless practice common in certain ethnic groups.
    B. problematic only if more nutritious food sources are left out of the diet and replaced by the nonfood substance.
    C. a way of providing select micronutrients not usually found in food products.
    D. potentially dangerous because of contaminants in the nonfood substance.

21. Examples of neural tube defects include all of the following except:

    A. anencephaly.
    B. spina bifida.
    C. encephalocele.
    D. omphalocele.

ANSWERS

11.	D	12.	C	13.	B
14.	B	15.	D	16.	D
17.	B	18.	A	19.	C
20.	D	21.	D		

DISCUSSION

The clinician should have knowledge of nutritional requirements during pregnancy to provide appropriate counseling. Folic acid deficiency is a teratogenic state, leading to an increased risk of neural tube defects (NTDs) and other defects in the developing pregnancy. NTDs are common serious fetal malformations in North America, second only to cardiac defects, with an incidence of 1.2 for every 1000 births. Examples of NTDs include anencephaly, spina bifida, and encephalocele. Correcting folic acid deficiency before pregnancy by increased dietary and supplement intake dramatically reduces this risk, and continuing this increased intake throughout pregnancy minimizes the mother's risk of developing folate deficiency anemia. Dietary-associated folic acid deficiency is rare unless severe malnutrition is present. A genetic contribution to NTDs is likely and is thought to be the result of a complex interaction of environment and heredity. As a result, if a woman has carried a pregnancy with an NTD, or there is a family history of NTD, recommended folic acid intake increases to 4 mg/d 1 month before pregnancy and during the first 3 months of gestation. Most prescription prenatal multivitamins contain 1 mg of folic acid.

Increased calcium intake is important to the development of bone and teeth; the required amount can usually be met by ensuring three to four servings of high-quality dairy products per day. Examples of a single dairy serving include 8 oz of milk, 1 oz of cheese, 1 cup of yogurt, or 1 cup of calcium-fortified juice. Although dietary sources of calcium are best, supplementation is sometimes required if a woman is lactose intolerant or is otherwise unable to meet these goals.

Maternal iron requirements increase in the second and third trimesters of pregnancy, in part because of the fetus's need for building iron stores. Iron deficiency is the most common form of anemia during pregnancy, with most cases occurring because the woman enters pregnancy with iron deficiency, rather than developing this problem because of increased iron requirements. Pregnancy-related iron requirements, given in terms of elemental iron, are as follows: in the absence of iron deficiency, 30 mg/d; with iron deficiency or in a multiple-gestation pregnancy, 60 to 100 mg/d; and with iron deficiency anemia, 200 mg/d. A 325-mg ferrous sulfate tablet contains 65 mg of elemental iron, whereas most prescription prenatal vitamins contain 30 to 65 mg.

Fetal alcohol syndrome (FAS) has most often been noted in the offspring of women who drank heavily throughout pregnancy. More commonly, infants whose mothers drink lightly or moderately are born with lesser degrees of alcohol-related problems. Given that FAS is the leading preventable cause of developmental disability and can be eliminated by avoiding alcohol consumption throughout pregnancy, no level of maternal alcohol intake during pregnancy is deemed safe. Maternal alcohol intake also increases the risk of miscarriage. Less is known about fetal risks when exposure occurs to other recreational drugs, such as marijuana, a substance often considered more benign and "natural" compared with alcohol. A safe level of maternal ingestion during pregnancy for marijuana and other intoxicating substances has not been established, and abstinence should be encouraged.

Pica is the ingestion of nonfood substances, such as clay, cornstarch, laundry starch, dry milk of magnesia, paraffin, coffee grounds, or ice. Although usually noted to be more common in select ethnic groups, pica is found in all socioeconomic groups. Certain pica habits are likely harmless, such as sucking on ice chips, and do little to replace intake of more nutritious substances. Most other pica forms contain potential risk, however, because nonfood substances are taken in preferably over more nutritious food sources. With the ingestion of clay, starches, and paraffin, there is risk of constipation, bowel obstruction, and nutritional deficiency. In particular, many common pica substances can be contaminated with heavy metals such as lead or mercury and other industrial pollutants that are particularly toxic to the mother and the developing fetus. The issue of pica should be raised with all pregnant women. Some women believe that pica is normal, or are encouraged to eat substances such as clay by well-meaning friends and family members as a way of relieving tension. Advice should be given recognizing this, but inform the woman about the potential risks of pica.

Discussion Sources

March of Dimes. http://www.marchofdimes.com/pnhec/159.asp, Pregnancy and Newborn Health Education Center, accessed 10/9/09.

National Clinical Clearinghouse. http://www.guideline.gov/summary/summary.aspx?doc_id=9789&nbr=5242&ss=6&xl=999, Routine prenatal and postnatal care, 2006, accessed 10/9/09.

QUESTIONS

22. to 34. Identify the following changes in a normal pregnancy as true (normal, anticipated finding) or false (not associated with normal pregnancy)

____ **22.** Blood volume increases by 40% to 50%, peaking at week 32.

____ **23.** Decrease in diastolic blood pressure most notable during second trimester.

____ **24.** S_1 heart sound becomes louder.

____ **25.** Physiologic systolic ejection murmur usually evident.

____ **26.** Dilation of renal collecting system.

____ **27.** Physiologic glucosuria and proteinuria common.

____ **28.** Decrease in transverse thoracic diameter and diaphragmatic contraction.

____ **29.** Lower esophageal sphincter more relaxed.

____ **30.** Increased intestinal motility.

____ **31.** Gallbladder doubles in size.

____ **32.** Insulin levels increase by 2-fold to 10-fold over prepregnancy levels.

____ **33.** Fasting plasma glucose increases slightly.

____ **34.** Thyroid decreases in size.

ANSWERS

22. True	**23.** True	**24.** True
25. True	**26.** True	**27.** True
28. False	**29.** True	**30.** False
31. True	**32.** True	**33.** False
34. False		

DISCUSSION

A woman's body changes dramatically throughout pregnancy. Knowledge of these normal physiological changes in pregnancy is crucial to providing safe and competent prenatal care (Table 16–3).

Discussion Source

Brown KP. Antenatal care. In: *Management Guidelines for Nurse Practitioners Working with Women*. 2nd ed. Philadelphia, PA: FA Davis; 2004:177–223.

QUESTIONS

35. The recommended frequency of prenatal visits in weeks 28 to 32 of pregnancy is every:

   A. 1 week.
   B. 2 weeks.
   C. 3 weeks.
   D. 4 weeks.

36. Testing for sexually transmitted infection should be initially obtained:

   A. as early as possible in pregnancy.
   B. during the second trimester.
   C. during the third trimester.
   D. as close to anticipated date of birth as possible.

TABLE 16–3
Physiological Adaptations During Pregnancy

Body Area	Physiological Adaptation
Uterus	Increases from ~10-mL capacity and 70-g weight prepregnancy to 5000-mL capacity and 1100-g weight at term. The uterine isthmus becomes soft and compressible (Hegar's sign)
Cervix	Color and texture change, becoming cyanotic (Chadwick's sign) and less firm (Goodell's sign)
Skin	Striae (stretch marks) in ~50%, melasma (pregnancy mask), linea nigra (hyperpigmented line on abdomen) appears or darkens as melanocytes are stimulated
Breast	Nipples and areolae darken and increase in size. Venous congestion noted. Breast tissue becomes more nodular because of proliferation of lactiferous glands
Blood	Blood volume increases by 40%–50%, peaking at week 32. Even with red blood cell production increase by 33%, but results in dilutional physiological anemia of pregnancy
Cardiovascular	Decrease in systolic blood pressure throughout pregnancy, with decrease in diastolic blood pressure most notable during second trimester. Cardiac output dependent on maternal position, with a noted decrease if in supine position because of reduced venous return caused by vena cava compression to an increase of 30%–50% with lateral recumbent position. S_1 heart sound becomes louder, physiological systolic ejection murmur usually evident. Heart is displaced, resulting in a left axis deviation
Renal	Increased renal blood flow, glomerular filtration rate, and dilation of renal collecting system. Physiologic glucosuria and proteinuria occur partly because of increase in glomerular filtration rate and resulting inability of renal tubules to reabsorb glucose and protein
Respiratory	Partly because of increased abdominal content, there is an increase in transverse thoracic diameter and diaphragmatic contraction, and costal angle widens. Tidal volume increases with reduced residual volume in later pregnancy
Digestive	Lower esophageal sphincter more relaxed while corresponding pressures increase, resulting in increased esophageal reflux. Decreased stomach and intestinal motility, allowing for greater nutrient absorption, but increased risk for constipation. (Increased progesterone levels influence aforementioned changes.) Gallbladder doubles in size with more dilute bile and less soluble cholesterol, increasing risk of stones
Metabolic/endocrine	Insulin levels increase by 2-fold to 10-fold over prepregnancy levels. Fasting plasma glucose decreases slightly. Thyroid and pituitary increase in size. Maternal weight changes account for weight gain in the first half of pregnancy, whereas uterine contents account for most weight gain in second half

Source: Brown KP. Antenatal care. In: *Management Guidelines for Nurse Practitioners Working with Women.* 2nd ed. Philadelphia, PA: FA Davis Co; 2004:177–223.

37. The "quad screen" should be obtained at about _____ weeks of pregnancy.
    A. 6 to 10
    B. 11 to 15
    C. 16 to 20
    D. 21 to 25

38. The "quad screen" is used to help detect increased risk for which of the following conditions in the fetus?
    A. trisomy 21 and open neural tube defects
    B. cystic fibrosis and Down syndrome
    C. Tay-Sachs disease and trisomy 18
    D. sickle cell anemia and beta-thalassemia major

39. Tina is a 26-year-old woman who is pregnant and has an abnormal "quad screen." When sharing this information with Tina, you consider that:
    A. this testing is diagnostic of specific conditions.
    B. further testing is recommended.
    C. the testing should be repeated.
    D. no further testing is required.

40. The rate of spontaneous fetal loss related to amniocentesis is approximately 1 in _____ procedures
    A. 75
    B. 200
    C. 300
    D. 500

41. All of the following can cause an elevated maternal alpha-fetoprotein (AFP) except:
    A. underestimated gestational age.
    B. open neural tube defect.
    C. meningomyelocele.
    D. Down syndrome.

42. Edwards syndrome is the clinical manifestation of trisomy ____.
    A. 13
    B. 15
    C. 18
    D. 21

43. In Edwards syndrome, which of the following statements is true?
    A. Edwards syndrome is more common than Down syndrome.
    B. Most affected infants die during the first year of life.
    C. Edwards syndrome is unlikely to cause developmental disability.
    D. Edwards syndrome is associated with elevated AFP.

44. In Down syndrome, which of the following is true?
    A. Most infants affected with Down syndrome are born to women older than age 35 years.
    B. Down syndrome is noted in about 1 in 10,000 live births.
    C. Down syndrome is associated with decreased maternal serum AFP level.
    D. Antenatal serum analysis is sufficient to make the diagnosis.

45. Down syndrome is the clinical manifestation of trisomy ____.
    A. 13
    B. 15
    C. 18
    D. 21

46. Components of the antenatal screening test known as the "quad screen" include all of the following except:
    A. AFP.
    B. hCG.
    C. unconjugated estriol.
    D. progesterone.

47. Elevated inhibin-A is noted when a pregnant woman is at increased risk of having an infant with:
    A. Down syndrome.
    B. Edwards syndrome.
    C. open neural tube defect.
    D. hemolytic anemia.

48. A 25-year-old woman presents in the 10th week of gestation requesting antenatal screening for Down syndrome. What advice should the NP give?
    A. Because of her age, no specific testing is recommended.
    B. She should be referred for second-trimester ultrasound.
    C. Screening that combines nuchal translucency measurement and biochemical testing is recommended.
    D. She should be referred to a genetic counselor.

49. To 51. Match the following at-risk ethnic groups for the following genetically based conditions.

____ 49. Tay-Sachs Disease   A. Ashkenazi Jewish ancestry

____ 50. Cystic Fibrosis   B. Northern European ancestry

____ 51. Sickle Cell Trait   C. African ancestry

ANSWERS

35.	B	36.	A	37.	C
38.	A	39.	B	40.	B
41.	D	42.	C	43.	B
44.	C	45.	D	46.	D
47.	A	48.	C	49.	A
50.	B	51.	C		

DISCUSSION

Numerous recommendations exist regarding frequency of prenatal care and associated laboratory and other testing (Tables 15–4, 15–5, and 15–6). These are simply guidelines for the care that is needed for a well woman with a pregnancy with low physiological and psychosocial risk. More frequent visits and testing are often indicated, but a minimum of 8 to 10 visits should be scheduled.

TABLE 16–4

Frequency of Prenatal Visits

Time in Pregnancy	Frequency of Visits
Up to 28 weeks	Every 4 weeks
28–36 weeks	Every 2 weeks
≥36 weeks	Every week

Source: National Guideline Clearinghouse: Routine prenatal care. Available at http://www.guideline.gov/summary/summary. aspx?doc_id=13010&nbr=6704&ss=6&xl=999, Accessed 12.28.09.

TABLE 16–5

Prenatal Care First Visit, Early in Pregnancy

Pap smear	Rubella, varicella, rubeola status if not previously known	Sexually transmitted infection screenings First trimester Down syndrome screening gonorrhea/chlamydia
CBC	Blood type, antibody screen	
Mantoux tuberculin skin test	Genetic screening as previously described if not previously obtained	Chorionic villus sampling as appropriate, requested (10–12 weeks)
HBsAg	Urinalysis, urine culture and sensitivity (treat asymptomatic bacteriuria)	Amniocentesis as appropriate, requested (15–18 weeks)

Source: National Guideline Clearinghouse: Routine prenatal care. Available at http://www.guideline.gov/summary/summary. aspx?doc_id=13010&nbr=6704&ss=6&xl=999. Accessed 12/28/09.
Source: Evidence-Based Prenatal Care. www.aafp.org/afp/20050401/1307.html, Part I: General prenatal care and counseling issues. Accessed 12/28/09.
Source: Evidence-Based Prenatal Care. www.aafp.org/afp/20050415/1555.html, Part II: Third-trimester care and prevention of infectious diseases. Accessed 12/28/09.

Prenatal screening and diagnostic procedures constitute an important clinical issue, although one that is often confusing, emotionally charged, and marked by disagreement among providers and patients. One point of confusion is the difference between screening and diagnostic tests. Commonly offered prenatal tests include maternal serum analysis for alpha-fetoprotein (AFP), human chorionic gonadotropin (hCG), inhibin-A, and unconjugated estriol levels, also known as the "quad (quadruple) screen." When the amounts of these substances are analyzed, increased risk of open neural tube defects (NTDs), trisomy 21 (Down syndrome), and trisomy 18 (Edwards syndrome) can be detected. An abnormal "quad screen" result is not diagnostic of any condition, however, and further testing is recommended including amniocentesis and level II ultrasound. Consultation with a perinatology specialist is also indicated.

Down syndrome is associated with developmental disability and an increased risk for cardiac and gastrointestinal malformation and early-onset Alzheimer disease. The risk of Down syndrome is approximately 1 in 1000 live births, with this number increasing to 1 in 270 in women 35 to 40 years old, and 1 in 100 in women older than 40 years; increased maternal age is a well-known risk factor for Down syndrome and other genetically based congenital anomalies. Although historically only pregnant women who would be 35 or older at the time of childbirth were offered the opportunity for prenatal diagnosis with amniocentesis or chorionic villus sampling, newer recommendations advise that all pregnant women, regardless of age, be offered the option of antenatal diagnostic testing, including evaluation for Down

TABLE 16–6

Prenatal Care Later in Pregnancy

Time of Testing	Test
16–20 weeks	"Quad marker/screen," ultrasound (little evidence of improved pregnancy outcomes with routine obstetric ultrasound in low physiological risk pregnancy)
24–28 weeks	1-hr glucose load to screen for gestational diabetes mellitus, Rh negative type and screen
28–32 weeks	Hg, STI testing as indicated (VDRL, HIV, HBsAg, gonorrhea, chlamydia), RhoGAM as indicated
32–36 weeks	Fetal presentation, kick count (fetal movements ≥4 in 1 hr, ≥10 in 2 hr)
35–37 weeks	Group B streptococcus culture (rectal and vaginal): Treat intrapartum with appropriate antibiotic to reduce risk of neonatal infection
40–42 weeks	Vaginal examination to assess cervical ripeness, fetal station (little evidence that results are predictive of labor onset)
≥41 weeks	Nonstress test, biophysical profile to check fetal status Biophysical profile consists of five components: fetal breathing movements, gross body movements, tone, amniotic fluid index, and nonstress test. Each component is scored as either 0 or 2, with a maximum score of 10

Source: National Guideline Clearinghouse: Routine prenatal care. Available at http://www.guideline.gov/summary/summary.aspx?doc_id= 13010&nbr=6704&ss=6&xl=999. Accessed 12/28/09.
Source: Evidence-Based Prenatal Care. www.aafp.org/afp/20050401/1307.html, Part I: General prenatal care and counseling issues.
Source: Evidence-Based Prenatal Care. www.aafp.org/afp/20050415/1555.html, Part II: Third-trimester care and prevention of infectious diseases, accessed 12.28.09.

syndrome. One of the factors leading to this recommendation is the finding that approximately 75% of all infants with Down syndrome are born to mothers younger than age 35. This finding is in part due to women in this age group being more likely to give birth compared with older women and to the lower rate of antenatal diagnostic testing such as amniocentesis being performed in younger women giving birth.

Edwards syndrome is much less common than Down syndrome, occurring in 1 in every 6000 births. Edwards syndrome is associated with low birth weight; developmental disability; and cranial, cardiac, and renal malformations. The complexity and severity of these problems are such that most affected infants die within the first year of life.

NTDs are second only to cardiac defects in frequency, with an incidence of NTDs of 1.2 for every 1000 births. Open NTDs such as meningomyelocele, anencephaly, and spina bifida carry risk of significant disability and the potential for shortened life span.

Alpha-fetoprotein is synthesized in the fetal yolk sac, gastrointestinal tract, and liver. Maternal levels can be elevated for many reasons, including an open NTD such as meningomyelocele, anencephaly, or spina bifida; fetal nephrosis; cystic hygroma; fetal gastrointestinal obstruction; omphalocele; intrauterine growth restriction; multiple fetuses; or fetal demise. Underestimated gestational age can also lead to a misinterpreted test because maternal AFP is higher in earlier pregnancy. The placenta, from precursors provided by the fetal adrenal glands, and the liver produces unconjugated estriol; maternal levels are decreased in trisomy 21 and trisomy 18. hCG is produced by trophoblast shortly after implantation into the uterine wall, with levels increasing rapidly in the first 8 weeks of pregnancy then steadily decreasing until week 20 when levels plateau. An increased hCG level appears to be a relatively sensitive marker for detecting trisomy 21, whereas a low hCG level is associated with trisomy 18. The hCG levels are typically normal in the presence of NTDs. Inhibin-A is a hormone produced by the placenta; levels of hCG and inhibin-A are higher than normal when a woman has an increased risk of carrying a fetus with Down syndrome. Lower than normal levels of estriol can also indicate that a woman is at high risk for carrying a fetus with Down syndrome

Interpreting the results of a "quad screen" requires knowledge of numerous factors, including the risk of false-positive and false-negative results, the significance of the results, and the woman's individual risk of having an affected pregnancy. In addition, all antenatal testing must be offered to a woman in a manner that allows her to make an informed decision to have or decline the test. Part of informed consent includes the information that the "quad screen" is simply that, a screening test that identifies higher risk situations, but is not diagnostic for the condition. With abnormal results, further testing is indicated; results that are normal do not ensure that no problem will occur with the pregnancy, but the risk is minimized.

As previously mentioned, if a "quad screen" yields abnormal results, further testing is indicated. For the detection of a genetic abnormality such as trisomy 18 or 21, the most commonly used test is amniocentesis, a procedure that carries a rate of spontaneous fetal loss of about 1 in every 200 procedures; the overall pregnancy loss after chorionic villi sampling is higher at approximately 3%. If a woman chooses not to have invasive testing, noninvasive follow-up evaluation after an abnormal "quad screen" often includes a level II ultrasound, a high-resolution study that can reveal fetal abnormalities such as an open NTD or increased nuchal folds and other anomalies often found in Down syndrome. Ultrasound can assist with diagnosis, but does not take the place of genetically based studies. When first-trimester testing is desired, screening using nuchal translucency as detected by ultrasound and serological testing for decreased pregnancy-associated plasma protein-A and increased free beta-hCG is effective in the general population and is more effective than nuchal translucency alone. Women found to be at increased risk of having an infant with Down syndrome with first-trimester screening should be offered genetic counseling and the option of chorionic villi sampling or mid-trimester amniocentesis.

Discussion Sources

American College of Obstetrics and Gynecology. Practice Bulletin #77: screening for fetal chromosomal abnormalities. *Obstet Gynecol.* 2007;109:217–228.

American Pregnancy Association. http://www.americanpregnancy. org/prenataltesting/cvs.html, Chronic villi sampling (CVS), accessed 10/8/09.

American Pregnancy Association. http://www.americanpregnancy. org/prenataltesting/quadscreen.html, Quad screen, accessed 10/8/09.

March of Dimes. http://www.marchofdimes.com/professionals/ 14332_1164.asp, Quick fact sheet: amniocentesis, accessed 10/8/09.

National Guideline Clearinghouse. http://www.guideline.gov/ summary/summary.aspx?doc_id=9789&nbr=5242&ss=6&xl=9 99, Routine prenatal and postnatal care, accessed 10/8/09.

QUESTIONS

52. Medications most commonly pass through the placenta via:

  A. facilitated transport.

  B. passive diffusion.

  C. capillary pump action.

  D. mechanical carrier state.

53. A drug with demonstrated safety for use in all trimesters of pregnancy is categorized as U.S. Food and Drug Administration (FDA) risk category:

  A. A.

  B. B.

  C. C.

  D. D.

54. A drug shown to cause teratogenic effects in human study, but the benefit of which could outweigh risk of use in a life-threatening situation, is assigned FDA risk category:
   A. A.
   B. B.
   C. C.
   D. D.

55. A drug that has not been shown to be harmful to the fetus in animal studies, but for which no human study is available is assigned FDA risk category:
   A. A.
   B. B.
   C. C.
   D. D.

56. A drug shown to cause teratogenic effect in animal studies, but for which no human study is available is assigned FDA risk category:
   A. A.
   B. B.
   C. C.
   D. D.

57. When treating a woman with a urinary tract infection who is 28 weeks pregnant, the NP prescribes:
   A. TMP-SMX.
   B. cefixime.
   C. ciprofloxacin.
   D. doxycycline.

58. According to Hale's Lactation Risk Category, a medication in which there is no controlled study on its use during lactation, or controlled study shows minimal, non–life-threatening risk, is listed as category:
   A. L2.
   B. L3.
   C. L4.
   D. L5.

59. According to Hale's Lactation Risk Category, a medication in which there is evidence of risk for its use in lactation, but it may be used if there is a maternal life-threatening situation, is listed as category:
   A. L2.
   B. L3.
   C. L4.
   D. L5.

60. In a pregnant woman with asthma, in what part of her pregnancy do symptoms and bronchospasm worsen?
   A. 6 to 14 weeks
   B. 15 to 23 weeks
   C. 24 to 33 weeks
   D. 29 to 36 weeks

61. In treating a pregnant woman with acute bacterial rhinosinusitis, the NP would likely avoid prescribing:
   A. amoxicillin.
   B. cefuroxime.
   C. azithromycin.
   D. levofloxacin.

62. The duration of antimicrobial therapy for treatment of urinary tract infection in a pregnant woman is:
   A. 3 days.
   B. 5 days.
   C. 7 days.
   D. 10 days.

63. Selective serotonin reuptake inhibitor (SSRI) withdrawal syndrome is best characterized as:
   A. bothersome but not life-threatening.
   B. potentially life-threatening.
   C. most often seen with medications with a longer half-life.
   D. associated with seizure risk.

64. The placenta is best described as:
   A. poorly permeable.
   B. an effective drug barrier.
   C. best able to transport lipophilic substances.
   D. capable of impeding substances with molecular weight equal to or less than 300 g/mol.

65. Preferred treatment options for a pregnant woman in the second trimester with migraine include:
   A. sumatriptan.
   B. codeine.
   C. aspirin.
   D. ibuprofen.

66. In counseling women about SSRI use during pregnancy, the NP considers that study reveals:
   A. a teratogenic pattern has been identified.
   B. the drugs have a negative effect on intellectual development.
   C. the use of paroxetine during pregnancy is associated with an increase in risk for congenital cardiac defect.
   D. increased rate of seizure disorder in exposed offspring.

67. Which SSRI has the longest half-life?
   A. paroxetine
   B. fluoxetine
   C. citalopram
   D. sertraline

68. Among the most commonly used medications by women in the first trimester of pregnancy are:

- **A.** antiepileptic drugs.
- **B.** antibiotics.
- **C.** antihypertensives.
- **D.** opioids.

69. Benzodiazepine withdrawal syndrome is best characterized as:

- **A.** bothersome but not life-threatening.
- **B.** not observed during pregnancy.
- **C.** most often seen with agents that have a long half-life.
- **D.** associated with seizure risk.

70. The cornerstone controller therapy for chronic persistent asthma during pregnancy is the use of:

- **A.** oral theophylline.
- **B.** mast cell stabilizers.
- **C.** short-acting beta$_2$-agonists.
- **D.** inhaled corticosteroids.

71. You examine a 24-year-old woman who is 24 weeks pregnant and has an acute asthma flare. Her medication regimen should be adjusted to include:

- **A.** theophylline.
- **B.** salmeterol (Serevent).
- **C.** prednisone.
- **D.** montelukast (Singulair).

72. For a pregnant woman with asthma, bronchospasm symptoms are often reported to improve usually during _____weeks of gestation.

- **A.** 8 to 13
- **B.** 20 to 26
- **C.** 29 to 36
- **D.** 36 to 40

73. Most SSRIs are FDA pregnancy risk category:

- **A.** B.
- **B.** C.
- **C.** D.
- **D.** X.

74. The benzodiazepines are FDA pregnancy risk category:

- **A.** B.
- **B.** C.
- **C.** D.
- **D.** X.

75. Bupropion is FDA pregnancy risk category:

- **A.** B.
- **B.** C.
- **C.** D.
- **D.** X.

76. Most tricyclic antidepressants are FDA pregnancy risk category:

- **A.** B.
- **B.** C.
- **C.** D.
- **D.** X.

77. An example of an antimicrobial that is FDA pregnancy risk category B is:

- **A.** clarithromycin.
- **B.** doxycycline.
- **C.** erythromycin.
- **D.** ofloxacin.

78. An antimicrobial that is FDA pregnancy risk category D is:

- **A.** amoxicillin.
- **B.** levofloxacin.
- **C.** tetracycline.
- **D.** TMP-SMX.

79. The penicillins are ranked as FDA pregnancy risk category:

- **A.** B.
- **B.** C.
- **C.** D.
- **D.** X.

80. All of the following uropathogens are capable of reducing urinary nitrates to nitrites except:

- **A.** *Escherichia coli.*
- **B.** *Proteus* species.
- **C.** *Klebsiella pneumoniae.*
- **D.** *Staphylococcus saprophyticus.*

81. Which of the following is FDA pregnancy risk category B until the 36th week of pregnancy?

- **A.** gentamicin
- **B.** nitrofurantoin
- **C.** clarithromycin
- **D.** ciprofloxacin

82. In a pregnant woman, asymptomatic bacteruria:

- **A.** should be treated only if bladder instrumentation or surgery is planned.
- **B.** needs to be treated to avoid complicated urinary tract infection (UTI).
- **C.** is a common, benign finding.
- **D.** is a risk factor for the development of hypertension.

83. Which of the following is the most common UTI organism in pregnant women?

- **A.** *Pseudomonas aeruginosa*
- **B.** *E. coli*
- **C.** *K. pneumoniae*
- **D.** *Proteus mirabilis*

84. Recommended length of antimicrobial therapy for a pregnant woman with asymptomatic bacteruria is:

   A. 1 to 3 days.
   B. 3 to 7 days.
   C. 8 to 10 days.
   D. 2 weeks.

ANSWERS

52.	B	53.	A	54.	D
55.	B	56.	C	57.	B
58.	B	59.	C	60.	D
61.	D	62.	C	63.	A
64.	C	65.	D	66.	C
67.	B	68.	B	69.	D
70.	D	71.	C	72.	D
73.	B	74.	C	75.	B
76.	D	77.	C	78.	C
79.	A	80.	D	81.	B
82.	B	83.	B	84.	B

DISCUSSION

Most women use more than three over-the-counter and prescription medications during the first trimester of pregnancy, but only about 40% of women report use of these drugs to their health-care provider. Certain medications are potentially teratogenic, or capable of inducing birth defects, and should be avoided or used with great caution during pregnancy. By definition, a teratogenic drug is a substance that has the potential to create a characteristic set of malformations in the fetus. The classic teratogenic period occurs in a specific time of fetal development, usually between day 31 and day 81 following the last menstrual period (LMP) when organogenesis is occurring. For a teratogen to exert its effect, the product must be taken at the point in the pregnancy when the affected organ system is developing. Lithium can cause a characteristic teratogenic cardiac defect when taken as the cardiac tube is forming; taken earlier or later in the organ development process, the drug likely has no effect on the heart. Fetal liver maturity also plays a role because 40% to 60% of fetal blood circulation goes through the liver. With increasing maturity, the fetus's hepatic enzymes become more capable of metabolizing drugs.

Before day 31 post-LMP, the pregnancy exists as a group of poorly differentiated cells with no discrete organ systems to damage. A teratogen could be taken at that point and no damage would result because there are no organ systems to disrupt. After day 81 post-LMP, the organs are formed, but still growing and developing. The likelihood of a substance exerting a teratogenic effect decreases.

Many factors influence drug transfer across the placenta, including the molecular weight of the substance, lipid solubility, and duration of exposure. Medications usually pass by passive diffusion, where the maternal drug level is greater than that of the fetus; more drug is passed when maternal levels are greatest. The degree of diffusion is influenced by many factors besides maternal drug levels including the drug's molecular weight and degree of lipophilicity. Drugs with a low molecular weight (<500 g/mol) cross the placental barrier more easily than drugs with a molecular weight greater than 500 g/mol, whereas drugs with a molecular weight greater than 1000 g/mol cross the placenta infrequently. The lower the molecular weight, the greater the potential for passage of the drug through the placenta. Alcohol and cocaine have low molecular weights (<100 g/mol) and are easily passed. Insulin and heparin (molecular weight >5000 g/mol) are examples of drugs that are poorly transported to the fetus and can be given with relative safety in pregnancy. Most oral over-the-counter and prescription medications have molecular weights of less than 500 g/mol and pass easily through the placenta. The placenta preferentially allows highly lipophilic drugs to pass through.

Not all drugs with the same therapeutic endpoint have the same lipid solubility. Diphenhydramine (Benadryl) is a highly lipophilic antihistamine and penetrates the placenta and maternal central nervous system easily, causing sedation. In contrast, loratadine (Claritin) is more hydrophilic and has fewer fetal or maternal effects. Drugs with a long half-life or with extended-release formulations are usually held in maternal circulation for protracted periods and have the potential to have a greater effect on the fetus than similar drugs with shorter half-lives or drugs metabolized more rapidly.

Table 16–7 describes the U.S. Food and Drug Administration (FDA) risk categories and provides examples for each. A quick way to remember the categories is as follows:

Category B for Best, as very few products are category A.

Category C for Caution, as these products have been shown to have risk in animal models.

Category D for Danger, as these products have been shown to have risk when used in human pregnancy, but are used occasionally in life-threatening maternal disease.

Category X for "Cross these drugs off the list," as these products have shown teratogenic risk and have no therapeutic indication for use during human pregnancy.

Pregnant women have similar incidence of acute and chronic illnesses as age-matched women who are not pregnant. An estimated 1% to 4% of all pregnancies are complicated by asthma, with a documented increase in maternal morbidity and mortality during pregnancy for women with the most severe asthma before conception. Most pregnant women with asthma have no change in their symptoms or experience an improvement in symptoms.

Bronchospasm symptoms are usually worse between 29 and 36 weeks of gestation because of esophageal irritation from gastroesophageal reflux disease. Symptoms usually

TABLE 16–7

Medication Use During Pregnancy

FDA risk category is assigned to all drugs. New drugs undergo animal study and perhaps a small number of inadvertent human exposures during clinical trials are considered; based on risk of drug exposure to human fetus: A–X

Risk Category	Outcomes	Example
Category A	Well-controlled human study: No fetal risk in first trimester No evidence of risk in second and third trimesters Risk to fetus seems remote	Vitamins at RDA • Vitamin A caution (risk factor X in doses >8000 IU/d) Levothyroxine
Category B B: Best because nothing is A	Animal studies do not show fetal risk, but no controlled study in humans, or Animal studies show adverse effect not shown in human study.	Beta-lactam antimicrobials • Penicillins, cephalosporins Select macrolides • Azithromycin, erythromycin Acetaminophen Ibuprofen • First and second trimesters only
Category C C: Caution	No controlled study in humans available Animal studies reveal adverse fetal effects	~⅔ of all prescription medications Select antimicrobials • Clarithromycin • Fluoroquinolones ("-floxacin" suffix) • TMP-SMX Commonly prescribed medications • Most SSRIs, corticosteroids, antihypertensives, others
Category D D: Danger	Positive evidence of human fetal risk Use in pregnant women occasionally acceptable despite risk	Gentamicin ACEI ("-pril" suffix), ARB ("-sartan" suffix) Ibuprofen • Third trimester only Tetracyclines • Doxycycline, minocycline Paroxetine
Category X Cross these off your list	Animal or human studies show fetal abnormality Evidence of fetal risk based on human study No therapeutic indication in pregnancy	Isotretinoin (Accutane), misoprostol (Cytotec), thalidomide

Source: Briggs G, Freeman R, Yaffee S. *Drugs in Pregnancy and Lactation*. Philadelphia, PA: Lippincott Williams & Wilkins; 2008.

improve late in gestation when gradual fetal descent occurs. Lifestyle changes that help improve symptoms of gastroesophageal reflux disease help with asthma management. Generally, the risk of fetal hypoxia is greater than the risk of medication exposure, so standard asthma medications should be continued. Most inhaled corticosteroids are FDA risk category C (with budesonide (Pulmicort) being the exception at risk category B), a designation that is based on high oral or parenteral doses given to laboratory animals, but seems to have little applicability in human use, which involves inhaled medications that have low rates of systemic absorption. Oral corticosteroids have the same designation, but should be used only to treat an asthma flare. Beta$_2$-agonist bronchodilators are also category C, based on study

on high oral doses in laboratory animals, and should be prescribed as a rescue drug for a pregnant woman with asthma. Leukotriene modifiers are newer medications and have not been studied as extensively in pregnant women and carry a risk category B or C.

Nausea and vomiting in pregnancy is often complicated by preexisting conditions such as gastritis. Although not yet conclusively established, more recent research has indicated that women with hyperemesis gravidarum have a higher incidence of *Helicobacter pylori* infection. Preconceptual treatment of *H. pylori* should be considered for women with history of a pregnancy complicated by severe nausea and vomiting or of recurrent gastrointestinal problems. Management is targeted toward relieving nausea by increasing rest and decreasing stress. Patients can make their own ginger or lemon aromatherapy "kit" by placing five ginger or lemon teabags in an airtight plastic tub. The tub is opened and the vapors inhaled when nausea occurs. Treating the concomitant gastritis that often accompanies severe nausea and vomiting during pregnancy with a chewable calcium antacid tablet every 2 hours for 2 to 3 days can be helpful. Taking vitamin B_6, 25 mg twice a day, has been noted to prevent future nausea and vomiting. A 5-HT_3-receptor antagonist, such as ondansetron (Zofran, pregnancy risk category B), can offer an effective therapeutic option for preventing severe morning sickness, but is not effective in managing acute symptoms.

Among women with a migraine history, most note fewer and less intense headaches during pregnancy. About 5% to 10% have worsening headaches, however. Treatment options include acetaminophen and nonsteroidal anti-inflammatory drugs (except at term because of potential risk of antiplatelet effect). Triptans are risk category C, partly because of the theoretical risk of vasoconstriction. No teratogenic effect in human pregnancy has been noted to date, however. Lidocaine 4% used as a nasal spray, applied to the nostril on the affected side of the head, can help attenuate headache symptoms with minimal system drug absorption.

Women are twice as likely to experience major depressive disorder (Table 16–8). Consequently, many women enter pregnancy in a depressed state or develop depression during the course of the pregnancy. Therapy for any mood disorder usually includes lifestyle changes, counseling, and drug therapy. Mood disorder treatment options include serotonin, norepinephrine, and dopamine receptor modulators; tricyclic antidepressants; and benzodiazepines. Although selective serotonin receptor inhibitors (SSRIs) are in risk category C (with the exception of paroxetine, which is risk category D), long-term observational study of children born to women who took these medications during pregnancy has failed to note significant differences compared with nonexposed matched controls. Bupropion is a dopamine receptor modulator and is also pregnancy risk category C. Serotonin-norepinephrine reuptake inhibitors such as venlafaxine (Effexor) and duloxetine (Cymbalta) are risk category C.

If a patient wishes to discontinue antidepressant therapy during pregnancy, she should be counseled about the risk of depression recurrence. A slow taper of approximately 25% of the total dose per week is required to avoid SSRI withdrawal syndrome. The withdrawal syndrome is bothersome, but not life-threatening. It includes jitteriness, nausea, and sleep disturbance, and is more severe with SSRIs with a shorter half-life such as paroxetine (T½ 26 hours) and less severe with SSRIs with longer half-life such as fluoxetine (T½ 24 to 72 hours and metabolite T½ up to 26 hours). If SSRIs are used late in the third trimester, fetal withdrawal can also occur, which is the reason for the common recommendation

TABLE 16–8
Postpartum Mood Disorders

Disorder	Incidence (%)	Presentation	Treatment
Postpartum blues	26–85	Often begins within days of giving birth, characterized by emotional lability, sleep disturbance, difficulty concentrating. 80% resolve by week 2; If persists >2 weeks, consider alternative diagnosis. 20% evolve to postpartum depression	Support and reassurance including recruiting helpers so mother can get more rest
Postpartum depression	10–20	Most common at 2–4 months postpartum, but can occur at any time in first year after giving birth. Characterized by depressed mood for ≥2 weeks with change in appetite, sleep disturbance, guilt, and worthlessness. As with all depression, greatest risk for death is suicide	Psychotherapy, psychopharmacological, medication therapy as indicated, recognizing all will be secreted in breast milk. Hospitalization as needed
Postpartum psychosis	0.2	Early onset usually by day 3 postpartum. Characterized by delusions, hallucinations, agitation, insomnia, confusion. Risk of infanticide, usually secondary to delusion about infant. Maternal suicide risk also increased	Hospitalization usually needed for safety of mother and infant. Psychopharmacological medication therapy as indicated (antipsychotics, mood stabilizers, benzodiazepines, antidepressants, others)

Source: Nonacs R. www.emedicine.com/med/topic3408.htm, Postpartum depression, accessed 9/28/09.

to taper a pregnant woman's SSRI dose over the last month of pregnancy. Neonatal effects are similar to maternal withdrawal and include irritability, protracted crying, and shivering; the timing of the onset of neonatal SSRI withdrawal symptoms is related to the drug's half-life and can occur within days to weeks of birth.

In an FDA advisory, results of domestic and European studies revealed that women who took paroxetine in early pregnancy had an approximately twofold increased risk for having an infant with a cardiac defect compared with the risk in the general population. The risk of a cardiac defect was about 2% in infants exposed to paroxetine versus 1% among all infants in one study, whereas a 1.5-fold increased risk for cardiac malformations and a 1.8-fold increased risk for congenital malformations overall in the infants exposed to paroxetine was noted in another study. Most of the cardiac defects reported in these studies were atrial or ventricular septal defects. As a result, the pregnancy risk category of paroxetine has been changed from C to D.

Tricyclic antidepressants and benzodiazepines are risk category D and are rarely prescribed during pregnancy. If an expectant mother has been on long-term benzodiazepine therapy, it is critical to taper doses gradually (25% per week) to avoid a withdrawal syndrome. Rapid withdrawal can lead to tremors, hallucinations, seizures, and a delirium tremens–like state, and is most common with the use of products with a shorter half-life. The onset of withdrawal symptoms occurs a few days after the last dose in a benzodiazepine with a shorter half-life (e.g., lorazepam) and up to 3 weeks in one with a longer half-life (e.g., clonazepam).

Pregnancy-related anatomic changes in the urinary tract, such as pressure on the bladder from enlarging uterus and increase in the size of the ureters, contribute to urinary reflux. Urinary tract infection (UTI) in a pregnant woman is a significant risk factor for low-birth-weight infants and prematurity.

Asymptomatic bacteriuria occurs in 5% to 9% of nonpregnant and pregnant women. If left untreated in pregnancy, progression of asymptomatic bacteriuria to symptomatic UTI including acute cystitis and pyelonephritis occurs in 15% to 45%, or fourfold higher than in nonpregnant women. This progression is due largely to the lower interleukin-6 levels and serum antibody responses to *E. coli* antigens that occur during pregnancy, resulting in less robust immune response.

Because asymptomatic bacteriuria, usually caused by aerobic gram-negative bacilli or *Staphylococcus saprophyticus,* can lead to UTI, a urine culture should be obtained from all women early in pregnancy, even in the absence of UTI symptoms. Approximately 20% to 40% of women with asymptomatic bacteriuria develop UTI during the course of the pregnancy; only 1% to 2% of women with a negative urine culture develop UTI. Asymptomatic bacteriuria should be treated with a 3- to 7-day course of antimicrobials, which reduces the risk of symptomatic UTI by 80% to 90%.

Options for the treatment of asymptomatic bacteriuria and symptomatic UTI during pregnancy are guided by pathogen susceptibility, and preferred antimicrobials include those with FDA pregnancy risk category B. Antimicrobials in pregnancy risk category B include beta-lactams (amoxicillin, cephalexin, cefpodoxime, cefixime, and amoxicillin/clavulanate) and nitrofurantoin. Nitrofurantoin has the advantage of sparing disruption of normal vaginal flora and consistent efficacy against *E. coli* and *S. saprophyticus.* Nitrofurantoin should be avoided after the 36th week of gestation because of the potential (although unlikely) risk for hemolysis if the fetus is glucose-6-phosphate dehydrogenase–deficient and in infections caused by *Proteus mirabilis.* Beta-lactam use usually fails to eradicate the offending pathogen from the periurethral and perivaginal area, increasing the risk of reinfection.

Women with symptomatic UTI during pregnancy should be treated for 7 days. When UTI is documented, monthly screening urine cultures should be obtained for the duration of the pregnancy. Daily antimicrobial prophylaxis with an appropriate agent should be considered with evidence of 2 days of a symptomatic UTI or persistent, unresolved bacteriuria despite effective antimicrobial therapy. Urological evaluation should also be considered to rule out structural abnormality.

Discussion Sources

Briggs G, Freeman R, Yaffe S, eds. *Drugs in Pregnancy and Lactation: A Reference for Fetal and Neonatal Risk*. 8th ed. Philadelphia, PA: Lippincott Williams & Wilkins; 2008.

Gilbert D, Moerlling R, Eliopoulos G, Chambers H, Saag M. *The Sanford Guide to Antimicrobial Therapy*. 39th ed. Sperryville, VA: Antimicrobial Therapy, Inc; 2009:30–31.

QUESTIONS

85. Risk factors for preeclampsia include all of the following except:

    A. low maternal weight.
    B. age younger than 16 years or older than 40 years.
    C. collagen vascular disease.
    D. first pregnancy with a new partner.

86. Blood pressure changes in preeclampsia include increases of blood pressure over normotensive baseline of ___ mm Hg systolic and ___ mm Hg diastolic or more.

    A. 10, 5
    B. 20, 10
    C. 30, 15
    D. 40, 20

87. Preeclampsia presentation is noted after the ___ week of pregnancy.

   A. 10
   B. 15
   C. 20
   D. 25

88. The components of HELLP syndrome include all of the following except:

   A. hepatic enzyme elevations.
   B. thrombocytosis.
   C. hemolysis.
   D. eclampsia.

89. Which of the following is the most important part of care of a woman with preeclampsia?

   A. antihypertensive therapy
   B. anticonvulsant therapy
   C. prompt recognition of the condition
   D. induction of labor

90. Regarding the risk for neonatal group B streptococcus (GBS) disease, the NP considers that:

   A. about 50% to 70% of all pregnant women harbor this organism.
   B. there is no risk of disease with cesarean birth.
   C. the organism is most often acquired by vertical transmission in the second trimester of pregnancy.
   D. intrapartum antimicrobials should be given to all women with evidence of GBS colonization.

91. GBS cultures should be obtained from:

   A. cervix.
   B. urethra.
   C. urine.
   D. lower vagina and rectum.

ANSWERS

85.	A	86.	C	87.	C
88.	B	89.	C	90.	D
91.	D				

DISCUSSION

Hypertensive disorders in pregnancy are usually divided into the following categories: chronic hypertension, or high blood pressure (BP) diagnosis that predates the pregnancy, and hypertensive disorders acquired during pregnancy. Hypertensive disorders acquired during pregnancy include gestational hypertension, preeclampsia, and eclampsia.

Preeclampsia risk factors include age (>40 years, <16 years), first pregnancy or first pregnancy with a new partner, pregestational diabetes mellitus, presence of collagen vascular disease, prepregnancy or primary hypertension, presence of renal disease, a family history of pregnancy-induced hypertension, or multiple gestation pregnancy.

An early or milder case presentation of preeclampsia is usually characterized by an increase in systolic BP of 30 mm Hg, an increase in diastolic BP of 15 mm Hg, or an absolute BP reading of 140 mm Hg/90 mm Hg in a pregnant woman with minimal proteinuria and pathological edema, with presentation after the 20th week of gestation. Additional problems include right upper quadrant abdominal pain, nausea, and vomiting. A systolic BP greater than 160 mm Hg or a diastolic BP greater than 110 mm Hg with significant proteinuria (>5 g/d) and evidence of hepatic, renal, or central nervous system end-organ damage indicate severe preeclampsia. Preeclampsia can progress to the syndrome of hemolysis with resulting anemia, elevated liver enzymes indicating hepatocellular damage, and low platelet count and eclampsia; this constellation is known as HELLP and is noted in 5% to 10% of patients with preeclamptic symptoms (Table 16–9).

The most important intervention in preeclampsia is maintaining a high index of suspicion in women with considerable risk and prompt recognition of the condition. When preeclampsia is recognized, expert obstetrical consultation should be obtained. Intervention includes rest, ongoing maternal and fetal monitoring, and antihypertensive or anticonvulsant medications or both; all of these measures have only a small effect on outcome. Birth is the definitive intervention and is usually the treatment of choice in later pregnancy.

Prenatal care in later pregnancy should include screening for group B streptococcus (GBS). Neonatal infection with GBS is a leading cause of newborn morbidity and mortality, resulting in an estimated 1600 early-onset cases and 80 deaths each year. Maternal lower genitourinary tract colonization with this organism is a major risk factor for early-onset, usually in the first week of life, GBS disease. The transmission of the organism from mother to fetus usually occurs after the onset of labor or membrane rupture. The lower gastrointestinal tract is the natural reservoir for this organism; this most likely contributes to GBS vaginal or rectal colonization in about 10% to 30% of pregnant women. GBS colonization is not considered to be a sexually transmitted infection and can be transient, chronic, or intermittent. Intrapartum antimicrobial chemoprophylaxis is currently the most effective intervention to help prevent infant GBS disease. As a result, GBS screening should be performed in all women at 35 to 37 weeks of pregnancy, including women who are to undergo cesarean birth because the organism can cause infection across intact membranes. The culture should be obtained by swabbing the lower vagina and vaginal introitus, followed by the rectum; insertion of the swab into the anal sphincter is needed for optimal results. The patient

TABLE 16–9

Hypertensive Disorders During Pregnancy

Category of Hypertensive Disorder during Pregnancy	Defining Characteristics of Disorder
Chronic hypertension	High blood pressure diagnosed before pregnancy, present before 20th week of pregnancy or persisting >6 weeks postpartum
Gestational hypertension	High blood pressure diagnosed after 20th week of pregnancy, but resolving within 6 weeks postpartum, without significant proteinuria or other signs of preeclampsia
Preeclampsia	High blood pressure diagnosed after 20th week of pregnancy, accompanied by significant proteinuria (>300 mg protein in 24-hour urine collection) that cannot be attributed to another cause. Usually accompanied by increased edema
Eclampsia	Presentation as in preeclampsia with tonic-clonic seizures or other alteration in mental status that cannot be attributed to another cause
HELLP syndrome	Preeclampsia accompanied by elevated hepatic enzymes and low platelets

Source: Gibson P. http://www.emedicine.com/MED/topic3250.htm, eMedicine: hypertension and pregnancy, accessed 10/6/09.

or health-care provider can obtain the culture. No vaginal speculum is needed and cervical cultures should not be obtained because these can be negative in the presence of heavy lower vaginal GBS colonization.

Discussion Sources

Gibson P. http://www.emedicine.com/MED/topic3250.htm, eMedicine: hypertension and pregnancy, accessed 10/6/09.

McFee J. Comprehensive prenatal care. In Bader T, ed. *OB/GYN Secrets*. Philadelphia, PA: Elsevier; 2005.

QUESTIONS

92. You note that a 28-year-old woman who is 4 months pregnant has bruises on her right shoulder. She states, "I fell up against the wall." The bruises appear finger-shaped. She denies that another person injured her. What is your best response to this?

    A. "Your bruises really look as if they were caused by someone grabbing you."
    B. "Was this really an accident?"
    C. "I notice the bruises are in the shape of a hand."
    D. "How did you fall?"

93. Which of the following statements is true concerning domestic violence during pregnancy?

    A. It is found largely among women of lower socioeconomic status.
    B. Women in an abusive relationship usually seek help.
    C. Routine screening is indicated during pregnancy.
    D. A predictable cycle of violent activity followed by a period of calm is the norm.

94. to 96. The following questions should be answered true or false.

    ____ 94. Domestic abuse is uncommon in same-sex relationships.
    ____ 95. Access to a firearm does not increase the rate of fatal episodes of domestic abuse.
    ____ 96. Child abuse is present in about half of all homes where partner mistreatment occurs.

ANSWERS

92.	C	**93.**	C	**94.**	False
95.	False	**96.**	True		

DISCUSSION

Interpersonal violence among family members (i.e., domestic violence) is found in all socioeconomic and ethnic groups. Because providers working with lower income and certain ethnic groups usually are more vigilant about domestic violence, however, there is often an appearance that the abuse is more of a problem in certain groups.

Domestic partner abuse can take many forms: psychological, financial, emotional, and physical. Acts of violence are typically thought to be against the victim, but may include destruction of property, intimidation, and threats. A cycle of tension building including criticism, yelling, and threats followed by violence and then a quieter period of apologies and promises to change is often seen. This cycle usually accelerates over time, with the violence being less predictable. Love for the perpetrator, hope that things will change, and fear of the consequences of leaving the relationship help to keep the victim in the relationship, particularly when the woman is pregnant with the perpetrator's child and fears abandonment. As a result, the victim often does not come forth asking for help.

As with counseling and screening for other health problems, using objective statements beginning with "I" is helpful. When a patient denies that finger-shaped bruises are caused by intentional injury by another person, the NP can simply state what is seen. This statement reinforces the assessment of abuse and allows the patient to offer more information. In a situation in which a patient is verbally abused in the presence of the NP, the NP should reinforce his or her role as patient advocate by stating that the behavior is unacceptable in the NP's presence. Some may fear that this assertive behavior could precipitate another episode of abuse; however, this is unlikely.

Applying the BATHE model is helpful in framing the problem and forming a therapeutic relationship and directing intervention. Developed by Stuart and Lieberman, this model provides a guide for gathering information, while helping the patient reflect on the issues at hand. The components :

- BATHE:
  - **B:** Background
    - How are things at home? At work? Has anything changed? Good or bad? Anything you wish would change?
- **A:** Affect, anxiety
  - How do you feel about home life? Work? School? Life in general?
- **T:** Trouble
  - What worries you the most? How stressed are you about this problem?
- **H:** Handling
  - How are you handling the problems in your life? How much support do you get at home or work? Who gives you support in dealing with problems?
- **E:** Empathy
  - "That sounds difficult."
- You may want to add SOAP to the BATHE:
  - **S:** Support
    - Normalize problems, but do not minimize.
    - "Many people struggle with the same (similar) problem."
    - "What supports or resources can you use to help deal with this?"
      - Some providers may use select self-disclosure for this. Self-disclosure usually works best in crises that are common and not of unusually tragic proportions, such as a timely death or job change.
  - **O:** Objectivity
    - Watch your reactions to the story. Maintain your professional composure without acting stonelike, but be mindful of "recoiling" gestures.
    - Help client with objectivity.
      - "What is the worst thing that can happen?"
      - "How likely is that?"
      - "Then what would happen?"

- Acceptance
  - Coach the client to personal acceptance.
    - "That is an understandable way to feel."
    - "I think you have done well considering the stress."
    - "I wonder if you are not being too hard on yourself."
- **A:** Acknowledge client priorities.
  - "It sounds like family is more important to you than your work."
- Acknowledge readiness or difficulty in making a change.
  - "Change is hard and sometimes very scary."
  - "It sounds to me like you are (not) ready to make a change."
- **P:** Present focus
  - Assist client in focusing on the present, without minimizing concerns of the past and future.
    - "How could you cope better?"
    - "What could you do differently?"
    - What to do after you have gathered this information:
  - Negotiate a problem-focused contract for behavioral change:
    - Repeat after me, "I promise not to harm myself or anyone else in any way between now and my next visit with _____."
  - Homework assignment with "I" messages:
    - "I would like more help with the children."
    - "I feel really unimportant to you when _____."
    - "I feel angry when _____."
- How do you keep this to 15 minutes?
  - Focus the client, using open and close-ended questions. Tell the client how much time you have, particularly with a revisit.
    - "We have ____ (fill in the blank) minutes to chat. What would you like to focus on?"
    - If the client cannot focus, ask, "If one problem in your life could just disappear, what would you choose?"

Interpersonal violence is likely as common in same-sex relationships as in opposite-sex relationships, but it is not as well studied. Violent behavior by a woman against a male partner is unlikely to result in injury as serious as a man's violence against a woman, partly because of the usual disparity in body size and lower likelihood of weapon use. In all socioeconomic groups, access to a firearm by a perpetrator is associated with increased risk of abuse with serious or fatal injury, however; this is also a risk for completed suicide. The NP is in an ideal position to direct the couple to appropriate resources for help in domestic violence, and should not attempt to provide this counseling because of the complexity of this type of care. Individual treatment is the rule as long as the violent behavior continues. Child abuse is present in about half of all households where there is partner abuse.

Discussion Sources

American Psychiatric Association. *Diagnostic and Statistical Manual of Mental Disorders.* 4th ed. Arlington, VA: American Psychiatric Publishing, Inc; 2000.

Stuart M, Lieberman J. *The 15-Minute Hour: Practical Therapeutic Intervention in Primary Care*. 3rd ed. Philadelphia, PA: Saunders; 2002.

QUESTIONS

97. Approximately ___% of all clinically recognized pregnancies end in spontaneous abortion.

   A. 10
   B. 20
   C. 30
   D. 40

98. Approximately __% of spontaneous abortions result from chromosomal defects.

   A. 20
   B. 40
   C. 60
   D. 80

99. The classic clinical triad of ectopic pregnancy includes all of the following except:

   A. abdominal pain.
   B. vaginal bleeding.
   C. large-for-gestational-age uterus.
   D. adnexal mass.

100. The classic clinical triad of ectopic pregnancy is found in no more than ___% of women presenting with this condition.

   A. 10
   B. 25
   C. 50
   D. 75

101. In the first weeks of a viable intrauterine pregnancy, serum quantitative hCG levels usually double every ___ hours.

   A. 24
   B. 48
   C. 72
   D. 96

102. In ectopic pregnancy, all of the following statements are true except:

   A. hCG is low for gestational age and is not increasing normally.
   B. Ultrasound evaluation fails to reveal abnormality in 20% to 30% of cases.
   C. Location of the pregnancy is often on the ovary or cervix.
   D. Risk factors include current pregnancy via assisted reproduction.

103. to 106. Match the clinical presentation of the following.

____ **103.** Complete abortion

____ **104.** Inevitable abortion

____ **105.** Threatened abortion

____ **106.** Incomplete abortion

   A. Uterine contents include a nonviable pregnancy that is in the process of being expelled.
   B. Some portion of the products of conception remain in the uterus, although the pregnancy is no longer viable.
   C. The products of conception have been completely expelled.
   D. Ultrasound evaluation shows a viable pregnancy, although vaginal bleeding is present.

ANSWERS

97.	B	98.	C	99.	C
100.	C	101.	B	102.	C
103.	C	104.	A	105.	D
106.	B				

DISCUSSION

Ectopic pregnancy is defined as any gestation that occurs outside of the uterus. Although reports of cervical, abdominal, and interstitial pregnancies exist, approximately 95% of all ectopic pregnancies are located in a fallopian tube; the term tubal pregnancy is nearly synonymous with ectopic pregnancy. Because the physiological and physical needs of the fetus cannot be met when pregnancy occurs outside the uterus, the pregnancy cannot progress beyond the earliest stages and will be lost. Most ectopic pregnancies resolve without intervention via miscarriage or involution of the gestation sac and reabsorption. Ectopic pregnancies that do not resolve pose a significant risk to the mother, however.

Risk factors for ectopic pregnancy include factors that can influence normal tubal motility and patency, such as a history of pelvic inflammatory disease, prior ectopic pregnancy, current intrauterine device (IUD) use, pregnancy achieved by means of *in vitro* fertilization or fertility drugs, prior tubal surgery (reconstruction or tubal ligation), and cigarette smoking (Table 16–10). Increasing age is also a risk factor for ectopic pregnancy.

The classic clinical triad of ectopic pregnancy—abdominal pain, vaginal bleeding, and an adnexal mass—is found in only 50% of women with the condition. Consequently, careful clinical assessment to support or disprove the diagnosis is critical. Diagnosis of ectopic pregnancy includes obtaining a

TABLE 16–10

Risk Factors for Ectopic Pregnancy

Strongest Evidence of Risk	Significant but Less Potent
History of salpingitis (most potent risk factor)	Progestin use
Prior ectopic pregnancy	Current IUD use
Tubal or pelvic surgery	Vaginal douching
Assisted reproduction	Tubal ligation failure (3% of all ectopic pregnancies)
Cigarette smoking	

beta hCG value. Urine and serum tests are usually positive, and a negative test rules out the diagnosis. Usually serum quantities of beta hCG in ectopic pregnancy at gestational weeks 6 to 10, the most common time for clinical presentation, are 1000 to 6000 IU/m; this compares with 40,000 IU/m or greater for a viable intrauterine pregnancy. The normal rapid increase in serum quantitative beta hCG noted in a viable intrauterine pregnancy is missing, and the value tends to stall. With a positive beta hCG level 1000 IU/mL or greater, a gestational sac should be identifiable within the uterus on transvaginal ultrasound with an intrauterine pregnancy; the presence of an intrauterine gestational sac effectively excludes the diagnosis of ectopic pregnancy (Tables 16–11 and 16–12).

Of women with ectopic pregnancy, 20% to 30% have a nondiagnostic ultrasound; a normal ultrasound scan does not rule out the condition. If ectopic pregnancy is suspected, a serum progesterone level is often obtained. Progesterone is a hormone produced by the developing chorion. A progesterone level less than 15 ng/mL is seen in only 11% of normal intrauterine pregnancies, but is noted in most ectopic pregnancies or with inevitable abortion. Occasionally, pelvic CT or MRI is indicated, recognizing the limitations of these studies in ectopic pregnancy but their utility in identifying other reasons for abdominal pain.

When the diagnosis of ectopic pregnancy is established, treatment depends on the patient's condition. If the patient is stable, evaluation for a concurrent (heterotopic) intrauterine pregnancy should be done because this can be found in 10% of women presenting with this condition. If the patient is hemodynamically unstable, immediate surgical intervention is warranted. Surgical or medical intervention is warranted according to the availability of treatment options if the patient is stable. Surgical treatments include salpingostomy, in which the tube is opened, and the pregnancy contents are removed. The tube is then repaired. Salpingectomy is usually performed when the tubal rupture has occurred, or tubal damage is severe, and repair is not possible.

TABLE 16–11

Clinical Presentation in Ectopic Pregnancy

Clinical Presentation	Laboratory Diagnosis	Ultrasound
Abdominal pain (nearly universal, often bilateral)	Serum progesterone (≤15 mg/mL, found in 81% ectopic pregnancy, 93% abnormal IUP, 11% normal IUP)	Consider diagnosis if transvaginal ultrasound fails to identify intrauterine gestational sac and hCG >1500 mIU/mL
Adnexal tenderness (75%)		
Menstrual irregularity (75%)		
Uterus size ≤ gestational age (90%)	Low for gestational age serum hCG (IUP <6000 mIU/mL, relatively stalled without normal hCG increases)	
Adnexal mass (53%)	Positive urine hCG (99% sensitivity and specificity)	

IUP, intrauterine pregnancy.

TABLE 16–12

Clinical Presentation in Intrauterine Pregnancy (IUP)

Transvaginal ultrasound	Gestational sac in normal IUP hCG ≥1000 mIU/mL
Transabdominal ultrasound	Gestational sac in normal IUP hCG ≥6500 mIU/mL

Medical therapy with methotrexate, a medication that inhibits cell division and causes the pregnancy to regress and resolve, is an option when ectopic pregnancy is diagnosed while the tube is intact, the patient is hemodynamically stable, there is no ultrasound evidence of fetal cardiac activity or free fluid in the cul-de-sac, and there are no contraindications for methotrexate use. A quantitative beta hCG of 15,000 IU/L, evidence of fetal cardiac activity, and free fluid in the cul-de-sac (a common finding in tubal rupture) are all contraindications to methotrexate use. Close follow-up is critical with medical management of ectopic pregnancy to ensure pregnancy resolution; surgical intervention is sometimes needed when this therapy fails. Compared with surgical therapy, tubal patency is usually better preserved with medical management. Regardless of the treatment modality in ectopic pregnancy, considerable emotional support is also needed because the woman has faced a potentially life-threatening illness and the loss of a pregnancy (Table 16–13).

Spontaneous abortion is defined as the natural ending of a pregnancy before 20 weeks of gestation. In about 60% of spontaneous abortions, chromosomal defects of maternal or paternal origin are responsible for the pregnancy loss. Maternal factors such as trauma, illness, or infection lead to the loss in about 15% of cases. In the remaining cases, no obvious cause can be found. With all threatened pregnancy loss, intervention is aimed at maintaining a stable hemodynamic state and providing considerable emotional support.

About 25% to 30% of women experience some vaginal bleeding in the first trimester, and at least 50% of these women have pregnancy loss. Four terms are usually used to modify the condition of spontaneous abortion: threatened, inevitable, incomplete, and complete.

Threatened abortion manifests as vaginal bleeding or brown spotting during early pregnancy with or without cramping, but without cervical dilation or change in cervical consistency. Ultrasound evaluation shows a viable pregnancy, and serum quantitative beta hCG is consistent with gestational age. Barring other complications, the pregnancy in threatened abortion progresses without problem. Intervention includes a few days of rest then resumption of normal activities, although even this commonsense treatment likely makes little difference in the pregnancy outcome. Less than one-half of women who have vaginal bleeding during the first trimester proceed to a complete abortion or miscarriage.

In inevitable abortion, the cervix is open, and the uterine contents are in the process of being expelled. The patient has cramping abdominal pain and usually brisk vaginal bleeding. Usually the uterine contents are expelled, and no further medical or surgical intervention is needed.

In incomplete abortion, some portion of the products of conception remains in the uterus. The os is usually closed, and minimal cramping is reported. Evacuation of the uterine contents by dilation and aspiration is one option for intervention. Expectant management, or "watch and wait" while the uterus completes the emptying process, and medical therapy to encourage uterine emptying are also appropriate options.

In a complete abortion, pregnancy-related uterine contents have been completely expelled. Quantitative hCG is low for gestational age, and the ultrasound fails to identify a pregnancy. On examination, the patient has minimal cramping, the cervical os is likely still slightly open, and the uterine size is returning to normal. Further medical or surgical intervention is usually not needed. As with all pregnancy loss, considerable emotional support is needed to help the woman and her family deal with this significant event.

Discussion Sources

Griebel C, Halvorsen J, Golemon T, May A. http://www.aafp.org/afp/20051001/1243.html, Management of spontaneous abortion. American Family Physician, 2005, accessed 10/8/09.

Lozeau AM, Potter B. http://www.aafp.org/afp/20051101/1707.html, Diagnosis and management of ectopic pregnancy, American Family Physician, 2005, accessed 10/8/09.

Sepilian V. http://www.emedicine.com/med/topic3212.htm, eMedicine: ectopic pregnancy, accessed 10/8/09.

TABLE 16–13
Ectopic Pregnancy Management

Most ectopic pregnancies resolve without intervention. No current reliable data are available on predictors of self-resolution

SURGICAL MANAGEMENT	Salpingostomy Salpingectomy
MEDICAL MANAGEMENT	Methotrexate therapy can be offered if following criteria are met • Conceptus <3.5 cm with no evidence of cardiac activity • Unruptured tube with no evidence of fluid in cul-de-sac • Beta hCG level <15,000 IU/L • Hemodynamically stable with no signs or symptoms of active bleeding or hemoperitoneum • Available for close follow-up

Sources: Erickson T. Ectopic pregnancy. In: Bader T, ed. *OB/GYN Secrets*. Philadelphia, PA: Elsevier; 2005:109–113.
Sepilia V. www.emedicine.com/med/topic3212.htm, Ectopic pregnancy, accessed 10/11/09.

QUESTIONS

107. First-time mothers usually have an average of _____ hours of active first-stage labor.

    A. 6 to 8
    B. 9 to 12
    C. 13 to 15
    D. 16 to 18

108. For women who have previously given birth vaginally, first-stage and second-stage labor usually lasts an average of _____ hours.

    A. 3 to 5
    B. 6 to 8
    C. 9 to 10
    D. 11 to 13

ANSWERS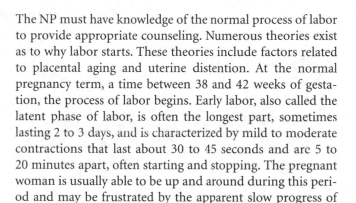

107.   B   108.   B

DISCUSSION

The NP must have knowledge of the normal process of labor to provide appropriate counseling. Numerous theories exist as to why labor starts. These theories include factors related to placental aging and uterine distention. At the normal pregnancy term, a time between 38 and 42 weeks of gestation, the process of labor begins. Early labor, also called the latent phase of labor, is often the longest part, sometimes lasting 2 to 3 days, and is characterized by mild to moderate contractions that last about 30 to 45 seconds and are 5 to 20 minutes apart, often starting and stopping. The pregnant woman is usually able to be up and around during this period and may be frustrated by the apparent slow progress of labor. During this time, the cervix usually dilates to around 3 cm, and the membranes are intact.

The first stage of active labor starts when the cervix is about 3 to 4 cm dilated and is complete when the cervix is fully dilated. Contractions become closer and more intense, culminating in transition when contractions occur every 2 to 3 minutes and last 50 to 70 seconds or more. The pregnant woman should be instructed to go to the hospital or birthing center when contractions are every 5 minutes and lasting 1 minute. During active labor, the woman often feels restless and excited by the impending birth, but is usually communicative between contractions. In transition, the woman is usually quite focused on getting through the birth process and may be distracted by the comments of others. The presence of a support person is important throughout the birth process.

The second stage of labor is the actual birth, a stage that can last a few minutes or a few hours. The mother often passes through this stage with a variety of emotions, from exhaustion to elation. The third stage of labor occurs when the placenta detaches and is expelled from the uterus.

First-time mothers usually have an average of 9 to 12 hours of first-stage labor, and second-stage labor lasts approximately 30 minutes to 2 hours. For women who have previously given birth, first-stage and second-stage labor usually lasts approximately 6 to 8 hours.

The pregnant woman and her labor support should be encouraged to attend childbirth and infant care class. Referral to these classes usually occurs during the second trimester of pregnancy.

Discussion Sources

American College of Nurse Midwives. http://www.mymidwife.org/labor.cfm, Labor and birth, accessed 10/8/09.

American Pregnancy Association. http://americanpregnancy.org/labornbirth/firststage.html, First stage of labor, accessed 10/8/09.

American Pregnancy Association. http://americanpregnancy.org/labornbirth/secondstage.html, Second stage of labor, accessed 10/8/09.

American Pregnancy Association. http://americanpregnancy.org/labornbirth/thirdstage.html, Third stage of labor, accessed 10/8/09.

APPENDIX A
Answers to Your Most Common Test-Taking Questions

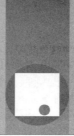

Are you preparing to take the NP certification examination? Are you confused about which organizations offer what kind of certification, or wondering about test content or focus? The answers to common questions about NP certification are provided here.

What are the agencies that offer adult, family, and gerontological NP certification examinations?

NP certification is offered by a variety of nongovernmental agencies.

- The American Nurses Credentialing Center (ANCC, www.nursecredentialing.org) offers year-round, computer-based testing for family, adult, and geriatric and select other NP certification.
- The American Academy of Nurse Practitioners (AANP, www.aanpcertification.org) offers year-round, computer-based testing for adult, family, and gerontological NP certification.

How many questions are on the NP certification examinations?

The ANCC examinations consist of 175 questions or test items. Of these, 150 items count toward your score, with the remaining 25 questions being sample items that might be used on future examinations but do not contribute to your examination score. The AANP examinations consist of 150 test items with 15 items as sample questions that do not contribute to your final score. One purpose of adding these items is to evaluate the question's validity and reliability before incorporating the item in the certification examination. These items are integrated throughout the examination, not listed in a separate section.

How are the NP certification examinations similar?

The content of all the NP certification examinations reflects the broad base of knowledge and the critical thinking skills necessary for entry-level NP practice. The largest sections are dedicated to assessment of and intervention for the health problems common to the chosen area of practice. Additional content area typically includes choice of the appropriate diagnostic studies and screening tests and the subsequent interpretation of findings. Content in the intervention section usually includes questions on pharmacological and nonpharmacological therapies and principles of therapeutic communication. The remainder of the examination is usually devoted to areas such as health promotion and disease prevention.

How do the NP examinations differ?

For both agencies, the family NP examination reflects the broad scope of knowledge necessary to care for patients of all ages, including pregnant women. The adult NP certification examinations focus on the care of patients who are 13 years old and older, whereas the gerontological NP test focuses on health care issues for adults 55 years old and older.

Are some of the NP examination questions about issues other than clinical issues?

The ANCC examinations contain a section on professional issues such as scope of practice, health-care ethics, reimbursement, and research; the AANP NP certification examination does not contain such a section. Check the respective agency's website for the current examination content outline.

How do I find out if I passed my NP certification examination?

The computer-based NP examinations provide your results on completion of the test. Before leaving the test site, you will know if you passed or failed your NP certification examination.

I am now a certified NP. Is there a special way to designate this?

The NP certification credential differs according to the certifying body. Following are the designations of the various certifying organizations.

The credentials for American Certification Credentialing Center (ANCC)–certified NPs is NP-BC (nurse practitioner–board certified) preceded by a letter indicating the particular specialty:

- Family nurse practitioner: FNP-BC
- Adult nurse practitioner: ANP-BC
- Gerontological nurse practitioner: GNP-BC

Here is an example of an ANCC-certified family NP:
Hugo Moreno, MS, FNP-BC

Family and adult NPs certified by the American Academy of Nurse Practitioners (AANP) are granted the designation of NP-C, or Nurse Practitioner–Certified. Here is an example:

Melissa Hammond, MSN, NP-C

How can I find out the pass rates of the NP certification examinations?

The pass rates of the NP certification examination are often posted by the agency. About 75% to 85% of the candidates successfully pass the NP certification examination. Put another way, about one in four to one in five NP certification candidates does not pass the examination.

What kind of questions will I find on the NP certification examinations?

The NP certification examinations comprise multiple-choice questions; there are no true/false, fill-in-the-blank, essay, or matching test items.

Are all of the examination questions at the same level of complexity or difficulty?

The examination questions are written on numerous levels of difficulty and depth, with the lowest level usually the fact-oriented or knowledge questions. This type of question tests generalizations, principles, and widely recognized theories. When answering this question, you might read the question and instantly recognize the correct answer from a piece of information that was memorized long ago. The following is an example of a fact-oriented question;

Pupillary constriction in reaction to light is in part a function of cranial nerve:

A. I.
B. II.
C. III.
D. IV.

(Correct answer: C)

Mnemonics or other memory aids can be helpful in answering a fact-oriented question. The certification examinations are likely to contain many more complex types of questions, however, that require application of clinical assessment and management skills. Examples of these include the comprehension question, where you must interpret the fact. An example of a comprehension question is as follows:

The person with Bell palsy has paralysis of cranial nerve:

A. V.
B. VI.
C. VII.
D. VIII.

(Correct answer: C)

To respond correctly to this question, you must know that Bell palsy is a condition where the facial nerve (cranial nerve VII) is affected.

Likely the most common question found on the certification examinations is application questions. In this type of question, you analyze the information then decide what is pertinent to the given situation. Look for key words in the stem (the question itself) that help set a priority. These include words such as "first," "initially," or "most important

action." If you are having difficulty ascertaining which action should be done first, particularly when the question poses many plausible actions, you should ask yourself, "What is the greatest risk in this situation?" Here is an example:

You are seeing Ms. Thomas, a 53-year-old woman who presents for a health examination. She smokes cigarettes with a 45-pack-years history, currently smoking 1.5 packs per day, and has a family history of premature heart disease. The most important part of her assessment is:

A. Chest x-ray
B. Auscultation for S_3 and S_4 heart sounds
C. Blood pressure measurement
D. Cervical examination with Pap testing

When looking at this question, you may think that you would certainly perform a cardiac examination and Pap test. With the limited amount of information available on this patient, no indication for chest x-ray is evident. So, how do you set the priority of the most important part of the assessment? Start with teasing out the facts and assumptions. In the information presented, Ms. Thomas has two risk factors for cardiovascular disease, cigarette smoking and family history of premature heart disease. In addition, heart disease is the leading cause of death in American women. Assume she is postmenopausal because the average woman reaches this stage by age 51 years. This gives her an additional cardiovascular risk factor. The stage is set for her to be at high risk for cardiovascular disease. Another assumption is that the best evaluation is one that detects early disease. Now, look at the answers given and think what you may expect for results.

In assessing Ms. Thomas, a chest x-ray could reveal lung cancer or findings consistent with tobacco-related lung disease. These changes would not be evident, however, until these diseases are advanced; in earlier disease, the chest x-ray is usually without specific findings. The presence of extra heart sounds would likely indicate systolic (S_3) or diastolic (S_4) cardiac dysfunction, again a marker of significant, usually advanced cardiac problems. Blood pressure measurement is critical, however, because it can detect hypertension in its asymptomatic, earliest state, and it increases Ms. Thomas' risk of heart disease. Although screening for cervical neoplasia is important, diagnosis and intervention in hypertension would be more likely to improve this woman's shorter term health. After pulling together the facts, the best answer is option C, blood pressure measurement.

How about some tips on answering multiple-choice questions?

A multiple-choice question has many components. Often, the first sentence is an introduction of a clinical scenario. Here is an example of a lengthy introduction, rich with information.

You see 18-year-old Sam, who was seen approximately 36 hours ago at a local walk-in center for treatment of ear pain. Diagnosed with (L) acute otitis media, amoxicillin was prescribed. Today, Sam states that he has taken 5 amoxicillin doses since the medication was prescribed, but continues to have discomfort in the affected ear. Left TM is red and immobile.

When responding to this question, remember that test questions are designed to have one best, although perhaps not perfect, answer. In clinical practice, you would likely gather more information than is given here. During the certification examination, you have to decide on the best response given the information in front of you while applying sound clinical judgment. Following are the clinical points as these relate to this particular question:

- Because no chronic health problems are mentioned, assume that Sam is a young adult who is typically in good health.
- Acute otitis media (AOM) is a common episodic illness usually caused by *S. pneumoniae, H. influenzae, M. catarrhalis,* or respiratory virus.
- A first-line antimicrobial for AOM treatment is amoxicillin. When given in an adequate dose, this antibiotic is effective against *S. pneumoniae* and non–beta-lactamase–producing *H. influenzae* and *M. catarrhalis.* Nearly all *M. catarrhalis* and about 30% of *H. influenzae* produce beta-lactamase, rendering amoxicillin ineffective. Clavulanate is a beta-lactamase inhibitor and when given in conjunction with amoxicillin is an effective treatment option when AOM fails to respond to amoxicillin alone.
- As inflammation and purulent exudate forms in the middle ear, a small space rich with pain receptors, otalgia is an expected finding in AOM. This usually resolves after 2 to 3 days of antimicrobial therapy.
- Tympanic membrane immobility is a cardinal sign of AOM that despite antimicrobial therapy does not resolve for many weeks. A patient report of otalgia is also needed to make the AOM diagnosis.

The next part is the statement that poses the question to be answered.

Your next best action is to:

- This is an action-oriented question, directing you to consider Sam's care and chief complaint.

  A. *Advise Sam to discontinue the current antimicrobial and start a course of amoxicillin with clavulanate*

- Choosing this response infers amoxicillin treatment failure. AOM antimicrobial treatment failure is usually defined, however, as persistent otalgia with fever after 72 hours of therapy. Sam has taken fewer than 2 days of therapy, too short an interval to assign continued symptoms to ineffective antimicrobial therapy.

  B. *Perform tympanocentesis and send a sample of the exudate for culture and sensitivity*

- AOM antimicrobial therapy is based on choosing an agent with activity against the most likely organisms, bearing in mind the most common resistant pathogens. Tympanocentesis is indicated only with treatment failure after 10 to 21 days of antimicrobial therapy with a second-line agent, with the goal of detecting a significantly resistant organism; at that point, culture and sensitivity of middle ear exudate would be appropriate. With fewer than 2 days of treatment, tympanocentesis is not indicated.

  C. *Have Sam return in 24 hours for re-evaluation.*

- If Sam's condition worsens in the next day, re-evaluation is prudent. However, choosing this option ignores Sam's complaint of pain, however.

  D. *Recommend that Sam take ibuprofen for the next 2 to 3 days.*

- Choosing option D response infers that treating Sam's pain is the most appropriate intervention. This is the best response and the correct answer.

  Now consider this question.

  Which of the following best describes asthma?

- No clinical scenario is presented; the question simply asks for a definition of a pathological state. When considering the options, the test-taker must recall that asthma is a chronic inflammatory disease of the airways involving an increase in bronchial hyperresponsiveness. This condition leads to a potentially reversible decrease in FEV1-to-FVC ratio.

  Here are your choices of answers.

  A. *Intermittent airway inflammation with occasional bronchospasm*

- Because asthma is a chronic, not intermittent, inflammatory airway disease, this option is incorrect.

  B. *A disease of bronchospasm leading to airway inflammation*

- Because asthma is first a chronic inflammatory airway disease that leads to airway hyperresponsiveness, this option is incorrect.

  C. *Chronic airway inflammation with superimposed bronchospasm*

- This option most closely matches the definition of asthma and is the best option.

  D. *Relatively fixed airway obstruction*

- Because the airway obstruction in asthma is largely reversible, this option is incorrect. This answer is more descriptive of chronic obstructive pulmonary disease.

  What about test anxiety?

  Everyone who sits for one of the certification examinations is anxious to some degree. This anxiety can be a helpful emotion, focusing the NP certification candidate on the task at hand, studying and successfully sitting for this important examination, a tangible end product of the candidate's graduate or post graduate education. When excessive, however, anxiety can get in the way of success.

  So, a little bit of anxiety is normal and helpful?

  Yes. Stress yields anxiety, anxiety yields stress; one can be viewed as the product of the other. The stress of preparing for an important examination triggers the sympathetic nervous system to Seyle's three phases of the general adaptation syndrome: alarm, resistance, and exhaustion. In the alarm stage, perhaps triggered by contemplating the preparation needed to achieve certification success, the hypothalamus activates the autonomic nervous system, triggering the pituitary and the body defenses, resulting in a heightened sense of awareness of surroundings, alertness, and focus. At this level of arousal, studying for and taking a test often yields great results. A well-prepared examination candidate is highly focused on what needs to be done to be successful on the examination. Distractions can be filtered out; extraneous information can be discarded in favor of the essentials. During the examination, this is where anxiety and knowledge intersect; information retrieval is facilitated, and examination questions are fluidly processed. Difficult examination items are usually put in perspective, with the test-taker recognizing that most items were answered with relative ease. The NP certification candidate emerges from the test feeling challenged but confident.

Can too much test anxiety be a problem?

Of course. Bringing together a sound knowledge base and a healthy dose of anxiety, most NP certification examination candidates proceed with confidence. Many candidates do not move through the examinations in this manner, however. The process of completing a rigorous course of graduate education and study can result in a protracted period of stress. Now the formerly helpful stress leads to the second stage of the general adaptation syndrome, resistance, where epinephrine is released to help counteract or escape from the stressor. At that time, the feeling of milder anxiety present in the first stage gives way to a sense of greater nervousness, often accompanied by uncomfortable physical sensations such as dry mouth, tachycardia, and tremor. Studying or test taking becomes difficult; information retrieval is inhibited. This stage is mentally and physically taxing and if left unchecked can lead to exhaustion, complicating the challenging task of successfully completing the certification examination.

What exactly is test-taking anxiety?

Although often described as test-taking anxiety, the problem usually includes an excessive dose of anxiety while attempting to study for the examination, and so can be termed studying-testing anxiety. Although the reaction is most severe at the time of the test, most people who have severe test-taking anxiety have a similar, although milder reaction with the deep study needed to prepare for a critical examination such as NP certification. The following scenario describes a person with a problematic case of studying-testing anxiety:

The NP examination candidate is having a tough day, with a work shift that stretched for 3 unexpected hours and an unusually long commute, all following a poor night's sleep resulting from a noisy neighborhood party. To counteract this, the NP candidate drank a few extra cups of strong coffee and drank an "energy drink," really nothing more than a can of sugar and caffeine. The NP candidate also skipped lunch and made a quick trip to a fast food restaurant for some fries as a snack. Studying was part of today's plan, however, so the NP candidate sits down to prepare for the examination with great intentions of reviewing critical information. Surrounded by great stacks of study material, the NP candidate thinks about what might be on the examination and ponders the wide scope and knowledge base needed to be successful. Now the NP candidate becomes aware of a

dry mouth, and tight feeling in the throat. Determined, the NP candidate sits down and decides to study about antimicrobial therapy. The words on the page seem to blur while the NP candidate tries to read about the spectrum of activity of an antibiotic, then, having difficulty keeping this information straight, decides to skip that and focuses on memorizing a few antibiotic doses. Even with repeated tries, the NP candidate cannot keep this information at hand and now feels even more anxious, feeling tension in the back of the neck and a rapidly beating heart. The NP candidate now tries a few practice examination questions, but answers three questions about the appropriate use of antimicrobial therapy in acute otitis media incorrectly. Now even the thought of sitting for the examination causes the NP candidate to freeze.

How can this situation be altered?

Although developing a study schedule is important, rescheduling the study time may be a good idea when a day has been particularly difficult. Trying to learn when exhausted and stressed by other influences is often counterproductive. Certain scents may be helpful for putting the NP candidate in the right frame of mind to study, particularly under less-than-ideal conditions. These include basil, cinnamon, lemon, and peppermint for mental alertness, and camomile, lavender, and orange for relaxation.

Learn a relaxation technique to use before studying or test taking. Start the session by reading or repeating a positive message about being successful on the examination. Avoid excessive amounts of caffeinated beverages, which can add to anxious feelings. Eat a light but nourishing meal containing complex carbohydrates, fruit or vegetables, and high-quality protein to feed the body and mind. Avoid refined sugars and excessive fat intake, which can sap energy and derail quality study.

The NP candidate's anxiety started when pondering the wide range of possible topics on the certification examination. Starting the session studying a narrowly focused topic with a specific outcome goal rather than simply studying might have averted this. Setting up a system of study can enhance the success of a study session further. One method is the SQ4R system, where one *surveys* the study information to establish goals; formulates *questions* about the information; and then *reads* to answer these questions, followed by *reciting* the responses to the original questions, and *reviewing* to see if the original goals were met. Study and test-taking anxiety can also be tamed with the help of a learning specialist who can work with the NP candidate to develop the needed skills. Learning specialists can usually be contacted through the academic support centers at universities.

What do NPs who have failed an NP certification examination offer for advice?

In the course of talking to candidates for certification, I often speak with NPs who do not pass the NP certification examination. I have learned from these conversations that this is a group of intelligent people who completed a course of rigorous graduate study. Despite this, they were unsuccessful at an examination that often dictates whether the NP can practice. This can be a devastating blow. In retrospect, most can say what it was, however, that got in the way of success. Here is what they have shared.

"I expected to read a question and instantly recognize the answer."

- Although this may happen with a low-level fact-oriented question, such as one identifying an anatomic landmark, you should not expect this to be the case for most of the questions. Most items test your ability to assess or develop a plan of intervention for a clinical situation. You should expect to apply clinical decision-making skills to the test question. Make sure you think through each question. In particular, bear in mind how the pathophysiology of the condition affects the presentation and treatment.

"I could not figure out what the question was asking."

- Sometimes identifying the verb in the question can help you determine the purpose of the question. In addition, look at the information presented, and then ask yourself, "Is this question a test of the ability to gather subjective or objective information? Is this question a test of the ability to develop a diagnosis or to plan a course of intervention?" This thinking helps focus your thought process as you choose the answer.

"More than one answer was applicable to the situation presented. I was not sure which response was correct."

- Take another look at the question, and then choose the response most specific to the given situation. Also, sometimes questions that relate to presentation of disease have more than one applicable answer. The response with the most common presentation is likely to be correct. For example, an adult with bacterial meningitis can present with nuchal rigidity and papilledema. Because nuchal rigidity is seen in the most adults with this diagnosis, and papilledema is found far less often, however, nuchal rigidity is a better choice. In addition, childhood development questions often have more than one correct response. A 4-month-old is expected to roll stomach to back and smile. Smiling is a developmental milestone achieved by age 2 months, however, whereas rolling is typically not seen until an infant is 4 months old. Rolling stomach to back is the best response.

"I work in an acute care setting. The scenarios and treatment options presented in the questions were quite different from what I am accustomed to seeing in my RN practice. I had a hard time choosing the best answer."

- Many new NP graduates are seasoned RNs. In the acute care setting, you are typically seeing the "worst-case scenario" of a disease state, rather than a typical presentation in primary care, the practice setting of most adult and family NPs. The NP certification examination is a test of entry-level NP knowledge. An acute care nurse is accustomed to seeing exceptions; the examination is likely to present situations that are more the rule. For example, chest pain associated with acute coronary syndrome or unstable angina can last for hours and is present often at rest. Because an acute care nurse likely has experience in caring for patients with unstable angina, this presentation may become the nurse's mind-set of the typical presentation of angina pectoris. A chest pain episode experienced by a community-dwelling elderly adult with stable angina pectoris is usually infrequent and lasts less than 10 minutes. Relief of symptoms usually occurs promptly with rest or cessation of the provoking activity. The test taker needs to apply primary care, not acute care, rules to the test.

How about some tips on approaching the certification examination?

Here are some certification examination *"dos"* and *"don'ts"*.

- *Do* read each question and all responses so that you mark your option choice only after you are sure you understand the concept being tested in the question. Answering a question quickly might lead to choosing a response that contains correct information about a given condition, but might not be the correct response for that particular question.
- *Do* be wary of options that include extreme words, such as "always," "never," "all," "best," "worst," "none." Seldom is anything absolute in health care.
- *Do* recall and jot down a few facts about the information if you are really stumped. Doing this may be enough to make the retrieval of information you need to respond to the question much easier. You will be supplied with some scratch paper and a pencil or pen at the certification testing center.
- *Do* remember that if the options cover a wide range of numerical values, a value at or near the middle is often correct.
- *Do* make sure that the extra information usually found in a particularly long answer is pertinent to the question and not simply a distractor.
- *Do* read the shortest answer with care before you reject it. Although the short option gives little detail, there still may be enough information to make it correct.
- *Do* notice if two options look similar. Usually one is the correct answer.
- *Do* note when two options convey the same information or have the same meaning. Usually both are wrong.
- *Do* read each option as if it were a true-false question, eliminating all the options that are false.
- *Do* expect to answer about 60 to 70 or more multiple-choice questions per hour. This means you will likely be spending less than a minute, on average, on each question. Some questions take only a few seconds, whereas others require more time for thought. Check yourself at 15- or 20-minute intervals to determine if you are progressing at an acceptable rate, setting a number of questions that you should have answered by a certain time.
- *Do* expect that the topics you studied will be presented in random order. A question on diabetes mellitus follows one on hypertension and can be preceded by a question on women's health.

- *Do* apply evidence-based and consensus-based practice to the examination. Expect that advice on health screenings and interventions is based on nationally recognized standards of care from authorities such as the American Diabetes Association, National Cholesterol Education Program, and American Cancer Society, not simply what you have observed being done in clinical practice.
- *Don't* forget that the computer-based test sites accommodate the needs of many different test candidates. You will see people taking a variety of tests besides the NP certification examination.
- *Don't* be misled by the close to correct option that often precedes the correct answer.
- *Don't* assume that an answer is correct because this is what you have observed in your current nursing practice. Apply evidence-based practice principles to all possible responses.
- *Don't* dismiss an option because it seems too obvious and simple to be correct. If you are well prepared for the examination, some if not most of the questions will appear very straightforward.
- *Don't* select an option just because it contains factually correct information about the clinical situation. You have to make sure that it is the "correct" or "best" answer to the question.
- *Don't* forget that as a result of your NP studies and certification preparation, you should be able to draw on your knowledge base and narrow choices to two options.
- *Don't* pick an answer just because it seems to make sense. You are answering from your knowledge of the course content, not just from your general knowledge and logic.
- *Don't* be taken in by the use of unfamiliar terms in the question. If you have studied the subject, few words should be unknown.
- *Don't* get bogged down on a question or questions part of the way through the examination. If you are stumped by a question, move on, with a plan to return to this item at the end of the test. Remind yourself that you have answered many questions with relative ease. Finish all of those questions that you can answer and then to come back later to process the problematic questions. The computer-based tests have a mechanism to highlight questions you want to revisit.
- *Don't* change an answer unless you first misinterpreted the question. If necessary, when looking over the questions again, change an answer only if you can logically justify the change.
- *Don't* respond to self-defeating thoughts that can creep into your mind, such as, "I did not study enough," or "This test is too hard." Recognize the time and energy you have put into your preparation.

When should I start studying for the NP certification examination?

I advise that you start at the beginning of your NP program! From your first day of NP study, think like an NP, whether in your NP clinical rotations or at your RN practice site, and work at developing the critical thinking and technical skills needed for success. The NP provides health care independently and as part of a health-care team, and assumes full accountability for clinical judgment. The content of the NP certification examinations reflects these fundamental components of NP practice.

How about some tips on how to prepare for NP practice after the certification examination?

Deep knowledge and appreciation of the pathophysiology and epidemiology of health problems inform NP practice. If you know what causes an illness, your job of figuring out how to help the person achieve health is greatly facilitated. Knowledge of disease epidemiology helps you to recognize the most likely health problems in given patient groups.

Clinical practice and certification tip: Remember that common disease occurs commonly, and that the uncommon presentation of a common disease is more common than the common presentation of an uncommon disease.

The fundamental tools of NP practice include the ability to procure comprehensively yet succinctly information needed to develop accurate diagnoses. Gathering the needed subjective and objective information in the care of a person with common acute, episodic, and chronic health problems is the most important skill the NP can develop. Develop the skill of taking a thorough yet concise health history that is pertinent to the patient's presenting complaint or health problem. As you proceed through the history, recall the rationale behind each question you ask and how a given response impacts the possible etiology of the patient's health problem. Know how to perform a thorough yet succinct symptom analysis. This is where the detective work of diagnosis starts. Use the physical examination to confirm the findings of the health history.

Clinical practice and certification tip: Remember that the physical examination is guided by the health history, not the other way around.

The advanced practice NP role includes the responsibility of arriving at a diagnosis, developing a treatment plan, and providing ongoing evaluation of response to treatment.

Clinical practice and certification tip: Learn to recognize the typical clinical presentation for the 10 most common health problems that present to your practice site, including chief complaint and physical examination findings, needed diagnostics, and intervention. Armed with this information, you can focus your study on a thorough knowledge of the assessment and treatment of these conditions. Continue to evaluate the patient's response to therapy.

Ask your preceptor to save laboratory results, EKGs, and other diagnostics for you to review at the next session. Do so with a clean eye, as if you were developing a plan of intervention or further diagnosis for the patient. This will help hone your skills. If you prescribed an intervention but will not have the opportunity to see the patient at a follow-up visit, ask your preceptor for an update.

Family, cultural, community, developmental, and environmental factors and lifestyle and health behaviors influence patient health and the NP-patient interaction. As an advanced practice nurse, the NP provides holistic, wellness-oriented care on an ongoing or episodic basis.

Clinical practice and certification tip: Remember to address a patient's primary, secondary and tertiary health care needs at every visit. Check for needed immunization, screening tests, and follow-up on previous health problems with every encounter. Think long-term. Envision working with patients during the years ahead and the health problems you may help a person avoid by working together. I have had the privilege of practicing in the same community for more than two decades. Having seen some of these families for more than 20 years, I can truly see the power of primary health care.

The health care provided by the NP is guided by health and wellness research. The NP is accountable for his or her ongoing learning and professional development and is a lifelong learner. The NP is also knowledgeable in accessing resources to guide evidence-based care.

Clinical practice and certification tip: Ask preceptors and peers what references are most helpful for that particular practice. Armed with this information, develop your own reference library that you can use with ease. Your investment of time and money to go gather these resources will pay off in your practice.

Reference

Nugent P, Vitale B. *Test Success: Test-Taking Techniques for Beginning Nursing Students*. 5th ed. Philadelphia, PA: FA Davis; 2008.

Index

Note: Page numbers followed by b, f, or t refer to Boxes, Figures or Table, respectively